IMMUNO BIOLOGY

THE IMMUNE SYSTEM IN HEALTH AND DISEASE

THIRD EDITION

P9-DYE-022

IMMUNO BIOLOGY

THE IMMUNE SYSTEM IN HEALTH AND DISEASE

THIRD EDITION

Charles A. Janeway, Jr.
Yale University Medical School

Paul Travers
Birkbeck College, London University

with the assistance of
Simon Hunt
Oxford University

Mark Walport
Royal Postgraduate Medical School, London

CURRENT BIOLOGY LIMITED ∎

Current Biology Ltd
London, San Francisco and New York

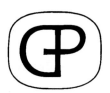

Garland Publishing Inc
New York and London

Text editors: Penelope Austin, Eleanor Lawrence,
Miranda Robertson
Project editors: Emma Hunt, Giles Montier,
Hazel Richardson
Illustrators: Celia Welcomme, Matthew McClements
Layout: Huw Woodman
Production: Kate Oldfield, Priya Gohil
Software support: Gary Brown
Proofreader: Melanie Paton
Indexer: Liza Weinkove

© 1997 by Current Biology Ltd./Garland Publishing Inc.
All rights reserved. No part of this publication may be
reproduced, stored in a retrieval system or transmitted in any
form or by any means—electronic, mechanical,
photocopying, recording or otherwise—without the prior
written permission of the copyright holders.

Distributors

Inside North America: Garland Publishing Inc., 717 Fifth
Avenue, New York, NY 10022, USA.
Inside Japan: Nankodo Co. Ltd., 42-6, Hongo 3-Chome,
Bunkyo-ku, Tokyo 113, Japan.
Outside North America and Japan: Churchill Livingstone,
Robert Stevenson House, 1-3 Baxter's Place, Leith Walk,
Edinburgh, EH1 3AF.

ISBN 0-8153-2818-4 (paperback) Garland
ISBN 0-443-05964-0 (paperback) Churchill Livingstone
ISBN 0-443-05995-0 (paperback) International Edition

A catalog record for this book is available from the British
Library.

Library of Congress Cataloging-in-Publication Data
Janeway, Charles.
    Immunobiology: the immune system in health and disease/
    Charles A. Janeway, Jr., Paul Travers.—Third ed.
        p. cm.
    Includes bibliographical references and index.
    ISBN 0-8153-2818-4 (pbk.).
    1. Immunity. I. Travers, Paul, 1956- .
II. Title
QR181.J37   1997
616. 07'9—dc21
                                        96-47915
                                        CIP

This book was produced using Corel Ventura Publisher 5.0
and CorelDRAW 5.0.

Printed in Singapore by Stamford Press.

Published by Current Biology Ltd., Middlesex House, 34-42
Cleveland Street, London W1P 6LB, UK and Garland
Publishing Inc., 717 Fifth Avenue, New York, NY 10022, USA.

Preface for the first edition

This book is intended as an introductory text for use in immunology courses for medical students, advanced undergraduate biology students, and graduate students. It attempts to present the field of immunology from a consistent viewpoint, that of the host's interaction with an environment containing myriad species of potentially harmful microbes. The justification for this particular approach is that the absence of components of the immune system is virtually always made clinically manifest by an increased susceptibility to infection. Thus, first and foremost, the immune system exists to protect the host from infection, and its evolutionary history must have been shaped largely by this challenge. Other aspects of immunology, such as allergy, autoimmunity, graft rejection, and immunity to tumors are treated as variations on this basic protective function in which the nature of the antigen is the major variable.

We have attempted to structure the book logically, focusing mainly on the adaptive immune response mediated by antigen-specific lymphocytes operating by clonal selection. The first part of the book summarizes our understanding of immunology in conceptual terms and introduces the main players—the cells, tissues, and molecules of the immune system. It also contains a 'toolbox' of experiments and techniques that form the experimental basis of immunology. The middle three parts of the book deal with three main aspects of adaptive immunity: how the immune system recognizes and discriminates among different molecules; how individual cells develop so that each bears a unique receptor directed at foreign, and not at self, molecules; and how these cells are activated when they encounter microbes whose molecular components bind their receptors, and the effector mechanisms that are used to eliminate these microbes from the body.

Having described the major features of lymphocytes and of adaptive immune responses, the last part of the book integrates this material at the level of the intact organism, examining when, how, and where immune responses occur, and how they fail in some instances. In this part of the book we also consider those aspects of host defense that do not involve clonal selection of lymphocytes, known as innate immunity or natural resistance. We then look at the role of the immune system in causing rather than preventing disease, focusing on allergy, autoimmunity, and graft rejection as examples. Finally, we consider how the immune system can be manipulated to the benefit of the host, emphasizing endogenous regulatory mechanisms and the possibility of vaccinating not only against infection, but also against cancer and immunological diseases. The book also contains a glossary of key terms, biographical notes on some immunologists, and summary tables of key molecules.

In preparing this textbook, we have striven for a coherent overall presentation of concepts supported by experiment and observation. We have had the chapters read by experts (see page ix) who have helped us to eliminate errors of fact and conclusion, to improve presentation, and to achieve better balance; we are sincerely grateful to them for their hours of hard work. Any shortcomings of the book are not their fault, but ours. We plan to keep this material current by revising the book each year, again relying on a panel of experts for each chapter. But the greatest help in improving the value of the book will come from its readers; we welcome your comments and criticisms, and we will work to incorporate your ideas into each new update. Thus, we plan to make this the first current textbook: we are attempting to do this because we believe that the field of immunology is advancing so rapidly at present that annual updating is essential.

There is no doubt that we have both omitted and included too much; the field of immunology covers such a broad area of interest that one of the most daunting challenges in writing this book has been in deciding what has to be discussed and what can be ignored. The judgements we have made are personal and so will not be shared exactly by anyone else. Again, we welcome your input and suggestions about places where this judgement is in clear error.

Finally, we want to thank the many people who have worked so hard to make this book possible. Our illustrator, Celia Welcomme, has brought her extraordinary talents to bear on the figures, while the book itself was edited by three highly skilled and knowledgeable individuals, Miranda Robertson, Rebecca Ward, and Eleanor Lawrence; led by Miranda, they questioned every word, sentence, comma and figure in the book, and made us tear our hair out in trying to be clear and accurate at the same time. If we have failed, it is not their fault. Peter Newmark and Vitek Tracz have provided intelligent and even inspirational guidance, motivated in no small part by the memory of our original publisher, the remarkable Gavin Borden, who sadly died young and never saw this book, into which he put so much, in print. Nothing would have been achieved without the diligence of Becky Palmer, who kept all of us organized over a long period, with the help of Emma Dorey, Sylvia Purnell, Gary Brown, and many other people at Current Biology Ltd. Charlie Janeway wants to thank several patient secretaries, especially Liza Cluggish, Anne Brancheau, Susan Morin, and Kara McCarthy for all their help. Finally, our families have suffered more than we have, from neglect, absence and fits of ill temper. Thus, we thank Kim Bottomly, Katie, Hannah and Megan Janeway, and Rose Zamoyska for their forbearance and support.

Charles A. Janeway Jr.   Paul Travers
Yale University School of Medicine   Birkbeck College
Howard Hughes Medical Institute   University of London

April 1994

Preface for the third edition

Immunology continues to accelerate its rate of progress, not only in the areas of the basic biology of adaptive immunity, but also in the study of host responses to various infectious agents, the understanding of allergy, rapid progress towards new vaccines, and other areas too numerous to mention. As we were preparing this third edition of our book, we again called on many experts to read chapters or parts of chapters in which they were greater experts than we are or could ever claim to be. They are acknowledged on page ix. As in the two previous editions, we would like to thank them for their earnest efforts, and to absolve them of responsibility for the final product, which is ours alone.

For this edition, we have added two new co-authors: Simon Hunt of Oxford University, who took responsibility for the chapters that deal with B-cell antigen recognition and B-cell development; and Mark Walport, who undertook the major overhaul of the chapters on the more clinical subjects of immunodeficiency, resistance of infectious agents to host responses, AIDS, allergy, autoimmunity, graft rejection, and manipulation of the immune response. Paul Travers and Charlie Janeway remain as lead authors, but the help of these two people has made their work much easier.

We have also modified our referencing for this edition. We generally cite one recent review and one or a few current papers under each concept heading, to serve as a starting point for students who wish to understand a particular topic in depth. Further references can be discovered by this process.

As for the first two editions of this book, we have again been helped by a very talented and tireless team of editors, illustrators, and publishers. Miranda Robertson continues to oversee the work as a whole, but Penny Austin in Washington DC skilfully undertook most of the editing of this edition, aided by Eleanor Lawrence in London. Matthew McClements has continued his wonderful work making good pictures from bad sketches. Emma Hunt, Hazel Richardson, and Giles Montier provided publishing and organizational support throughout the process of putting the book together, with Huw Woodman producing the final layout.

Again, we want to thank our publishers for their continuing support of our effort to remain current: Peter Newmark and Vitek Tracz of Current Biology Ltd., and Libby Borden of Garland Publishing.

Now that the Jenner Bicentenial is behind us, it seems fitting to draw a breath and then push harder than we ever have in the past. The challenges ahead of us are even greater than those we have met over the two hundred years since Jenner first successfully attempted to use vaccination to prevent smallpox. Now that we are beginning to understand the immune system and how it works, future challenges will come more than ever from trying to use it to promote human health all over the world. Nowhere is this more apparent than in the battle against AIDS. Recent discoveries of new receptors for this vicious virus give hope for novel blockers of these receptors, while drug treatments promise a respite from the deadly progress of this disease. But these are stopgap measures at best, and it is our belief that a vaccine should remain the top priority. Vaccines for many other debilitating diseases are also being developed, and there is now also discussion of vaccinating against autoimmune diseases and cancer. We are confident that this will eventually be achieved, just as Jenner showed the world over two hundred years ago that he could prevent smallpox by vaccinating a boy with cowpox. The only real question is when.

Finally, we would like to thank our long-suffering families and the members of our respective laboratories for the hours of neglect we have inflicted on them over the past year. Charlie Janeway wants to thank Kim Bottomly for her unflagging support, and also his children, Katie, Hannah, and Megan for being at least understanding of the pre-occupation of their father with something as abstruse as modern immunobiology. Paul Travers thanks Rose Zamoyska for her continuing support and encouragement. Mark Walport thanks Julia for her loving support, and his children, Louise, Robert, Emily, and Fiona for coping with their father's abstraction by matters immunological. Simon Hunt wants to thank his many pupils who unknowingly personified his readership, especially PK and JW; thanks his whole family, particularly H, A, and L for their support and diversions; and is grateful to DO who critically read some of the drafts.

Charles A. Janeway Jr.
Yale University School of Medicine
Howard Hughes Medical Institute

Simon Hunt
University of Oxford

Paul Travers
Birkbeck College
University of London

Mark Walport
Royal Postgraduate Medical School

Acknowledgements

Text

We would like to thank the following experts who read parts or the whole of the chapters indicated and provided us with invaluable advice.

Chapter 1: J. J. Cohen, University of Colorado; J. Howard, University of Cologne; E. V. Rothenburg, California Institute of Technology.

Chapter 2: J. Frelinger, University of Rochester Cancer Center; J. Goding, Monash University; R.R. Hardy, Fox Chase Cancer Center; A. Munro, Cambridge University.

Chapter 3: F. Alt, Howard Hughes Medical Institute Children's Hospital, Boston; J. Cambier, National Jewish Center for Immunology and Respiratory Medicine, Denver; A. DeFranco, University of California, San Francisco; R. Mariuzza, Center for Advanced Research in Biotechnology, Rockville, Maryland; V. Tybulewicz, National Institute for Medical Research, London.

Chapter 4: P.M. Allen, Washington University School of Medicine; D. Campbell, University of Oxford; P. Cresswell, Howard Hughes Medical Institute, Yale University School of Medicine; A. DeFranco, University of California, San Francisco; R.N. Germain, National Institute of Allergy and Infectious Disease, Bethesda; B. Malissen, INSERM-CNRS de Marseille-Luminy.

Chapter 5: F. Alt, Howard Hughes Medical Institute Children's Hospital, Boston; S. Desiderio, Howard Hughes Medical Institute, John Hopkins University, Baltimore; C. Goodnow, Howard Hughes Medical Institute, Stanford University; P.W. Kincade, Oklahoma Medical Research Foundation; K. Rajewsky, University of Cologne.

Chapter 6: M.J. Bevan, Howard Hughes Medical Institute, University of Washington; K. Shortman, Walter and Eliza Hall Institute of Medical Research, Melbourne; A. Singer, National Cancer Institute, Bethesda.

Chapter 7: J. Allison, University of California, Berkeley; G.M. Griffiths, University College, London; A. Sher, National Institute of Allergy and Infectious Disease, Bethesda; T. Springer, Center for Blood Research, Harvard Medical School.

Chapter 8: D.T. Fearon, University of Cambridge School of Medicine; G. Kelsoe, University of Maryland, Baltimore; J-P. Kinet, Harvard Medical School; I. MacLennan, University of Birmingham; P. Parham, Stanford University; K. Rajewsky, University of Cologne.

Chapter 9: G. Bancroft, London School of Hygiene and Tropical Medicine; A. Bendelac, Princeton University; K. Karre, Karolinska Institute, Stockholm; A. Livingstone, Imperial College of Science, Technology, and Medicine, London; I. MacLennan, University of Birmingham; C.F. Nathan, Cornell University Medical College; P. Scott, University of Pennsylvania; E. Skamene, McGill Center for the study of Host Resistance, Montreal General Hospital; T. Springer, Center for Blood Research, Harvard Medical School.

Chapter 10: A. McMichael, Institute of Molecular Medicine, Oxford; P.M. Murphy, National Institute of Allergy and Infectious Disease, Bethesda; F.R. Rosen, Harvard Medical School; A.D. Webster, Royal Free Hospital School of Medicine, London; R.A. Weiss, Institute of Cancer Research, London.

Chapter 11: H. Auchinloss, Jr., Harvard Medical School; R.S. Geha, Boston Children's Hospital; A.B. Kay, National Heart and Lung Institute, London; R. Lechler, Royal Postgraduate Medical School, London; Y.W. Loke, University of Cambridge; J. Sprent, Scripps Research Institute, La Jolla; D. Wraith, Univerity of Bristol.

Chapter 12: G. Ada, John Curtin Medical School, Australian National University, Canberra; B.R. Bloom, Howard Hughes Medical Institute, Albert Einstein College of Medicine, New York; G. Dougan, Imperial College of Science, Technology, and Medicine, London; M. Liu, Merck Research Laboratories, West Point, Philadelphia.

Pedagogic: L. Berg, University of Harvard; J. Danska, Hospital for Sick Children, Toronto; J. Frelinger, University of Rochester Cancer Center; M.E. Perry, United Medical and Dental Schools, London.

Appendix: N. Barclay, MRC Center, University of Oxford.

First and second editions A.K. Abbas, Harvard Medical School; H. Acha-Orbea, Ludwig Institute for Cancer Research; K. Arai, University of Tokyo; J.P. Allison, University of California, Berkeley; P. Beverley, Ludwig Institute for Cancer Research; T. Boon, Ludwig Institute for Cancer Research; F.M. Brodsky, University of California, San Francisco; M.P. Cancro, University of Pennsylvania School of Medicine; S. Corey, Walter and Eliza Hall Institute, Melbourne; R. Corley, Duke University Medical Center, Durham, N.C.; A. Coutinho, Institute Pasteur, Paris; G. Crabtree, Howard Hughes Medical Institute, Stanford University; S.C. Crebe, The American University, Washington, D.C.; M. Davis, Howard Hughes Medical Institute, Stanford University; W. Dunnick, University of Michigan; T. Fauci, National Institute of Allergy and Infectious Diseases, Bethesda; M. Feinberg, Office of AIDS Research, Bethesda; A. Gann, Ludwig Institute for Cancer Research, London; S. Gillis, Immunex Research and Development Corporation; P. Golstein, INSERM-CNRS de Marseille-Luminy; L. Gooding, Emory University School of Medicine, S. Gordon, University of Oxford; H. Gould, Randall Institute, University of London; D. Gray, Royal Postgraduate Medical School, London; K. Grimnes, Alma College, Alma. J. Groopman, New England Deaconess Hospital, Boston; R. Handschumacher, Yale University of Medicine; E.R. Heise, Bowman Gray School of Medicine, Winston-Salem; P. Holt, West Australian Research Institute for Child Health; J. Howard, Babraham Institute, Cambridge, U.K.; E.J. Jenkinson, University of Birmingham, U.K.; K. Joiner, Yale University School of Medicine; G. Kelsoe, University of Maryland; C. Kinnon, Institute of Child Health, London; J. Ledbetter, Bristol Myers Squibb Pharmaceutical Research Institute; I. Mellman, Yale University School of Medicine; B. Moss, National Institute of Allergy and Infectious Diseases, Bethesda; D.B. Murphy, New York State Department of Health; R.J. Noelle, Dartmouth Medical School; D. Pardoll, John Hopkins University School of Medicine; P. Parham, Stanford University Medical Center; W.E. Paul, National Institute of Allergy and Infectious Diseases, Bethesda;

D. Paulnock, University of Wisconsin Medical School; B. M. Peterlin, Howard Hughes Medical Institute, University of California, San Francisco; G.A. Petsko, Brandeis University; L. Picker, University of Texas Southwestern Medical Centre; S.K. Pierce, Northwestern University; R. Poljak, Institute Pasteur, Paris; M. Ptashne, Harvard University; M. Neuberger, MRC Center, Cambridge; T.B. Nutman, National Institute of Allergy and Infectious Diseases, Bethesda; D.H. Raulet, University of California, Berkeley; K.B.M. Reid, University of Oxford; D. Richman, University of California, San Diego; J.J. van Rood, University Hospital, Leiden; N.R. Rose, John Hopkins University School of Hygiene and Public Health, Baltimore; D.H. Sachs, Massachussetts General Hospital; D. Schatz, Howard Hughes Medical Institute, Yale University School of Medicine; E. Sercarz, University of California, Los Angeles; S. Shaw, National Cancer Institute, Bethesda; R. Steinman, Rockefeller University; A. Strasser, Walter and Eliza Hall Institute, Melbourne; J. W. Streilein, University of Miami School of Medicine; I. Tomlinson, MRC Center, Cambridge; J. Tooze, Imperial Cancer Research Fund, London; J. Uhr, University of Texas Southwestern Medical School; H. Weiner, Harvard Medical School; I. Wilson, Scripps Research Institute; S. Wain Hobson, Unite de Retrovirologie Moleclaire; H. Waldmann, University of Oxford; M. Walport, Royal Postgraduate Medical School, University of London; S. Wright, Rockefeller University.

Photographs

The following photographs have been reproduced with the kind permission of the journal in which they were originally published.

Chapter 1.

Fig 1.8 from the *Journal of Experimental Medicine*, 1972, **135**:200–219, by copyright permission of The Rockefeller University Press.
Fig 1.24 from the *Journal of Experimental Medicine*, 1987, **169**:893–907, by copyright permission of the Rockefeller University Press.

Chapter 3.

Fig 3.1 from *Nature,* 1992, **360**:369-372. © 1992 Macmillan Magazines Limited.
Fig 3.5 from *Advances in Immunology* 1969, **11**:1–30.
Fig 3.9, top panel from *Science* 1990, **248**:712–719. © 1990 by the AAAS. Middle panel, from *Structure* 1993, 1:83–3. © Current Biology Ltd.
Fig 3.11 from *Science* 1986, **233**:747–53. © 1990 by the AAAS.
Fig 3.22, top panel from the *European Journal of Immunology* 1988, **18**:1001–1008

Chapter 4.

Fig 4.11 from *Science* 1995, **268**:533–539. © 1995 by the AAAS.
Fig 4.13, model structure from *Cell* 1996, **84**:505. © 1996 by Cell Press.
Fig 4.14 from *Science* 1994, **266**:1566–1569. © 1994 by the AAAS.
Fig 4.28 from *Science* 1996, **274**:209–219. © 1996 by the AAAS.

Chapter 5.

Fig 5.4, right panel from the *European Journal of Immunology* 1987, **17**:1473–1484.

Chapter 6.

Fig 6.5 from *Nature*, 1994, **372**:100–103. © 1994 Macmillan Magazines Limited.
Fig 6.18 from *Science* 1990, **250**:1720–723. © 1990 by the AAAS.

Chapter 7.

Fig 7.28, panel c from *Second International Workshop on Cell Mediated Cytotoxicity*. Eds. P.A. Henkart and E. Martz. New York, Plenum Press 1985, 99–119.
Fig 7.36 from the *European Journal of Immunology*. 1989, **19**:1253–1259
Fig 7.37, panels a and b from *Second International Workshop on Cell Mediated Cytotoxicity*. Eds. P.A. Henkart and E. Martz. New York, Plenum Press 1985, 99–119, panel c from *Immunology Today* 1985, **6**:21–27

Chapter 8.

Fig 8.18 from *Nature*, 1994, **372**:336–383. © 1994 Macmillan Magazines Limited.
Fig 8.34 from *Essays in Biochemistry* 1986. **22**:27–68.
Fig 8.35, planar conformation from the *European Journal of Immunology* 1988, **18**:1001–1003.
Fig 8.49 from *Blut* 1990, **60**:309–318.

Chapter 9.

Fig 9.15, top panel from *Nature*, 1994, 367: 338–345. Copyright 1994 Macmillan Magazines Limited. Bottom panel from the *Journal of Immunology* 1990, 144: 2287–2294. © 1990, the *Journal of Immunology*.
Fig 9.36, panel a from the *Journal of Immunology* 1985, **134**:1349–1359. © 1985, the *Journal of Immunology*. Panels b and c from *Annual Reviews in Immunology* 1989, **7**:91–109. © 1989, Annual Reviews Inc.

Chapter 10.

Fig 10.6, top left panel from International Review of Experimental Pathology 1986, **28**:45–78. © 1986, Academic Press.

Chapter 12.

Fig 12.28 from the *Journal of Experimental Medicine*, 1992, **176**:1355–1364, by copyright permission of the Rockefeller University Press.

Chapter 13.

Fig 13.16 from *Mechanisms of Cytotoxicity by Natural Killer cells*. R.B. Herberman (Ed.) Academic Press, New York. 1985, 195. © 1985, Academic Press.

CONTENTS

EXPANDED CONTENTS

Part IV   THE ADAPTIVE IMMUNE RESPONSE

Part V   THE IMMUNE SYSTEM IN HEALTH AND DISEASE

List of Headings

Part II — THE RECOGNITION OF ANTIGEN

Chapter 3: Structure of the Antibody Molecule and Immunoglobulin Genes

Chapter 4: Antigen Recognition by T Lymphocytes

The major histocompatibility complex of genes: organization and polymorphism.

The T-cell receptor complex.

Part III   THE DEVELOPMENT OF LYMPHOCYTE REPERTOIRES

Chapter 5: The Development of B Lymphocytes

Generation of B cells.

Selection of B cells.

B-cell heterogeneity.

Chapter 6: The Thymus and the Development of T Lymphocytes

The development of T cells in the thymus.

Part IV	THE ADAPTIVE IMMUNE RESPONSE

Chapter 7: T-Cell Mediated Immunity

Part V THE IMMUNE SYSTEM IN HEALTH AND DISEASE

Chapter 9: Host Defense Against Infection

Chapter 12:   Immune Response in the Absence of Infection

Chapter 13:   Manipulation of the Immune Response

PART I

AN INTRODUCTION TO IMMUNOBIOLOGY

Basic Concepts in Immunology

1

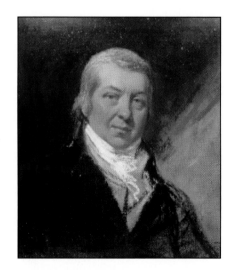

Fig. 1.1 Edward Jenner. Portrait by John Raphael Smith. Reproduced courtesy of the Yale Historical Medical Library.

Immunology is a relatively new science. Its origin is usually attributed to Edward Jenner (Fig. 1.1) who discovered in 1796 that cowpox, or vaccinia, induced protection against human smallpox, an often fatal disease. Jenner called his procedure vaccination, and this term is still used to describe the inoculation of healthy individuals with weakened or attenuated strains of disease-causing agents to provide protection from disease. Although Jenner's bold experiment was successful, it took almost two centuries for smallpox vaccination to become universal, an advance that

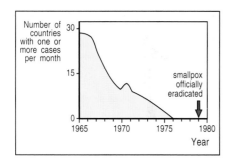

Fig. 1.2   The eradication of smallpox by vaccination. After a period of 3 years in which no cases of smallpox were recorded, The World Health Organization was able to announce in 1979 that smallpox had been eradicated.

[handwritten note:]
Adaptive Immune Response:
1. Specific
2. Adaptive rsp   5. lymphocytes
3. AB to specific pathogen
4. life-long immunity

Innate Immunity:
1. macrophages + other phagocytes = granulocytes
   - immed. available
   - fights wide-range bact. w/o prior expos.

enabled the World Health Organization to announce in 1979 that smallpox had been eradicated (Fig. 1.2), arguably the greatest triumph of modern medicine.

When Jenner introduced vaccination he knew nothing of the infectious agents that cause disease: it was not until late in the 19th century that Robert Koch proved that infectious diseases are caused by **microorganisms**, each one responsible for a particular disease, or **pathology**. We now recognize four broad categories of disease-causing microorganisms, or **pathogens**: these are **viruses**; **bacteria**; pathogenic **fungi**; and other relatively large and complex eukaryotic organisms collectively termed **parasites**.

The discoveries of Koch and other great 19th century microbiologists stimulated the extension of Jenner's strategy of vaccination to other diseases. In the 1880s, Louis Pasteur devised a vaccine against cholera in chickens, and developed a rabies vaccine that proved a spectacular success upon its first trial use in a boy bitten by a rabid dog. These practical triumphs led to a search for the mechanism of protection and the development of the science of immunology. In 1890, Emil von Behring and Shibasaburo Kitasato discovered that the serum of vaccinated individuals contained substances—which they called **antibodies**—that specifically bound to the relevant pathogen.

A specific **immune response**, such as the production of antibodies to a particular pathogen, is known as an **adaptive immune response**, because it occurs during the lifetime of an individual as an adaptive response to infection with that pathogen. In many cases, an adaptive immune response confers life-long protective **immunity** to re-infection with the same pathogen. This distinguishes such responses from **innate immunity**, which, at the time von Behring and Kitasato discovered antibodies, was known chiefly through the work of the great Russian immunologist Elie Metchnikoff. Metchnikoff discovered that many microorganisms could be engulfed and digested by **phagocytic cells**, which he called **macrophages**. These cells are immediately available to combat a wide range of bacteria without requiring prior exposure, and act in the same way in all normal individuals. Antibodies, by contrast, are produced only in response to specific infections, and the antibodies present in a given individual directly reflect the infections to which he or she has been exposed.

Indeed, it quickly became clear that specific antibodies can be induced against a vast range of substances. These are known as **antigens** because they can stimulate the generation of antibodies, although we shall see that not all adaptive immune responses entail the production of antibodies, and the term antigen is now used in a rather broader sense, to describe any substance capable of being recognized by the adaptive immune system.

Both innate immunity and adaptive immune responses depend upon the activities of white blood cells, or **leukocytes**. Innate immunity is mediated largely by granulocytes, so called because they contain prominent cytoplasmic granules. Granulocytes are a diverse collection of cells that include the macrophages championed by Metchnikoff, as well as other phagocytic cells that are able to engulf and destroy microorganisms. Adaptive immune responses depend upon **lymphocytes**, which provide the life-long immunity that can follow exposure to disease or vaccination. The innate and adaptive immune systems together provide a remarkably effective defense system that ensures that, although we spend our lives surrounded by potentially pathogenic microorganisms, we become ill only relatively rarely, and when infection occurs it is usually met successfully and is followed by lasting immunity.

The main focus of this book will be on the diverse mechanisms of adaptive immunity, whereby specialized classes of lymphocytes recognize and target pathogenic microorganisms or cells infected with them. We shall see, however, that all the cells that mediate innate immune responses also participate in adaptive immune responses, and indeed most of the actions of the adaptive immune system depend upon them.

In this chapter, we first introduce the cells of the immune system, and the tissues in which they develop and through which they circulate or migrate. In later sections, we outline the specialized functions of the different types of cells and the mechanisms whereby they eliminate infection.

The components of the immune system.

The cells of the immune system originate in the **bone marrow**, where many of them also mature. They then migrate to patrol the tissues, circulating in the blood and in a specialized system of vessels called the **lymphatic system**.

1-1   The white blood cells of the immune system derive from precursors in the bone marrow.

All the cellular elements of blood, including the red blood cells that transport oxygen, the platelets that trigger blood clotting in damaged tissues, and the white blood cells of the immune system, derive ultimately from the same **progenitor** or precursor cells, the **hematopoietic stem cells** in the bone marrow. As these stem cells can give rise to all of the different types of blood cells, they are often known as pluripotent hematopoietic stem cells. They give rise, in turn, to stem cells of more limited potential, which are the immediate progenitors of red blood cells, platelets, and the two main categories of white blood cells. The different types of blood cells and their lineage relationships are summarized in Fig. 1.3. We shall be concerned here only with the cells derived from the **myeloid progenitor** and the **common lymphoid progenitor**.

The myeloid progenitor is the precursor of the granulocytes and macrophages of the immune system. Macrophages are one of the two types of phagocytes of the immune system and are distributed widely in the body tissues where they play a critical part in innate immunity. They are the mature form of **monocytes**, which circulate in the blood and differentiate continuously into macrophages upon migration into the tissues.

The **granulocytes** are so called because they have densely staining granules in their cytoplasm; they are also sometimes called **polymorphonuclear leukocytes** because of their oddly shaped nuclei. There are three types of granulocytes. **Neutrophils**, which comprise the other phagocytic cell of the immune system, are the most numerous and most important cellular component of the innate immune response: hereditary deficiencies in neutrophil function lead to overwhelming bacterial infection, which is fatal if untreated. **Eosinophils** are thought to be important chiefly in defense against parasitic infections; they are activated by the lymphocytes of the adaptive immune response and we shall discuss their functions in Chapters 8 and 11. The function of **basophils** is

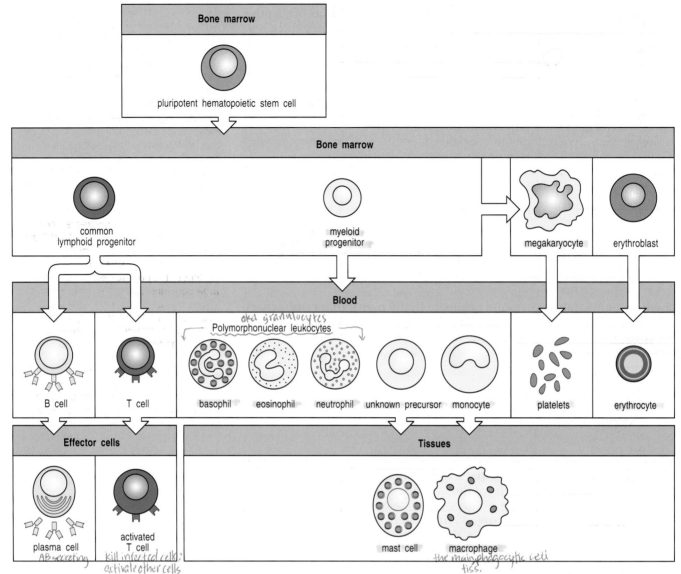

Fig. 1.3 **All the cellular elements of blood, including the lymphocytes of the adaptive immune system, arise from hematopoietic stem cells in the bone marrow.** These pluri-potent cells divide to produce two more specialized types of stem cells, a lymphoid stem cell (lymphoid progenitor), which gives rise to T and B lymphocytes, and a myeloid stem cell (myeloid progenitor), which gives rise to leukocytes, erythrocytes (red blood cells that carry oxygen), and the megakaryocytes that produce platelets, which are important in blood clotting. Although we have illustrated only one progenitor cell for the T and B lymphocytes, an alternative that has not been ruled out is that both T- and B-cell lineages arise directly from the pluripotent stem cell. The T and B lymphocytes are distinguished by their site of differentiation, T cells in the thymus and B cells in the bone marrow, and by their antigen receptors. B lymphocytes differentiate on activation into antibody-secreting plasma cells, and T lymphocytes differentiate into cells that can kill infected cells or activate other cells of the immune system.

The leukocytes that derive from the myeloid stem cell are the monocytes, and the basophils, eosinophils, and neutrophils, which are collectively termed either polymorphonuclear leukocytes, because of their irregularly shaped nuclei, or granulocytes, because of the cytoplasmic granules whose characteristic staining gives them a distinctive appearance in blood smears. Monocytes differentiate into macrophages in the tissues and these are the main tissue phagocytic cell of the immune system. Neutrophils, the most important phagocytic cells, have functions similar to those of macrophages but remain in the bloodstream; eosinophils are blood-borne cells that are involved mainly in inflammation, while basophils are found in blood and are similar in some ways to mast cells but arise from a separate lineage. Mast cells also arise from precursors in bone marrow but complete their maturation in tissues, although it is not known how they migrate there; they are important in allergic responses.

probably similar to that of **mast cells**, which are believed to play a part in protecting the mucosal surfaces of the body and are the cells that release substances that affect vascular permeability. The cells of the myeloid lineage are shown in Fig. 1.4.

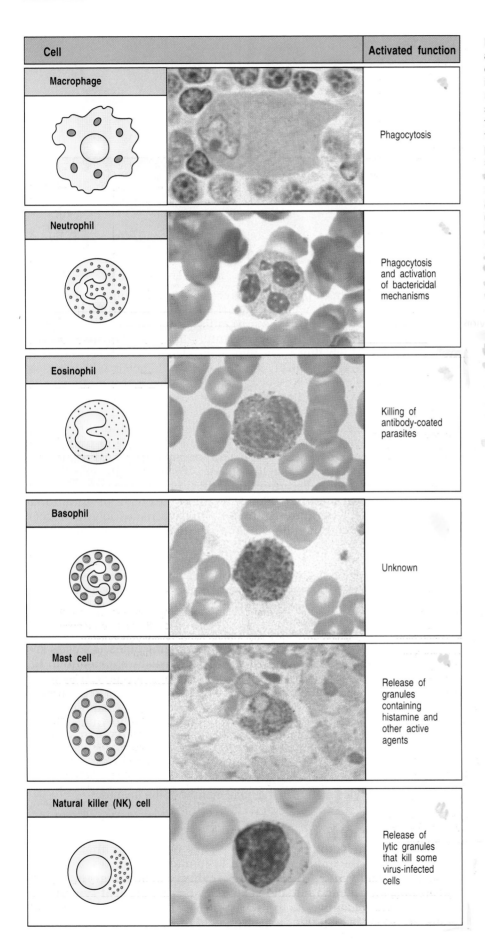

Cell		Activated function
Macrophage		Phagocytosis
Neutrophil		Phagocytosis and activation of bactericidal mechanisms
Eosinophil		Killing of antibody-coated parasites
Basophil		Unknown
Mast cell		Release of granules containing histamine and other active agents
Natural killer (NK) cell		Release of lytic granules that kill some virus-infected cells

Fig. 1.4   Myeloid cells in innate and adaptive immunity. Several different cell types of the myeloid lineage perform important functions in the immune response; these cells are shown schematically in the left column in the form in which they will be represented throughout the rest of the book. A photomicrograph of each cell type is shown in the center column. Macrophages and neutrophils, or polymorphonuclear neutrophilic leukocytes, are primarily phagocytic cells that engulf antibody-coated pathogens, which they destroy in intracellular vesicles after pathogen uptake. The other myeloid accessory effector cells are primarily secretory cells, which release the contents of their prominent granules upon binding to antibody-coated particles. Eosinophils are thought to be involved in attacking large parasites such as worms, while the function of basophils is unclear. Mast cells are tissue cells that trigger a local inflammatory response by releasing substances that act on local blood vessels when they are activated by antigen binding to IgE. Natural killer (NK) cells are large granular lymphocytes with important functions in viral infection and innate immunity. Photographs courtesy of N Rooney and B Smith.

Fig. 1.5 Small lymphocytes are cells whose main feature is inactivity. The left panel shows a light micrograph of a small lymphocyte. Note the condensed chromatin of the nucleus, indicating little transcriptional activity, the relative absence of cytoplasm, and the small size. The right panel shows a transmission electron micrograph of a small lymphocyte. Note the condensed chromatin, the scanty cytoplasm, the absence of rough endoplasmic reticulum, and other evidence of functional activity. Photographs courtesy of N Rooney.

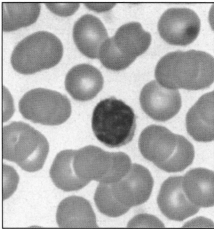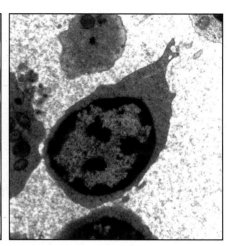

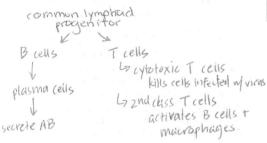

The common lymphoid progenitor gives rise to the lymphocytes, with which most of this book will be concerned. There are two major types of lymphocytes: **B lymphocytes or B cells**, which when activated differentiate into **plasma cells** that secrete antibodies; and **T lymphocytes or T cells**, of which there are two main classes. One class consists mainly of **cytotoxic T cells**, which kill cells infected with viruses, while the second class of T cells includes cells that activate other cells, such as B cells and macrophages.

Most lymphocytes are small, featureless cells with much of the nuclear chromatin inactive, as shown by its condensed state, and by the few cytoplasmic organelles (Fig. 1.5). This appearance is typical of inactive cells and it is not surprising that textbooks as recently as the early 1960s could describe these cells, now the central focus of immunology, as having no known function. Indeed, lymphocytes have no functional activity until they encounter antigen, which is necessary to trigger their proliferation and the differentiation of their specialized functional characteristics.

Both T and B lymphocytes bear on their surface highly diverse **receptors**. Each lymphocyte is equipped with a receptor specific for a particular antigen. Together, the receptors of all the different lymphocytes are capable of recognizing a very wide diversity of antigens. The **antigen receptor** of B lymphocytes is a membrane-bound form of the antibody that they will secrete when activated. Antibody molecules as a class are now generally known as **immunoglobulins**, usually shortened to **Ig**, and the antigen receptor of B lymphocytes is known as **surface immunoglobulin**. Immunoglobulin molecules are discussed in detail in Chapter 3, and the development of B lymphocytes is described in Chapter 5. The **T-cell antigen receptor** is related to immunoglobulin but quite distinct from it, and we shall describe the T-cell receptor for antigen in detail in Chapter 4 and T cell development in Chapter 6.

1-2   **Lymphocytes mature in the bone marrow or the thymus.**

The **lymphoid organs** are organized tissues where lymphocytes interact with non-lymphoid cells, which are important either to their maturation or to the initiation of adaptive immune responses. They can be divided broadly into primary or **central lymphoid organs**, where lymphocytes are generated, and secondary or **peripheral lymphoid organs**, where adaptive immune responses are initiated. The central lymphoid organs are the bone marrow and the **thymus**, a large organ

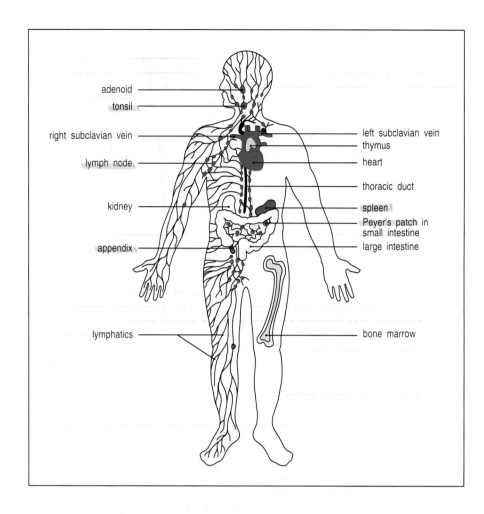

*Fig. 1.6   The distribution of lymphoid
tissues in the body*. Lymphocytes
arise from stem cells in bone marrow,
and differentiate in the central lymphoid
organs (yellow): B cells in bone marrow
and T cells in the thymus. They migrate
from these tissues through the bloodstream to the peripheral lymphoid tissues
(blue), the lymph nodes, spleen, and
lymphoid tissues associated with mucosa,
like the gut-associated lymphoid tissues
such as tonsils, Peyer's patches, and
appendix. These are the sites of
lymphocyte activation by antigen.
Lymphatics drain extracellular fluid as
lymph through the lymph nodes and into
the thoracic duct, which returns the
lymph to the bloodstream by emptying
into the left subclavian vein. Lymphocytes
that circulate in the bloodstream enter
the peripheral lymphoid organs, and are
eventually carried by lymph to the
thoracic duct where they re-enter the
bloodstream. Lymphoid tissue is also
associated with other mucosa such as
the bronchial linings (not shown).

in the upper chest: the location of the thymus, with the other lymphoid
organs, is shown schematically in Fig. 1.6.

Both B and T lymphocytes originate in the bone marrow but only B lymphocytes mature there: T lymphocytes migrate to the thymus to undergo maturation. Thus B lymphocytes are so called because they are bone marrow
derived, and T lymphocytes because they are thymus derived. Once
they have completed their maturation, both types of lymphocytes enter
the bloodstream, from which they migrate to the peripheral lymphoid organs.

1-3   The peripheral lymphoid organs are specialized to trap antigen and allow the initiation of adaptive immune responses.

Pathogens can enter the body by many routes and set up infections
anywhere but antigen and lymphocytes will eventually encounter each
other in the peripheral lymphoid organs—the lymph nodes, the spleen,
and mucosal lymphoid tissues (see Fig. 1.6). Lymphocytes are continually recirculating through these tissues, to which antigen is also carried
from all sites of infection and where it is trapped by specialized cells.

The **lymph nodes** are highly organized lymphoid structures that are
the sites of convergence of an extensive system of vessels that collect the
extracellular fluid from tissues and return it to the blood. The fluid is
called **lymph**, and the vessels that carry it **lymphatic vessels**, or
sometimes just **lymphatics** (see Fig. 1.6). The **afferent lymphatic
vessels**, which drain fluid from the tissues, also carry cells bearing

antigens from sites of infection in most parts of the body to the lymph nodes, where they are trapped. In the lymph nodes, B lymphocytes are localized in **follicles**, with T cells more diffusely distributed in surrounding **paracortical areas** also referred to as T-cell zones. Some of the B-cell follicles include **germinal centers**, where B cells are undergoing intense proliferation after encountering their specific antigen and helper T cells (Fig. 1.7). B and T lymphocytes are segregated in similar fashion in the other peripheral lymphoid tissues, and we shall see when we come to discuss the adaptive immune response that this organization promotes the crucial interactions that occur between B and T cells upon encountering antigen.

The **spleen** is a fist-sized organ just behind the stomach (see Fig. 1.6) that collects antigen from the blood. It also collects and disposes of senescent red blood cells. Its organization is shown schematically in Fig. 1.8. The bulk of the spleen is composed of **red pulp**, which is the site of red blood cell disposal. The lymphocytes surround the arterioles entering the organ, forming areas of **white pulp**, the inner region of which is divided into a **periarteriolar lymphoid sheath (PALS)** containing mainly T cells, and a flanking **B-cell corona**.

The **gut-associated lymphoid tissues (GALT)**, which include the **tonsils, adenoids**, and **appendix**, and specialized structures called **Peyer's patches** in the small intestine, collect antigen from the epithelial surfaces of the gastrointestinal tract. In Peyer's patches, which are the most important and highly organized of these tissues, the antigen is collected by specialized epithelial cells called **M cells**.

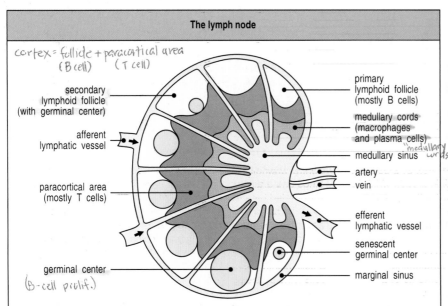

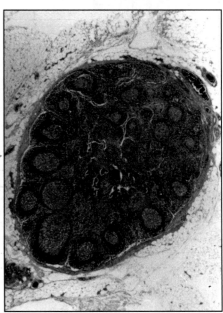

Fig. 1.7   A schematic view and a light micrograph of a lymph node. A lymph node consists of an outermost cortex and an inner medulla. The cortex is composed of an outer cortex of B lymphocytes organized into lymphoid follicles, and deep or paracortical areas made up mainly of T lymphocytes and specialized cells known as dendritic cells. Some of the B-cell follicles contain central areas of intense B-cell proliferation called germinal centers. These follicles are known as secondary lymphoid follicles. Lymph draining the extracellular spaces of the body carries antigens from the tissues to the lymph node via the afferent lymphatics. Lymph leaves by the efferent lymphatic in the medulla. The medulla consists of strings of macrophages and antibody-secreting plasma cells known as the medullary cords. Naive lymphocytes enter the node from the bloodstream through specialized post-capillary venules (not shown) and leave with the lymph through the efferent lymphatic. The photograph shows a section through a lymph node, with prominent follicles containing germinal centers. Photograph (x 7) courtesy of N Rooney.

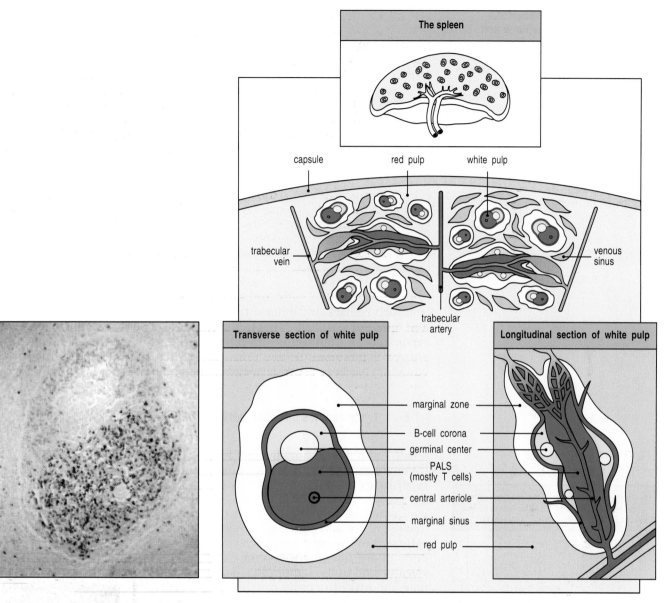

Fig. 1.8　Schematic views and light micrograph of a section of spleen. The spleen consists of red pulp (pink areas), which is a site of red blood cell destruction, interspersed with lymphoid white pulp (yellow and blue areas in the lower panels). The center panel shows an enlargement of a small section of the spleen showing the arrangement of discrete areas of white pulp around central arterioles. Most of the white pulp is shown in transverse section, with one portion shown in longitudinal section. The bottom two diagrams show enlargements of a transverse section (lower left) and longitudinal section (lower right) of white pulp. In each area of white pulp, blood carrying lymphocytes and antigen flows from a trabecular artery into a central arteriole. Cells and antigen then pass into a marginal sinus and drain into a trabecular vein. The marginal sinus is surrounded by a marginal zone of lymphocytes. Within the marginal sinus and surrounding the central arteriole is the periarteriolar lymphoid sheath (PALS), made up of T cells (stained darkly in the micrograph, which shows a transverse section of white pulp). The lymphoid follicles consist mainly of B cells (lightly stained), including germinal centers (the unstained cells lying between the B- and T-cell areas in the micrograph). While the organization of the spleen is similar to that of a lymph node, antigen enters the spleen from the blood rather than from the lymph. Photograph courtesy of J C Howard.

The lymphocytes form a follicle consisting of a large central dome of B lymphocytes surrounded by smaller numbers of T lymphocytes (Fig. 1.9). Similar but more diffusely organized aggregates of lymphocytes protect the respiratory epithelium, where they are known as **bronchial-associated lymphoid tissue** (**BALT**), and other mucosa, where they are known simply as **mucosal-associated lymphoid tissue** (**MALT**).

Fig. 1.9   Typical gut-associated lymphoid tissue in schematic and light microscopic views. The antigen enters across a specialized epithelium made up of so-called M cells. The bulk of the lymphoid tissue is B cells, organized in a large and highly active domed follicle. T cells occupy the areas between follicles. Although this tissue looks very different from other lymphoid organs, the basic divisions are maintained. The photograph shows a section of the gut wall. The dome of gut-associated lymphoid tissue can be seen lying beneath the epithelial tissues. Photograph (x 16) courtesy of N Rooney.

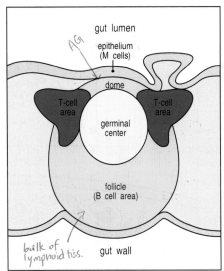
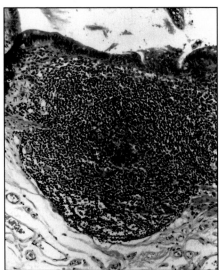

Although remarkably different in appearance, the lymph nodes, spleen, and mucosal-associated lymphoid tissues all share the same basic architecture. Each of these tissues operates on the same principle, trapping antigen from sites of infection and presenting it to migratory small lymphocytes, thus inducing adaptive immune responses.

1-4   Lymphocytes circulate between blood and lymph.

Small T and B lymphocytes that have matured in the bone marrow and thymus but have not yet encountered antigen are referred to as **naive lymphocytes**. These cells circulate continually from the blood into the peripheral lymphoid tissues, which they enter by means of specialized adhesive interactions with the capillaries supplying these tissues that allow them to squeeze between the endothelial cells. They are then returned to the blood via the lymphatic vessels (Fig. 1.10). In the presence of an infection, lymphocytes that recognize the infectious agent are arrested in the lymphoid tissue where they proliferate and differentiate into **effector cells** capable of combating the infection.

When an infection occurs in the periphery, for example, large amounts of antigen are taken up by phagocytic cells, which then travel from the site of infection through the afferent lymphatic vessels into the lymph nodes (see Fig. 1.10). In the lymph nodes, these cells display the antigen to recirculating lymphocytes, which they also help to activate. Once these specific lymphocytes have undergone a period of proliferation and differentiation, they leave the lymph nodes as effector cells through the **efferent lymphatic vessel** (see Fig. 1.7).

All the lymphoid tissues operate on the same principle, trapping cells arriving from sites of infection that present antigen to migratory small lymphocytes to stimulate adaptive immune responses. The lymphoid tissues are thus not static structures but vary quite dramatically depending upon whether or not infection is present. The diffuse mucosal lymphoid tissues may appear and disappear in response to infection, while the architecture of the more organized tissues changes in a defined way during an infection. For example, the B-cell follicles of the lymph nodes expand as B lymphocytes proliferate to form germinal centers (see Fig. 1.7), and the entire lymph node enlarges, a phenomenon familiarly known as swollen glands.

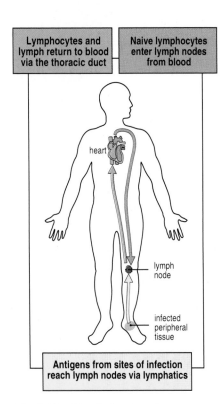

Fig. 1.10   Circulating lymphocytes encounter antigen in peripheral lymphoid tissues.

Summary.

Immune responses are mediated by leukocytes, which derive from precursors in the bone marrow. These give rise to the polymorpho-nuclear leukocytes and the macrophages of the innate immune system, and also the lymphocytes of the adaptive immune system. There are two major types of lymphocytes: B lymphocytes, which mature in the bone marrow; and T lymphocytes, which mature in the thymus. The bone marrow and thymus are thus known as the central lymphoid organs. Monocytes and mast-cell precursors migrate to the body tissues where they mature, while all the other cells of the immune system circulate in the blood. Lymphocytes recirculate continually from the bloodstream through the peripheral lymphoid organs, where antigen is trapped, returning to the bloodstream through the lymphatic vessels. The three major types of peripheral lymphoid tissue are the spleen, which collects antigens from the blood, the lymph nodes, which collect antigen from sites of infection in the tissues, and the gut-associated lymphoid tissue (GALT), which collects antigens from the gut. Other epithelia also have diffuse lymphoid tissue associated with them: these are known collectively with the GALT as mucosal-associated lymphoid tissue. Adaptive immune responses are initiated in the peripheral lymphoid tissues.

Principles of innate and adaptive immunity.

The phagocytes of the innate immune system provide a first line of defense against many common microorganisms and are essential to the control of common bacterial infections. However, they cannot always eliminate infectious organisms, and there are many pathogens that they cannot recognize. The lymphocytes of the adaptive immune system have evolved to provide a more versatile means of defense that, in addition, provides an increased level of protection from a subsequent re-infection with the same pathogen. The cells of the innate immune system play a crucial part in the initiation and subsequent direction of adaptive immune responses. Moreover, since there is a delay of 4-7 days before the initial adaptive immune response takes effect, the innate immune response has a critical role in controling infections during this period.

innate immune system
- *1st line of defense*
- *common bact. infections*
- *initiation + direction of adaptive immune rsp*
- *immediate (first few days crucial)*

1-5 Many bacteria activate phagocytes and trigger inflammatory responses.

Macrophages and neutrophils have surface receptors that have evolved to recognize and bind common constituents of many bacterial surfaces. Bacterial molecules binding to these receptors trigger the cells to engulf ① the bacterium and also induce the ② secretion of chemical mediators by these phagocytes. Among these are substances known as cytokines, which are defined as chemical mediators released by cells that affect the behavior of other cells. The cytokines released by phagocytes in response to bacterial constituents have a range of effects that are collectively known as **inflammation**. Inflammation is traditionally defined by the four Latin words *calor*, *dolor*, *rubor*, and *tumor*, meaning heat, pain, redness, and swelling, all of which reflect the effects of cytokines on the local blood vessels (Fig. 1.11). Dilation and increased permeability of the blood vessels during inflammation lead to increased local blood flow

Fig. 1.11 Bacterial infection triggers an inflammatory response. Macrophages encountering bacteria in the tissues are triggered to release cytokines that increase the permeability of blood vessels, allowing fluid and proteins to pass into the tissues. The stickiness of the endothelial cells of the blood vessels is also changed, so that cells adhere to the blood vessel wall and are able to crawl through it; macrophages and neutrophils are shown here entering the tissue from a blood vessel. The accumulation of fluid and cells at the site of infection causes the redness, swelling, heat, and pain, known collectively as inflammation. Macrophages and neutrophils are the principal inflammatory cells. Later in an immune response, activated lymphocytes may also contribute to inflammation.

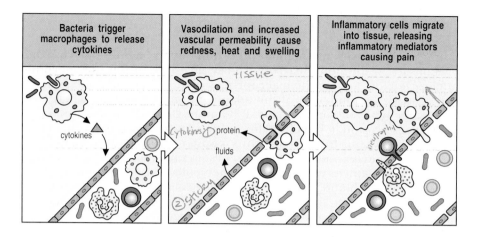

and the leakage of fluid, and account for the heat, redness and swelling. Cytokines also have important effects on the adhesive properties of the endothelium, causing circulating leukocytes to stick to the endothelial cells of the blood vessel wall and migrate through them to the site of infection, to which they are attracted by yet other cytokines. The migration of cells into the tissue and their local actions account for the pain. The main cell types seen in an inflammatory response in its initial phases are neutrophils, followed by macrophages; these are therefore known as **inflammatory cells**.

Inflammatory responses later in an infection involve the lymphocytes of the adaptive immune response, which have meanwhile been activated by antigen draining from the site of infection via the afferent lymphatics. The activation of lymphocytes depends critically on interactions with phagocytic cells, and bacterial constituents induce changes in the surface molecules expressed by these cells that are crucial to the central part they play in the induction of adaptive immune responses; we shall discuss these in detail in Chapter 9.

1-6 Lymphocytes are activated by antigen to give rise to clones of antigen-specific cells that mediate adaptive immunity.

The defense systems of innate immunity are effective in combating many pathogens but they are limited to those that bear surface molecules that are common to many pathogens and have remained unchanged in the course of evolution so that they can be recognized by neutrophils and macrophages in vertebrates. Not surprisingly, many bacteria have evolved capsules that enable them to conceal these molecules and thereby avoid provoking phagocytic cells. Viruses carry no such unvarying molecules and are rarely recognized by phagocytic cells. Moreover, the surface molecules of pathogens evolve much faster than could any ordinary vertebrate recognition system. The recognition mechanism used by the lymphocytes of the adaptive immune response has evolved to overcome these problems.

Instead of bearing several receptors each specifically recognizing a conserved surface molecule of a pathogen, each naive lymphocyte entering the bloodstream bears receptors of only a single specificity. However, the specificity of these receptors is determined by a unique genetic mechanism that operates during the development of lymphocytes in the bone marrow and thymus to generate hundreds of different variants of the genes encoding the receptor molecules. Thus, although the individual lymphocyte carries receptors of only one specificity, the

Fig. 1.12 The clonal selection hypothesis. During its normal course of development, each lymphocyte progenitor is able to give rise to many lymphocytes, each bearing a distinct antigen receptor. Many lymphocytes with receptors that bind ubiquitous self antigens are eliminated early in development before they become able to respond, assuring tolerance to such self antigens. When antigen interacts with the receptor on a mature lymphocyte, that cell is activated to become a blast cell (lymphoblast) and then starts to divide. It gives rise to a clone of identical progeny, all of whose receptors bind the same antigen. Antigen specificity is thus maintained as the progeny proliferate and differentiate into effector cells. Once antigen is eliminated by these effector cells, the immune response ceases.

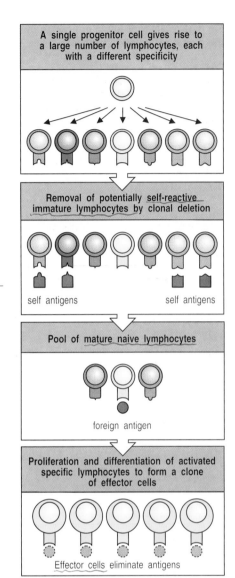

A single progenitor cell gives rise to a large number of lymphocytes, each with a different specificity

Removal of potentially self-reactive immature lymphocytes by clonal deletion

self antigens   self antigens

Pool of mature naive lymphocytes

foreign antigen

Proliferation and differentiation of activated specific lymphocytes to form a clone of effector cells

Effector cells eliminate antigens

specificity of each lymphocyte is different, and thus the millions of lymphocytes in the body give rise to millions of different specificities (Fig. 1.12). These lymphocytes then undergo a process akin to natural selection during the lifetime of an individual: only those lymphocytes that encounter an antigen to which their receptor binds will be activated to proliferate and differentiate into effector cells.

This selective mechanism was first proposed in the 1950s by F. McFarlane Burnet to explain why antibodies, which can be induced in response to virtually any antigen, are produced in each individual only to those antigens to which he or she is exposed. He postulated the pre-existence in the body of many different potential antibody-producing cells, each having the ability to make antibody of a different specificity and displaying on its surface a membrane-bound version of the antibody serving as a receptor for antigen. On binding antigen, the cell is activated to proliferate and produce many identical progeny, known as **clones**, which now secrete antibodies with a specificity identical to that of the surface receptor. McFarlane Burnet called this the **clonal selection theory**.

1-7 Clonal selection of lymphocytes is the central principle of adaptive immunity.

Remarkably, at the time that McFarlane Burnet formulated his theory, nothing was known of the antigen receptors of lymphocytes and indeed the function of lymphocytes themselves was still obscure. Lymphocytes did not take center stage until the early 1960s, when James Gowans discovered that removal of the small lymphocytes from rats resulted in the loss of all known immune responses. The immune responses were restored when the lymphocytes were replaced. This led to the realization that lymphocytes must be the units of clonal selection, and their biology became the focus of the new field of **cellular immunology**.

Clonal selection of lymphocytes with diverse receptors elegantly explained adaptive immunity but it raised one significant intellectual problem. If the antigen receptors of lymphocytes are generated randomly during the lifetime of an individual, how are lymphocytes prevented from recognizing antigens on the tissues of the body and attacking them? Peter Medawar had shown, in 1953, that if exposed to foreign tissues during embryonic development, animals become immunologically **tolerant** to these tissues and will not subsequently make immune responses to them. Burnet proposed that developing lymphocytes that are potentially self-reactive are removed before they can mature. He has since been proved right in this too, although the mechanisms of tolerance are still being worked out, as we shall see when we discuss the development of lymphocytes in Chapters 5 and 6.

Fig. 1.13 The four basic principles of the clonal selection hypothesis.

Postulates of the clonal selection hypothesis
Each lymphocyte bears a single type of receptor with a unique specificity
Interaction between a foreign molecule and a lymphocyte receptor capable of binding that molecule with high affinity leads to lymphocyte activation
The differentiated effector cells derived from an activated lymphocyte will bear receptors of identical specificity to those of the parental cell from which that lymphocyte was derived
Lymphocytes bearing receptors specific for ubiquitous self molecules are deleted at an early stage in lymphoid cell development and are therefore absent from the repertoire of mature lymphocytes

Clonal selection of lymphocytes is the single most important principle in adaptive immunity. It is shown schematically in Fig. 1.12, and its four basic postulates are listed in Fig. 1.13. The last of the problems posed by the clonal selection theory—that of how the diversity of lymphocyte antigen receptors is generated—was solved in the 1970s when advances in molecular biology made it possible to clone the genes encoding antibody molecules.

1-8 The structure of antibody molecules illustrates the problem of lymphocyte antigen receptor diversity.

Antibodies, as discussed above, are the secreted form of the B-cell antigen receptor. Since they are produced in very large quantities in response to antigen, they can be studied by traditional biochemical techniques; indeed their structure was understood long before recombinant DNA technology made it possible to study the membrane-bound antigen receptors of lymphocytes. The startling feature that emerged from the biochemical studies was that antibody molecules as a class are composed of two distinct regions: a **constant region**, that can take one of only four or five biochemically distinguishable forms; and a **variable region** that can take an apparently infinite variety of subtly different forms that allow it to bind specifically to an equally vast variety of different antigens.

This division is illustrated in the simple schematic diagram in Fig. 1.14, where the antibody is depicted as a Y-shaped molecule, with the constant region shown in blue and the variable region in red. The variable region determines the antigen-binding specificity of the antibody, and the constant region determines how the antibody disposes of the antigen once it is bound.

Each of the two antigen-binding regions of the antibody molecule is, in fact, composed of two chains, each having both a constant and a variable region (Fig. 1.15); the variable regions combine to form the antigen-binding site and both chains contribute to the antigen-binding specificity of the antibody molecule. The antibody molecule itself, therefore, is composed of four chains. The structure of antibody molecules will be described in detail in Chapter 3, where we shall also discuss the structural and genetic basis for the different functional properties of antibodies conferred by their constant regions. For the time being we are concerned only with the properties of immunoglobulin molecules as antigen receptors, and the central issue of how the diversity of the variable regions is generated.

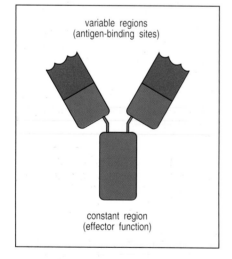

variable regions
(antigen-binding sites)

constant region
(effector function)

Fig. 1.14 Structure of the antibody molecule. The two arms of the Y-shaped antibody molecule contain the variable regions that form the two identical antigen-binding sites. The stem can take one of only a limited number of forms and is known as the constant region. It is the region that engages the effector mechanisms that antibodies activate to eliminate pathogens.

| 1-9 | **Each developing lymphocyte generates a unique receptor by rearranging its receptor genes.** |

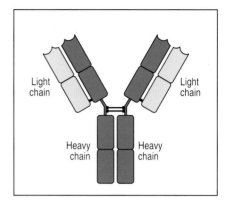

How are antigen receptors with an almost infinite range of specificities encoded by a finite number of genes? This question was answered in 1976, when Susumu Tonegawa discovered that the genes for immunoglobulin variable regions are inherited as sets of **gene segments** each encoding a part of the variable region of one of the polypeptide chains that make up an immunoglobulin molecule (Fig. 1.16). As B lymphocytes differentiate in the bone marrow, these gene segments are joined to form a stretch of DNA that codes for an entire variable region. Since there are many different segments in each set, and different gene segments are joined in different cells, each cell generates a unique gene for the variable region of each chain of the antibody molecule.

This mechanism has three important consequences. First it enables a limited number of gene segments to generate a very diverse set of proteins. Second, as each cell assembles a different set of gene segments to encode its antigen receptor, each cell expresses a unique receptor specificity. Third, as gene rearrangement involves an irreversible change in a cell's DNA, all the progeny of that cell will inherit genes encoding the same receptor specificity. This general scheme was later confirmed for the genes encoding the antigen receptor on T lymphocytes. The main distinctions between B and T lymphocyte receptors are that the cell-surface immunoglobulin molecule that serves as the B-cell receptor has two identical antigen recognition sites and can be secreted, while the **T-cell receptor** has a single antigen recognition site and is always a cell-surface molecule. We shall see later that these receptors also recognize antigen in very different ways.

The potential diversity of lymphocyte receptors generated in this way is enormous. Just a few hundred different gene segments can combine in different ways to generate thousands of different receptor chains. The diversity of lymphocyte receptors is further amplified by the fact that each receptor is made by pairing two different variable chains, each encoded in distinct sets of gene segments. A thousand different chains of each type could generate 10^6 distinct antigen receptors through this **combinatorial diversity**. Thus a small amount of genetic material can encode a truly staggering diversity of receptors; there are lymphocytes of at least 10^8 different specificities in an individual at any one time. Once gene rearrangement is complete, the antigen receptor is expressed on the surface of the developing lymphocyte, which is now ready to interact with antigen.

Fig. 1.15 Antibodies are made up of four chains. There are two types of chains in an antibody molecule: a larger chain called the heavy chain (green), and a smaller one called the light chain (yellow). Each chain has both a variable and a constant region, and there are two light chains and two heavy chains in each antibody molecule.

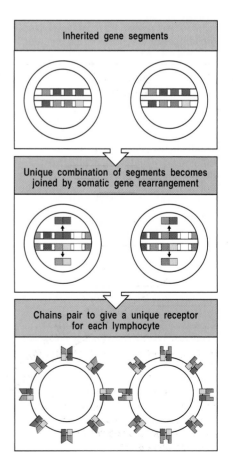

Fig. 1.16 The diversity of lymphocyte antigen receptors is generated by somatic gene rearrangements. Different parts of the variable region of antigen receptors are encoded by sets of gene segments. During a lymphocyte's development, one member of each set of gene segments is joined randomly to the others by an irreversible process of DNA recombination. The juxtaposed gene segments make up a complete gene encoding the variable part of one chain of the receptor, which is unique to that cell. This random process is repeated for the other set of gene segments, giving rise to the other chain. The expressed rearranged genes produce the two types of polypeptide chains that come together to form the unique antigen receptor on the lymphocyte surface. Once the two required recombination events have occurred, further gene rearrangement is prohibited. Thus, the receptor specificity of a lymphocyte cannot change once it has been determined, and the lymphocyte can only express one receptor specificity. Each lymphocyte bears many copies of its unique receptor.

1-10   **Lymphocytes proliferate in response to antigen in peripheral lymphoid tissue.**

Since each lymphocyte has a different antigen-binding specificity, the fraction of lymphocytes that can bind and respond to any given antigen is very small. To generate sufficient specific effector lymphocytes to fight an infection, an activated lymphocyte must proliferate before its progeny finally differentiate into effector cells. This **clonal expansion** is a feature of all adaptive immune responses.

Lymphocyte activation and proliferation is initiated in the lymphoid tissues where phagocytic cells carrying antigen are trapped. These display the antigen to the naive recirculating lymphocytes as they migrate through the lymphoid tissue before returning to the bloodstream via the lymph.

Fig. 1.17 Transmission electron micrographs of lymphocytes at various stages of activation to effector function. Small resting lymphocytes (upper panel) have not yet encountered antigen. Note the small amount of cytoplasm, with no rough endoplasmic reticulum, indicating an inactive cell. This cell could be either a T cell or a B cell. Small circulating lymphocytes are trapped in lymph nodes when their receptors encounter antigen on antigen-presenting cells. Stimulation by antigen induces the lymphocyte to become an active lymphoblast. This cell undergoes clonal expansion by repeated division, which is followed by differentiation to effector function. The central micrograph shows an activated lymphoblast responding to antigen. Note the large size, the nucleoli, the enlarged nucleus with diffuse chromatin, and the active cytoplasm; again, T and B cells are similar in appearance. The lower panels show effector T and B lymphocytes. Note the large amount of cytoplasm, the nucleus with prominent nucleoli, abundant mitochondria and the presence of rough endoplasmic reticulum, all hallmarks of active cells. The rough endoplasmic reticulum is especially prominent in antibody-secreting B cells, usually called plasma cells, which synthesize and secrete very large amounts of antibody protein. Photographs courtesy of N Rooney.

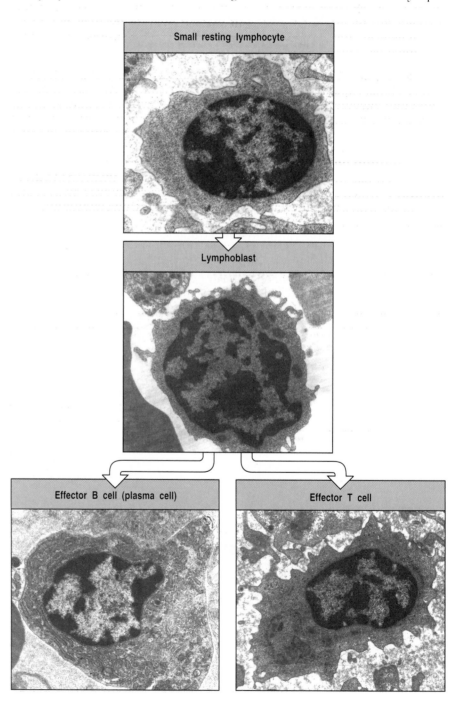

Small resting lymphocyte

Lymphoblast

Effector B cell (plasma cell)

Effector T cell

On recognizing its specific antigen, the small lymphocyte stops migrating and enlarges. The chromatin in its nucleus becomes less dense, nucleoli appear, the volume of cytoplasm increases, and new RNA and protein synthesis are induced. Within a few hours, the cell looks completely different, and activated cells at this stage are called **lymphoblasts** (Fig. 1.17).

The antigen-specific cells now begin to divide, normally duplicating two to four times every 24 hours for 3–5 days, so that one naive lymphocyte gives rise to a clone of around 1000 daughter cells of identical specificity. These then differentiate into effector cells able to secrete antibody, in the case of B cells, or in the case of T cells, to destroy infected cells or activate other cells of the immune system. These changes also affect the recirculation of lymphocytes—because of changes in the expression of specialized adhesion molecules on their surface, they cease circulating through the blood and lymph and instead migrate through the endothelial cells at sites of infection, signaled by the cytokines released by inflammatory cells at these sites.

After a lymphocyte has been activated, it takes 4–5 days of proliferation before clonal expansion is complete and the lymphocytes have differentiated into effector cells. That is why adaptive immune responses occur only after a delay of several days. Effector cells have only a limited lifespan and, once antigen is removed, most of the antigen-specific cells generated by the clonal expansion of small lymphocytes undergo **programmed cell death**, or **apoptosis**. However, some persist after the antigen has been eliminated. This is the basis of **immunological memory**, which ensures a more rapid and effective response on a second encounter with a pathogen and thereby provides lasting immunity.

The characteristics of immunological memory are observed readily by comparing the antibody response of an individual to a first or **primary immunization** with the response elicited in the same individual by a **secondary** or **booster immunization** with the same antigen. As detailed in Fig. 1.18, the **secondary antibody response** occurs after a shorter lag phase, achieves a markedly higher plateau level, and produces antibodies of higher affinity. We shall describe the mechanisms of these remarkable changes in Chapters 8 and 9. The cellular basis of

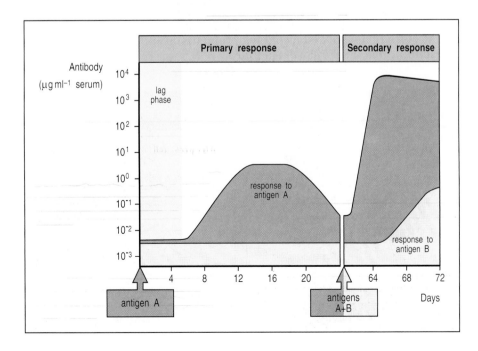

Fig. 1.18 The course of a typical antibody response. Antigen A introduced at time zero encounters little specific antibody in the serum. After a lag phase, antibody to antigen A (blue) appears and its concentration rises to a plateau, and then declines. When the serum is tested for antibody against another antigen, B (yellow), there is none present, demonstrating the specificity of the antibody response. When the animal is later challenged with a mixture of antigens A and B, a very rapid and intense response to A occurs. This illustrates immunological memory, the ability of the immune system to make a second response to the same antigen more efficiently and effectively, providing the host with specific defense against infection. Note that the response to B resembles the initial or primary response to A, as this is the first encounter of the host with antigen B.

immunological memory is the clonal expansion and clonal differentiation of cells specific for the eliciting antigen, and it is therefore entirely antigen specific.

It is immunological memory that allows successful vaccination and prevents re-infection with pathogens that have been repelled successfully by an adaptive immune response. Immunological memory is perhaps the most important biological consequence of the development of adaptive immunity based on clonal selection, although its cellular and molecular basis is still not fully understood, as we shall see in Chapter 9.

1-11 | Interaction with other cells as well as with antigen are necessary for lymphocyte activation.

Peripheral lymphoid tissues are specialized not only to trap phagocytic cells that ingest antigen but also to promote the interactions between cells that are necessary for the initiation of adaptive immune responses. The spleen and lymph nodes in particular are highly organized for the latter function.

We have already mentioned that one of the functions of T cells is to stimulate the production of antibody by B cells. In fact, all lymphocyte responses to antigen require a second signal from another cell. For most B-cell responses, the signal comes from a T cell (Fig. 1.19, left panel); for T cells (see Fig. 1.19, right panel), the second signal may be delivered by any of three cell types: **dendritic cells**, macrophages, and B cells. Mature dendritic cells are cells with a distinctive branched morphology found exclusively in the T-cell areas of lymphoid tissue. The precursors of these cells trap antigen in the periphery and migrate to lymphoid tissues where they present antigens to T cells. Because of this and their ability to deliver activating signals, they, with macrophages and B cells, are known as **professional antigen-presenting cells**, or often just **antigen-presenting cells**. The three cell types that can present antigen to T cells are illustrated in Fig. 1.20. Dendritic cells are the most important antigen-presenting cell of the three, playing a central part in the initiation of adaptive immune responses while macrophages mediate innate immune responses directly and make a crucial contribution to the effector phase of the adaptive immune response.

Antigen born by antigen-presenting cells may be swept into the spleen by the blood or into the lymph nodes by the lymph, or be taken up by the **M cells** of the gut-associated lymphoid tissue and trapped by antigen-presenting cells already present there.

Fig. 1.19 Two signals are required for lymphocyte activation. As well as receiving a signal through their antigen receptor, mature lymphocytes must also receive a second signal in order to become activated. For B cells (left panel), the second signal is usually delivered by a T cell. For T cells (right panel) it is delivered by a professional antigen-presenting cell, shown here as a dendritic cell.

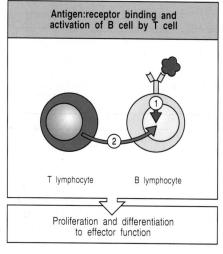

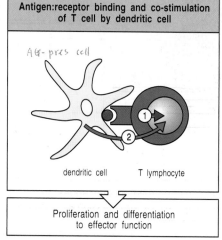

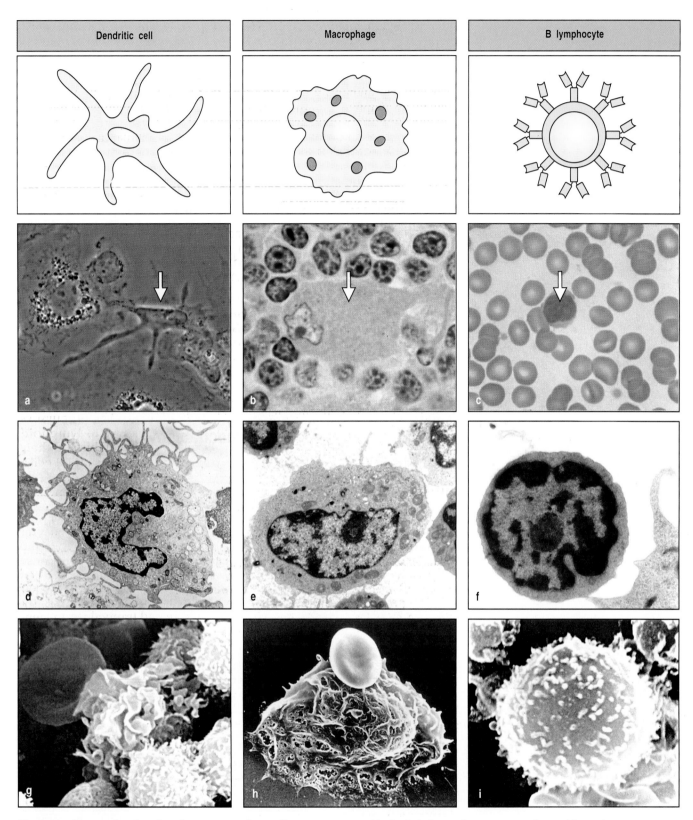

Fig. 1.20   The professional antigen-presenting cells.
The three types of professional antigen-presenting cell are shown in the form in which they will be depicted throughout this book (top row), as they appear in the light microscope (second row), by transmission electron microscopy (third row) and by scanning electron microscopy (bottom row). Dendritic cells are found in lymphoid tissues and are thought to have a critical role in immunity to many antigens. Macrophages are specialized to internalize and present particulate antigens, and B cells have antigen-specific receptors that allow them to internalize large amounts of specific antigen and present it to T cells. Photographs courtesy of R M Steinman (a); N Rooney (b, c, e, f); S Knight (d, g); P F Heap (h, i).

Summary.

The early innate systems of defense, which depend on invariant responses to common features of pathogens, are important but they cannot confer protection from novel types of pathogens and do not lead to immunological memory. These are the unique features of adaptive immunity based on clonal selection of lymphocytes bearing specific receptors.

The clonal selection of lymphocytes provides a theoretical framework for understanding all the key features of adaptive immunity. Each lymphocyte carries cell-surface receptors of a single specificity, generated by random recombination of variable receptor gene segments and the pairing of different variable chains. This produces lymphocytes each bearing a distinct receptor, so that the total **repertoire** of receptors can recognize virtually any antigen. If the receptor on a lymphocyte is specific for a ubiquitous self antigen, the cell is eliminated by encountering the antigen early in development. When a recirculating lymphocyte encounters foreign antigen in lymphoid tissues, it is induced to proliferate and its progeny then differentiate into effector cells that can eliminate a specific infectious agent. A subset of these proliferating lymphocytes differentiates into memory cells, ready to respond rapidly to the same pathogen if it is encountered again. The details of these processes of recognition, development, and differentiation form the main material of the middle three parts of this book.

Recognition and effector mechanisms of adaptive immunity.

Clonal selection describes the basic operating principle of the adaptive immune response but not its mechanisms. In the last section of this chapter, we outline the mechanisms by which pathogens are detected by lymphocytes and eventually destroyed in a successful adaptive immune response. Different pathogens have distinct lifestyles that require different mechanisms not only to ensure their destruction but also for their detection and recognition (Fig. 1.21). We have already seen that there are two different

Fig. 1.21   The major pathogen types confronting the immune system and some of the diseases they cause.

The immune system protects against four classes of pathogens		
Type of pathogen	Examples	Diseases
Extracellular bacteria, parasites, fungi	*Streptococcus pneumoniae* *Clostridium tetani* *Trypanosoma brucei*	Pneumonia Tetanus Sleeping sickness
Intracellular bacteria, parasites	*Mycobacterium leprae* *Leishmania donovani* *Plasmodium falciparum*	Leprosy Leishmaniasis Malaria
Viruses (intracellular)	Variola Influenza Varicella	Smallpox Flu Chickenpox
Parasitic worms (extracellular)	*Ascaris* *Schistosoma*	Ascariasis Schistosomiasis

kinds of antigen receptors: the surface immunoglobulin of B cells, and the smaller antigen receptor of T cells. These surface receptors are adapted to recognize antigen in two different ways: B cells recognize antigen outside cells, where, for example, most bacteria are found; T cells, by contrast, can detect antigens generated inside cells, for example by viruses.

The **effector mechanisms** that operate to eliminate pathogens in an adaptive immune response are essentially identical to those of innate immunity. Indeed, it seems likely that specific recognition by clonally distributed receptors evolved as a late addition to existing innate effector mechanisms to produce the present-day adaptive immune response. We begin by outlining the effector actions of antibodies, which depend almost entirely on recruiting cells and molecules of the innate immune system.

1-12	**Extracellular pathogens and their toxins are eliminated by antibodies.**

Antibodies, which were the first specific product of the immune response to be identified, are found in the fluid component of blood, or **plasma**, and in extracellular fluids. Since body fluids were once known as humors, immunity mediated by antibody is known as **humoral immunity**.

B cells → AB

As we have seen in Fig. 1.14, antibodies are Y-shaped molecules whose arms form two identical antigen-binding sites that are highly variable from one molecule to another, providing the diversity required for specific antigen recognition. The stem of the Y, which defines the **class** of the antibody and determines its functional properties, takes one of only five major forms, or **isotypes**. Each of the five antibody classes engages a distinct set of effector mechanisms for disposing of antigen once it is recognized. We shall describe the isotypes and their actions in detail in Chapters 3 and 8.

The simplest way in which antibodies can protect from pathogens or their toxic products is by binding to them and thereby blocking their access to cells they may infect or destroy (Fig. 1.22, left panels). This is known as **neutralization** and is important for protection against bacterial toxins and against pathogens such as viruses, which can thus be prevented from entering cells and replicating.

AB bind to pathogen

Binding by antibodies, however, is not sufficient on its own to arrest the replication of bacteria that multiply outside cells. In this case, one role of antibody is to enable a phagocytic cell to ingest and destroy the bacterium. This is important for the many bacteria that are resistant to direct recognition by phagocytes; instead, the phagocytes recognize the constant region of the antibodies coating the bacterium (see Fig. 1.22, middle panels). The coating of pathogens and foreign particles in this way is known as **opsonization**.

*AB coats bac...
phagocytes ingest*

The third function of antibodies is to activate a system of plasma proteins known as **complement**. The complement system, which we shall discuss in detail in Chapter 8, can directly destroy bacteria, and this is important in a few bacterial infections (see Fig. 1.22, right panels). Its main function, however, like that of antibodies themselves, is to enable phagocytes to engulf and destroy bacteria they would otherwise not recognize. Complement also enhances the bactericidal actions of phagocytes; indeed it is so called because it complements the activities of antibodies.

AB activate plasma (P) = complement

Antibodies of different isotypes are found in different compartments of the body and differ in the effector mechanisms they recruit, but all

Fig. 1.22 Antibodies can participate in host defense in three main ways. The left panels show antibodies binding to and neutralizing a bacterial toxin, preventing it from interacting with host cells and causing pathology. Unbound toxin can react with receptors on the host cell, whereas the toxin:antibody complex cannot. Antibodies also neutralize complete virus particles and bacterial cells by binding to them and inactivating them. The antigen:antibody complex is eventually scavenged and degraded by macrophages. Antibodies coating an antigen render it recognizable as foreign by phagocytes (macrophages and polymorphonuclear leukocytes), which then ingest and destroy it; this is called opsonization. The middle panels show opsonization and phagocytosis of a bacterial cell. The right panels show activation of the complement system by antibodies coating a bacterial cell. Bound antibodies form a receptor for the first protein of the complement system, which eventually forms a protein complex on the surface of the bacterium that, in some cases, can kill the bacterium directly but more generally favors the uptake and destruction of the bacterium by phagocytes. Thus, antibodies target pathogens and their products for disposal by phagocytes.

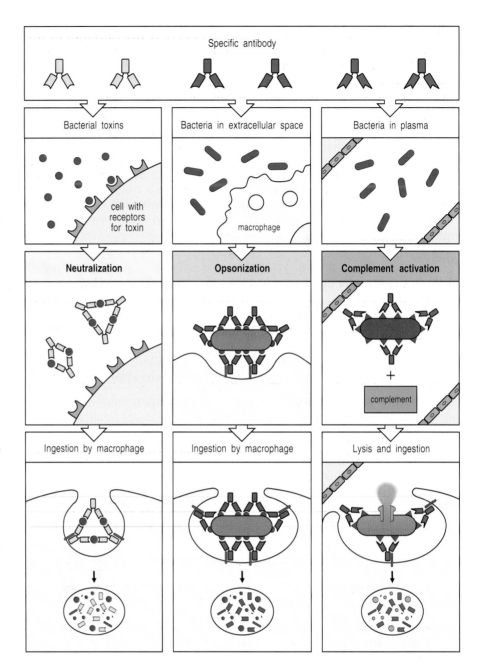

pathogens and particles bound by antibody are eventually delivered to phagocytes for ingestion, degradation, and removal from the body (see Fig. 1.22, bottom panels).

The complement system and the phagocytes that antibodies recruit are not themselves antigen-specific; they depend upon antibody molecules to mark the particles as foreign. Antibodies are the sole contribution of B cells to the adaptive immune response. T cells, by contrast, have a variety of effector actions.

1-13   T cells are needed to control intracellular pathogens and to activate B-cell responses to most antigens.

Pathogens are accessible to antibodies only in the blood and the extracellular spaces. However, some bacterial pathogens and parasites, and all viruses, replicate inside cells where they cannot be detected by antibodies. The destruction of these invaders is the function of the T lymphocytes, or T cells, which are responsible for the **cell-mediated immune responses** of adaptive immunity.

Cell-mediated reactions depend on direct interactions between T lymphocytes and cells bearing the antigen the T cells recognize. The actions of cytotoxic T cells are the most direct. These cells recognize body cells infected with viruses, which replicate inside cells using the synthetic machinery of the cell itself. The replicating virus eventually kills the cell, releasing the new virus particles. Antigens derived from the replicating virus, however, are meanwhile displayed on the surface of infected cells, where they are recognized by cytotoxic T cells and these may then control the infection by killing the cell before viral replication is complete (Fig. 1.23).

T lymphocytes are also important in the control of intracellular bacterial infections. Some bacteria grow only in the vesicles of macrophages; an important example is *Mycobacterium tuberculosis*, the pathogen that causes tuberculosis (Fig. 1.24). Bacteria entering macrophages are usually destroyed in the lysosomes, which contain a variety of enzymes and bactericidal substances. Intracellular bacteria survive because the vesicles they occupy do not fuse with the lysosomes. These infections can be controlled by a second type of T cell, known as a **T$_H$1 cell**, which activates macrophages, inducing the fusion of their lysosomes with the vesicles containing the bacteria and at the same time stimulating other antibacterial mechanisms of the phagocyte. T$_H$1 cells also release cytokines that attract macrophages to the site of infection.

T cells destroy intracellular pathogens by killing infected cells and by activating macrophages but they also play a central part in the destruction of extracellular pathogens by activating B cells. This is the specialized

(Handwritten margin notes: T cells; intracellular viral; intracellular bac.; extracellular via B cell activatn)

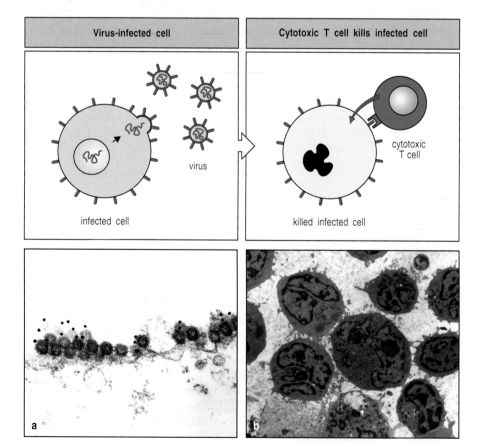

Virus-infected cell — infected cell — virus

Cytotoxic T cell kills infected cell — cytotoxic T cell — killed infected cell

a

b

Fig. 1.23 Mechanism of host defense against intracellular infection by viruses. Cells infected by viruses are recognized by specialized T cells called cytotoxic T cells, which kill the infected cells directly. The killing mechanism involves the activation of nucleases in the infected cell, which cleave host and viral DNA. Panel a is a transmission electron micrograph showing the plasma membrane of a Chinese hamster ovary (CHO) cell infected with influenza virus. Many virus particles can be seen budding from the cell surface. Some of these have been labeled with a monoclonal antibody that is specific for a viral protein and that is coupled to gold particles, which appear as the solid black dots in the micrograph. Panel b is a transmission electron micrograph of a virus-infected cell surrounded by reactive T lymphocytes. Note the close apposition of the membranes of the virus-infected cell and the T cell in the upper left corner of the micrograph, and the clustering of the cytoplasmic organelles between the nucleus and the point of contact with the infected cell. Panel a courtesy of M Bui and A Helenius. Panel b courtesy of N Rooney.

Fig. 1.24 Mechanism of host defense against intracellular infection by mycobacteria. Mycobacteria infecting macrophages live in cytoplasmic vesicles that resist fusion with lysosomes and consequent destruction of the bacteria by macrophage bactericidal activity. However, when a specific T$_H$1 cell recognizes an infected macrophage, it releases macrophage-activating molecules or cytokines that induce lysosomal fusion and the activation of macrophage bactericidal activities. The elimination of mycobacteria from the vesicles of activated macrophages can be seen in the light micrographs (bottom row) of resting (left) and activated (right) macrophages infected with *M. tuberculosis*. The cells have been stained with an acid-fast red dye to reveal the presence of the mycobacteria, which are prominent as red-staining rods in the resting macrophages but have been eliminated from the activated macrophages. Photographs courtesy of G Kaplan.

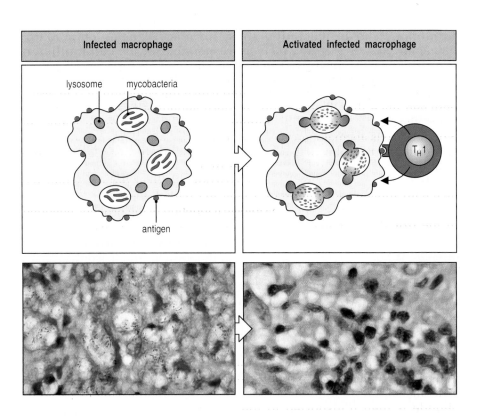

role of a third subset of T cells, called **helper T cells** or **T$_H$2 cells**. We shall see in Chapter 8 when we discuss the humoral immune response in detail that only a few antigens, that have special properties, are capable of activating naive B lymphocytes on their own. Most antigens require an accompanying signal from T$_H$2 cells before they can stimulate B cells to proliferate and differentiate into cells capable of secreting antibody (see Fig. 1.19). The ability of T cells to activate B cells was discovered long before it was recognized that a largely distinct class of T cells exists that activate macrophages, and the term helper T cell was originally coined to describe T cells that activate B cells. Although the designation 'helper' was later extended to T cells that activate macrophages (hence the H in T$_H$1), we consider this usage confusing and we will, in the remainder of this book, reserve the term helper T cells for T cells that activate B cells.

1-14   T cells are specialized to recognize foreign antigens as peptide fragments bound to proteins of the major histocompatibility complex.

All the effects of T lymphocytes depend upon interactions with cells containing foreign proteins. In the case of cytotoxic T cells and T$_H$1 cells, the proteins are produced by pathogens infecting the target cell or that have been ingested by it. Helper T cells, on the other hand, recognize and interact with B cells that have bound and internalized foreign antigen via their surface immunoglobulin. In all cases, T cells recognize their targets by detecting peptide fragments derived from these foreign proteins and bound to specialized cell-surface molecules on the infected host cells, on phagocytes, or on B cells. The molecules that display peptide antigen to T cells are membrane glycoproteins encoded in a cluster of genes bearing the cumbersome name **major histocompatibility complex**, abbreviated to **MHC**.

The human **MHC molecules** were first discovered as the result of attempts to use skin grafts from donors to repair badly burned pilots and bomb victims during World War II. The patients rejected the grafts, and eventually genetic experiments on inbred mice led to the identification of a complex of genes that would cause the rejection of skin grafts between mice that differed only at these genetic loci and at no other. Since they control the compatibility of tissue grafts, these genes, of which there is an analogous set in humans, became known as the histocompatibility complex of genes. It is called the major histocompatibility complex because proteins encoded by other genes can have minor effects on tissue compatibility, for reasons we shall discuss when we deal with antigen recognition by T cells in Chapter 4 and transplantation of tissues in Chapter 12. The physiological function of the proteins encoded by the MHC did not emerge until many years after their discovery.

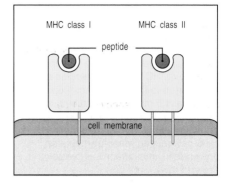

Fig. 1.25   MHC molecules display peptide fragments of antigens on the surface of cells. MHC molecules are membrane proteins whose outer extracellular domains form a cleft in which a peptide fragment can bind. These fragments, which are derived from proteins degraded inside the cell, including foreign protein antigens, are bound by the newly synthesized MHC molecule before it reaches the surface. There are two kinds of MHC molecules, MHC class I molecules and MHC class II molecules, which differ in structure and function.

1-15   Two major types of T cells recognize peptides bound by two different classes of MHC molecule.

It is now known that there are two types of MHC molecules, called MHC class I and MHC class II, which differ in subtle ways but share most of their major structural features. The most important of these structural features is the outer extracellular domains that form a long cleft in which peptide fragments are trapped during the synthesis and assembly of the MHC molecule inside the cell. The MHC molecule bearing its cargo of peptide is then transported to the cell surface where it displays the bound peptide to T cells (Fig. 1.25). The antigen receptors of T lymphocytes are specialized to recognize foreign antigenic peptide fragments bound to an MHC molecule.

The most important differences between the two classes of MHC molecules lie not in their structure but in the source of the peptides they trap and carry to the cell surface. **MHC class I molecules** collect peptides derived from proteins synthesized in the cytosol, and are thus able to display fragments of viral proteins on the cell surface (Fig. 1.26). **MHC class II molecules** bind peptides derived from proteins in intracellular membrane-bound vesicles, and thus display peptides derived from pathogens living in macrophage vesicles or internalized by phagocytic cells or B cells (Fig. 1.27). We shall see in Chapter 4 exactly how peptides from these different origins are made differentially accessible to the two types of MHC molecules.

Once they reach the cell surface with their cargo of antigenic peptides, the two classes of MHC molecules are recognized by different functional

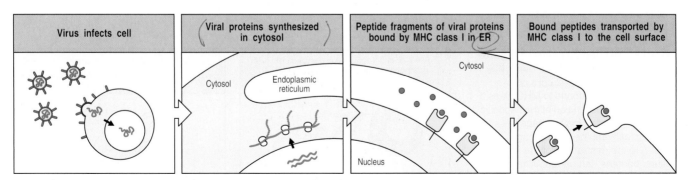

Fig. 1.26   MHC class I molecules present antigen derived from proteins in the cytosol. In cells infected with viruses, viral proteins are synthesized in the cytosol. Peptide fragments of viral proteins are transported into the endoplasmic reticulum where they are bound by MHC class I molecules, which then deliver the peptides to the cell surface.

Fig. 1.27   MHC class II molecules present antigen originating in intracellular vesicles. Some bacteria infect cells and grow in intracellular vesicles. Peptides derived from such bacteria are bound by MHC class II molecules and transported to the cell surface (top row). MHC class II molecules also bind and transport peptides derived from antigen that has been bound and internalized by B-cell antigen receptor-mediated endocytosis into intracellular vesicles (bottom row).

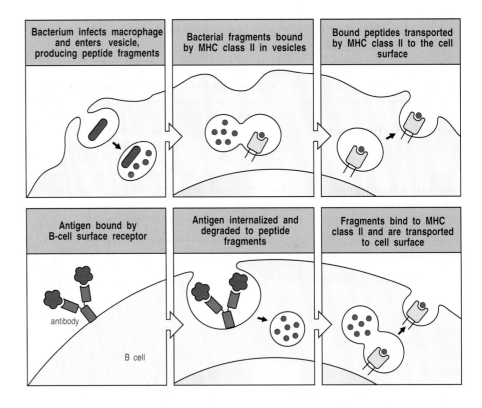

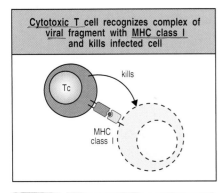

Fig. 1.28   Cytotoxic T cells recognize antigen presented by MHC class I molecules and kill the cell. The peptide:MHC class I complex on virus-infected cells is detected by antigen-specific cytotoxic T cells. Cytotoxic T cells are pre-programmed to kill cells.

classes of T cells. MHC class I molecules bearing viral peptides are recognized by cytotoxic T cells, which kill the infected cell (Fig. 1.28); MHC class II molecules bearing peptides derived from pathogens living in the vesicles of macrophages or taken up by B cells are recognized by the TH1 or TH2 cells (Fig. 1.29). How the differential recognition of the two types of MHC molecules becomes coupled to the distinct functions of the different classes of T cells during their development is a central problem in immunology and will be a major topic of Chapter 6.

On recognizing their targets, the three types of T cells are stimulated to release different sets of effector molecules that directly affect their target cells in ways we shall discuss in Chapter 7, and help to recruit other effector cells, as we shall see in Chapter 9 where we discuss the integration of various responses to infection. We shall see that many cytokines are included in these effector molecules; these play a crucial part in clonal expansion of lymphocytes as well as in innate immune responses and in the effector actions of most immune cells, and are thus central to the understanding of the immune system.

Fig. 1.29   TH1 and TH2 cells recognize antigen presented by MHC class II molecules. TH1 and TH2 cells both recognize peptides bound to MHC class II molecules. On recognition of their specific antigen on infected macrophages, TH1 cells activate the macrophage, leading to the destruction of the intracellular bacteria (left panel). When TH2 cells recognize antigen on B cells, helper T cells activate these cells to proliferate and differentiate into antibody-producing plasma cells (right panel).

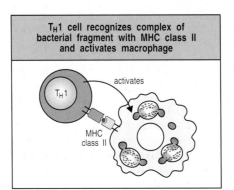
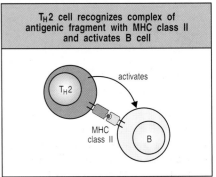

1-16 Specific infectious diseases result from immune deficiencies or specialized strategies of pathogens.

We tend to take for granted the ability of our immune systems to free our bodies of infection and prevent its recurrence. In some people, however, parts of the immune system fail. In the most severe of these **immunodeficiency diseases**, adaptive immunity is completely eliminated, and death occurs in infancy from overwhelming infection unless heroic measures are taken. Other less catastrophic failures lead to specific recurrent infections, and much has been learned about the functions of the different components of the immune system through the study of these diseases.

Eighteen years ago, a devastating form of immunodeficiency appeared, the **acquired immune deficiency syndrome**, or **AIDS**, which is itself caused by an infectious agent. This disease destroys the T_H1 and T_H2 cells that play a central part in most immune responses, leading to infections caused by intracellular bacteria and other pathogens normally controlled by macrophages activated by these T cells. Such infections are the major cause of death from this increasingly prevalent immunodeficiency disease.

AIDS is caused by a virus, the **human immunodeficiency virus**, or **HIV**, that has evolved several strategies whereby it not only evades but also subverts the protective mechanisms of the adaptive immune response. We discuss in Chapter 10 the devices that have evolved to allow many bacteria and parasites, as well as viruses, to avoid destruction by the immune system. The conquest of many of the world's leading causes of disease, including malaria and the various diarrheal diseases (the leading killers of children), as well as of the more recent threat from AIDS, may depend upon a better understanding of the interactions of these pathogens with the cells of the immune system.

1-17 Understanding adaptive immune responses is important for the control of allergies, autoimmune disease, and organ graft rejection, and for vaccination.

Many medically important diseases are associated with immune responses directed against inappropriate antigens, often in the absence of infectious disease. Normal immune responses in the absence of infection occur in **allergy**, where the antigen is an innocuous foreign substance, in **autoimmune disease**, where the response is to a self antigen, and in **graft rejection**, where the antigen is borne by a foreign cell. What we call an immune response or its failure, and whether the response is considered harmful or beneficial to the host, depends not on the response itself but on the nature of the antigen (Fig. 1.30).

Allergies, which include asthma, are an increasingly common cause of disability in the developed world, and many important diseases are now recognized as autoimmune. An autoimmune response directed against pancreatic β cells is the leading cause of diabetes in the young. In allergies and autoimmune diseases, the powerful protective mechanisms of the adaptive immune response are the cause of serious damage to the host.

Immune responses to harmless antigens, to body tissues, or to organ grafts, like all other immune responses, are highly specific. At present, the usual way to treat these responses is with **immunosuppressive drugs**, which inhibit all immune responses, desirable or undesirable. If, instead, it were possible to suppress only those lymphocyte clones

Fig. 1.30   Immune responses can be beneficial or harmful depending on the nature of the antigen. Beneficial responses are shown in white, harmful responses in shaded boxes. Where the response is beneficial, its absence is harmful.

Antigen	Effect of response to antigen	
	Normal response	Deficient response
Infectious agent	Protective immunity	Recurrent infection
Innocuous substance	Allergy	No response
Grafted organ	Rejection	Acceptance
Self organ	Autoimmunity	Self tolerance
Tumor	Tumor immunity	Cancer

responsible for the unwanted response, the disease could be cured (or the grafted organ protected) without impeding protective immune responses. Although antigen-specific suppression of immune responses can be induced experimentally, the molecular basis of suppression is unknown. If one could achieve control of the immune response, then the dream of antigen-specific **immunoregulation** to control unwanted immune responses could become a reality. We shall see in Chapter 9 how the mechanisms of immune regulation are beginning to emerge from a better understanding of the functional subsets of lymphocytes and the cytokines that control them, and we shall discuss the present state of understanding of allergies, autoimmune disease, graft rejection, and of immunosuppressive drugs in Chapters 11, 12, and 13.

1-18   Specific stimulation of adaptive immune responses is the most effective way to prevent infectious disease.

While the specific suppression of immune responses must await advances in basic research on immune regulation and its application, immunology has, in the two centuries since Jenner's pioneering experiment, achieved its greatest practical successes in the results of vaccination.

Mass immunization programs have led to the virtual eradication of several diseases that used to be associated with significant mortality and morbidity (Fig. 1.31). Immunization is considered so safe and so important that most states in the USA require children to be immunized against up to seven common childhood diseases. Impressive as these accomplishments are, there are still many diseases for which we lack effective vaccines, and even where a vaccine such as measles or polio can be used effectively in developed countries, technical and economic problems may prevent its widespread use in developing countries, where mortality from these diseases is still high. The tools of modern immunology and molecular biology are being applied to develop new vaccines and improve old ones, and we shall discuss these advances in Chapter 13. The prospect of controlling these important diseases is tremendously exciting. The guarantee of good health is a critical step towards population control and economic development. At a cost of pennies per person, great hardship and suffering can be alleviated.

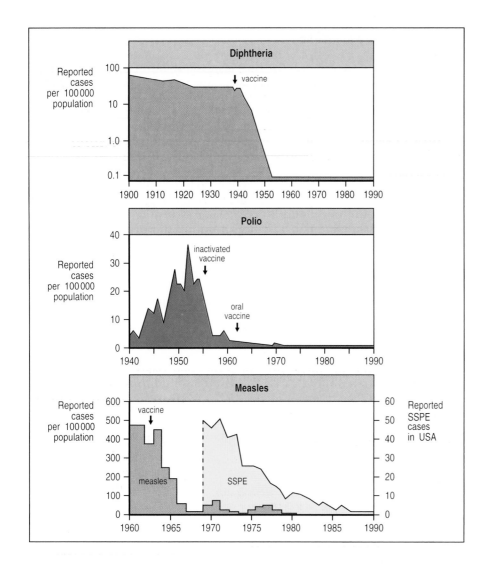

Fig. 1.31 Successful vaccination campaigns. Diphtheria, polio, and measles and its consequences have been virtually eliminated in the USA, as shown in these three graphs. SSPE stands for subacute sclerosing panencephalitis, a brain disease that is a late consequence of measles infection in a few patients. When measles was prevented, SSPE disappeared 10–15 years later. However, as these diseases have not been eradicated worldwide, immunization must be maintained in a very high percentage of the population to prevent their reappearance.

Summary.

Lymphocytes have two distinct recognition systems specialized for detection of extracellular and intracellular pathogens. B cells have cell-surface immunoglobulin molecules as receptors for antigen and, upon activation, secrete the immunoglobulin as soluble antibody that provides defense against pathogens in the extracellular spaces of the body. T cells have receptors that recognize peptide fragments of intracellular pathogens transported to the cell surface by the glycoproteins of the major histo-compatibility complex (MHC). Two classes of MHC molecules transport peptides from different intracellular compartments to present them to distinct types of effector T cells: cytotoxic T cells that kill infected target cells, and T_H1 and T_H2 cells that mainly activate macrophages and B cells. Thus, T cells are crucially important for both the humoral and cell-mediated responses of adaptive immunity. The adaptive immune response appears to have engrafted specific antigen recognition by highly diversified receptors onto innate defense systems. These play a central part in the effector actions of both B and T lymphocytes. The antigen-specific suppression of adaptive immune responses is the goal of treatment for important human diseases involving inappropriate activation of lymphocytes, while the specific stimulation of adaptive immune responses is the basis for successful vaccination campaigns.

Summary to Chapter 1.

The immune system defends the host against infection. Innate immunity serves as a first line of defense but lacks the ability to recognize certain pathogens and to provide the specific protective immunity that prevents re-infection. Adaptive immunity is based on the clonal selection of lymphocytes bearing highly diverse antigen-specific receptors, which allow the immune system to recognize any foreign antigen. In the adaptive immune response, antigen-specific lymphocytes proliferate and differentiate into effector cells that eliminate pathogens. Host defense requires different recognition systems and a wide variety of effector mechanisms to seek out and destroy the wide variety of pathogens in their various habitats within the body and at its surface. Not only can the adaptive immune response eliminate a pathogen but, in the process, it also generates increased numbers of differentiated memory lymphocytes through clonal section and this allows a more rapid and effective response upon re-infection. The regulation of immune responses, whether to suppress them when unwanted or to stimulate them in the prevention of infectious disease, is the major medical goal of research in immunology.

General references.

Historical background

Silverstein, A.M.: *History of Immunology*, 1st edn. London, Academic Press, 1989.

Landsteiner, K.: *The Specificity of Serological Reactions*, 3rd edn. Boston, Harvard University Press, 1964.

Burnet, F.M.: *The Clonal Selection Theory of Acquired Immunity*. London, Cambridge University Press, 1959.

Metchnikoff, E.: *Immunity in the Infectious Diseases*, 1st edn. New York, Macmillan Press, 1905.

Gowans, J.L.: *The Lymphocyte—a disgraceful gap in medical knowledge*. *Immunol. Today*, 1996, **17**:288-291.

Biological background

Alberts, B., Bray, D., Lewis, J., Raff, M., Roberts, K., and Watson, J.D.: *Molecular Biology of the Cell*, 3rd edn. New York, Garland Publishing, 1994.

Ryan, K.J., (ed): *Medical Microbiology*, 3rd edn. East Norwalk, CT, Appleton-Lange, 1994.

Stryer, L.: *Biochemistry*, 4th edn. New York, Freeman, 1995.

Primary journals devoted solely or primarily to immunology

Immunity
Journal of Immunology
European Journal of Immunology
International Immunology
Journal of Experimental Medicine
Immunology
Thymus
Clinical and Experimental Immunology
Regional Immunology
Comparative and Developmental Immunology
Infection and Immunity
Immunogenetics
Autoimmunity

Primary journals with frequent papers in immunology

Nature
Science
Proceedings of the National Academy of Sciences, USA
Cell
EMBO Journal
Current Biology
Journal of Clinical Investigation
Journal of Cell Biology
Journal of Biological Chemistry
Molecular Cell Biology

Review journals in immunology

Current Opinion in Immunology
Immunological Reviews
Annual Reviews in Immunology
The Immunologist
Immunology Today
Seminars in Immunology
Contemporary Topics in Microbiology and Immunology
Research in Immunology
Proceedings of the International Congress of Immunology: Progress in Immunology, **1–8**, 1971–1992.

The Immunologist, **3**: Proceedings Issue, 9th International Congress of Immunol.

Advanced textbooks in immunology, compendia, etc.

Lachmann, P.J., Peters, D.K., Rosen, F.S., Walport, M.J. (eds): *Clinical Aspects of Immunology*, 5th edn. Oxford, Blackwell Scientific Publications, 1993.

Paul, W.E. (ed): *Fundamental Immunology*, 3rd edn, New York, Raven Press, 1993.

Roitt, I.M., and Delves, P.J. (eds): *Encyclopedia of Immunology*, 3rd edn. London/San Diego, Academic Press, 1992.

Rosen, F.S., Geha, R.S: *Case Studies in Immunology: A Clinical Companion*. New York, Garland Publishing/Current Biology, 1996.

The Induction, Measurement, and Manipulation of the Immune Response

2

 STOP Before you read further, a word from the authors about this chapter. We have written it to be read when it is needed to understand a particular method; later chapters reference Chapter 2 as appropriate. Although it is also written so that it can be read from start to finish, most students will want to dip into this toolbox of methods when they encounter a reference to it in later chapters, rather than tackling it now. To make the sections relevant to later chapters easy to identify, the edges of the paper in this chapter are colored, and the most useful methods for any part of the book are color coded to the part in which they are needed. However, we recommend that you read the first six sections of Chapter 2 before continuing with the rest of the book.

The description of the immune system outlined in Chapter 1 is drawn from the results of many different kinds of experiment and from the study of human disease. Immunologists have devised a wide variety of techniques for inducing, measuring, and characterizing immune responses, and for altering the immune system through cellular, molecular, and genetic manipulation. Before we examine the cellular and molecular basis of host defense described in the remainder of this book, we shall look at how the immune system is studied and introduce the specialized language of immunology. In this chapter, we also describe many basic immunological phenomena that experimental immunologists seek to explain in terms of the cellular and molecular features of the immune system. Since genetics plays an important role in the analysis of the immune system and of human disease, the genetic analysis of the immune system is also discussed here, including recently developed techniques for genetic manipulation that have had a tremendous impact on all areas of biology. We also describe clinical tests used to assess immune function in patients with immunological disorders.

Immunological techniques are also widely applied in many other areas of biology and medicine. The use of antibodies to detect specific molecules in complex mixtures and in tissues is of particular importance. We therefore devote an entire section of this chapter to the antibody-based methods used by immunologists, by basic scientists in many other biological disciplines, and by clinicians. These methods illustrate the specificity and utility of antibodies, whose structure and generation form an important theme in subsequent parts of this book.

Related
to Part I

The induction and detection of immune responses.

Most of the material in this book focuses on **adaptive immunity**, that is, on immune responses of lymphocytes to foreign materials, most importantly the antigens borne by various pathogenic microorganisms. However, experimental immunologists, in developing our understanding of the immune response, have mainly examined responses induced by simple non-living antigens. Thus, we shall begin our consideration of how the immune system is studied by discussing how such adaptive immune responses are induced and detected. The deliberate induction of an immune response is known as **immunization**. Experimental immunizations are carried out routinely by injecting the test antigen into the animal or human subject, and we shall see that the route, dose, and form in which antigen is administered can profoundly affect whether a response occurs and the type of response that is produced. To determine whether an immune response has occurred and to follow its course, the immunized individual is monitored for the appearance of immune reactants directed at the specific antigen. Immune responses to most antigens elicit the production of both specific antibodies and specific effector T cells. Monitoring the antibody response often involves analysis of relatively crude preparations of **antiserum** (plural: **antisera**). This is the fluid phase of clotted blood (the **serum**), which, in an immunized individual, is called antiserum because it contains specific antibodies against the immunizing antigen as well as other soluble serum proteins. To study immune responses mediated by T cells, blood lymphocytes or cells from lymphoid organs are tested; T-cell responses are more commonly studied in experimental animals than in humans.

Any substance that can elicit an immune response is said to be **immunogenic** and is called an **immunogen**. There is a clear operational distinction between an immunogen and an antigen. An antigen is defined as any substance that can bind to a specific antibody. All antigens therefore have the potential to elicit specific antibodies but some need to be attached to an immunogen in order to do so. This means that although all immunogens are antigens, not all antigens are immunogenic.

The following sections describe some of the most commonly used techniques for inducing, detecting, and measuring adaptive immune responses. These techniques are used to address many questions in immunology. What determines whether a particular substance will be immunogenic or not? How does one raise antibodies against substances that are not by themselves immunogenic? And what determines which type of response will be provoked by a particular immunization? We shall first examine the nature of antigens and the features that make a substance immunogenic, before turning to a general consideration of how the response is detected.

2-1 Antibodies can be produced against almost any substance.

When antibodies were first discovered as the agents of resistance to infection, it was thought likely that their ability to bind pathogens had been selected over evolutionary time because of their importance to survival. However, Karl Landsteiner soon showed that antibodies could be elicited against a virtually limitless range of molecules, including synthetic chemicals never found in the natural environment. This demonstrated unequivocally that the repertoire of possible antibodies in any

Fig. 2.1 Antibodies can be elicited by small chemical groups called haptens only when the hapten is linked to a protein carrier. Three types of antibodies are produced. One set (blue) binds the carrier protein alone and is called carrier-specific. One set (red) binds to the hapten on any carrier or to free hapten in solution and is called hapten-specific. One set (purple) only binds the specific conjugate of hapten and carrier used for immunization, apparently binding to sites at which the hapten joins the carrier, and is called conjugate-specific. The amount of antibody of each type in this serum is shown schematically in the graphs at the bottom; note that the original antigen binds more antibody than the sum of anti-hapten and anti-carrier owing to the additional binding of conjugate-specific antibody.

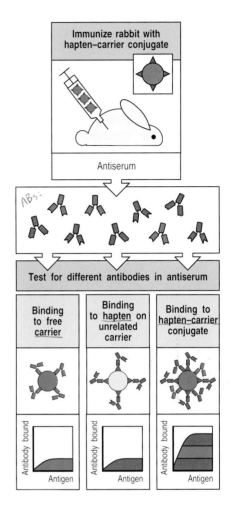

Related to Part I

individual is essentially unlimited, and that the genes encoding individual antibodies could not have been selected for their action against pathogens. This radically changed the way that immunologists thought about the antibody response, forcing them to the conclusion that evolution must have selected not for specific antibody structures but rather for the ability to generate an open repertoire of antibodies of diverse structure, a subject we shall focus on in Chapter 3. This meant that no two individuals are likely to make the same response to any antigen. It also alerted immunologists to the potential utility of antibodies for detecting and measuring almost any substance in a complex mixture of molecules.

In order to determine the range of antibodies that could be produced, Landsteiner studied the immune response to small organic molecules, such as arsonates and nitrophenyls. Although these simple structures do not provoke antibodies when injected by themselves, Landsteiner found that antibodies could be raised against them if the molecule was attached covalently to a protein carrier. He therefore termed them **haptens** (from the Greek *haptein*, to fasten). Animals immunized with a hapten–carrier conjugate produced three distinct sets of antibodies (Fig. 2.1). One set comprised hapten-specific antibodies that reacted with the hapten on any carrier, as well as with free hapten. The second set of antibodies was specific for the carrier protein, as shown by their ability to bind both the hapten-modified and unmodified carrier protein. Finally, some antibodies reacted only with the specific conjugate of hapten and carrier used for immunization. Landsteiner studied mainly the antibody response to the hapten, as these small molecules could be synthesized in many closely related forms. As can be seen in Fig. 2.2, antibodies raised against a particular hapten bind that hapten but, in general, fail to bind even very closely related chemical structures. The binding of haptens by anti-hapten antibodies has played an important part in defining the precision of antigen binding by antibody molecules. Anti-hapten antibodies are also important medically as they mediate allergic reactions to penicillin and other compounds that elicit antibody responses when they attach to self proteins (see Section 11-10).

Antisera contain many different antibody molecules that bind to the immunogen in slightly different ways (see Fig. 2.1 and Fig. 2.2). Some of the antibodies in an antiserum are cross-reactive. A **cross-reaction** is defined as the binding of an antibody to an antigen other than the immunogen; most cross-react with closely related molecules but some are specific for antigens having no clear relationship to the immunogen.

Fig. 2.2 Anti-hapten antibodies can distinguish small changes in hapten structure. Antibodies raised to the *meta* substituted azobenzenearsonate ring react predominantly with the *meta* form, and have limited or no cross-reactivity with the *ortho* and *para* forms. The particular antibody shown here fits the *meta* form perfectly, weakly binds to the *ortho* form, and does not bind the *para* form.

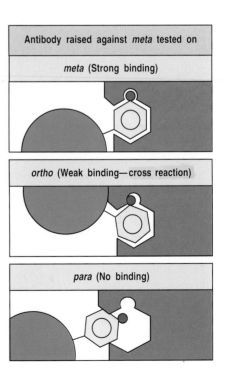

Related
to Part I

These cross-reacting antibodies can create problems when the antiserum is used for detection of specific antigen using the techniques outlined in the next part of this chapter. They can be removed from an antiserum by **absorption** with the cross-reactive antigen, leaving behind the antibodies that bind only to the immunogen. This can be performed using immobilized antigen by affinity chromatography, which is also used for purification of antibodies or antigens (see Section 2-7). The problems resulting from the heterogeneity of the antibodies present in an antiserum can be avoided by making monoclonal antibodies, which are homogeneous antibodies derived from a single antibody-producing cell (see Section 2-11). These can be selected for lack of cross-reactivity and their binding properties can be defined more reliably.

The antigens used most frequently in experimental immunology are proteins, and antibodies to proteins are of enormous utility in experimental biology and medicine. Therefore, in this chapter we shall focus on the production and use of anti-protein antibodies. While antibodies can also be made to haptens, to carbohydrates, to nucleic acids, and to other structural classes of antigen (see Chapter 8), their induction generally requires the attachment of the antigen to a protein carrier. Thus, the immunogenicity of protein antigens determines the outcome of virtually every immune response.

| 2-2 | **The immunogenicity of a protein depends on its presentation to T cells.** |

Although any structure can be recognized by antibody as an antigen, usually only proteins elicit fully developed adaptive immune responses because of their ability to engage the T cells which contribute to inducing most antibody responses and which are required for immunological memory. Proteins engage T cells because the T cells recognize antigens

Fig. 2.3   Intrinsic properties and extrinsic factors that affect the immunogenicity of proteins.

Factors that influence the immunogenicity of proteins		
Parameter	**Increased immunogenicity**	**Decreased immunogenicity**
Size	Large	Small (MW<2 500)
Dose	Intermediate	High or low
Route	Subcutaneous > intraperitoneal > intravenous or intragastric	
Composition	Complex	Simple
Form	Particulate	Soluble
	Denatured	Native
Similarity to self protein	Multiple differences	Few differences
Adjuvants	Slow release	Rapid release
	Bacteria	No bacteria
Interaction with host MHC	Effective	Ineffective

as peptide fragments of proteins bound to major histocompatibility complex (MHC) molecules (see Section 1-14). An adaptive immune response that includes immunological memory can only be induced by other classes of antigen when they are attached to a protein carrier that can engage the necessary T cells. Immunological memory is produced as a result of the initial or **primary immunization**. This is also known as **priming**, as the animal or person is now primed to mount a more potent response to subsequent challenges by the same antigen. The response to each challenge is increasingly intense, so that **secondary**, **tertiary**, and subsequent responses are of increasing magnitude. Repetitive injection of antigen to achieve a heightened state of immunity is known as **hyperimmunization**.

Certain properties of a protein that favor the priming of an adaptive immune response have been defined by studying antibody responses to simple natural proteins like hen egg-white lysozyme and, more importantly, to synthetic polypeptide antigens (Fig. 2.3). The larger and more complex a protein, and the more distant its relationship to self proteins, the more likely it is to elicit a response. This is because such responses depend on the protein being degraded into peptides that can bind to MHC molecules, and on the subsequent recognition of these peptide: MHC complexes by T cells that have survived a process of selection against responsiveness to self. Particulate or aggregated antigens are more immunogenic because they are taken up more efficiently by the specialized antigen-presenting cells responsible for initiating a response (see Section 1-11); indeed small soluble proteins are unable to induce a response unless they are made to aggregate in some way. As we shall see in Sections 2-3 and 2-4, the way in which protein antigens are administered can greatly influence the induction and character of the immune response. For the purposes of this chapter we are focusing on empirical observations relevant to the practice of immunization. A clearer understanding of how these various parameters determine immunogenicity will become evident when the priming of T cells is described in Chapter 7.

2-3   The response to a protein antigen is influenced by dose, form, and route of administration.

The magnitude of the immune response depends on the dose of immunogen administered. Below a certain threshold dose, most proteins do not elicit an immune response. Above the threshold dose, there is a gradual increase in the response with increasing dose to a broad plateau level, followed by a decline at very high antigen doses (Fig. 2.4). As most infectious agents enter the body in small numbers, immune responses are generally elicited only by pathogens that multiply to a level sufficient to exceed the antigen dose threshold. The broad-response optimum allows the system to respond to infectious agents across a wide range of doses. At very high antigen doses the immune response is inhibited, which may be important in maintaining tolerance to abundant self proteins, such as plasma proteins. In general, secondary and subsequent immune responses occur at lower antigen doses and achieve higher plateau values, which is a sign of immunological memory. However, under some conditions, very low or very high doses of antigen may induce specific unresponsive states, known respectively as acquired **low-zone** or **high-zone tolerance**.

The route by which antigen is administered also affects both the magnitude and the type of response obtained. Antigens injected subcutaneously generally elicit the strongest responses, while antigens injected or transfused directly into the bloodstream, especially those freed of aggregates

Related to Part I

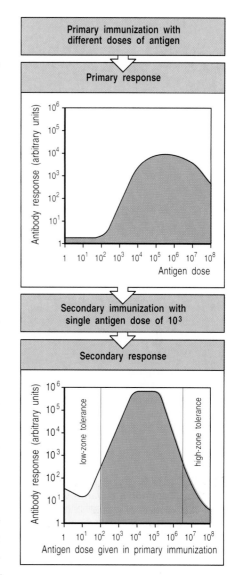

Fig. 2.4   The dose of antigen used in an initial immunization affects the primary and secondary antibody response. The typical antigen dose–response curve shown here illustrates the influence of dose on both a primary antibody response (amounts of antibody produced expressed in arbitrary units) and the effect of the dose used for priming on a secondary antibody response elicited by a dose of antigen of 10^3 arbitrary mass units. Very low doses of antigen do not cause an immune response at all. Slightly higher doses appear to inhibit specific antibody production, an effect known as low-zone tolerance. Above these doses there is a steady increase in the response with antigen dose to reach a broad optimum. Very high doses of antigen also inhibit immune responsiveness to a subsequent challenge, a phenomenon known as high-zone tolerance.

that are readily taken up by antigen-presenting cells, tend to induce unresponsiveness or tolerance unless they bind to host cells. Antigens administered solely to the gastrointestinal tract have distinctive effects, frequently eliciting a local antibody response in the intestinal lamina propria, while at the same time producing a state of systemic tolerance that manifests as a diminished response to the same antigen if it is administered in immunogenic form elsewhere in the body. This 'split tolerance' may be important in avoiding allergy to antigens in food, as the local response prevents food antigens from entering the body. The inhibition of systemic immunity helps to prevent formation of IgE antibodies, which are the cause of such allergies (see Chapter 11). By contrast, protein antigens that enter the body through the respiratory epithelium tend to elicit allergic responses, for reasons that are not clear.

2-4 Immunogenicity can be enhanced by administration of proteins in adjuvants.

Most proteins are poorly immunogenic or non-immunogenic when administered by themselves. Strong adaptive immune responses to protein antigens almost always require that the antigen be injected in a mixture known as an **adjuvant**. An adjuvant is any substance that enhances the immunogenicity of substances mixed with it. Adjuvants differ from protein carriers in that they do not form stable linkages with the immunogen. Furthermore, adjuvants are needed primarily in initial immunizations, whereas carriers are required to elicit not only primary but also subsequent responses to haptens. Commonly used adjuvants are listed in Fig. 2.5.

Adjuvants can enhance immunogenicity in two different ways. First, adjuvants convert soluble protein antigens into particulate material,

Fig. 2.5 Common adjuvants and their use. Adjuvants are mixed with the antigen and usually render it particulate, which helps to retain the antigen in the body and promotes macrophage uptake. Most adjuvants include bacteria or bacterial components that stimulate macrophages, aiding in the induction of the immune response. ISCOMs (immune stimulatory complexes) are small micelles of the detergent Quil A; when viral proteins are placed in these micelles, they apparently fuse with the antigen-presenting cell, allowing the antigen to enter the cytosol and stimulate a response to the protein, much as a virus infecting these cells would stimulate an anti-viral response.

Adjuvants that enhance immune responses		
Adjuvant name	Composition	Mechanism of action
Incomplete Freund's adjuvant	Oil-in-water emulsion	Delayed release of antigen; enhanced uptake by macrophages
Complete Freund's adjuvant	Oil-in-water emulsion with dead mycobacteria	Delayed release of antigen; enhanced uptake by macrophages; induction of co-stimulators in macrophages
Freund's adjuvant with MDP	Oil-in-water emulsion with muramyldipeptide (MDP), a constituent of mycobacteria	Similar to complete Freund's adjuvant
Alum (aluminum hydroxide)	Aluminum hydroxide gel	Delayed release of antigen; enhanced macrophage uptake
Alum plus Bordetella pertussis	Aluminum hydroxide gel with killed B. pertussis	Delayed release of antigen; enhanced uptake by macrophages; induction of co-stimulators
Immune stimulatory complexes (ISCOMs)	Matrix of Quil A containing viral proteins	Delivers antigen to cytosol; allows induction of cytotoxic T cells

which is more readily ingested by antigen-presenting cells, such as macrophages. The antigen can be adsorbed on particles of the adjuvant (such as alum) or made particulate by emulsification in mineral oils. This enhances immunogenicity somewhat, but such adjuvants are relatively weak unless they also contain bacteria or bacterial products, the second means by which adjuvants enhance immunogenicity. Although the exact contribution of the microbial constituents to enhancing immunogenicity is unknown, they are clearly the more important component of an adjuvant. Microbial products may signal macrophages or dendritic cells to become more effective antigen-presenting cells, and their role is considered in more detail in Chapter 7. The bacterial constituents in most adjuvants induce the production of inflammatory cytokines and potent local inflammatory responses; this effect is probably intrinsic to their activity in enhancing responses, but precludes their use in humans. Nevertheless, purified constituents of the bacterium *Bordetella pertussis*, which is the causal agent of whooping cough, are used as both antigen and adjuvant in the triplex DPT (diphtheria, pertussis, tetanus) vaccine against these diseases.

Related
to Part I

2-5   B-cell responses are detected by antibody production.

B cells contribute to adaptive immunity by secreting antibodies, and the response of B cells to an injected immunogen is usually measured by analyzing the specific antibody produced in a **humoral immune response**. This is most conveniently achieved by assaying the antibody that accumulates in the fluid phase of the blood or **plasma**; such antibodies are known as circulating antibodies. Circulating antibody is usually measured by collecting blood, allowing it to clot, and then isolating the serum from the clotted blood. The amount and characteristics of the antibody in the resulting antiserum are then determined using the assays we shall describe in the next part of this chapter.

The most important characteristics of an antibody response are the specificity, amount, isotype (class), and affinity of the antibodies produced. The specificity determines the ability of the antibody to distinguish the immunogen from other antigens. The amount of antibody can be determined in many different ways and is a function of the number of responding B cells, their rate of antibody synthesis, and the persistence of the antibody after production. The persistence of an antibody in the plasma and extracellular fluid bathing the tissues is determined by its isotype (see Chapter 3); each isotype has a different half-life *in vivo*. The isotypic composition of an antibody response also determines the biological functions these antibodies can perform and the sites in which antibody will be found. Finally, the strength of binding of the antibody to its antigen is termed its **affinity**. Binding strength is important, since the higher the affinity of the antibody for its antigen, the less antibody is required to eliminate the antigen, as antibodies with higher affinity will bind at lower antigen concentrations. All these parameters of the humoral immune response help to determine the capacity of that response to protect the host from infection.

2-6   T-cell responses are detected by their effects on other cells or by the cytokines they produce.

The measurement of antibody responses in humoral immunity is fairly simple; by contrast, immunity that is mediated by T cells, called **cell-mediated immunity**, is technically far more difficult to measure. This is principally because T cells do not make a secreted antigen-binding

Related
to Part II

product, so there is no simple binding assay for their antigen-specific responses. T-cell activity can be divided into an induction phase, in which T cells are activated to divide and differentiate, and an effector phase, in which their function is expressed. Both phases require an interaction between two cells, in which the T cell recognizes specific antigen displayed in the form of peptide:MHC complexes on the surface of the interacting cell. In the induction phase, the interaction must be with an antigen-presenting cell able to deliver co-stimulatory signals, whereas, in the effector phase, the appropriate target cell depends on the type of armed effector T cell that has been activated. Most commonly, the presence of T cells that have responded to a specific antigen is detected by their subsequent *in vitro* proliferation when re-exposed to the same antigen. However, T-cell proliferation only indicates that cells able to recognize that antigen have been activated previously; it does not reveal what effector function they mediate. The effector function of a T cell is assayed by its effect on an appropriate target cell. As we learned in Chapter 1, several basic effector functions have been defined for T cells. Cytotoxic CD8 T cells can kill infected target cells, thus preventing further replication of obligate intracellular pathogens, while CD4 T cells can activate either B cells or macrophages in ways that are determined largely by the cytokines they produce (see Section 7-17). The different T-cell effector responses that can be elicited by immunization determine the functional outcome of an immune response. However, no general principles that allow one to predict the type of immune response produced by a particular immunization regimen have emerged. The ability to control the type of immune response produced remains a central goal of immunology as we shall see in Chapters 9–13.

Summary.

Adaptive immunity is studied by eliciting a response through deliberate infection or, more commonly, by injection of antigens in an immunogenic form, and by measuring the outcome in terms of humoral and cell-mediated immunity. Intrinsic properties of the antigen determine its immunogenic potential. However, the elicitation of an immune response is heavily influenced by the dose and route of antigen administration and by the adjuvants used to administer it. The main parameters of the antibody response are the amount, affinity, isotype, and specificity of the antibody produced, the isotype determining the functional capabilities of the humoral immune response to a given antigen. The main parameters of the cell-mediated immune response are the numbers of T cells able to respond and their functional properties.

The measurement and use of antibodies.

Antibody molecules are highly specific for their corresponding antigen, being able to detect one molecule of a protein antigen out of more than 10^8 similar molecules. This makes antibodies both easy to isolate and study, and invaluable as probes of biological processes. While standard chemistry would have great difficulty in distinguishing two such closely related proteins as human and pig insulin, antibodies can be made that discriminate between these two structures absolutely. The utility of antibodies as molecular probes has stimulated the development of many sensitive and highly specific techniques to measure their presence, to determine their specificity and affinity for a range of antigens, and to ascertain their functional capabilities. Many standard techniques used throughout biology exploit the specificity and stability of antigen binding by antibodies. Comprehensive guides to the conduct of these antibody assays are available in many books on immunological methodology; we shall illustrate here only the most important techniques, especially those used in studying the immune response itself. These examples also illustrate the unique properties of antibody molecules that are explained by their structure and genetic origin, as we shall see in Chapter 3.

2-7 | **The amount and specificity of an antibody can be measured by its direct binding to antigen.**

The presence of specific antibody can be detected using many different assays. Some measure the direct binding of the antibody to its antigen. Such assays are based on **primary interactions** and we shall describe several in this section. Others determine the amount of antibody present by the changes it induces in the physical state of the antigen, such as the precipitation of soluble antigen or the clumping of antigenic particles; these are called **secondary interactions** and will be described in the next section. Both types of assay can be used to measure the amount and specificity of the antibodies produced after immunization, and both can be applied to a wide range of other biological problems. Here, we shall describe several of these assays that are commonly used in immunology, biology, and medicine. As such assays were originally conducted using sera from immune individuals, or antisera, they are commonly referred to as **serological assays**, and the use of antibodies is often called **serology**. The amount of antibody is usually determined by titration of the antiserum by serial dilution, and the point at which binding falls to 50% of the maximum is usually referred to as the **titer** of an antiserum.

Two commonly used direct binding assays are **radioimmunoassay (RIA)** and **enzyme-linked immunosorbent assay (ELISA)**. For these one needs a pure preparation of a known antigen or antibody, or both. In a radioimmunoassay, a pure component (antigen or antibody) is radioactively labeled, usually with ^{125}I. For the ELISA, an enzyme is linked chemically to the antibody or antigen. The unlabeled component (again either antigen or antibody) is attached to a solid support, such as the wells of a plastic multiwell plate, which will adsorb a certain amount of any protein. Most commonly, the antigen is attached to the solid support and the binding of labeled antibody is assayed. The labeled antibody is allowed to bind to the unlabeled antigen, under conditions where non-specific adsorption is blocked, and any unbound antibody and other proteins are washed away. Antibody binding is measured directly in terms of the amount of radioactivity retained by the coated wells in radioimmunoassay, while in ELISA, binding is detected by a reaction that converts a colorless substrate into a colored reaction product (Fig. 2.6). The color change can be read directly in the reaction tray, making data collection very easy, and ELISA also avoids the hazards of radioactivity. This makes ELISA the preferred method for most direct-binding assays.

These assays illustrate two crucial aspects of all serological assays. First, at least one of the reagents must be available in a pure, detectable form in order to obtain quantitative information. Second, there must be a means of separating the bound fraction of the labeled reagent from the unbound, free fraction so that specific binding can be determined. Normally, this separation is achieved by having the unlabeled partner

Related to Part II

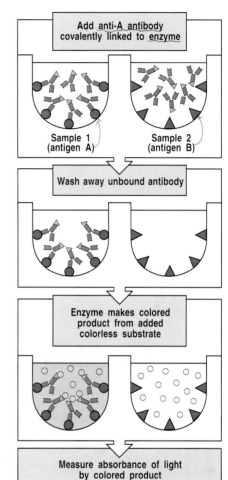

Add anti-A antibody covalently linked to enzyme

Sample 1 (antigen A)   Sample 2 (antigen B)

Wash away unbound antibody

Enzyme makes colored product from added colorless substrate

Measure absorbance of light by colored product

Fig. 2.6   The principle of the enzyme-linked immunosorbent assay (ELISA). To detect antigen A, purified antibody specific for antigen A is linked chemically to an enzyme. The samples to be tested are coated onto the surface of plastic wells to which they bind non-specifically; residual sticky sites on the plastic are blocked by adding irrelevant proteins (not shown). The labeled antibody is then added to the wells under conditions where non-specific binding is prevented, so that only binding to antigen A causes the labeled antibody to be retained on the surface. Unbound labeled antibody is removed from all wells by washing, and bound antibody is detected by an enzyme-dependent color-change reaction. This assay allows arrays of wells known as microtiter plates to be read in fiberoptic multichannel spectrometers, greatly speeding the assay. Modifications of this basic assay allow antibody or antigen in unknown samples to be measured as shown in Figs. 2.7 and 2.34 (see also Section 2-9).

Related
to Part II

trapped on a solid support, allowing the labeled partner that binds to be separated from the unbound labeled molecules by washing. In Fig. 2.6, the unlabeled antigen is attached to the well and the labeled antibody is trapped by binding to it. This separation of bound from free is an essential step in every assay that uses antibodies.

These assays do not allow one to measure directly the amount of antigen or antibody in a sample of unknown composition, as both depend on binding of a pure labeled antigen or antibody. There are various ways around this problem, one of which is to use a competitive inhibition assay, as shown in Fig. 2.7. In this type of assay, the presence and amount of a particular antigen in an unknown sample is determined by its ability to compete with a labeled reference antigen for binding to an antibody attached to a plastic well. By adding varying amounts of a known, unlabeled standard preparation, a standard curve is constructed, and the assay can then measure the amount of antigen in unknown samples by comparison to the standard. The competitive binding assay can also be used for measuring antibody in a sample of unknown composition by attaching the appropriate antigen to the plate and measuring the ability of the test sample to inhibit the binding of a labeled specific antibody.

All the assays described so far rely on pure preparations of an antibody. However, antibody to any one antigen makes up a very small percentage

Fig. 2.7   Competitive inhibition assay for antigen in unknown samples.
A fixed amount of unlabeled antibody is attached to a set of wells, and a standard reference preparation of a labeled antigen is bound to it. Unlabeled standard or test samples are then added in varying amounts and the displacement of labeled antigen is measured, generating characteristic inhibition curves. A standard curve is obtained using known amounts of unlabeled antigen identical to that used as the labeled species, and comparison with this curve allows the amount of antigen in unknown samples to be calculated. The green line on the graph represents a sample lacking any substance that reacts with anti-A antibodies.

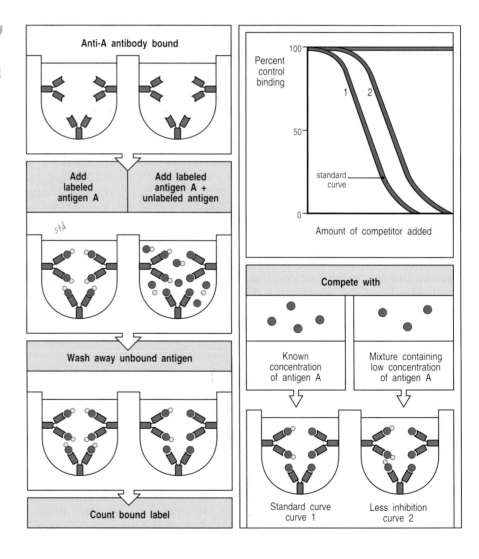

Fig. 2.8   Affinity chromatography uses antigen:antibody binding to purify antibodies or antigens. To purify a specific antibody from serum, antigen is attached to an insoluble matrix, such as chromatography beads, and the serum is passed over the matrix. The specific antibody binds, while other antibodies and proteins are washed away. Specific antibody is then eluted by altering the pH, which can usually disrupt antigen:antibody bonds. In this way, antibodies can be purified from highly complex mixtures of proteins. Antigens can be purified in the same way on beads coupled to antibody (not shown).

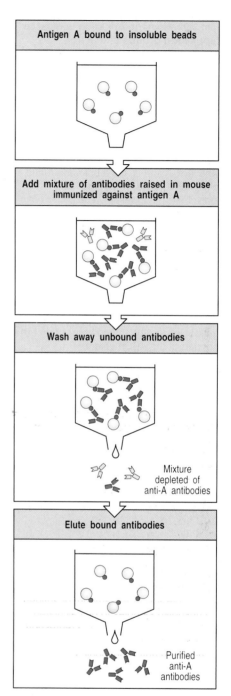

Antigen A bound to insoluble beads

Add mixture of antibodies raised in mouse immunized against antigen A

Wash away unbound antibodies

Mixture depleted of anti-A antibodies

Elute bound antibodies

Purified anti-A antibodies

Related to Part II

of the total protein in an antiserum, even after repeated immunizations. Therefore, antibody must be purified before it can be labeled. Specific antibody can be isolated from an antiserum using **affinity chromatography**, which exploits the specific binding of antibody to antigen held on a solid matrix (Fig. 2.8). Antigen is bound covalently to small, chemically reactive beads, which are loaded into a column, and the antiserum is allowed to pass over the beads. The specific antibodies bind, while all the other proteins in the serum, including antibodies to other substances, can be washed away. The specific antibodies are then eluted, typically by lowering the pH to 2.5 or raising it to greater than 11. This demonstrates that antibodies bind stably under physiological conditions of salt concentration, temperature, and pH, but that the bonds are non-covalent since the binding is reversible. Affinity chromatography can also be used to purify antigens from complex mixtures by coating the beads with specific antibody. The technique is known as affinity chromatography because it separates molecules on the basis of their affinity for one another.

2-8   Antibody binding can be detected by changes in the physical state of the antigen.

The direct measurement of antibody binding to antigen is used in most quantitative serological assays. However, some important assays are based on the ability of antibody binding to alter the physical state of the antigen it binds to. These **secondary interactions** can be detected in a variety of ways. For instance, when the antigen is displayed on the surface of a large particle like a bacterium, antibodies can cause the bacteria to clump or **agglutinate**. The same principle applies to the reactions used in blood typing, only here the target antigens are on the surface of red blood cells and the clumping reaction caused by antibodies against them is called **hemagglutination** (from the Greek, *haima*, blood).

This procedure is used to determine the ABO blood group of blood donors and transfusion recipients by inducing clumping or agglutination with antibodies (agglutinins) anti-A or anti-B that bind to the A or B blood group substances respectively (Fig. 2.9). These blood-group antigens are arrayed in many copies on the surface of the red blood cell, causing the cells to agglutinate when crosslinked by antibodies. Since agglutination involves the crosslinking of blood cells by simultaneous binding of antibody molecules to identical antigens on different cells, this reaction demonstrates that each antibody molecule has at least two identical antigen-binding sites.

When sufficient quantities of antibody are mixed with soluble macromolecular antigens, a visible precipitate consisting of large aggregates of antigen crosslinked by antibody molecules can form. The amount of

Related to Part II

Fig. 2.9 Hemagglutination is used to type blood groups and match compatible donors and recipients for blood transfusion. Common gut bacteria bear antigens that are similar or identical to blood group antigens, and these stimulate the formation of antibodies to these antigens in individuals who do not bear the corresponding antigen on their own red blood cells (left column); thus, type O individuals, who lack A and B, have both anti-A and anti-B antibodies, while type AB individuals have neither. The pattern of agglutination of the red blood cells of a transfusion donor or recipient with anti-A and anti-B antibodies reveals the individual's ABO blood group. Before transfusion, the serum of the recipient is also tested for antibodies that agglutinate the red blood cells of the donor, and vice versa, a procedure called a cross-match, which may detect potentially harmful antibodies to other blood groups that are not part of the ABO system.

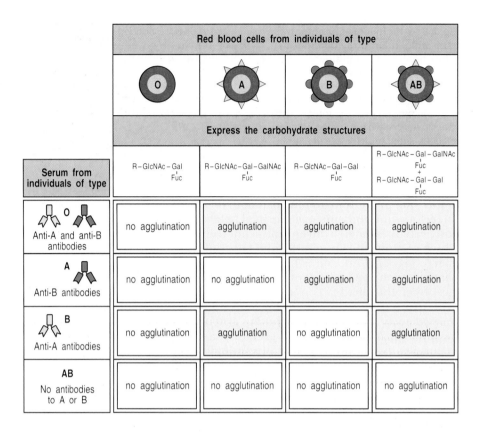

Red blood cells from individuals of type			
O	A	B	AB
Express the carbohydrate structures			
R–GlcNAc–Gal ‖ Fuc	R–GlcNAc–Gal–GalNAc ‖ Fuc	R–GlcNAc–Gal–Gal ‖ Fuc	R–GlcNAc–Gal–GalNAc ‖ Fuc + R–GlcNAc–Gal–Gal ‖ Fuc

Serum from individuals of type				
O — Anti-A and anti-B antibodies	no agglutination	agglutination	agglutination	agglutination
A — Anti-B antibodies	no agglutination	no agglutination	agglutination	agglutination
B — Anti-A antibodies	no agglutination	agglutination	no agglutination	agglutination
AB — No antibodies to A or B	no agglutination	no agglutination	no agglutination	no agglutination

precipitate depends on the amounts of antigen and antibody, and on the ratio between them (Fig. 2.10). This **precipitin reaction** provided the first quantitative assay for antibody but is now seldom used in immunology. However, it is important to understand the interaction of antigen with antibody that leads to this reaction, as the production of antigen:antibody complexes (**immune complexes**) *in vivo* occurs in almost all immune responses and occasionally can cause significant pathology (see Chapters 11 and 12).

In the precipitin reaction, varying amounts of soluble antigen are added to a fixed amount of serum containing antibody. As the amount of antigen added increases, the amount of precipitate generated also increases up to a maximum and then declines (see Fig. 2.10). When small amounts of antigen are added, antigen:antibody complexes are formed under conditions of antibody excess so that each molecule of antigen is bound extensively by antibody and crosslinked to other molecules of antigen. When large amounts of antigen are added, only small antigen:antibody complexes can form and these are often soluble in this zone of antigen excess. Between these two zones, all of the antigen and antibody is found in the precipitate, generating a zone of equivalence. At equivalence,

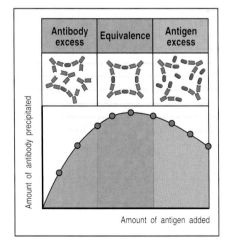

Fig. 2.10 Antibody can precipitate soluble antigen to generate a precipitin curve. Different amounts of antigen are added to a fixed amount of antibody, and precipitates form by antibody crosslinking of antigen molecules. The precipitate is recovered and the amount of precipitated antibody measured, while the supernatant is tested for residual antigen or antibody. This defines zones of antibody excess, equivalence, and antigen excess. At equivalence, the largest antigen:antibody complexes form. In the zone of antigen excess, some of the immune complexes are too small to precipitate. These soluble immune complexes can cause pathological damage to small blood vessels when they form *in vivo* (see Chapter 12).

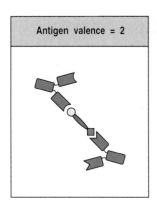 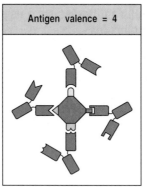 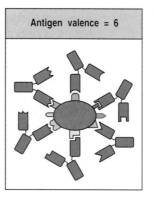

| Antigen valence = 2 | Antigen valence = 4 | Antigen valence = 6 |

Fig. 2.11 Different antibodies bind to distinct epitopes on an antigen molecule. The surface of an antigen possesses many potential antigenic determinants or epitopes, distinct sites to which an antibody can bind. The number of antibody molecules that can bind to a molecule of antigen at one time defines the antigen's valence. Steric considerations can limit the number of different antibodies that bind to the surface of an antigen at any one time (right panel) so that the number of epitopes on an antigen (here 8) is always greater than or equal to its valence (here 6).

Related to Part II

very large lattices of antigen and antibody are formed by crosslinking. The small, soluble immune complexes formed in the zone of antigen excess are the cause of pathology *in vivo*.

Antibody can only precipitate antigen molecules that have several antibody-binding sites, so that large antigen:antibody complexes can be formed. Macromolecular antigens have a complex surface to which antibodies of many different specificities can bind. The site to which each distinct antibody molecule binds is called an **antigenic determinant** or an **epitope**. As a result of the complexity of macromolecular surfaces, a single molecule of antigen has many different epitopes. However, steric considerations limit the number of distinct antibody molecules that can bind to a molecule of antigen at any one time, since antibody molecules binding to epitopes that partially overlap will compete for binding. For this reason, the **valence** of an antigen, which is the number of antibody molecules that can bind to a molecule of the antigen at saturation, is almost always less than the number of epitopes on the antigen (Fig. 2.11).

The precipitation of antigen by antibody can be exploited to characterize the antigen:antibody mixtures by carrying out the reaction in a clear gel. When antigen is placed in one well cut in the gel and the antibody is placed in an adjacent well, they diffuse into the gel and form a line of visible precipitate where they meet at equivalence (Fig. 2.12). The same principle is used in other assays that we shall learn about in subsequent sections.

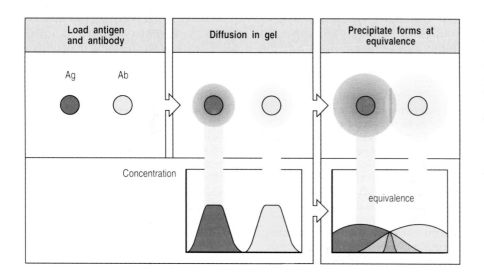

| Load antigen and antibody | Diffusion in gel | Precipitate forms at equivalence |

Fig. 2.12 Ouchterlony gel-diffusion assay for antigen:antibody binding. Antigen and antibody are placed in different wells of an agar gel. They diffuse toward each other and precipitate where they meet at equivalence, forming a visible band. When serum samples in two wells are tested against the same well of antigen, the relatedness of the samples can be determined by the shape of the precipitin line formed (not shown).

Related to Part II

Related to Part V

2-9   Anti-immunoglobulin antibodies are a useful tool for detecting bound antibody molecules.

As we learned in Section 2-7, antibody can be detected by the direct binding of labeled antibody to antigen coated on plastic surfaces. A more general approach that avoids the need to label each preparation of antibody molecule is to detect bound, unlabeled antibody with a labeled antibody specific for all immunoglobulins. Immunoglobulins, like all other proteins, are immunogenic when used to immunize individuals of another species. The majority of **anti-immunoglobulin antibodies** raised in this way recognize conserved features of antibodies shared by all immunoglobulin molecules. These anti-immunoglobulin antibodies can be purified using affinity chromatography, then labeled, and used as a general probe for bound antibody. Anti-immunoglobulin antibodies were first developed by Robin Coombs to study **hemolytic disease of the newborn**, or **erythroblastosis fetalis**, and the test for this disease is still called the Coombs test. Hemolytic disease of the newborn occurs when a mother makes IgG antibodies specific for the **Rhesus** or **Rh blood group antigen** expressed on the red blood cells of her fetus. Rh-negative mothers make these antibodies when they are exposed to Rh-positive fetal red blood cells bearing the paternally inherited Rh antigen. Maternal IgG antibodies are normally transported across the placenta to the fetus where they protect the newborn infant against infection. However, IgG anti-Rh antibodies coat the fetal red blood cells, which are then destroyed by phagocytic cells in the liver, causing a hemolytic anemia in the fetus and newborn infant.

Since the Rh antigens are widely spaced on the red blood cell surface, the IgG anti-Rh antibodies cannot fix complement and cause lysis of red blood cells *in vitro*. Furthermore, for reasons that are not fully understood, antibodies to Rh blood group antigens do not agglutinate red blood cells as do antibodies to the ABO blood group antigens. Thus detecting these antibodies was difficult until anti-human immunoglobulin antibodies were developed. With these, maternal IgG antibodies bound to the fetal red blood cells can be detected after washing the cells to remove unbound immunoglobulin in the serum that interferes with detection of bound antibody. Adding anti-human immunoglobulin antibodies to the washed fetal red blood cells agglutinates any cells to which maternal antibodies are bound. This is the **direct Coombs test** (Fig. 2.13), so called because it directly detects antibody bound to the surface of the patient's red blood cells. An **indirect Coombs test** is used to detect non-agglutinating anti-Rh antibody in serum; the serum is first incubated with Rh-positive red blood cells, which bind the anti-Rh antibody, after which the antibody-coated cells are washed to remove unbound immunoglobulin and are then agglutinated with anti-immunoglobulin antibody (see Fig. 2.13). The indirect Coombs test allows

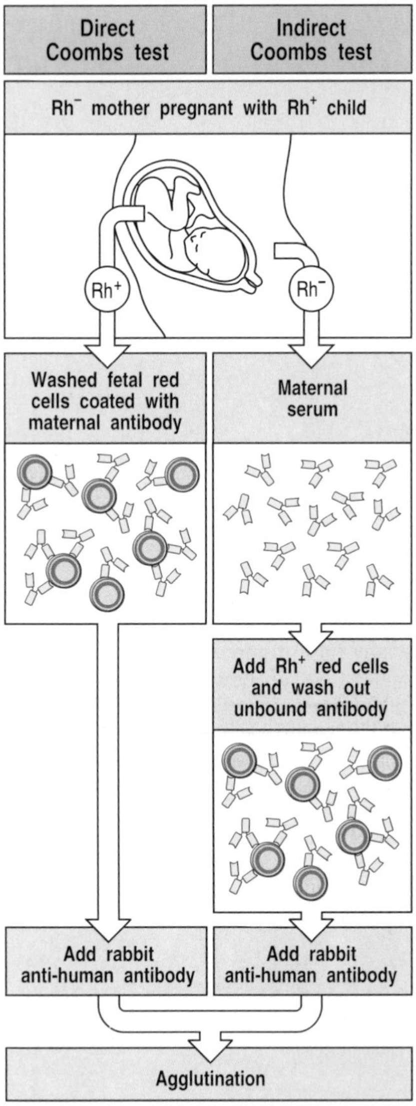

Direct Coombs test	Indirect Coombs test
Rh⁻ mother pregnant with Rh⁺ child	

Rh⁺ ... Rh⁻

| Washed fetal red cells coated with maternal antibody | Maternal serum |

Add Rh⁺ red cells and wash out unbound antibody

| Add rabbit anti-human antibody | Add rabbit anti-human antibody |

Agglutination

Fig. 2.13   The Coombs direct and indirect anti-globulin tests for antibody to red blood cell antigens. A Rh⁻ mother of a Rh⁺ fetus can become immunized to fetal red blood cells that enter the maternal circulation at the time of delivery. In a subsequent pregnancy with a Rh⁺ fetus, IgG anti-Rh antibodies can cross the placenta and damage the fetal red blood cells. In contrast to anti-Rh antibodies, anti-ABO antibodies are of the IgM isotype and cannot cross the placenta, and so do not cause harm. Anti-Rh antibodies do not agglutinate red blood cells but their presence on the fetal red cell surface can be shown by washing away unbound immunoglobulin and then adding antibody to human immuno- globulin, which agglutinates the antibody-coated cells. Anti-Rh antibodies can be detected in the mother's serum in an indirect Coombs test; the serum is incubated with Rh⁺ red blood cells, and once the antibody binds, the red cells are treated as in the direct Coombs test.

Rh incompatibilities that might lead to hemolytic disease of the newborn to be detected and this knowledge allows the disease to be prevented, as we shall see in Chapter 9.

Anti-immunoglobulin antisera have found many uses in clinical medicine and biological research since their introduction. Labeled anti-immunoglobulin antibodies can be used in radioimmunoassay or ELISA to detect binding of unlabeled antibody to antigen-coated plates. The ability of anti-immunoglobulins to react with antibodies of all specificities demonstrates that antibody molecules have constant features recognizable by the anti-immunoglobulin, in addition to the variability required for antibodies to discriminate between a myriad of antigens. The presence of both constant and variable features in one protein posed a genetic puzzle for immunologists, the solution to which is described in Chapter 3.

Some anti-immunoglobulin antibodies made in rabbits react with only a subset of human immunoglobulin molecules. It was this property of anti-immunoglobulin antibodies that led to the discovery that several distinct sets of antibodies, the immunoglobulin isotypes, are present in human serum. The different immunoglobulin isotypes can be seen, along with other serum proteins, by combining electrophoresis, which separates the proteins by charge, with immunodiffusion to detect individual proteins as precipitin arcs. This is achieved by placing an antiserum against whole human serum in a trough that is cut parallel to the direction of electrophoresis, so that each antibody forms an arc of precipitation with a particular serum protein. This technique is called **immunoelectrophoresis** (Fig. 2.14).

Related to Part II

Related to Part V

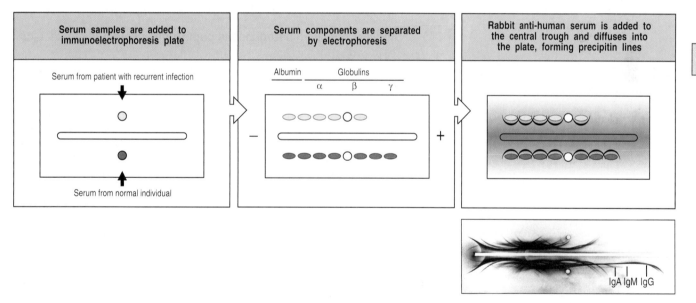

Fig. 2.14   Immunoelectrophoresis reveals the presence of several distinct immunoglobulin isotypes in normal human serum. Serum samples from a normal control and from a patient with recurrent bacterial infection caused by an absence of antibody production, as reflected in an absence of gamma globulins, are separated by electrophoresis on an agar coated slide. Antiserum raised against whole normal human serum and containing antibodies to many of its different proteins is put in a trough down the middle, and each antibody forms an arc of precipitation with the protein it recognizes (see Fig. 2.12). The position of each arc is determined by the electrophoretic mobility of the serum protein; immunoglobulins migrate to the gamma globulin region of the gel. The absence of immunoglobulins in a patient who has X-linked agammaglobulinemia, a form of immune deficiency in which no antibodies of any isotype are formed, is shown in the photograph at the bottom, where several arcs are missing from the patient's serum (upper set). These are IgM, IgA, and several subclasses of IgG, each recognized in normal serum (lower set) by antibodies in the antiserum against human serum proteins. Photograph from the collection of the late C A Janeway Snr.

Related
to Part II

Serum from rare individuals, who demonstrate increased susceptibility to infection, show no precipitin lines in the region where precipitin arcs for the immunoglobulin isotypes now known as IgM, IgA, and several subclasses of IgG are normally detected. As proteins migrating in this region of a serum protein electrophoresis were originally called **gamma globulins**, the failure to make immunoglobulins, which is the result of a single-gene defect on the X chromosome and so occurs mainly in males, is called **X-linked agammaglobulinemia**; its cause has recently been discovered, as we shall see in Chapter 10.

Anti-immunoglobulins specific for each isotype can be produced by immunizing an animal of a different species with a pure preparation of one isotype and then removing those antibodies that cross-react with immunoglobulins of other isotypes using affinity chromatography (see Fig. 2.8). Anti-isotype antibodies can be used to measure how much antibody of a particular isotype in an anti-serum reacts with a given antigen. This reaction is particularly important for detecting small amounts of specific IgE antibodies, which are responsible for most allergies. IgE binding to an antigen correlates with allergic reactions to that antigen.

An alternative approach to detecting bound antibodies exploits bacterial proteins that bind to immunoglobulins with high affinity and specificity. One of these, **Protein A** from the bacterium *Staphylococcus aureus*, has been exploited widely in immunology for the affinity purification of immunoglobulin and for detection of bound antibody.

The use of standard second reagents such as labeled anti-immunoglobulin or Protein A to detect antibody bound specifically to its antigen allows great savings in reagent labeling costs, and also provides a standard detection system so that results in different assays can be compared directly.

2-10   Antisera contain heterogeneous populations of antibody molecules.

The antibodies generated in a natural immune response or after immunization in the laboratory are a mixture of molecules of different specificities and affinities. Some of this heterogeneity results from the production of antibodies that bind to different epitopes on the immunizing antigen, but even antibodies directed at a single antigenic determinant such as a hapten can be markedly heterogeneous. This heterogeneity is detectable by **isoelectric focusing**. In this technique, proteins are separated on the basis of their isoelectric point, the pH at which their net charge is zero. By electrophoresing proteins in a pH gradient for long enough, each molecule migrates along the pH gradient until it reaches the pH at which it is neutral, and is thus concentrated (focused) at that point. When antiserum containing anti-hapten antibodies is treated in this way and then transferred to a solid support such as nitrocellulose paper, the anti-hapten antibodies can be detected by their ability to bind labeled hapten (Fig. 2.15). The binding of antibodies of varying isoelectric points to the hapten shows that even antibodies that bind the same antigenic determinant are heterogeneous.

Antisera are valuable for many biological purposes but they have certain disadvantages that relate to the heterogeneity of the antibodies they contain. First, each antiserum is different from all other antisera, even if raised in a genetically identical animal using the identical preparation of antigen and the same immunization protocol. Second, antisera can only be produced in limited volumes, and thus it is impossible to use the identical serological reagent in a long or complex series of experiments or clinical tests. Finally, even antibodies purified by affinity chromatography (see Section 2-7) may include minor populations of antibodies that give

Fig. 2.15 Isoelectric focusing of antiserum reveals the heterogeneity of antibodies specific for a given antigen. The heterogeneity of antibodies specific for a hapten can be shown by gel electrophoresis of antiserum in a pH gradient generated by ampholytes. The serum proteins migrate to a pH equivalent to their isoelectric point, where they become uncharged and cease to migrate. The proteins are transferred to nitrocellulose paper, which is then treated with the enzyme-coupled hapten, which binds the hapten-specific antibodies in the antiserum. These antibodies are then detected by an enzymatic reaction, which produces a colored product from a colorless substrate, as in ELISA. Even antibodies to a single hapten can be very heterogeneous, as seen here, because of differences in their amino acid sequence.

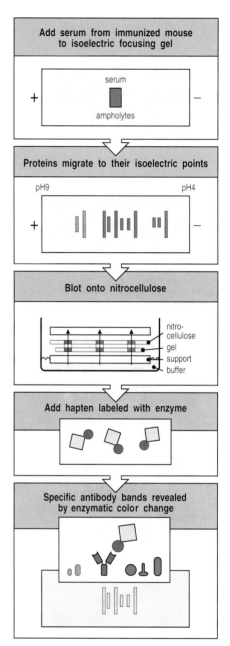

Related to Part II

unexpected cross-reactions, which confound the analysis of experiments. For this reason, an unlimited supply of antibody molecules of homogeneous structure and known specificity would be very desirable. This has been achieved through the production of monoclonal antibodies from hybrid antibody-forming cells or, more recently, by genetic engineering, as we shall see in the next section.

2-11   Monoclonal antibodies have a homogeneous structure and can be produced by cell fusion or by genetic engineering.

Biochemists in search of a homogeneous preparation of antibody that they could subject to detailed chemical analysis turned first to proteins produced by patients with multiple myeloma, a common tumor of plasma cells. It was known that antibodies are normally produced by plasma cells and since this disease is associated with the presence of large amounts of a homogeneous gamma globulin called a **myeloma protein** in the patient's serum, it seemed likely that myeloma proteins would serve as models for normal antibody molecules. Thus, much of the early knowledge of antibody structure came from studies on myeloma proteins. These studies showed that monoclonal antibodies could be obtained from immortalized plasma cells. However the antigen-specificity of most myeloma proteins was unknown, which limited their usefulness as objects of study, or as immunological tools.

This problem was solved by Georges Köhler and Cesar Milstein, who devised a technique for producing a homogeneous population of antibodies of known antigenic specificity. They did this by fusing spleen cells from an immunized mouse to cells of a mouse myeloma to produce hybrid cells that both proliferated indefinitely and secreted antibody specific for the antigen used to immunize the spleen cell donor. The spleen cell provides the ability to make specific antibody, while the myeloma cell provides the ability to grow indefinitely in culture and secrete immunoglobulin continuously. By using a myeloma cell partner that produces no antibody proteins itself, the antibody produced by the hybrid cells comes only from the immune spleen cell partner. After fusion, the hybrid cells are selected using drugs that kill the myeloma parental cell, while the unfused parental spleen cells have a limited lifespan and soon die, so that only hybrid myeloma cell lines or **hybridomas** survive. Those hybridomas producing antibody of the desired specificity are then identified and cloned by regrowing the cultures from single cells. Since each hybridoma is a **clone** derived from fusion with a single B cell, all the antibody molecules it produces are identical in structure, including their antigen-binding site and isotype. Such antibodies are therefore called **monoclonal antibodies** (Fig. 2.16). This technology has revolutionized the use of antibodies by providing a limitless supply of antibody of a single and known specificity and a homogeneous structure. Monoclonal antibodies are now used in most serological assays as diagnostic probes, and as therapeutic agents.

Recently, a novel technique for producing antibody-like molecules has been introduced. Gene segments encoding the antigen-binding variable or V domains of antibodies are fused to genes encoding the coat protein of a bacteriophage. Bacteriophage containing such gene fusions are used to infect bacteria, and the resulting phage particles have coats that express the antibody-like fusion protein, with the antigen-binding domain displayed on the outside of the bacteriophage. A collection of recombinant phage, each displaying a different antigen-binding domain on its surface, is known as a **phage display library**. In much the same way that antibodies specific for a particular antigen can be isolated from a complex mixture using affinity chromatography (see Section 2-7), phage expressing antigen-binding domains specific for a particular antigen can be isolated by selecting the phage in the library for binding to that antigen. The phage particles that bind are recovered and used to infect fresh bacteria. Each phage isolated in this way will produce a monoclonal antigen-binding particle analogous to a monoclonal antibody (Fig. 2.17). The genes encoding the antigen-binding site, which are unique to each phage, can then be recovered from the phage DNA and used to construct genes for a complete antibody molecule by joining them to gene segments that encode the invariant parts of an antibody. When these reconstructed antibody genes are introduced into a suitable host cell line, such as the non-antibody producing myeloma cells used for hybridomas, the transfected cells secrete antibodies with all the desirable characteristics of monoclonal antibodies produced from hybridomas. This technique may ultimately replace the traditional route of cell fusion for production of monoclonal antibodies.

Related to Part II

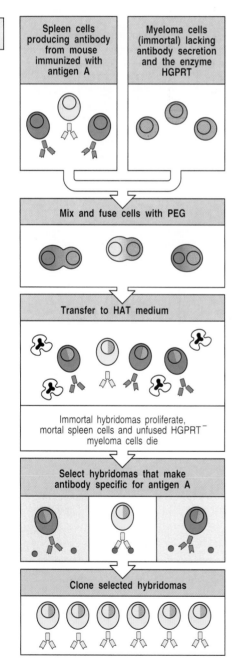

Fig. 2.16 The production of monoclonal antibodies. Mice are immunized with antigen A and given an intravenous booster immunization three days before they are killed in order to produce a large population of spleen cells secreting specific antibody. Spleen cells die after a few days in culture. In order to produce a continuous source of antibody they are fused with immortal myeloma cells using polyethylene glycol (PEG) to produce a hybrid cell line called a hybridoma. The myeloma cells are selected beforehand to ensure that they are not secreting antibody themselves and that they are sensitive to the hypoxanthine-aminopterin-thymidine (HAT) medium that is used to select hybrid cells because they lack the enzyme hypoxanthine:guanine phosphoribosyl transferase (HGPRT). The HGPRT gene contributed by the spleen cell allows hybrid cells to survive in the HAT medium, and only hybrid cells can grow continuously in culture because of the malignant potential contributed by the myeloma cells. Therefore, unfused myeloma cells and unfused spleen cells die in the HAT medium, as shown here by cells with dark, irregular nuclei. Individual hybridomas are then screened for antibody production, and cells that make antibody of the desired specificity are cloned by growing them up from a single antibody-producing cell. The cloned hybridoma cells are grown in bulk culture to produce large amounts of antibody. As each hybridoma is descended from a single cell, all the cells of a hybridoma cell line make the same antibody molecule, which is called a monoclonal antibody.

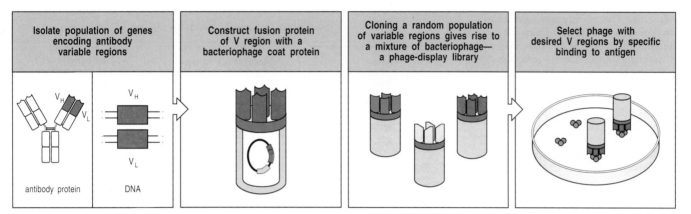

| Isolate population of genes encoding antibody variable regions | Construct fusion protein of V region with a bacteriophage coat protein | Cloning a random population of variable regions gives rise to a mixture of bacteriophage— a phage-display library | Select phage with desired V regions by specific binding to antigen |

Fig. 2.17 The production of antibodies by genetic engineering. Short primers to consensus sequences in heavy- and light-chain variable or V regions of immunoglobulin genes are used to generate a library of heavy- and light-chain V-region cDNAs by the polymerase chain reaction (see Fig. 2.44) using spleen mRNA as the starting material. These heavy- and light-chain V-region genes are cloned randomly into a filamentous phage such that each phage expresses one heavy- and one light-chain V region as a surface fusion protein with antibody-like properties. The resulting phage display library is expanded in bacteria, and the phage are then bound to a surface coated with antigen. The unbound phage are washed away, while the bound phage are recovered and again bound to antigen. After a few cycles only specific high-affinity antigen-binding phage are left. These can be used like antibody molecules, or their V genes can be recovered and engineered into antibody genes to produce genetically engineered antibody molecules (not shown). This technology may replace the hybridoma technology for producing monoclonal antibodies and has the advantage that any species can be used as the source of the initial mRNA.

Related to Part II

2-12 The affinity of an antibody can be determined directly by measuring binding to small monovalent ligands.

The **affinity** of an antibody is the strength of binding of a monovalent ligand to a single antigen-binding site. The affinity of an antibody that binds small antigens, such as haptens that can diffuse freely across a dialysis membrane, can be determined directly by the technique of **equilibrium dialysis**. A known amount of antibody, whose molecules are too large to cross a dialysis membrane, is placed in a dialysis bag and offered varying amounts of antigen. Molecules of antigen that bind to the antibody are no longer free to diffuse across the dialysis membrane, so only the unbound molecules of antigen equilibrate across it. By measuring the concentration of antigen inside the bag and in the surrounding fluid, one can determine the amount of the antigen that is bound as well as the amount that is free when equilibrium has been achieved. Given that the amount of antibody present is known, the affinity of the antibody and the number of specific binding sites for the antigen per molecule of antibody can be determined from this information. The data is usually analyzed using **Scatchard analysis** (Fig. 2.18); such analyses were used to demonstrate that a molecule of IgG has two identical antigen-binding sites.

While affinity measures the strength of binding of an antigenic determinant to a single antigen-binding site, an antibody reacting with an antigen that has multiple identical epitopes or with the surface of a pathogen will often bind the same molecule or particle with both of its antigen-binding sites. This increases the apparent strength of binding, since both binding sites must release at the same time in order for the two molecules to dissociate. This is often referred to as **cooperativity** in binding, but it should not be confused with the cooperative binding found in a protein such as hemoglobin in which binding of ligand at one site enhances the affinity of a second binding site for its ligand. The overall strength of binding of an antibody molecule to an antigen or particle is called its

Related to Part II

Fig. 2.18 The affinity and valence of an antibody can be determined by equilibrium dialysis. A known amount of antibody is placed in the bottom half of a dialysis chamber and exposed to different amounts of a diffusible monovalent antigen, such as a hapten. At each concentration of antigen added, the fraction of the antigen bound is determined from the difference in concentration of total antigen in the top and bottom chambers. This information can be transformed into a Scatchard plot as shown here. In Scatchard analysis, the ratio of r/c, where r = moles of antigen bound per mole of antibody and c = molar concentration of free antigen, is plotted against r. The number of binding sites per antibody molecule can be determined from the value of r at infinite free-antigen concentration, where r/free = 0, in other words at the x-axis intercept. The analysis of a monoclonal IgG antibody molecule in which there are two identical antigen-binding sites per molecule is shown in the left panel. The slope of the line is determined by the affinity of the antibody molecule for its antigen; if all the antibody molecules in a preparation are identical, as for this monoclonal antibody, then a straight line is obtained whose slope is equal to $-K_a$, where K_a is the association (or affinity) constant and the dissociation constant $K_d = 1/K_a$. However, antisera raised even against a simple antigenic determinant such as a hapten containing heterogeneous populations of antibody molecules (see Section 2-10). Each antibody molecule would, if isolated, make up part of the total and give a straight line whose x-axis intercept is less than two, as it contains only a fraction of the total binding sites in the population (middle panel). As a mixture, they give curved lines with an x-axis intercept of two for which an average affinity ($\overline{K}_a$) can be determined from the slope of this line at a concentration of antigen where 50% of the sites are bound, or at $x = 1$ (right panel). The association constant determines the equilibrium state of the reaction Ag + Ab = Ag:Ab, where antigen = Ag and antibody = Ab, and $K_a = [Ag:Ab]/[Ag][Ab]$. This constant reflects the 'on' and 'off' rates for antigen binding to the antibody; with small antigens like haptens, binding is usually as rapid as diffusion allows, while differences in off rates determine the affinity constant. However, with larger antigens the 'on' rate may also vary as the interaction becomes more complex.

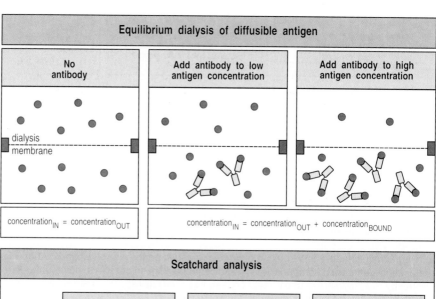

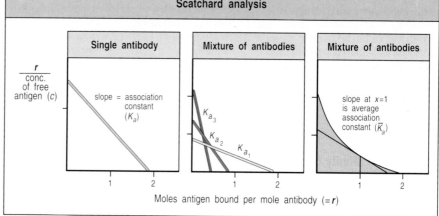

avidity (Fig. 2.19). For IgG antibodies, bivalent binding can significantly increase avidity; in IgM antibodies, which have ten identical antigen-binding sites, the affinity of each site for a monovalent antigen is usually quite low, but the avidity of binding of the whole antibody to a surface such as a bacterium that displays multiple identical epitopes can be very high.

| 2-13 | **Antibodies can be used to identify antigen in cells, tissues, and complex mixtures of substances.** |

Since antibodies bind stably and specifically to antigen, they are invaluable as probes for identifying a particular molecule in cells, tissues, or biological fluids. They are used in this way to study a wide range of biological processes and clinical conditions. In this section, a few techniques that are used to study the immune system, as well as in cell biology generally, will be described; a complete treatment of this subject can be found in any of the excellent methodology books available.

Antibody molecules can be used to locate their target molecules accurately in single cells or in tissue sections by a variety of different labeling techniques. As in all serological tests, the antibody binds stably to its antigen, allowing unbound antibody to be removed by thorough washing. As antibodies to proteins recognize the surface features of the native, folded protein, the native structure of the protein being sought usually

Fig. 2.19 The avidity of an antibody is its strength of binding to intact antigen. When an IgG antibody binds a ligand with multiple identical epitopes, both binding sites can bind the same molecule or particle. The overall strength of binding, called avidity, is greater than the affinity, the strength of binding of a single site, since both binding sites must dissociate at the same time for the antibody to release the antigen. This property is very important in the binding of antibody to bacteria, which usually have multiple identical epitopes on their surfaces.

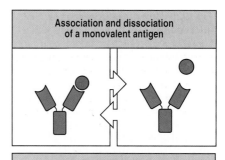

Association and dissociation of a monovalent antigen

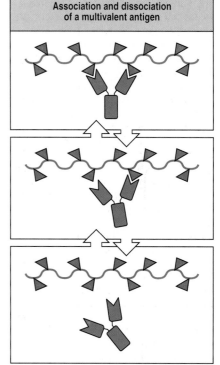

Association and dissociation of a multivalent antigen

Related to Part II

needs to be preserved, either by gentle fixation techniques or by using frozen tissue sections that are fixed only after the antibody reaction has been performed. Some antibodies, however, bind proteins even if they are denatured, and such antibodies will bind specifically even to protein in fixed tissue sections.

The bound antibody can be visualized using a variety of sensitive techniques, and the specificity of antibody binding coupled to sensitive detection provides remarkable detail about the structure of cells. One very powerful technique for identifying antibody-bound molecules in cells or tissue sections is **immunofluorescence**, in which a fluorescent dye is attached directly to the specific antibody. More commonly, bound antibody is detected by fluorescent anti-immunoglobulin, a technique known as **indirect immunofluorescence**. The dyes chosen for immunofluorescence are excited by light of one wavelength, usually blue or green, and emit light of a different wavelength in the visible spectrum. By using selective filters, only the light coming from the dye or fluorochrome used is detected in the fluorescence microscope (Fig. 2.20). Although Albert Coons first devised this technique to identify the plasma cell as the source of antibody, it can be used to detect the distribution of any protein. By attaching different dyes to different antibodies, the distribution of two or more molecules can be determined in the same cell or tissue section (see Fig. 2.20). An alternative method of detecting a protein in tissue sections is to use **immunohistochemistry**, in which the antibody is chemically coupled to an enzyme that converts a colorless substrate into a colored reaction product whose deposition can be directly observed under a light microscope. This technique is analogous to the ELISA assay described in Section 2-7.

The recent development of the confocal fluorescent microscope, which uses computer-aided techniques to produce an ultrathin optical section of a cell or tissue, gives very high resolution immunofluorescence microscopy, without the need for elaborate sample preparation. To examine cells at even higher resolution, similar procedures can be applied to ultrathin sections examined in the transmission electron microscope. Antibodies labeled with gold particles of distinct diameter enable two or more proteins to be studied simultaneously. The difficulty with this technique is in staining the ultrathin section, as few molecules of antigen will be present in each section.

In order to raise antibodies against membrane proteins and other cellular structures that are difficult to purify, mice are often immunized with whole cells or crude cell extracts. Antibodies to the individual molecules are then obtained by preparing monoclonal antibodies that bind to the cell used for immunization. To characterize the molecules identified by these antibodies, cells of the same type are labeled with radioisotopes and dissolved in non-ionic detergents that disrupt cell membranes but do not interfere with antigen:antibody interactions. This allows the labeled protein to be isolated by binding to the antibody. The antibody is usually attached to a solid support, such as the beads used in affinity chromatography. Cells can be labeled in two main ways for this **immunoprecipitation analysis**. All of the proteins in a cell

Related to Part II

Fig. 2.20 Immunofluorescence microscopy. Antibodies labeled with a fluorescent dye such as fluorescein (green triangle) are used to reveal the presence of their corresponding antigens in cells or tissues. The stained cells are examined in a microscope that exposes them to blue or green light to excite the fluorescent dye. The excited dye emits light at a characteristic wavelength, which is captured by viewing the sample through a selective filter. This technique is applied widely in biology to determine the location of molecules in cells and tissues. Different antigens can be detected in tissue sections by labeling antibodies with dyes of distinctive color. Here, antibodies to the protein glutamic acid decarboxylase (GAD) coupled to a green dye are shown to stain the β cells of pancreatic islets of Langerhans, while the α cells, labeled with antibodies to the hormone glucagon coupled with an orange fluorescent dye, do not have this enzyme. GAD is an important auto-antigen in diabetes, an autoimmune disease in which the insulin-secreting β cells of the islets of Langerhans are destroyed. Photograph courtesy of M Solimena and P De Camilli.

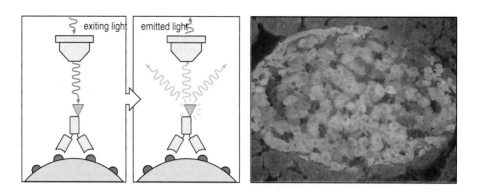

can be labeled metabolically by growing the cell in radioactive amino acids that are incorporated into cellular protein (Fig. 2.21). Alternatively, one can label only the cell-surface proteins by radioiodination under conditions that prevent iodine from crossing the plasma membrane and labeling proteins inside the cell, or by a reaction that labels only membrane proteins with biotin, a small molecule that binds covalently with proteins and is detected readily by its reaction with labeled avidin.

Once the labeled proteins have been isolated by the antibody, they can be characterized in several ways. The most common is polyacrylamide gel electrophoresis (PAGE) of the proteins once they have been dissociated from antibody in the strong ionic detergent, sodium dodecyl sulfate (SDS), a technique generally abbreviated as **SDS-PAGE**. SDS binds relatively homogeneously to proteins, conferring a charge that allows the electrophoretic field to drive protein migration through the gel. The rate of

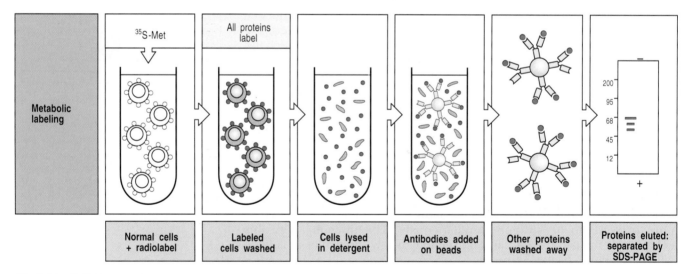

Fig. 2.21 Cellular proteins reacting with an antibody can be characterized by immunoprecipitation of labeled cell lysates. All actively synthesized cellular proteins can be labeled metabolically by incubating cells with radioactive amino acids (shown here for methionine) or one can label just the cell-surface proteins by using radioactive iodine in a form that cannot cross the cell membrane or by a reaction with the small molecule biotin, detected by its reaction with labeled avidin (not shown). Cells are lysed with detergent and individual labeled cell-associated proteins can be precipitated with a monoclonal antibody attached to beads. After washing away unbound proteins, the bound protein is eluted in the detergent sodium dodecyl sulfate (SDS), which dissociates it from the antibody and also coats the protein with a strong negative charge, allowing it to migrate according to its size in polyacrylamide gel electrophoresis (PAGE). The positions of the labeled proteins are determined by autoradiography using X-ray film. This technique of SDS-PAGE can be used to determine the molecular weight and subunit composition of a protein. Patterns of protein bands observed using metabolic labeling are usually more complex than those revealed by radioiodination, owing to the presence of precursor forms of the protein (right panel). The mature form of a surface protein can be identified as being the same size as that detected by surface iodination or biotinylation (not shown).

Fig. 2.22 Two-dimensional gel electrophoresis of MHC class II molecules. Proteins in mouse spleen cells have been labeled metabolically (see Fig. 2.20), precipitated with a monoclonal antibody against the mouse MHC class II molecule H2-A, and separated by isoelectric focusing in one direction and SDS-PAGE in a second direction at right angles to the first, hence the term two-dimensional gel. This allows one to distinguish molecules of the same molecular weight on the basis of their charge. The separated proteins are detected using auto-radiography. The MHC molecules are composed of two chains, α and β, and in the different MHC class II molecules these have different isoelectric points (compare upper and lower panels). The MHC genotype of mice is indicated by lower case superscripts (k,p). Actin, a common contaminant, is marked a. Photograph courtesy of J F Babick.

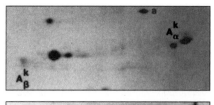

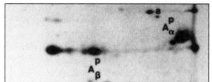

Related to Part II

migration is controlled mainly by protein size (see Fig. 2.21). However, this technique does not separate proteins that are of similar size but differ in charge as a result of having different amino acid sequences, such as major histocompatibility complex (MHC) proteins. Proteins of different charge can be separated using isoelectric focusing (see Section 2-10). This technique can be combined with SDS-PAGE in a procedure known as **two-dimensional gel electrophoresis**. For this, the immuoprecipitated protein is eluted in urea, a non-ionic solubilizing agent, and run on an isoelectric focusing gel in one direction in a narrow tube of polyacrylamide. This first-dimensional isoelectric focusing gel is then placed across the top of an SDS-PAGE slab gel, which is then run vertically to separate the proteins by molecular weight. Two-dimensional gel electrophoresis is a powerful technique that allows many hundreds of proteins in a complex mixture to be distinguished from one another (Fig. 2.22).

An alternative approach that avoids the problem of radiolabeling cells is to solubilize all cellular proteins by placing unlabeled cells directly in detergent and running the lysate on SDS-PAGE. The size-separated proteins are then transferred from the gel to a stable support such as nitrocellulose paper. Specific proteins are detected by antibodies (mainly those that react with denatured sequences) and their position revealed by anti-immunoglobulin that is labeled with radioisotopes or an enzyme. This procedure is called **immunoblotting** or **Western blotting**. (The latter term arose because the comparable technique for detecting specific DNA sequences is known as Southern blotting, after Ed Southern who devised it, which in turn provoked the name Northern for blots of size-separated RNA). Western blots are used in many applications in basic research and clinical diagnosis, for example to detect antibodies to different constituents of HIV (Fig. 2.23).

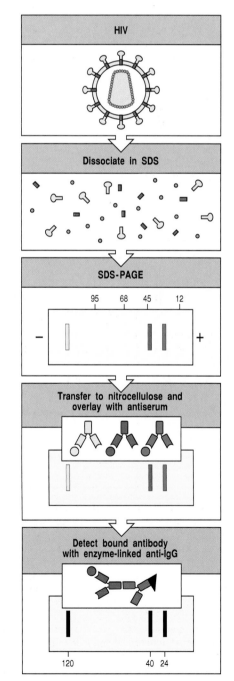

Fig. 2.23 Western blotting is used to identify antibodies to the human immunodeficiency virus (HIV) in serum from infected individuals. The virus is dissociated into its constituent proteins by treatment with the detergent SDS, and its proteins separated using SDS-PAGE. The separated proteins are transferred to a nitrocellulose sheet and reacted with the test serum. Anti-HIV antibodies in the serum bind to the various HIV proteins and are detected using enzyme-linked anti-human immunoglobulin, which deposits colored material from a colorless substrate. This general methodology will detect any combination of antibody and antigen and is used widely, although the denaturing effect of SDS means that the technique works most reliably with antibodies that recognize the antigen when it is denatured.

Related
to Part II

| 2-14 | **Antibodies can be used to isolate protein antigens for further characterization.** |

Immunoprecipitation and Western blotting are useful for determining the molecular weight and isoelectric point of a protein. These characteristics can then help to distinguish it from other proteins and provide a means of recognizing it on an electrophoretic gel. The protein's abundance, distribution, and whether, for example, it undergoes changes in molecular weight and isoelectric point as a result of processing within the cell can thus be determined. However, these techniques do not provide a definitive characterization of the protein.

To do this, the protein must be isolated and purified. Antibodies specific for the protein can be used to isolate it using affinity chromatography (see Section 2-7), but this does not usually yield sufficient protein for a full characterization. Often, this small amount of purified protein is used to obtain amino acid sequence information from the protein's amino-terminal end or from proteolytic peptide fragments of the protein. These amino acid sequences are used to generate a set of synthetic oligonucleotides capable of encoding these peptides, which are then used as probes to isolate the gene encoding the protein from either a library of DNA sequences complementary to mRNA (a cDNA library) or a genomic library. The full amino acid sequence of the protein can be deduced from the nucleotide sequence of its cDNA, and this often gives clues to the nature of the protein and its biological properties. The nucleotide sequence of the gene and its regulatory regions can be determined from genomic DNA clones. The gene can be manipulated and introduced into cells by transfection for larger-scale production and functional studies. This approach has been used to characterize many immunologically important proteins, such as the MHC glycoproteins.

| 2-15 | **Antibodies can be used to identify genes and their products.** |

An alternative approach uses antibodies directly to identify and isolate a gene encoding a cell-surface protein. A specific antibody is used to detect the expression of the protein on the surface of a cell type that does not normally express it, after the cell has been transfected with the gene in the form of a cDNA. A suitable cDNA library is prepared from total mRNA isolated from a cell type known to express the protein. The cDNA library is then cloned into special vectors, called expression vectors, which are constructed to allow the genes they carry to be expressed upon transfection into cultured mammalian cells. These vectors drive expression of the gene in the transfected cells without integrating into the host cell DNA. Cells expressing the protein are isolated by binding to antibody (see Section 2-17), and the vector is recovered by lysing the cells (Fig. 2.24).

The vector is then introduced into bacterial cells where it replicates rapidly, and these amplified vectors are used in a second round of transfection in mammalian cells. After several cycles of transfection, isolation, and amplification in bacteria, single colonies of bacteria expressing the vector are picked and used in a final transfection to identify a cloned vector carrying the cDNA of interest, which is then isolated and characterized. This methodology has been used to isolate many genes encoding cell-surface molecules. It cannot, however, be used to isolate genes for proteins that remain within the cell, as these cannot be detected by surface antibody binding, nor can it be used to isolate the genes for proteins that are only expressed on the cell surface as parts of multichain arrays, as these would require the simultaneous expression of several different cDNAs in the same cell to produce a detectable cell-surface molecule.

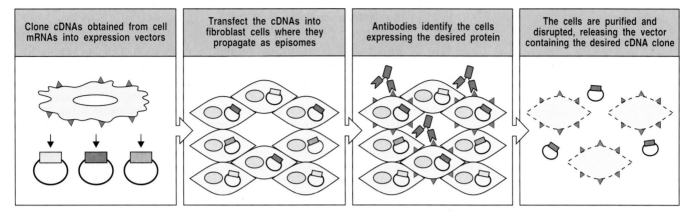

| Clone cDNAs obtained from cell mRNAs into expression vectors | Transfect the cDNAs into fibroblast cells where they propagate as episomes | Antibodies identify the cells expressing the desired protein | The cells are purified and disrupted, releasing the vector containing the desired cDNA clone |

Fig. 2.24 The gene encoding a cell-surface molecule can be isolated by expressing it in fibroblasts and detecting its protein products with monoclonal antibodies. Total mRNA from a cell line or tissue expressing the protein is isolated, converted into cDNA, and cloned as a cDNA in a vector designed to direct expression of the cDNA in fibroblasts. The entire cDNA library is used to transfect cultured fibroblasts. Fibroblasts that have taken up cDNA encoding a cell-surface protein express the protein on their surface; they can be isolated by binding a monoclonal antibody against that protein. The vector containing the gene is isolated from these cells and used for more rounds of transfection and re-isolation until uniform positive expression is obtained, ensuring that the correct gene has been isolated. The cDNA insert can then be sequenced to determine the sequence of the protein it encodes and can also be used as the source of material for large-scale expression of the protein for analysis of its structure and function. The method illustrated is limited to cloning genes for single-chain proteins (i.e. those encoded by only one gene) that can be expressed in fibroblasts. It has been used to clone many genes of immunological interest such as that for CD4.

Related to Part II

The converse approach is taken to identify the unknown protein product of a cloned gene. The gene sequence is used to construct synthetic peptides of 10–20 amino acids that are identical to part of the deduced protein sequence, and antibodies are then raised against these peptides by coupling them to carrier proteins; the peptides behave as haptens. These anti-peptide antibodies often bind the native protein and so can be used to identify its distribution in cells and tissues to isolate it and to try to ascertain its function (Fig. 2.25). This approach is often called reverse genetics as it works from gene to phenotype rather than from phenotype to gene, which is the classical genetic approach. The great advantage of reverse genetics over the classical approach is that it does not require a phenotypic genetic trait for identifying a gene. The main disadvantage of reverse genetics is that often there is no mutant phenotype of the gene so that its functional importance may be difficult to infer. However, mutant genes can be produced by the technique of *in vitro* mutagenesis and then inserted into cells and animals in order to test for their effects. In addition, as it is now possible to inactivate genes deliberately in cells and animals, mutant phenotypes can be generated directly from the gene (see Section 2-37).

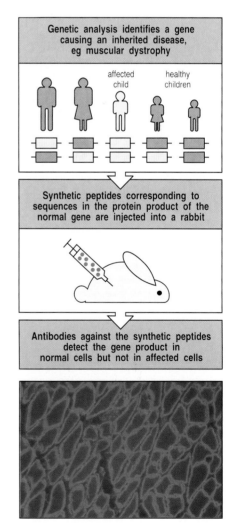

Fig. 2.25 The use of antibodies to detect the unknown protein product of a known gene is called reverse genetics. When the gene responsible for a genetic disorder such as Duchenne muscular dystrophy is isolated, the amino acid sequence of the unknown protein product of the gene can be deduced from the nucleotide sequence of the gene and synthetic peptides representing parts of this sequence can be made. Antibodies are raised against these peptides and purified from the antiserum by affinity chromatography on a peptide column (see Fig. 2.8). Labeled antibody is used to stain tissue from individuals with the disease and from unaffected individuals to determine differences in the presence, amount, and distribution of the normal gene product. The product of the dystrophin gene is present in normal mouse skeletal muscle cells, as shown in the bottom panel (red fluorescence); but is missing in the cells of mice bearing the mutation *mdx*, the mouse equivalent of Duchenne muscular dystrophy (not shown). Photograph (x15) courtesy of H G W Lidov and L Kunkel.

Summary.

The interaction of an antibody molecule with its ligand serves as the paradigm for immunological specificity, an essential concept in immunology. This is best understood by studying the binding of antibodies to antigens, which illustrates their tremendous power to discriminate between related antigens and their high affinity of binding to particular structures. The behavior of antibodies in serological assays shows that antibody molecules are highly diverse, symmetrically bivalent, and have both constant and variable structural features. How the immune system produces the millions of different antibody molecules found in serum while maintaining their overall structural identity that allows anti-immunoglobulin antibodies to detect any antibody molecule, is the main subject of Chapter 3. In Chapter 8, we will learn about the production of antibody by B cells and why the amount, specificity, isotype, and affinity of antibody molecules are important in humoral immunity; here, we have learned how these attributes can be measured in a wide variety of distinct assays, each giving its own type of information about the antibody response. Since antibodies can be raised to any structure, can bind it with high affinity and specificity, and can be made in unlimited amounts through monoclonal antibody production, they are particularly powerful tools of investigation. Many different techniques using antibodies have been devised and they have played a central role in both clinical medicine and biological research.

Related
to Part III

The study of lymphocytes.

The analysis of immunological specificity has focused largely on the antibody molecule as the most easily accessible agent of adaptive immunity. However, all adaptive immune responses are mediated by lymphocytes, so an understanding of immunology must be based on an understanding of lymphocyte behavior. To study and assay lymphocyte behavior the cells must be isolated and the distinct functional lymphocyte subpopulations identified and separated. This section emphasizes studies on T lymphocytes, as the only known effector function of B cells is to produce antibodies, the subject of the preceding part of this chapter.

2-16 Lymphocytes can be isolated from blood, bone marrow, lymphoid organs, epithelia, and sites of inflammation.

The first step in studying lymphocytes is to isolate them so that their behavior can be analyzed *in vitro*. Human lymphocytes can be isolated most readily from peripheral blood using density centrifugation over a step gradient consisting of a mixture of the carbohydrate polymer Ficoll™ and the dense iodine-containing compound metrizamide. This yields a population of mononuclear cells at the interface that has been depleted of red blood cells and most polymorphonuclear leukocytes or granulocytes (Fig. 2.26). The resulting population, called **peripheral blood mononuclear cells**, consists mainly of lymphocytes and monocytes. Although this population is readily accessible, it is not necessarily representative of the lymphoid system, as only recirculating lymphocytes can be isolated from blood. In experimental animals, and occasionally in humans, lymphocytes can be isolated from lymphoid organs, such as spleen, thymus, bone marrow, lymph nodes, or mucosal-associated lymphoid tissues, most commonly the palatine tonsils

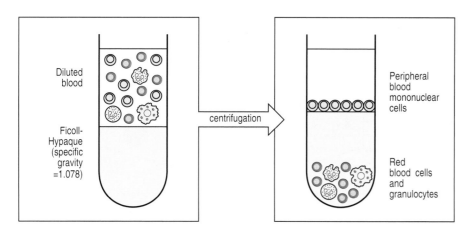

Fig. 2.26 Peripheral blood mono-nuclear cells can be isolated from whole blood using Ficoll-Hypaque™ centrifugation. Diluted anti-coagulated blood (left panel) is layered over Ficoll-Hypaque and centrifuged. Red blood cells and polymorphonuclear leukocytes or granulocytes are more dense and centrifuge through the Ficoll-Hypaque, while mononuclear cells consisting of lymphocytes together with some monocytes band over it and can be recovered at the interface (right panel).

in humans (see Fig. 1.6). A specialized population of lymphocytes resides in surface epithelia; these cells are isolated by fractionating the epithelial layer after its detachment from the basment membrane. Finally, in situations where local immune responses are prominent, lymphocytes can be isolated from the site of the response itself. For example, in order to study the autoimmune reaction that is thought to be responsible for rheumatoid arthritis, an inflammatory response in joints, lymphocytes are isolated from the fluid aspirated from the inflamed joint space.

2-17 Lymphocyte populations can be purified and characterized by antibodies specific for cell-surface molecules.

Resting lymphocytes present a deceptively uniform appearance to the investigator, all being small round cells with a dense nucleus and little cytoplasm (see Fig. 1.5). However, these cells comprise many functional subpopulations, which are usually identified and distinguished from each other on the basis of their differential expression of cell-surface proteins, which can be detected using specific antibodies (Fig. 2.27). B and T lymphocytes, for example, are identified unambiguously and separated from each other by antibodies to the constant regions of the B- and T-cell antigen receptors. T cells are further subdivided on the basis of expression of the co-receptor proteins CD4 and CD8.

An immensely powerful tool for defining and enumerating lymphocytes is the **flow cytometer**, which detects and counts individual cells passing in a stream through a laser beam. A flow cytometer equipped to separate the identified cells is called a **fluorescence-activated cell sorter** (**FACS**). These instruments are used to study the properties of cell subsets identified with monoclonal antibodies to cell-surface proteins. Individual cells within a mixed population are first tagged by treatment with specific monoclonal antibodies labeled with fluorescent dyes, or by specific antibodies followed by labeled anti-immunoglobulin. The mixture of labeled cells is then forced with a much larger volume of saline through a nozzle, creating a fine stream of liquid containing cells spaced singly at intervals. As each cell passes through a laser beam it scatters the laser light, and any dye molecules bound to the cell will be excited and will fluoresce. Sensitive photomultiplier tubes detect both the scattered light, which gives information on the size and granularity of the cell, and the fluorescence emissions, which give information on the binding of the labeled monoclonal antibodies and hence on the expression of cell-surface proteins by each cell (Fig. 2.28).

In the cell sorter, the signals passed back to the computer are used to generate an electric charge, which is passed from the nozzle through the liquid stream at the precise time the stream breaks up into droplets,

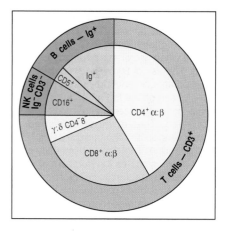

Fig. 2.27 The distribution of lympho-cyte subpopulations in human peripheral blood. As shown on the outside, lymphocytes can be divided into T cells bearing T-cell receptors, detected with anti-CD3 antibodies, B cells bearing immunoglobulin receptors, detected with anti-immunoglobulin, and null cells including natural killer (NK) cells that label with neither. Further divisions of the T-cell and B-cell populations are shown inside. Using anti-CD4 and anti-CD8 antibodies, α:β T cells can be subdivided into two populations, while γ:δ T cells are identified with antibodies against the γ:δ T-cell receptor and mainly lack CD4 and CD8. A minority population of B cells express CD5 on their surface (see Section 5-14).

Related to Part III

Fig. 2.28 The FACS™ allows individual cells to be identified by their cell-surface antigens and to be sorted. Cells to be analyzed by flow cytometry are labeled with fluorescent dyes (top panel). This can either be achieved directly using dye-coupled antibodies specific for cell-surface antigens (as shown here), or indirectly using a dye-coupled anti-immunoglobulin reagent to detect unlabeled cell-bound antibody. The cells are forced through a nozzle in a single-cell stream that passes through a laser beam (second panel). Photomultiplier tubes (PMTs) detect the scattering of light, which is a sign of cell size and granularity, and emissions from the different fluorescent dyes. This information is then analyzed using a computer. By examining many cells in this way, the number of cells with a specific set of characteristics can be counted and levels of expression of various molecules on these cells can be measured. As shown in the bottom left panels, use of a single antibody can indicate the percentage of a cell population bearing the molecule detected by that antibody, and the amount of that molecule expressed by each cell. This information can be presented as a one-color histogram (lower middle panels). Two-color contour profiles (bottom panels) are employed mainly when two or more antibodies are used. The use of two different dye-coupled specific antibodies (bottom right panels) can define four populations of cells: those expressing either molecule alone (red or green), those expressing both (orange), and those expressing neither (gray). The size and intensity of each circle indicates the numbers of cells with these characteristics. The same information is often portrayed in black and white by representing each cell with a dot.

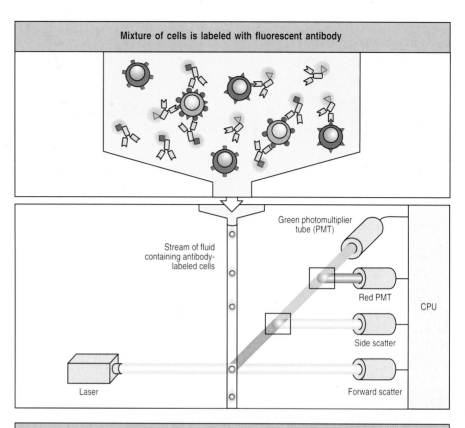

Mixture of cells is labeled with fluorescent antibody

Green photomultiplier tube (PMT)

Stream of fluid containing antibody-labeled cells

Red PMT

CPU

Side scatter

Laser

Forward scatter

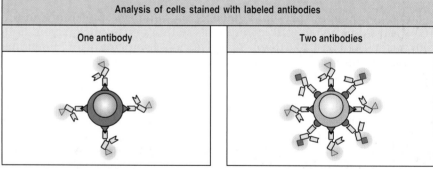

Analysis of cells stained with labeled antibodies

One antibody

Two antibodies

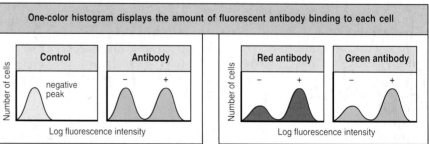

One-color histogram displays the amount of fluorescent antibody binding to each cell

Number of cells

Control

negative peak

Antibody

− +

Log fluorescence intensity

Number of cells

Red antibody

− +

Green antibody

− +

Log fluorescence intensity

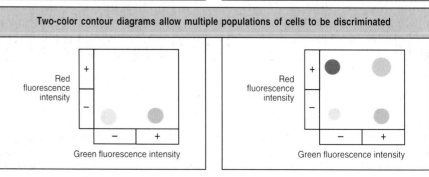

Two-color contour diagrams allow multiple populations of cells to be discriminated

Red fluorescence intensity

+

−

− +

Green fluorescence intensity

Red fluorescence intensity

+

−

− +

Green fluorescence intensity

each containing no more than a single cell; droplets containing a charge can then be deflected from the main stream of droplets as they pass between plates of opposite charge, so that positively charged droplets are attracted to a negatively charged plate, and vice versa.

When cells are labeled with a single fluorescent antibody, the data from flow cytometers are usually displayed in the form of a histogram of fluorescence intensity versus cell numbers. If two or more antibodies are used, each coupled to different fluorescent dyes, then the data are more usually displayed in the form of a two-dimensional scatter diagram or as a contour diagram, where the fluorescence of one dye-labeled antibody is plotted against that of a second, with the result that a population of cells labeling with one antibody can be further subdivided by its labeling with the second antibody (see Fig. 2.28). By examining large numbers of cells, flow cytometry can give quantitative data on the percentage of cells bearing different molecules, such as surface immunoglobulin, which characterizes B cells, the T-cell receptor-associated molecules known as CD3, and the CD4 and CD8 co-receptor proteins that distinguish the major T-cell subsets. Likewise, FACS analysis has been instrumental in defining stages in the early development of B and T cells. FACS analysis has been applied to a broad range of problems in immunology; indeed, it played a vital role in the early identification of AIDS as a disease in which T cells bearing CD4 are depleted selectively (see Chapter 10).

Although the FACS is superb for isolating small numbers of cells in pure form, when large numbers of lymphocytes must be prepared quickly, mechanical means of separating cells are preferable. A powerful and accurate way of isolating lymphocyte populations is to expose them to paramagnetic beads coated with a monoclonal antibody that recognizes a distinguishing surface molecule. The tube containing the cells is then placed in a strong magnetic field, the cells attached to the beads are retained and cells lacking the surface molecule recognized by the monoclonal antibody can be decanted off, leaving behind only the bound cells that express that protein (Fig. 2.29). The bound cells are positively selected for expression of the determinant, while the unbound cells are

Related
to Part III

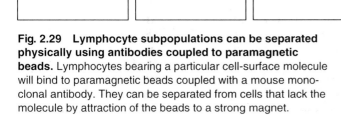

Fig. 2.29 Lymphocyte subpopulations can be separated physically using antibodies coupled to paramagnetic beads. Lymphocytes bearing a particular cell-surface molecule will bind to paramagnetic beads coupled with a mouse monoclonal antibody. They can be separated from cells that lack the molecule by attraction of the beads to a strong magnet. Unbound cells are decanted to yield a population that is said to be negatively selected for absence of the antigen recognized by the monoclonal antibody. Bound cells are recovered by warming or other treatments that disrupt antigen:antibody binding; they are said to be positively selected for presence of the antigen recognized by the antibody.

negatively selected for its absence. Cells have also been isolated by binding to antibody-coated plastic surfaces, a technique known as panning, or by killing cells bearing a particular molecule with specific antibody and complement (see Fig. 2.39). All these techniques can also be used as a pre-purification step prior to sorting out large numbers of highly purified populations by FACS.

The main conclusion reached from studies on isolated lymphocyte populations is that lymphocytes bearing particular combinations of cell-surface proteins represent distinct developmental stages that have particular functions, which suggested that these proteins must be involved directly in the function of the cell. For this reason, such surface molecules were originally called **differentiation antigens**. When groups of monoclonal antibodies were found to recognize the same differentiation antigen, they were said to define **clusters of differentiation**, abbreviated to **CD**, followed by an arbitrarily assigned number. This is the origin of the CD nomenclature for lymphocyte cell-surface antigens. The known CD antigens are listed in Appendix I.

2-18   **Lymphocytes can be stimulated to grow by polyclonal mitogens or by specific antigen.**

To function in adaptive immunity, rare antigen-specific lymphocytes must proliferate extensively before they differentiate into functional effector cells, in order to generate sufficient numbers of effector cells of a particular specificity. Thus, the analysis of induced lymphocyte proliferation is a central issue in their study. However, it is difficult to detect the proliferation of normal lymphocytes in response to specific antigen, because only a minute proportion of cells will be stimulated to divide. Enormous impetus was given to the field of lymphocyte culture by the finding that certain substances induce many or all lymphocytes of a given type to proliferate. These substances are referred to collectively as **polyclonal mitogens** because they induce mitosis in lymphocytes of many different specificities or clonal origins. T and B lymphocytes are stimulated by different polyclonal mitogens (Fig. 2.30). Polyclonal mitogens seem to trigger essentially the same growth response mechanisms as antigen. Lymphocytes normally exist as resting cells in the G_0 phase of the cell cycle. When stimulated with polyclonal mitogens, they rapidly enter the G_1 phase and progress through the cell cycle. In most studies, lymphocyte proliferation is most simply measured by the incorporation of ^{3}H-thymidine into DNA. This assay is used clinically for assessing the ability of lymphocytes from patients with suspected immunodeficiencies to proliferate in response to a non-specific stimulus (see Section 2-31).

Related to Part IV

Fig. 2.30 Polyclonal mitogens, many of plant origin, stimulate lymphocyte proliferation in tissue culture. Many of these mitogens are used to test the ability of lymphocytes in human peripheral blood to proliferate.

Mitogen	Abbreviation	Source	Responding cells
Phytohemagglutinin	PHA	*Phaseolus vulgaris* (red kidney beans)	T cells
Concanavalin A	ConA	*Canavalia ensiformis* (Jack bean)	T cells
Pokeweed mitogen	PWM	*Phytolacca americana* (pokeweed)	T and B cells
Lipopolysaccharide	LPS	*Escherichia coli*	B cells (mouse)

Fig. 2.31 Antigen-specific T-cell proliferation is used frequently as an assay for T-cell responses. T cells from mice or humans that have been immunized with an antigen (A) proliferate when they are exposed to antigen A and antigen-presenting cells but not to unrelated antigens to which they have not been immunized (antigen B). Proliferation can be measured by incorporation of ^{3}H-thymidine into the DNA of actively dividing cells. Antigen-specific proliferation is a hallmark of specific CD4 T-cell immunity.

Once lymphocyte culture had been optimized using the proliferative response to polyclonal mitogens as an assay, it became possible to detect antigen-specific T-cell proliferation in culture by measuring ^{3}H-thymidine uptake in response to an antigen to which the T-cell donor had been previously immunized (Fig. 2.31). This is the assay most commonly used for assessing T-cell responses after immunization, but it reveals little about the functional capabilities of the responding T cells. These must be ascertained by functional assays, as described in the next section.

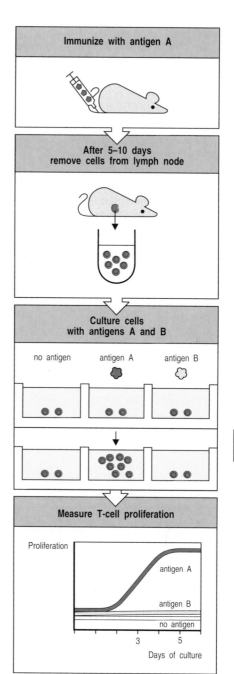

Immunize with antigen A

After 5–10 days remove cells from lymph node

Culture cells with antigens A and B

no antigen   antigen A   antigen B

Measure T-cell proliferation

Proliferation

antigen A

antigen B

no antigen

3   5

Days of culture

Related to Part IV

2-19   T-cell effector functions can be measured in four ways—target-cell killing, macrophage activation, B-cell activation, or lymphokine production.

As we learned in Section 2-6, effector T cells are detected by their effects on target cells displaying antigen, or the secretion of specific cytokines that act on such target cells. Measuring these effector functions forms the basis for T-cell bioassays used to assess both T-cell specificity for antigen and T-cell effector functions.

Activated CD8 T cells generally kill any cells that display the specific peptide:MHC class I complex they recognize. Therefore CD8 T-cell function can be determined using the simplest and most rapid T-cell bioassay—the killing of a target cell by a cytotoxic T cell. This is usually detected in a ^{51}Cr-release assay. Live cells will take up, but do not spontaneously release, radioactively labeled sodium chromate, Na$_2$^{51}CrO$_4$. When these labeled cells are killed, the radioactive chromate is released and its presence in the supernatant of mixtures of target cells and cytotoxic T cells can be measured (Fig. 2.32). In a similar assay, proliferating target cells such as tumor cells can be labeled with ^{3}H-thymidine, which is incorporated into the replicating DNA. On attack by a cytotoxic T cell, the DNA of the target cells is rapidly fragmented and released into the supernatant, and one can measure either the release of these fragments or the retention of ^{3}H-thymidine in chromosomal DNA. These assays provide a rapid, sensitive, and specific measure of the activity of cytotoxic T cells.

The fragmentation of the DNA of cells killed by cytotoxic T cells results from the induction of a process of programmed cell death, or apoptosis,

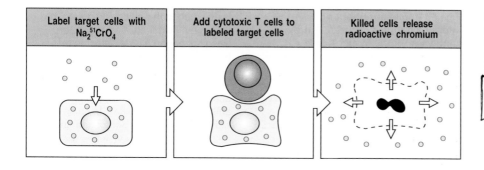

Label target cells with Na$_2$^{51}CrO$_4$

Add cytotoxic T cells to labeled target cells

Killed cells release radioactive chromium

Fig. 2.32 Cytotoxic T-cell activity is often assessed by chromium release from labeled target cells. Target cells are labeled with radioactive chromium as Na$_2$^{51}CrO$_4$ and exposed to cytotoxic T cells. Cell destruction is measured by the release of radioactive chromium into the medium, detectable within 4 hours of mixing target cells with T cells.

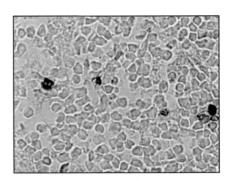

| The DNA in apoptotic cells is extensively nicked | The enzyme TdT adds biotinylated nucleotides to the free 3′ ends of the nicked DNA | Enzymes coupled to streptavidin bind to the labeled bases; the enzyme generates a colored reaction product |

Fig. 2.33   Fragmented DNA can be labeled by terminal deoxyribonucleotidyl transferase (TdT) to reveal apoptotic cells. When cells undergo programmed cell death, or apoptosis, their DNA becomes fragmented (left panel). The enzyme TdT is able to add nucleotides to the ends of DNA fragments; in this assay, biotin-labeled dUTP is added (second panel). The biotinylated DNA can be detected using streptavidin, which binds to biotin, coupled to enzymes that convert a colorless substrate into a colored insoluble product (third panel). Cells stained in this way can be detected by light microscopy, as shown in the photograph of apoptotic cells (stained red, right panel). Photograph courtesy of R Budd and J Russell.

within the target cell. The characteristic cleavage of the DNA in cells undergoing programmed cell death has been used as the basis for an assay to identify apoptotic cells *in situ*. Nucleotides tagged with biotin are added to the cells, along with the enzyme terminal deoxyribonucleotidyl transferase (TdT) which can add the biotin-tagged nucleotides to the free 3′ ends of the DNA fragments produced by apoptosis. Reporter enzymes coupled to avidin or streptavidin will bind to the tagged nucleotides and can be used to identify apoptotic cells by converting a colorless substrate into a colored insoluble product (Fig. 2.33), in much the same way that such reagents are used in immunohistochemical staining (see Section 2-13). The labeled nucleotide most commonly used in this assay is dUTP, coupled to biotin. Hence the assay is often called the TdT-dependent dUTP–biotin nick end labeling, or **TUNEL assay**.

CD4 T-cell functions usually involve the activation rather than the killing of cells bearing specific antigen, which for CD4 cells is a specific peptide: MHC class II complex. The activating effects of CD4 T cells on B cells or macrophages are mediated in large part by non-specific mediator proteins called cytokines, which are released by the T cell when it recognizes antigen (see Chapter 7). Thus, CD4 T-cell function is usually studied by measuring the type and amount of these released proteins. As different effector T cells release different amounts and types of cytokines, one can learn about the effector potential of that T cell by measuring the proteins it produces. Cytokines can be detected by their activity in biological assays of cell growth, where they serve either as growth factors or growth inhibitors, or more specifically by a modification of ELISA, known as a **capture** or **sandwich ELISA**. In this assay, the cytokine is characterized by its ability to bridge between two monoclonal antibodies reacting with different epitopes on the cytokine molecule (Fig. 2.34). Sandwich ELISA can also be carried

Related to Part IV

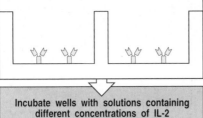

Coat plastic wells with antibody to IL-2

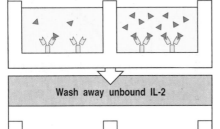

Incubate wells with solutions containing different concentrations of IL-2

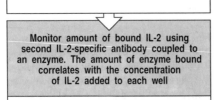

Wash away unbound IL-2

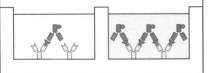

Monitor amount of bound IL-2 using second IL-2-specific antibody coupled to an enzyme. The amount of enzyme bound correlates with the concentration of IL-2 added to each well

Fig. 2.34   Measurement of interleukin-2 (IL-2) production by sandwich ELISA. When T cells are activated with a mitogen or antigen they usually release the T-cell growth factor IL-2. The IL-2 can be measured by induction of growth of an IL-2 responsive indicator cell (not shown); however, assay for IL-2 by sandwich ELISA is far more accurate and specific. In this assay, one unlabeled anti-IL-2 antibody is attached to the plastic, and then the IL-2-containing fluid is added. After washing, bound IL-2 is detected by binding a second, labeled anti-IL-2 antibody directed at a different epitope. This assay is highly specific because antigens that cross-react with one antibody are very unlikely to cross-react with the other. It can detect and quantify IL-2 and many other cytokines with great sensitivity and precision.

out by placing the cells themselves on a surface coated with antibody to a cytokine. After a short incubation, the cytokine released by each cell is trapped on the antibody coat and the presence of cytokine-secreting cells can be revealed when the cells are washed off and a labeled second anti-cytokine antibody is added. The cytokine released by each cell makes a distinct spot in this assay, which is therefore known as an **ELISPOT assay**. ELISPOT can also be used to detect specific antibody secretion by B cells, in this case using antigen-coated surfaces to trap specific antibody, and labeled anti-immunoglobulin to detect the bound antibody. Sandwich ELISA avoids a major problem of cytokine bioassays, the ability of different cytokines to stimulate the same response in a bioassay. Bioassays must always be confirmed by inhibition of the response with monoclonal antibodies against the cytokine.

An alternative method is to identify cytokine mRNA, either in a cell population by reverse transcriptase-polymerase chain reaction (RT-PCR) or by *in situ* hybridization of single cells. Reverse transcriptase is an enzyme that is used by RNA viruses, like the human immunodeficiency virus that causes Acquired Immune Deficiency Syndrome (AIDS), to convert an RNA genome into a DNA copy, or cDNA. By harvesting mRNA from T cells stimulated with antigen, one can make cDNA copies, which are then amplified selectively using cytokine-specific primers by the polymerase chain reaction (see Fig. 2.44). The amount of product is proportional to its representation in the RNA in the responding cell. *In situ* hybridization uses labeled anti-sense RNA probes to hybridize with sense RNA in single cells, either isolated from culture or directly in tissue sections. This allows the number of cells making RNA encoding a particular cytokine to be determined.

2-20	**Homogeneous T lymphocytes can be obtained as T-cell hybrids, cloned T-cell lines, or T-cell tumors.**

Just as the analysis of antibody specificity and structure has been aided greatly by the development of hybridomas making monoclonal antibodies, the analysis of specificity and effector function in T cells has depended heavily on monoclonal populations of T lymphocytes. These can be obtained in three ways. First, as for hybridomas, normal T cells proliferating in response to specific antigen can be fused to malignant T-cell lymphoma lines to generate **T-cell hybrids**. The hybrids express the receptor of the normal T cell, but proliferate indefinitely owing to the cancerous state of the lymphoma parent. T-cell hybrids can be cloned to yield a population of cells all having the same T-cell receptor. These cells can be stimulated by specific antigen to release biologically active mediator molecules such as the T-cell growth factor interleukin-2, and the production of cytokines is used to assess the specificity of the T-cell hybrid.

T-cell hybrids are excellent tools for the analysis of T-cell specificity, as they grow readily in suspension culture. However, they cannot be used to analyze the regulation of specific T-cell proliferation in response to antigen because they are continually dividing. T-cell hybrids cannot be transplanted into an animal to test for function *in vivo* because they would give rise to tumors, and functional analysis of T-cell hybrids is also confounded by the fact that the malignant partner cell affects their behavior in functional assays. Therefore, the regulation of T-cell growth and the effector functions of T cells must be studied using cloned T-cell lines, derived from single T cells, whose growth is dependent on periodic restimulation with specific antigen and, frequently, the addition of T-cell growth factors (Fig. 2.35). Such cells are more tedious to grow but,

Related to Part IV

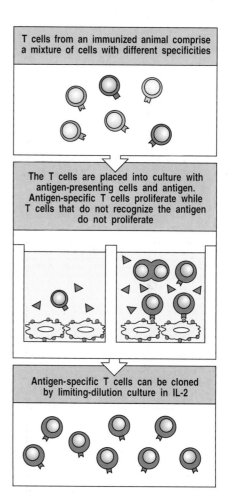

T cells from an immunized animal comprise a mixture of cells with different specificities

The T cells are placed into culture with antigen-presenting cells and antigen. Antigen-specific T cells proliferate while T cells that do not recognize the antigen do not proliferate

Antigen-specific T cells can be cloned by limiting-dilution culture in IL-2

Fig. 2.35 Production of cloned T-cell lines. T cells from an immune donor, comprising a mixture of cells with different specificities, are activated with antigen and antigen-presenting cells. Single responding cells are cultured by limiting dilution (see Fig. 2.36) in the T-cell growth factor interleukin-2 (IL-2). From these single cells, cloned lines specific for antigen are identified and can be propagated by culture with antigen, antigen-presenting cells, and IL-2.

because their growth depends on specific antigen recognition, they maintain antigen specificity, which is often lost in T-cell hybrids. Cloned T-cell lines can be used for studies of effector function both *in vitro* and *in vivo*. In addition, the proliferation of T cells, a critical aspect of clonal selection, can only be characterized in cloned T-cell lines where such growth is dependent on antigen recognition. Thus, both types of mono-clonal T-cell line have valuable applications in experimental studies.

In studies of human T cells, T-cell clones have proven of greatest value because a suitable fusion partner for making T-cell hybrids has not been identified. However, a human T-cell lymphoma line, called Jurkat, has been characterized extensively because it secretes interleukin-2 when its antigen receptor is crosslinked with anti-receptor monoclonal anti-bodies. This simple assay system has yielded much information about signal transduction in T cells. One of the Jurkat cell line's most interesting features, shared with T-cell hybrids, is that it stops growing when its antigen receptor is crosslinked. This has allowed mutants lacking the receptor or having defects in signal transduction pathways to be selected simply by culturing the cells with anti-receptor antibody and selecting those that continue to grow. Thus, T-cell tumors, T-cell hybrids, and cloned T-cell lines all have valuable applications in experimental immunology.

| 2-21 | **Limiting dilution measures the frequency of lymphocytes specific for a particular antigen.** |

Related to Part IV

The response of a lymphocyte population is a measure of the overall response, but the frequency of specific lymphocytes able to respond to an antigen can only be determined by limiting dilution culture. This assay makes use of the Poisson distribution, a statistical function that describes how objects are distributed at random. For instance, when different numbers of T cells are distributed into a series of culture wells, some wells will receive no specific T cells, some will receive one specific T cell, some two and so on. The T cells are activated with specific anti-gen, antigen-presenting cells (APCs), and growth factors. After allowing several days for their growth and differentiation, the cells in each well are tested for a response to antigen, such as cytokine release or the ability to kill specific target cells. The logarithm of the proportion of wells in which there is no response is plotted against the linear number of cells initially added to the well. If cells of one type, typically antigen-specific T cells because of their rarity, are the only limiting factor for obtaining a response, then a straight line is obtained. From the Poisson distribution, it is known that there is, on average, one antigen-specific cell per well when the proportion of negative wells is 37%. Thus, the frequency of antigen-specific cells in the population equals the reciprocal of the number of cells added to the wells when 37% of the wells are negative. After priming, the frequency of specific cells goes up substant-ially, reflecting the antigen-driven proliferation of antigen-specific cells (Fig. 2.36). The limiting dilution assay can also be used to measure the frequency of B cells that can make antibody to a given antigen.

| | **Summary.** |

The cellular basis of adaptive immunity is the clonal selection of lympho-cytes by antigen. Therefore, to study adaptive immune responses, one must isolate lymphocytes and characterize them. Lymphocytes can be divided into subpopulations using antibodies that detect cell-surface

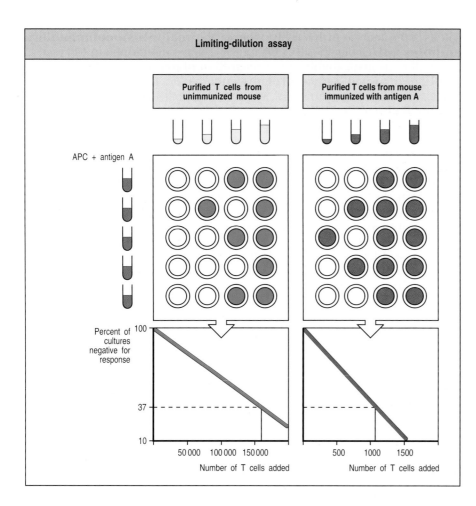

Fig. 2.36 The frequency of specific lymphocytes can be determined using limiting dilution assay. Varying numbers of lymphoid cells from normal or immunized mice are added to individual culture wells and stimulated with antigen and antigen-presenting cells (APCs) or polyclonal mitogen and added growth factors. After several days, the wells are tested for a specific response to antigen, such as cytotoxic killing of target cells. Each well that initially contained a specific T cell will make a response to its target, and from the Poisson distribution one can determine that when 37% of the cultures are negative, each well contained, on average, one specific T cell at the beginning of the culture. In the example shown, for the unimmunized mouse 37% of the wells are negative when 160 000 T cells have been added to each well; thus the frequency of antigen-specific T cells is 1 in 160 000. When the mouse is immunized, 37% of the wells are negative when only 1100 T cells have been added; hence the frequency of specific T cells after immunization is 1 in 1100, an increase in responsive cells of 150 fold.

Related to Part IV

molecules expressed selectively on cells of a given type. Subsets defined in this way also differ functionally, suggesting that the cell-surface molecules detected are important for the function of that cell. Antibodies to cell-surface antigens can be used to separate lymphocytes physically, using magnetic beads, or by fluorescence-activated cell sorting, which also allows quantitative analysis of cell subpopulations. The functional capabilities of these isolated populations can then be tested *in vitro* and *in vivo*. Individual T cells can also be cloned, either as T-cell hybridomas or as continuously growing lines of normal T cells, which are valuable for analyzing the specificity, function, and signaling properties of T cells.

Immunogenetics: the major histocompatibility complex.

Immunogenetics includes the use of antibodies, and more recently of T cells, to detect genetic differences or polymorphisms within a population. The first polymorphic system to be studied by immunogenetics was the ABO blood group system defined by Karl Landsteiner, and virtually all blood typing is carried out using immunogenetic techniques (see Fig. 2.9). In no area has immunogenetics played such a vital

Related
to Part II

role as in the analysis of the highly polymorphic **major histocompatibility complex (MHC)** of genes (see Chapter 4). As we mentioned in Chapter 1, all T-cell responses involve the recognition of peptide fragments of antigen bound to cell-surface proteins encoded in the MHC (MHC molecules), making the analysis of the MHC a central concern of immunologists. The MHC in humans is the most polymorphic cluster of human genes known, and this polymorphism is of interest to immunologists because it affects antigen recognition by T cells (see Chapter 4). Its role in T-cell development (see Chapter 6), the rejection of tissue grafts (see Chapter 12), and susceptibility to many immunological disorders (see Chapters 11 and 12), provides a strong clinical impetus to the analysis of the MHC in humans. The MHC is also of great interest to students of evolution who study polymorphism in an effort to measure genetic history of particular genes or the role of natural selection in maintaining polymorphism. Here, we shall look at the techniques used to analyse MHC genetics and function. We will start by describing the graft rejection responses that are caused by MHC polymorphism and that first drew the attention of biologists to its existence.

2-22 ## Tissues grafted between unrelated individuals are rejected.

The existence of a highly polymorphic MHC was first inferred from the rejection of grafted tissues. Blood transfusion had proved very successful once the genetics of the ABO blood group system had been deciphered, and this led to the idea that solid tissues could similarly be replaced by surgical transplantation. The first attempts to do so all failed: graft rejection was rapid and total, most grafts functioning for a brief period before becoming infiltrated with lymphocytes and dying (Fig. 2.37).

Skin was the favored tissue for experimental transplants, as the graft could be examined directly on a regular basis. The genetic basis of graft rejection was first shown by the successful grafting of skin between individuals of an inbred mouse strain. Inbred mice have been specially bred so that they are homozygous at all loci. All members of an inbred strain carry identical alleles at each locus. These mice are equivalent to monozygotic human twins, and tissues can be grafted between monozygotic twins without rejection as well. Skin transplanted to inbred mice from members of other inbred strains or from other species was invariably rejected (Fig. 2.38). It was soon appreciated that the skin graft rejection was caused by an immune response against the grafted tissue. Graft rejection showed specific immunological memory, and immunodeficient mice did not reject grafts. However, the immunological and genetic basis of graft rejection remained to be worked out.

To analyze the genetic basis of this response, two inbred strains that mutually reject skin grafts were bred with each other, so that their F1 hybrid offspring had one set of alleles from each parental strain. When grafts were made between the F1 hybrid offspring and the parental strains, the F1 hybrid accepted skin from both parental strains, while the skin of the F1 hybrid was rejected by both parents. This showed that all the antigens involved in transplant rejection are expressed in the F1 hybrid mouse, as both parents reject its skin; and that its immune system is tolerant of all such antigens, as it accepts grafts from each parental strain. What was of particular interest was that half the offspring of F1 mice backcrossed to one parental strain rapidly rejected grafts of the other parental strain, starting about 8 days after grafting, indicating that a single genetic locus must control rapid graft rejection. This locus was later found to be composed of a cluster of related genes, and was

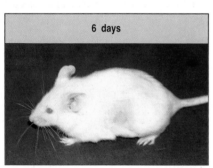

6 days

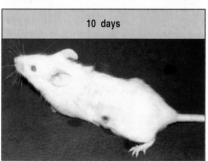

10 days

Fig. 2.37 The immune response to a skin graft causes its rejection by the recipient. Skin from mice of one genotype is grafted to a mouse of a different genotype. Six days after grafting, the skin is healthy (top panel). However, ten days after grafting, an adaptive immune response to the foreign antigens on the graft leads to its destruction (bottom panel).

Fig. 2.38 The terminology of transplantation. Grafts from one site to another on the same individual are termed autologous grafts or autografts and are accepted. Grafts between genetically identical individuals, including those between members of the same inbred strain or between identical twins, are called syngeneic grafts, behave as autografts, and are also accepted. Grafts between genetically non-identical or allogeneic members of the same species are called allografts and are rejected. Grafts between the members of different species are called xenografts and are rejected.

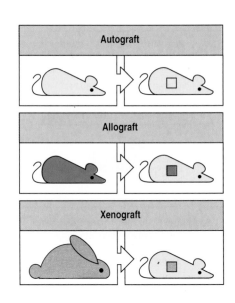

Related to Part II

termed the major histocompatibility complex (MHC) because it is the major determinant of graft survival. The genetic locus determining rapid graft rejection was found to segregate precisely with an antigen detected by an antibody that reacted with mouse red blood cells. This antigen was known as antigen-2, and the locus it defined was named histocompatibility-2 or **H-2**, the genetic designation for the mouse MHC. Subsequently, it was discovered that grafts between mice identical at H-2 were also rejected, although rejection generally occurred longer after grafting. These mice were shown to differ at other genetic loci encoding **minor histocompatibility (H) antigens**.

As genetic matching at H-2 led to prolonged survival of tissue grafts, it was believed that identification of a similar genetic complex might allow tissue grafting in humans. The human MHC was studied first using antibody reactions with white blood cells (Fig. 2.39) and is now called the **human leukocyte antigen**, or **HLA**, system. Unfortunately, the remarkable polymorphism of HLA in the outbred human population makes the identification of HLA-identical individuals enormously difficult. Furthermore, the presence of minor H antigens in humans means that it is only possible to to achieve the perfect matching that is available in genetically identical members of an inbred mouse strain when the human donor and recipient are monozygotic twins (see Chapter 12).

2-23 | MHC congenic, recombinant, and mutant inbred mouse strains are essential tools for analyzing MHC function.

The MHC is a complex of many closely linked genes, and most of the genes that encode MHC molecules that present antigens to T cells are highly polymorphic in both mice and humans. To study the function of the MHC and the effect of MHC polymorphism on immune responses, animals are needed that differ genetically only at the MHC. To produce such animals, George Snell took advantage of the observation that a tumor transplanted from one mouse would grow progressively in another mouse only if the recipient mouse carried the same MHC genes expressed by the tumor. Under these conditions, the recipient is tolerant to the tumor's MHC antigens and fails to reject it, so the tumor grows and kills the recipient mouse. One tumor used by Snell arose in mice of strain A and would therefore grow in and kill any strain A mouse it was injected into, so Snell crossed strain A mice (MHC genotype H-2^a) with mice of a different MHC genotype, such as strain C57BL/6 (MHC genotype H-2^b), to generate F1 hybrid mice (H-2^{axb}), which were then intercrossed to generate F2 mice. The F2 generation was injected with the tumor,

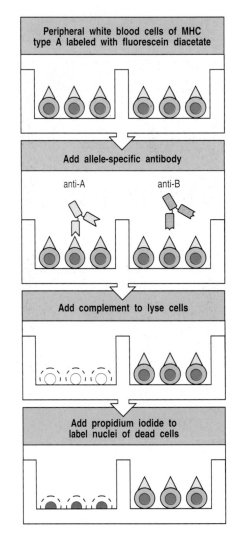

Peripheral white blood cells of MHC type A labeled with fluorescein diacetate

Add allele-specific antibody

anti-A   anti-B

Add complement to lyse cells

Add propidium iodide to label nuclei of dead cells

Fig. 2.39 The microcytotoxicity assay is used in histocompatibility testing. Leukocytes labeled with the vital dye fluorescein diacetate, which stains viable cells green, are exposed to antibody specific for allelic variants of MHC proteins and then exposed to complement. If the antibody reacts with the MHC proteins on a cell, this activates the complement so that the cell is killed, as seen by loss of green cells and the appearance of cells labeled by uptake of the dye propidium iodide (red), which only enters dead cells.

Related
to Part II

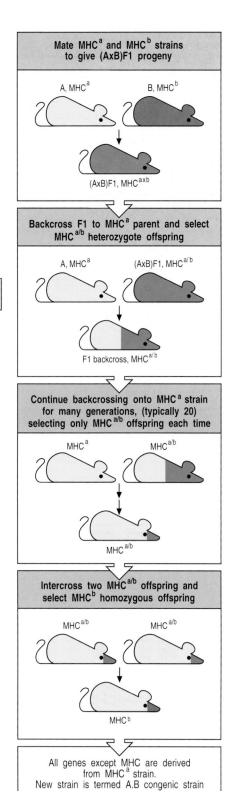

Mate MHC^a and MHC^b strains
to give (AxB)F1 progeny

A, MHC^a B, MHC^b

(AxB)F1, MHC^{axb}

Backcross F1 to MHC^a parent and select
MHC$^{a/b}$ heterozygote offspring

A, MHC^a (AxB)F1, MHC$^{a/b}$

F1 backcross, MHC$^{a/b}$

Continue backcrossing onto MHC^a strain
for many generations, (typically 20)
selecting only MHC$^{a/b}$ offspring each time

MHC^a MHC$^{a/b}$

MHC$^{a/b}$

Intercross two MHC$^{a/b}$ offspring and
select MHC^b homozygous offspring

MHC$^{a/b}$ MHC$^{a/b}$

MHC^b

All genes except MHC are derived
from MHC^a strain.
New strain is termed A.B congenic strain

Fig. 2.40   The production of MHC congenic mouse strains. Mice of two strains, strain A with MHC genotype a (yellow) and strain B with MHC genotype b (blue) are crossed, and their F1 hybrid offspring, which are heterozygous at all loci including MHC^{axb} (green), are backcrossed to parental strain A. The F1 backcross progeny, which are homozygous A at 50% of their loci (yellow) are selected for expression of the other parental MHC^b and those that are MHC^{axb} are backcrossed again to strain A. This continues for 10–30 backcross generations, after which the mice are homozygous A at virtually all loci except MHC, where they are a/b (green). These mice are intercrossed and selected for homozygosity at the MHC for alleles of donor origin (MHC^b) (blue). Virtually all the rest of the genome is derived from strain A to which the MHC genotype MHC^b has been introgressively backcrossed. These mice are strain A co-isogeneic or congenic for MHC^b, and are designated A.B. They can be used to determine if genetic traits that differ between strain A and strain B map to the MHC.

and the one mouse in four that was homozygous H-2^b survived because it was intolerant of H-2^a. These mice were then backcrossed to strain A and the progeny again intercrossed and challenged with the tumor. After 10 backcross/intercross generations, Snell obtained a mouse that was genetically 99% strain A but was homozygous for the MHC of the other parent in the initial cross, in this case H-2^b. These are called **congenic resistant** (to the strain A tumor) or **MHC congenic** mice, and are designated A.B, where B denotes the strain designation of the parent donating the MHC genes, in this case B6. This experiment illustrates not only MHC genetics and function but also that the immune system can combat tumors provided that they express recognizable antigens. We shall return to tumor immunity as a potential therapy for naturally occurring cancers in Chapter 13.

Congenic resistant mice have been crucial to our understanding of the role of the MHC in immunobiology. Fortunately there are now easier ways of producing them. For instance, antibodies to allelic variants of MHC proteins can be used to identify offspring that inherit the new MHC genes being bred onto strain A. One can therefore simply select the mice at each backcross generation that carry these genes, speeding the derivation of the new strains by avoiding the intercross generation (Fig. 2.40). During this process, it is also possible to detect mice that have undergone recombination within the MHC, such that only some MHC alleles are inherited from the donor parent. These are called **MHC recombinant strains**. These intra-MHC recombinant mice allow one to map a particular phenotype to a particular region of the MHC, further refining the genetic map. Although the molecular structure of the MHC is now well defined, *in vivo* analysis of MHC function still depends largely on such recombinant and congenic mice. For example, one can map traits to a single locus in the MHC using **MHC mutant** strains of mice (inbred mice differing only at a single MHC locus), or by using transgenic or gene knock-out mice, as we shall see in Section 2-37.

2-24   T lymphocytes respond strongly to MHC polymorphisms.

Graft rejection is carried out by T cells that recognize foreign MHC molecules and destroy the graft. Although this process can be studied *in vivo*, experimental analysis, especially in humans, required the development of *in vitro* correlates of graft rejection. One such assay is provided by the **mixed lymphocyte reaction** (MLR), in which T cells are co-cultured with so-called stimulator cells (Fig. 2.41). These are usually irradiated peripheral blood lymphocytes, together with some antigen-presenting cells from an unrelated individual who is therefore likely to

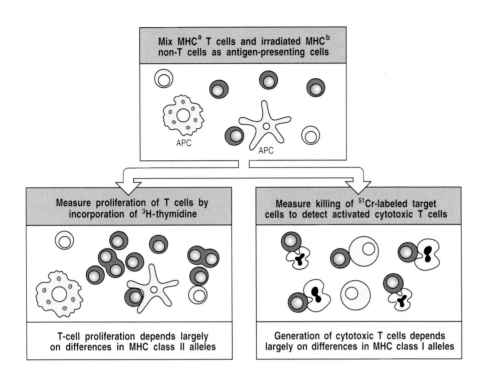

Related
to Part II

Fig. 2.41 The mixed lymphocyte reaction (MLR) can be used for detecting histoincompatibility.
Lymphocytes from two people are isolated from the peripheral blood. Cells of one person serve as the responders (blue), while the cells of the other donor (yellow) are used as stimulator cells. The non-T cells, which will include antigen-presenting cells, are irradiated or treated with the antibiotic mitomycin C before culture to block DNA synthesis and cell division. Between three to seven days after mixing the cells, the cultures are assessed for T-cell proliferation by measuring the uptake of ^{3}H-thymidine, which is mainly the result of CD4 T cells recognizing differences in MHC class II genes, and for the generation of cytotoxic CD8 T cells that respond to differences MHC class I genes by the chromium-release assay on labeled target cells.

be MHC disparate. The T cells are stimulated to proliferate and differentiate into effector cells; the irradiation of the stimulator cells prevents them from responding back. The T cells respond because they recognize MHC molecules on the stimulating cells that are different from their own MHC molecules.

The strong T-cell proliferative response in mixed lymphocyte culture reflects the high frequency of responding T cells. By limiting dilution assay (see Fig. 2.36), normal lymphocytes that respond to MHC differences are estimated to be present at between 1 cell in 500 and 1 cell in 20. The reason for this will be discussed in Chapters 4 and 6. The proliferative response is largely the result of CD4 T-cell recognition of MHC class II polymorphisms (see Fig. 2.41; lower left panel), while the cytotoxic T cells that result are predominantly CD8 T cells recognizing MHC class I polymorphisms (see Fig. 2.41, lower right panel). This *in vitro* correlate of graft rejection is very useful in screening for histoincompatibility between potential donors and recipients, as it is extremely sensitive and more closely related to the actual graft rejection response than is the microcytotoxicity assay carried out with antibodies (see Fig. 2.39). Unfortunately, it is also more cumbersome and expensive to carry out, and takes several days to produce an answer.

2-25   Antibodies to MHC molecules inhibit T-cell responses.

MHC polymorphism not only accounts for graft rejection but also has profound effects on antigen recognition by T cells, as we shall learn in Chapter 4. As the MHC encodes several different proteins that present antigen to T cells, it is often difficult using genetics alone to determine which MHC molecule a T cell is recognizing.

An alternative approach is to use monoclonal antibodies that bind to a given MHC molecule and prevent its recognition by the T-cell receptor (Fig. 2.42). Thus, proliferative responses of CD4 T cells in mixed lymphocyte reactions are largely inhibited by antibodies to MHC class II molecules, while antibodies to MHC class I molecules

Related to Part II

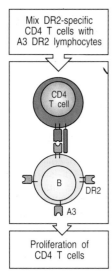

Mix DR2-specific CD4 T cells with A3 DR2 lymphocytes

Proliferation of CD4 T cells

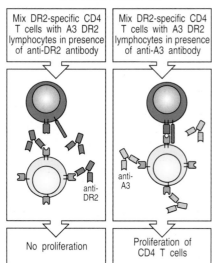

Mix DR2-specific CD4 T lymphocytes in presence of anti-DR2 antibody

Mix DR2-specific CD4 T lymphocytes in presence of anti-A3 antibody

No proliferation

Proliferation of CD4 T cells

Fig. 2.42   Antibody to specific MHC molecules can inhibit the mixed lymphocyte reaction. A CD4 T-cell response to the MHC Class II molecule HLA-DR2 is inhibited by anti-HLA-DR2 antibodies, which compete with the T-cell receptor for binding to HLA-DR2. However, antibodies to the MHC Class I molecule HLA-A3 do not inhibit the response of CD4 T cells to HLA-DR2, even though they bind to the stimulator cell surface. This shows that antibodies that bind the stimulator cells inhibit specific recognition events and are not interfering with the response non-specifically.

block the cytolytic response of CD8 T cells in the same culture. Similarly, antibodies to MHC molecules can be used to define which MHC molecule is presenting peptides to an antigen-specific T cell. Antibodies to other structures crucial for cell interactions likewise inhibit these responses, so the use of monoclonal antibodies to inhibit T-cell responses has played a critical role in our understanding of these processes.

2-26   Antibodies to MHC molecules can be used to define the MHC genotype.

Although T cells can be used to detect MHC variability, routine genetic typing for MHC uses antibodies that distinguish between the numerous different allelic variants of any MHC molecule. Most of our information about MHC genetics has been, and continues to be, generated in this way. Antibody typing has defined multiple gene loci within the MHC, each with a large number of alleles in the two species studied most extensively, humans and mice. These loci comprise a tightly linked complex of genes on chromosome 6 in humans and chromosome 17 in mice. As the MHC genes are close together on the chromosome, genetic recombination rarely occurs within the MHC, and most individuals will inherit an intact set of parental alleles from each parent; such a set of linked genes is referred to as a **haplotype**, the MHC genes found in one haploid genome. The tight genetic linkage of MHC genes can be documented readily by genotyping family members (Fig. 2.43).

Population and family studies have revealed a striking association of HLA genotype with the incidence of a number of immune-mediated diseases. For some of these diseases, susceptibility was linked to a particular MHC class I genotype, but the majority were affected more strongly by genotype at the MHC class II locus. This linkage has stimulated the analysis of MHC polymorphism because the accuracy of disease-association analyses depends on how precisely the HLA genotypes of unrelated people can be determined and compared. Fortunately, the molecular analysis of MHC alleles is now possible, as we shall see in the next section.

2-27   Accurate MHC genotyping requires direct analysis of DNA sequence.

Although serological analysis is the main method for HLA genotyping humans, the reagents used are not specific enough to determine the precise structural identity of MHC molecules in unrelated individuals, who may have inherited closely related but distinct genes. Thus, while

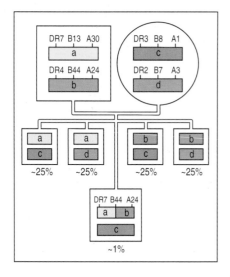

DR7 B13 A30   a
DR4 B44 A24   b
DR3 B8 A1   c
DR2 B7 A3   d

a c ~25%   a d ~25%   b c ~25%   b d ~25%

DR7 B44 A24   a b   c   ~1%

Fig. 2.43   The inheritance of MHC haplotypes in families. Each parent contributes genes from one of their two haplotypes, usually designated as a, b, c, and d. Most offspring inherit a complete MHC haplotype from each parent and can be designated simply a/c, a/d, b/c, or b/d; recombination within MHC haplotypes occurs at a frequency of only 1–2% (bottom panel).

Fig. 2.44 The polymerase chain reaction. To amplify a specific region of genomic DNA, such as a polymorphic exon of an MHC gene, synthetic oligonucleotide primers complementary to the DNA sequence flanking that region are made. The genomic DNA is denatured in the presence of an excess of these two oligonucleotide primers so that after reannealing, the primers have bound their complementary sequence in genomic DNA. The DNA polymerase Taq from the bacterium *Thermus aquaticus*, which is stable at the high temperatures used to denature DNA between replication cycles, elongates the primer using the genomic DNA between the two primers as a template. The replicated DNA is separated into single strands by heating and then the mixture is cooled so that a new cycle of primer annealing and replication can commence. The first extension products are random in length but as the reaction continues, the products that are delimited by the primers accumulate and hence are of the same length.

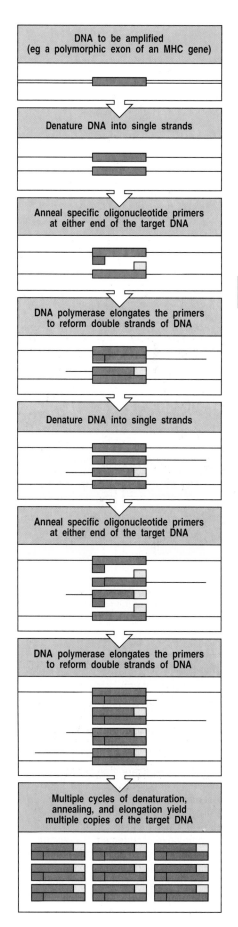

Related to Part II

serological typing can accurately predict genotype in family members for shared MHC alleles, the identity of MHC alleles in unrelated individuals can be established only by direct structural analysis of their genes. This is now most conveniently performed using the **polymerase chain reaction** (**PCR**), a rapid method of selectively replicating a particular stretch of genomic DNA *in vitro* (Fig. 2.44). Once enough DNA is produced from the gene being amplified, it can be sequenced. Sequence analysis has shown that serologically identical alleles actually comprise several closely related alleles. There are now many known sequence variants of most serologically defined MHC alleles, which are quite similar to each other but differ by one or a few amino acids, whereas the proteins of different serologically determined alleles differ from one another by many amino acids.

Once the DNA sequence of a given allele has been determined, oligonucleotide probes can be constructed from the regions where differences from other alleles occur, and these differences can be detected by direct hybridization of the probe to PCR-amplified genomic DNA. This provides a rapid, cheap, and sensitive means of defining MHC gene structure. The application of this technique to MHC genetics has allowed the accurate determination of associations between MHC genes and several immunological diseases, and should help ultimately in determining the mechanism by which certain MHC alleles confer genetic susceptibility to particular diseases.

Summary.

The cell-surface glycoproteins encoded by the MHC play a central role in immunology. As we learned in Chapter 1, their main function is to deliver peptide fragments of antigen to the cell surface where the peptide: MHC complex can be recognized by T cells. However, the MHC was originally discovered as the major genetic barrier to transplantation, because the strong response of T cells to foreign MHC molecules causes graft rejection. T-cell recognition of peptide antigens is also influenced profoundly by MHC polymorphism. Thus, the analysis of this polymorphism is essential in immunology. It is also important in clinical medicine, not only as a way to match graft donors with recipients but also for studying the role of MHC genotype in determining susceptibility to many human allergic and autoimmune diseases. Such studies require reliable genotyping of the MHC in humans, which is best carried out using DNA analysis. Experimental studies of MHC polymorphism are facilitated greatly by specialized MHC congenic, recombinant and mutant strains of mice. These clinical and experimental tools are essential for examining the impact of MHC polymorphism on immunity and immunological diseases.

Analyzing immune responses in intact or manipulated organisms.

The ultimate goal of immunology is to understand the immune response *in vivo* and to control it. To do so, techniques to study immunity in live animals and in human patients are essential. The following sections describe how immunity is measured and characterized in the intact organism, be it a mouse or a human being. From these observations much is learned about the functioning of the intact immune system. The cellular and molecular basis for these observed functions is the subject of much of this book. Experimental animals, and in particular inbred mice, can also be manipulated by various means for the purposes of studying immune functions. This can be achieved by transfering lymphocytes or antibodies, or by altering the genome, either by inserting new genes to create transgenic animals, or deleting genes using gene knock-out techniques.

2-28   Protective immunity can be assessed by challenge with infectious agents.

An adaptive immune response against a pathogen often confers long-lasting immunity against infection with that pathogen; successful vaccination achieves the same end. The very first experiment in immunology, Jenner's successful vaccination against smallpox, is still the model for assessing the presence of such protective immunity. The assessment of protective immunity conferred by vaccination has three essential steps. First, an immune response is elicited by immunization with a candidate vaccine. Second, the immunized individuals, along with unimmunized controls, are challenged with the infectious agent. Finally, the prevalence and severity of infection in the immunized individual is compared with the course of the disease in the unimmunized controls (Fig. 2.45). For obvious reasons, such experiments are usually carried out first in animals, if a suitable animal model for the infection exists. However, eventually a trial must be carried out in humans. In this case, the infectious challenge is usually provided naturally by carrying out the trial in a region where the disease is prevalent. The efficacy of the vaccine is determined by assessing the prevalence and severity of new infections in the immunized and control populations. Such studies necessarily give less precise results than a direct experiment but, for most diseases, they are the only way of assessing a vaccine's ability to induce protective immunity in humans.

2-29   Immunity can be transferred by antibodies or by lymphocytes.

The tests described in the previous section show that protective immunity has been established but cannot show whether it involves humoral immunity, cell-mediated immunity, or both. When these studies are carried out in immunized or previously infected inbred mice, the nature of protective immunity can be determined by transferring serum or lymphoid cells from an immunized donor to an unimmunized syngeneic recipient (that is, a genetically identical animal of the same inbred strain) (Fig. 2.46). If protection against infection can be conferred by the transfer of serum, the immunity is provided by circulating antibodies and is called **humoral immunity**. Transfer of immunity by antiserum or purified antibodies provides immediate protection against many pathogens and against toxins such as those of tetanus and snake venom. However,

Related to Part V

Inject saline solution | Inject killed pathogen (test vaccine)

After 10 days challenge with lethal dose of live pathogen

Animal dies | Animal remains healthy

Non-immune control | Active immunization

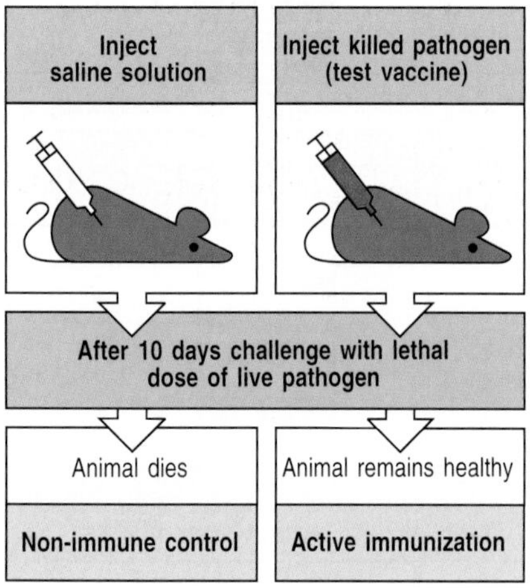

Fig. 2.45 *In vivo* assay for the presence and nature of protective immunity after vaccination in animals. Mice are injected with the test vaccine or a control such as saline solution. Different groups are then challenged with lethal or pathogenic doses of the test pathogen or with an unrelated pathogen as a specificity control (not shown). Unimmunized animals die or become severely infected. Successful vaccination is seen as specific protection of immunized mice against infection with the test pathogen. This is called active immunity and the process is called active immunization.

Fig. 2.46 Immunity can be transferred by antibodies or by lymphocytes. Successful vaccination leads to a long-lived state of protection against the specific immunizing pathogen. If this immune protection can be transferred to a normal syngeneic recipient with serum from an immune donor, then immunity is mediated by antibodies; such immunity is called humoral immunity and the process is called passive immunization. If immunity can only be transferred by infusing lymphoid cells from the immune donor into a normal syngeneic recipient, then the immunity is called cell-mediated immunity and the transfer process is called adoptive transfer or adoptive immunization. Passive immunity is short-lived, as antibody is eventually catabolized, but adoptively transferred immunity is mediated by immune cells, which can survive and provide longer-lasting immunity.

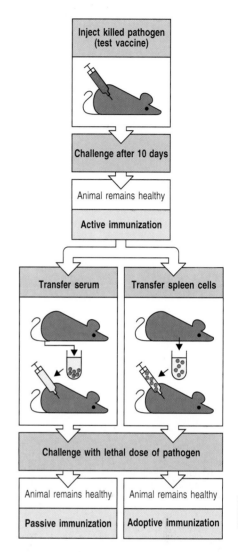

although protection is immediate, it is temporary, lasting only so long as the transferred antibodies remain active in the recipient's body. This type of transfer is therefore called **passive immunization**. Only **active immunization** with antigen can provide lasting immunity.

Protection against many diseases cannot be transferred by serum but can be transferred by lymphoid cells from immunized donors. The transfer of lymphoid cells from an immune donor to a normal syngeneic recipient is called **adoptive transfer** or **adoptive immunization**, and the immunity transferred is called **adoptive immunity**. Immunity that can be transferred only with lymphoid cells is called cell-mediated immunity. Such cell transfers must be between genetically identical donors and recipients, such as members of the same inbred strain of mouse, so that the donor lymphocytes are not rejected by the recipient and do not attack the recipient's tissues. Adoptive transfer of immunity is not used clinically in humans except in experimental approaches to cancer therapy or as an adjunct to bone marrow transplantation.

2-30   Local responses to antigen can indicate the presence of active immunity.

Active immunity is often studied *in vivo*, especially in humans, by injecting antigens locally in the skin. If a reaction appears, this indicates the presence of antibodies or immune lymphocytes that are specific for that antigen; the **tuberculin test** is an example of this. When people have had tuberculosis they develop cell-mediated immunity that can be detected as a local response when their skin is injected with a small amount of tuberculin, an extract of *Mycobacterium tuberculosis*, the pathogen that causes tuberculosis. The response typically appears a day or two after the injection and consists of a raised, red, and hard (or indurated) area in the skin, which then disappears as the antigen is degraded.

The immune system can also make less desirable responses, such as the hypersensitivity reactions responsible for allergies (see Chapter 11). Local intracutaneous injections of minute doses of the antigens that cause allergies are used to determine what antigen triggers a patient's allergic reactions. Local responses that happen in the first few minutes after antigen injection in immune recipients are called **immediate hypersensitivity reactions**, and they can be of several forms, one of which is the wheal-and-flare response described in Chapter 11. Immediate hypersensitivity reactions are mediated by specific antibodies of the IgE class formed as a result of earlier exposures to the antigen. Responses that take hours to days to develop, such as the tuberculin test, are referred to as **delayed-type hypersensitivity** responses and are caused by pre-existing immune T cells. This latter type of response was observed by Jenner when he tested vaccinated individuals with a local injection of vaccinia virus.

Related to Part V

These tests work because the local deposit of antigen remains concentrated in the initial site of injection, eliciting responses in local tissues. They do not cause generalized reactions if sufficiently small doses of antigen are used. However, local tests carry a risk of systemic allergic reactions, and they should be used with caution in people with a history of hyper-sensitivity.

| 2-31 | **The assessment of immune responses and immunological competence in humans.** |

The methods used for testing immune function in humans are necessarily more limited than those used in experimental animals, but many different tests are available, some of which have been mentioned already. They fall into several groups depending on the reason the patient is being studied.

Assessment of protective immunity in humans generally relies on tests conducted *in vitro*. To assess humoral immunity, specific antibody levels in the patient's serum are assayed using the test microorganism or a purified microbial product as antigen. To test for humoral immunity against viruses, antibody production is often measured by the ability of serum to neutralize the infectivity of live virus for tissue culture cells. In addition to providing information about protective immunity, the presence of antibody to a particular pathogen indicates that the patient has been exposed to it, making such tests of crucial importance in epidemiology. At present, testing for antibody to HIV is the main screening test for infection, critical both for the patient and in blood banking, where blood from infected donors must be excluded from the supply. Essentially similar tests are used in investigating allergy, where allergens are used as the antigens in tests for specific IgE antibody by ELISA or radioimmunoassay (see Section 2-7), which may be used to confirm the results of skin tests.

Cell-mediated immunity to infectious agents can be tested either by skin test with extracts of the pathogen, as in the tuberculin test (see Section 2-30), or by the ability of the pathogen or an extract from it to stimulate T-cell proliferative responses *in vitro* (Section 2-18). These tests provide information about the exposure of the patient to the disease and also about their ability to mount an adaptive immune response to it.

Patients with immune deficiency (see Chapter 10) are usually detected clinically by a history of recurrent infection. To determine the competence of the immune system in such patients, a battery of tests is usually conducted (Fig. 2.47); these focus with increasing precision as the nature of the defect is narrowed down to a single element. The presence of the various cell types in blood is determined by routine hematology, often followed by FACS analysis (see Section 2-17) of lymphocyte subsets, and the measurement of serum immunoglobulins. The phagocytic competence of freshly isolated polymorphonuclear leukocytes and monocytes is tested, and the efficiency of the complement system (see Chapter 8) is determined by testing the dilution of serum required for lysis of 50% of antibody-coated red blood cells (CH_{50}).

In general, if such tests reveal a defect in one of these broad compartments of immune function, more specialized testing is then needed to determine the precise nature of the defect. Tests of lymphocyte function are often valuable, starting with the ability of polyclonal mitogens to induce T-cell proliferation and B-cell secretion of immunoglobulin in tissue culture (see Section 2-18). These tests eventually pinpoint the cellular defect in immunodeficiency.

Related to Part V

Evaluation of the cellular components of the human immune system

	B cells	T cells	Phagocytes
Normal numbers ($\times 10^9$ per liter of blood)	Approximately 0.3	Total 1.0–2.5 CD4 0.5–1.6 CD8 0.3–0.9	Monocytes 0.15–0.6 Polymorphonuclear leukocytes Neutrophils 3.00–5.5 Eosinophils 0.05–0.25 Basophils 0.02
Measurement of function *in vivo*	Serum Ig levels Specific antibody levels	Skin test	–
Measurement of function *in vitro*	Induced antibody production in response to pokeweed mitogen	T-cell proliferation in response to phytohemagglutinin or to tetanus toxoid	Phagocytosis Nitro blue tetrazolium uptake Intracellular killing of bacteria
Specific defects	See Fig. 10.8	See Fig. 10.8	See Fig. 10.8

Evaluation of the humoral components of the human immune system

	Immunoglobulins				Complement
Component	IgG	IgM	IgA	IgE	
Normal levels	600–1400 mg dl^{-1}	40–345 mg dl^{-1}	60–380 mg dl^{-1}	0–200 IU ml^{-1}	CH$_{50}$ of 125–300 IU ml^{-1}

Fig. 2.47 The assessment of immunological competence in humans. Both humoral and cell-mediated aspects of host defense can be checked, usually in a prescribed sequence, to identify the presence of an immune response or the causes of immunological incompetence. The initial screen consists of measuring levels of immunoglobulin and complement, and counting lymphocytes and phagocytic cells. (IgE is present, if at all, at very low levels and is measured in international units (IU) per ml; the CH$_{50}$ of complement is the dilution at which 50% of antibody-coated red blood cells are lysed.) This initial screen usually indicates whether a defect in humoral or T-cell mediated immunity is present, and also whether it affects the induction or mediation of a response. In Chapter 10, defects in host defense known as immunodeficiency diseases are described in detail.

Related to Part V

In patients with autoimmune diseases (see Chapter 12), the same parameters are usually analyzed to determine whether there is a gross abnormality in the immune system. However, most patients with such diseases show few abnormalities in general immune function. To determine whether a patient is producing antibody against their own cellular antigens, the most informative test is to react their serum with tissue sections, which are then examined for bound antibody by indirect immunofluorescence using fluorescent-labeled anti-human immunoglobulin (see Section 2-13). Most autoimmune diseases are associated with the production of broadly characteristic patterns of autoantibodies directed at self tissues. These patterns aid in the diagnosis of the disease and help to distinguish autoimmunity from tissue inflammation due to infectious causes.

2-32 Irradiation kills lymphoid cells, allowing the study of immune function by adoptive transfer and the study of lymphocyte development in bone marrow chimeras.

Ionizing radiation from X-ray or γ-ray sources kills lymphoid cells at doses that spare the other tissues of the body. This makes it possible to eliminate immune function in a recipient animal before attempting to restore immune function by adoptive transfer, and allows the effect of the adoptively-transferred cells to be studied in the absence of other lymphoid cells. James Gowans originally used this technique to prove the role of the lymphocyte in immune responses. He showed that all active immune responses could be transferred to irradiated recipients by small lymphocytes from immunized donors. This technique can be refined by transferring only certain lymphocyte subpopulations, such as B cells, CD4 T cells, and so on. Even cloned T-cell lines have been tested for their ability to transfer immune function, and have been shown to confer adoptive immunity to their specific antigen. Such adoptive transfer studies are a cornerstone in the study of the intact immune system, as they can be carried out rapidly, simply, and in any strain of mouse.

Somewhat higher doses of irradiation eliminate all cells of hematopoietic origin, allowing replacement of the entire hematopoietic system, including lymphocytes, from donor bone marrow stem cells. The resulting animals are called **radiation bone marrow chimeras** from the Greek word *chimera*, a mythical animal that had the head of a lion, the tail of a serpent and the body of a goat. This technique is used to examine the development of lymphocytes as opposed to their effector functioning, and it has been particularly important in studying T-cell development, as we shall see in Chapter 6. Essentially the same technique is used in humans to replace bone marrow when it fails, as in aplastic anemia or after nuclear accidents, or to eradicate the bone marrow and replace it with normal marrow in the treatment of certain cancers.

2-33   Genetic defects can prevent the development of all lymphocytes.

There are several inherited immunodeficiencies in humans that are described as severe combined immune deficiency, or SCID, because they are characterized by defects in both humoral and cell-mediated immunity (we shall describe these various syndromes further in Chapter 10). Patients with these disorders suffer from a lack of lymphocytes, or lymphocyte function, and are remarkably susceptible to infection with a wide range of agents: most can survive only if completely isolated from their surroundings. Some SCID patients can be treated by bone marrow transplantation. SCID individuals are a dramatic illustration of the importance of lymphocytes in host defense and of the origin of all lymphocytes from a bone marrow progenitor.

Related
to Part V

In the mouse, a recessive mutation called *scid* prevents lymphocyte differentiation (see Chapter 10). Such mice have normal microenvironments for both B- and T-lymphocyte differentiation from stem cells, so grafting normal bone marrow into homozygous *scid/scid* mice can generate an intact immune system. Individual components of the mature immune system can also be transferred to *scid/scid* mice to generate animals expressing only the functions of particular subpopulations of lymphocytes. *Scid* mice are useful for distinguishing those immune functions that are innate (see Chapter 9) as opposed to those that require adaptive immunity mediated by specific lymphocytes. More recent studies use mice mutant in the *RAG-1* and *RAG-2* genes. These mice are completely devoid of functional T and B cells, whereas *scid* mice produce some lymphocytes as they age.

2-34   T cells can be eliminated selectively by removal of the thymus or by the *nude* mutation.

The importance of T-cell function *in vivo* can be ascertained in mice with no T cells of their own. Under these conditions, the effect of a lack of T cells can be studied, and T-cell subpopulations can be restored selectively to analyze their specialized functions. T lymphocytes originate in the thymus, and neonatal **thymectomy**, the surgical removal of the thymus of a mouse at birth, prevents T-cell development from occurring because the export of most functionally mature T cells only occurs after birth in the mouse. Alternatively, adult mice can be thymectomized and then irradiated and reconstituted with bone marrow; such mice will develop all hematopoietic cell types except mature T cells.

The recessive *nude* mutation in mice, which in homozygous form causes hairlessness and absence of the thymus, is also associated with failure to develop T cells from bone marrow progenitors. Grafting thymectomized or *nude/nude* mice with thymic epithelial elements depleted of lymphocytes allows the graft recipients to develop normal mature T cells. This procedure allows the role of the non-lymphoid thymic stroma to be examined; it has been crucial in determining the role of thymic stromal cells in T-cell development (see Chapter 6).

2-35	**B cells are depleted selectively in agammaglobulinemic humans and genetically manipulated mice.**

There is no single site of B-cell development in mice, so techniques such as thymectomy cannot be applied to the study of B-cell function and development in rodents. Nor are there mutations equivalent to *nude* that provide one with mice that have T cells but no B cells. However, such mutations exist in humans, leading to a failure to mount humoral immune responses or make antibody. The diseases produced by such mutations are called **agammaglobulinemias**, as they were originally detected as the absence of gamma globulins (see Section 2-9). The genetic basis for one form of this disease in humans has now been established (see Chapter 10), and some features of the disease can be reproduced in mice by targeted disruption of the corresponding gene (see Section 2-37). Several different mutations in crucial regions of immunoglobulin genes have already been produced by gene targeting and have provided mice lacking B cells.

2-36	**Individual genes can be introduced into mice by transgenesis.**

The function of genes has traditionally been studied by observing the effects of spontaneous mutations in whole organisms and, more recently, by analyzing the effects of targeted mutations in cultured cells. The advent of gene cloning and *in vitro* mutagenesis now make possible the analysis of specific mutations within whole animals. Mice with extra copies or altered copies of a gene in their genome can be generated by **transgenesis**, which is now a well established procedure. To produce **transgenic** mice, a cloned gene is introduced into the mouse genome by micro-injection into the male pronucleus of a fertilized egg, which is then implanted into the uterus of a pseudopregnant female mouse. In some of the eggs, the injected DNA becomes integrated randomly into the genome, giving rise to a mouse that has an extra genetic element of known structure, the **transgene** (Fig. 2.48). This technique allows one to study the impact of a new gene on development, to identify the regulatory regions of a gene required for its normal tissue specific expression, to determine the effects of its overexpression or expression in inappropriate tissues,

Related to Part V

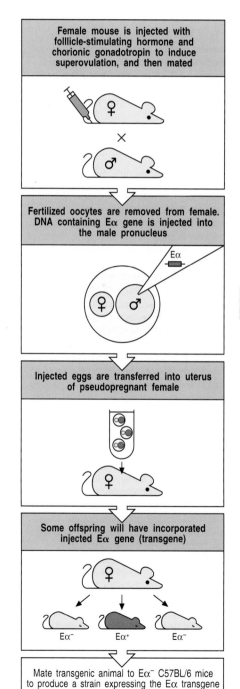

Fig. 2.48 The function and expression of genes can be studied *in vivo* using transgenic mice. DNA encoding a gene of interest, here the mouse MHC class II gene Eα, is purified and microinjected into the male pronucleus of fertilized ova. The ova are then implanted into pseudopregnant female mice. The resulting offspring are screened for the presence of the transgene in their cells, and positive mice are used as founders that transmit the transgene to their offspring, establishing a line of transgenic mice that carry one or more extra genes. The function of the Eα gene used here is tested by breeding the transgene into C57BL/6 mice that carry an inactivating mutation in their endogenous Eα gene.

and to find out the impact of mutations on gene function. Transgenic mice have been particularly useful in studying the role of T-cell and B-cell receptors in lymphocyte development, as will be described in Chapters 5 and 6.

2-37 The role of individual genes can be studied *in vivo* by gene knock-out.

In many cases, the functions of a particular gene can only be fully understood if a mutant animal that does not express the gene can be obtained. While genes used to be discovered through identification of mutant phenotypes, it is now more common to discover and isolate the normal gene and then determine its function by replacing it *in vivo* with a defective copy. This procedure is known as **gene knock-out**, and it has been made possible by two fairly recent developments: a powerful strategy to select for targeted mutation by homologous recombination, and the development of continuously growing lines of pluripotent **embryonic stem cells** (**ES cells**).

The technique of **gene targeting** takes advantage of the phenomenon known as **homologous recombination** (Fig. 2.49). Cloned copies of the target gene are altered to make them non-functional and are then introduced into the ES cell where they recombine with the homologous gene in the cell's genome, replacing the normal gene with a non-functional copy. Homologous recombination is a rare event in mammalian cells,

Fig. 2.49 The deletion of specific genes can be accomplished by homologous recombination. When pieces of DNA are introduced into cells, they can integrate into cellular DNA in two different ways. If they randomly insert into sites of DNA breaks, the whole piece is usually integrated, often in several copies. However, extrachromosomal DNA can also undergo homologous recombination with the cellular copy of the gene, in which case only the central, homologous region is incorporated into cellular DNA. Inserting a selectable marker gene such as resistance to neomycin (neo^r) into the coding region of a gene does not prevent homologous recombination, and it achieves two goals. First, it protects any cell that has integrated the injected DNA from the neomycin-like antibiotic G418. Second, when the gene recombines with homologous cellular DNA, the neo^r gene disrupts the coding sequence of the modified cellular gene. Homologous recombinants can be discriminated from random insertions if the gene for herpes simplex virus thymidine kinase (HSV-tk) is placed at one or both ends of the DNA construct, which is often known as a 'targeting construct' because it targets the cellular gene. In random DNA integrations, HSV-tk is retained. HSV-tk renders the cell sensitive to the anti-viral agent ganciclovir. However, as HSV-tk is not homologous to the target DNA, it is lost from homologous integrants. Thus, cells that have undergone homologous recombination are uniquely both neo^r- and ganciclovir-resistant, and survive in a mixture of the two antibiotics. The presence of the disrupted gene has to be confirmed by Southern blotting or by the polymerase chain reaction (PCR) using primers in the neo^r gene and in cellular DNA lying outside the region used in the targeting construct. By using two different resistance genes one can disrupt the two cellular copies of a gene, making a deletion mutant (not shown).

Related to Part V

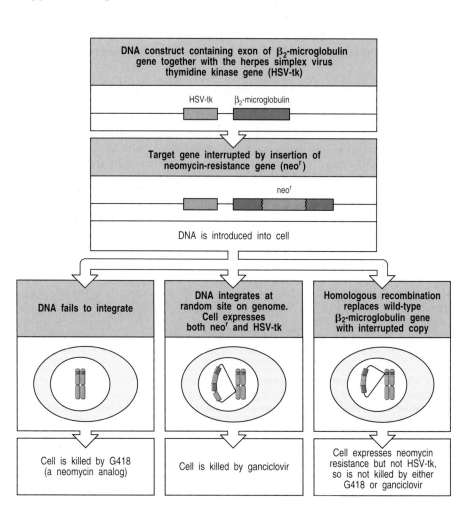

and thus a powerful selection strategy is required to detect those cells in which it has occurred. Most commonly, the introduced gene construct has its sequence disrupted by an inserted antibiotic-resistance gene such as that for neomycin resistance. If this construct undergoes homologous recombination with the endogenous copy of the gene, the endogenous gene is disrupted but the antibiotic-resistance gene remains functional, allowing cells that have incorporated the gene to be selected in culture for resistance to the neomycin-like drug G418. Antibiotic resistance on its own shows only that the cells have taken up and integrated the neomycin-resistance gene. To select for those cells in which homologous recombination has occurred, the ends of the construct usually carry the thymidine kinase gene from the herpes simplex virus (HSV-tk). Cells that incorporate DNA randomly usually retain the entire DNA construct including HSV-tk, whereas homologous recombination between the construct and cellular DNA, the desired result, involves the exchange of homologous DNA sequences so that the non-homologous HSV-tk genes at the ends of the construct are eliminated. Cells carrying HSV-tk become sensitive to the anti-viral drug, ganciclovir, and so cells with homologous recombinations have the unique feature of being resistant to both neomycin and ganciclovir, allowing them to be selected efficiently when these drugs are added to the cultures (see Fig. 2.49).

This technique can be used to produce homozygous mutant cells in which the effects of knocking-out a specific gene can be analyzed. Diploid cells in which both copies of a gene have been mutated by homologous recombination can be selected·after transfection with a mixture of constructs in which the gene to be targeted has been disrupted by one or other of two different antibiotic resistance genes. Having obtained a mutant cell with a functional defect, the defect can be ascribed definitively to the mutated gene if the mutant phenotype can be reverted with a copy of the wild-type gene transfected into the mutant cell. Restoration of function means that the defect in the mutant gene has been complemented by the wild-type gene's function. This technique is very powerful, since it allows the gene that is being transferred to be mutated in precise ways to determine which parts of the protein are required for function.

Related
to Part V

To knock out a gene *in vivo*, it is only necessary to disrupt one copy of the cellular gene in an embryonic stem cell. Embryonic stem cells carrying the mutant gene are produced by targeted mutation (as in Fig. 2.49), and injected into a blastocyst which is re-implanted into the uterus. The mutated cells become incorporated into the developing embryo and contribute to all tissues of the resulting chimeric offspring including the germline. The mutated gene can therefore be transmitted to some of the offspring of the original chimera, and further breeding of the mutant gene to homozygosity produces mice that completely lack the expression of that particular gene product (Fig. 2.50). The effects of the absence of the gene's function can then be studied. In addition, the parts of the gene that are essential for its function can be identified by determining whether function can be restored by introducing different mutated copies of the gene back into the genome by transgenesis. The manipulation of the mouse genome by gene knock-out and transgenesis is revolutionizing our understanding of the role of individual genes in lymphocyte development and function, as we shall see throughout this book.

A problem with gene knock-outs arises when the function of the gene is essential for the survival of the animal; in such cases the gene is termed a **recessive lethal gene** and homozygous animals cannot be produced. However, by making chimeras with mice that are deficient in B and T cells, it is possible to analyze the function of recessive lethal genes in lymphoid cells. To do this, ES cells with homozygous lethal loss-of-function mutations are injected into blastocysts of mice lacking the ability to

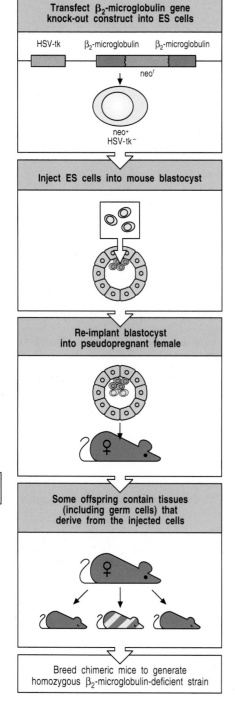

Related to Part V

Fig. 2.50 Gene knock-out in embryonic stem (ES) cells enables mutant mice to be produced. Specific genes can be inactivated by homologous recombination in tissue cultures of cells known as embryonic stem cells, which, on implantation into a blastocyst, can give rise to all cell lineages in a chimeric mouse. The technique of homologous recombination is carried out as described in Fig. 2.48. In this example, the gene for β₂-microglobulin is disrupted by homologous recombination of a targeting construct in ES cells. Only a single copy of the gene needs to be disrupted. ES cells in which homologous recombination has taken place are injected into mouse blastocysts. If the mutant ES cells give rise to germ cells in the resulting chimeric mice (striped in the figure), then the mutant gene can be transferred to their offspring. By breeding the mutant gene to homozygosity, a mutant phenotype is generated. In this case, the homozygous mutant mice lack MHC class I molecules on their cells, as MHC class I molecules have to pair with β₂-microglobulin for surface expression. The β₂-microglobulin-deficient mice can then be bred with mice transgenic for subtler mutants of the deleted gene, allowing the effect of such mutants to be tested *in vivo*.

rearrange their antigen receptor genes because of a mutation in their recombinase-activating genes (*RAG* knock-out mice). As these chimeric embryos develop, the *RAG*-deficient cells can compensate for any developmental failure resulting from the gene knock-out in the ES cells, in all but the lymphoid lineage. So long as the mutated ES cells can develop into hematopoietic progenitors in the bone marrow, the embryos will survive, and all the lymphocytes in the resulting chimeric mouse will be derived from the mutant ES cells (Fig. 2.51).

A second, powerful technique achieves tissue-specific or developmentally regulated gene deletion by employing the DNA sequences and enzymes used by bacteriophage P1 to excise itself from a host cell's genome. The integrated phage DNA is flanked by recombination signal sequences, called *loxP* sites. A recombinase, Cre, recognizes these sites, cuts the DNA and joins the two ends, thus excising the intervening DNA in the form of a circle. This mechanism can be adapted to allow the deletion of specific genes in a transgenic animal only in certain tissues or at certain times in development. First, *loxP* sites flanking a gene, or perhaps just a single exon, are introduced by homologous recombination (Fig. 2.52). Usually, the introduction of these sequences into flanking or intronic DNA does not disrupt the normal function of the gene. Mice containing such *loxP* mutant genes are then mated with mice made transgenic for the Cre recombinase, under the control of a tissue-specific or inducible promoter. When the Cre recombinase is active, either in the appropriate tissue or when induced, it excises the DNA between the inserted *loxP* sites, thus inactivating the gene or exon. Thus, using a T-cell specific promoter to drive expression of the Cre recombinase, a gene can be deleted only in T cells, while remaining functional in all other cells of the animal. This is an extremely powerful genetic technique that is still in its infancy and is certain to yield exciting results in the future.

Summary.

The measurement of immune function in intact organisms is essential to a full understanding of the immune system in health and disease. The ability of an immunized individual to resist infection is still the standard assay for protective immunity conferred by infection or vaccination. Local reactions to antigens injected into the skin can provide information

Fig. 2.51 The role of recessive lethal genes in lymphocyte function can be studied using *RAG*-deficient chimeric mice. Embryonic stem (ES) cells carrying the lethal mutation are injected into a *RAG*-deficient blastocyst (top panel). The *RAG*-deficient cells can give rise to all the tissues of a normal mouse except lymphocytes, and so can compensate for any deficiency in the developmental potential of the mutant ES cells (middle panel). If the mutant ES cells are capable of differentiating into hematopoietic stem cells, that is, if the gene function that has been deleted is not essential for this developmental pathway, then all the lymphocytes in the chimeric mouse will be derived from the ES cells (bottom panel), as *RAG*-deficient mice cannot make lymphocytes of their own.

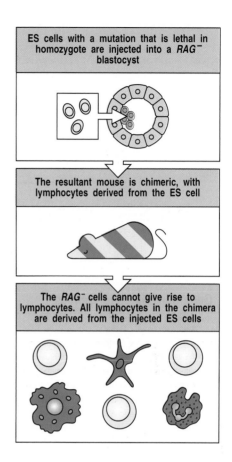

about antibody and T-cell responses to the antigen, a procedure that is particularly important in testing for allergic reactions. Finally, many *in vitro* assays such as the analysis of specific antibody in serum and the proliferative responses of T cells to mitogens and specific antigen are used to assess immune function in human patients.

Manipulation of the immune system *in vivo* reveals the need for each of its components. Using irradiation or mutation to eliminate lymphocytes or particular lymphocyte lineages, and then adoptively transferring mature lymphocytes, isolated subpopulations, cloned T-cell lines, or bone marrow stem cells allows one to study the functions and development of individual normal or immune cell types in an *in vivo* setting. The role of individual genes in lymphocyte development and function can be studied *in vivo* by manipulating the mouse genome, adding genes by transgenesis or eliminating them through gene knock-out. These two techniques can be combined to give detailed information about structure–function relationships in genes and their protein products, either in cultured cells or *in vivo*. These powerful techniques are increasing our understanding of immunobiology at an astonishing rate. The use of mutant mice in the study of host defenses to specific pathogens should provide a new understanding of these highly complex processes.

Related to Part V

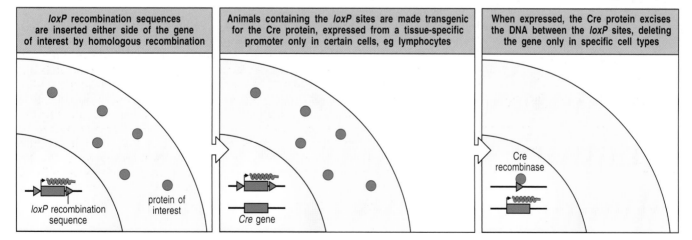

Fig. 2.52 The P1 bacteriophage recombination system can be used to eliminate genes in particular cell lineages. The P1 bacteriophage protein Cre will excise DNA that is bounded by recombination signal sequences called *loxP* sequences. These sequences can be introduced at either end of a gene by homologous recombination (left panel). Animals carrying *loxP*-flanked genes can also be made transgenic for the gene for the Cre protein, which is placed under the control of a tissue-specific promoter so that it is only expressed in certain cells or at certain times during development (middle panel). In the cells in which the Cre protein is expressed, it recognises the *loxP* sequences and excises the DNA lying between them (right panel). Thus, individual genes cen be deleted only in certain cell types or only at certain times. In this way, genes that are essential for the normal development of a mouse may be deleted from, for example, T cells, and the role of such genes in T-cell function studied. Genes are shown as boxes, RNA as squiggles, and proteins as coloured balls.

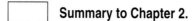 **Summary to Chapter 2.**

The immune system is very complex. To analyze it properly, it must be broken down into its individual components, and these must be studied both in isolation and in the context of the larger system. In this chapter we have described how immune responses are induced and measured, and how the immune system can be manipulated experimentally. An appreciation of the methodologies and findings described in this chapter is essential for a full understanding of immunobiology, and many of the techniques included here are used routinely in the experiments described in subsequent chapters. Some, especially the use of monoclonal antibodies for identifying molecules in cells and tissues and the manipulation of the mouse genome, also have general applications in biology.

General methods references.

Weir, D. (ed): *The Handbook of Experimental Immunology, vol 1.*, 5th edn. Oxford, Blackwell Scientific Publications, 1996.

Coligan, J.E.: *Current Protocols in Immunology*, 1st edn. New York, Greene Publishing Associates and Wiley Interscience, 1991. Continuous updates added.

Ausubel, M.: *Current Protocols in Molecular Biology*, 1st edn. New York, Greene Publishing Associates and Wiley Interscience, 1987. Continuous updates added.

Sambrook, J., Fritsch, E.F., Maniatis, T.: *Molecular Cloning: A Laboratory Manual*, 2nd edn. Cold Spring Harbor, NY, Cold Spring Harbor Laboratory Press, 1989.

Harlow, E. and Lane, D.: *Antibodies: a Laboratory Manual.* Cold Spring Harbor, NY, Cold Spring Harbor Laboratory Press, 1988.

Green, M.C. (ed): *Genetic Variant and Strains of the Laboratory Mouse*, 1st edn. New York, Gustav Fischer Verlag, 1981.

Rose, N.R., Conway de Macario, E., Fahey, J.L., Friedman, H., Penn, G.M. (eds): *Manual of Clinical Laboratory Immunology*, 4th edn. Washington DC, American Society of Microbiology, 1992.

Journals and Series:
Journal of Immunological Methods
Cytometry
Methods in Enzymology

Specific techniques.

Radbruch, A., Recktenwald, D.: **Detection and isolation of rare cells.** *Curr. Opin. Immunol.* 1995, **7**:270-273.

Yeung, R.S.M., Penninger, J., Mak, T.W.: **T-cell development and function in gene-knockout mice.** *Curr. Opin. Immunol.* 1994, **6**:298-307.

Chen, J., Shinkai, Y., Young, F., Alt, F.W.: **Probing immune functions in RAG-deficient mice.** *Curr. Opin. Immunol.* 1994, **6**:313-319.

Mueller, R., Sarvetnick, N.: **Transgenic/knockout mice—tools to study autommunity.** *Curr. Opin. Immunol.* 1995, **7**:799-803.

PART II   THE RECOGNITION OF ANTIGEN

Structure of the Antibody Molecule and Immunoglobulin Genes

3

Antibodies are the antigen-specific products of B cells, and the production of antibody in response to infection is the main contribution of B cells to adaptive immunity. Antibodies were the first of the molecules that participate in specific immune recognition to be characterized and are still the best understood. Collectively, antibodies form a family of plasma proteins known as the immunoglobulins, whose basic building block, the immunoglobulin fold or immunoglobulin domain, is used in various forms in many molecules of both the immune system and other biological recognition systems.

The antibody molecule has two separable functions: one is to bind specifically to molecules from the pathogen that elicited the immune response; the other is to recruit other cells and molecules to destroy the pathogen once the antibody is bound to it. These functions are structurally separated in the antibody molecule, one part of which specifically recognizes antigen, while the other engages the effector mechanisms that will dispose of it. The antigen-binding region varies extensively between antibody molecules and is thus known as the **variable region** or **V region**. The variability of antibody molecules allows each molecule to recognize a particular antigen, and the total repertoire of antibodies made by a single individual is large enough to ensure that virtually any structure can be bound. The region of the antibody molecule that engages the effector functions of the immune system does not vary in the same way and is thus known as the **constant region** or **C region**, although it has in fact five main forms, or isotypes, which are specialized for activating different immune effector mechanisms.

The remarkable diversity of antibody molecules is the consequence of a highly specialized mechanism by which the antibody genes expressed in any given cell are assembled by DNA rearrangements that join together two or three different gene segments to form a variable-region gene during the development of the B cell. Subsequent DNA rearrangement can attach the assembled variable-region gene to any constant-region gene and thus produce antibodies of any of the five isotypes.

B cells do not secrete antibody until they have been stimulated by specific antigen, which they recognize by means of membrane-bound immunoglobulin molecules which serve as their antigen receptors. Antigen binding to these surface receptors is a crucial step in inducing the B cell to proliferate and differentiate into an antibody-secreting cell. In this chapter, we will describe the structural and functional properties of antibody molecules and explain the specialized genetic processes that generate antibody diversity and produce functional versatility, ending with an account of the mechanisms whereby antigen binding to surface immunoglobulin molecules on the B cell signals them to become activated.

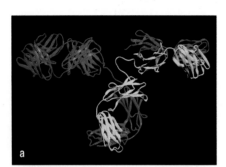

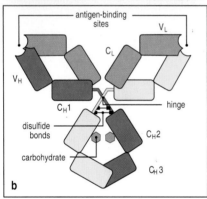

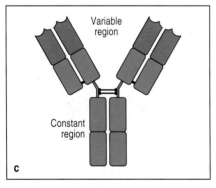

Fig. 3.1 Structure of an antibody molecule. Panel a: a ribbon diagram based on the X-ray crystal structure shows the course of the backbone polypeptide chain. Three globular regions form a Y. The two antigen-binding sites are at the tips of the arms, which are tethered to the trunk of the Y by a flexible hinge region. Panel b: a schematic representation of the structure shown in a, illustrating the four-chain composition and the separate domains comprising each chain. Panel c: a simplified schematic representation that will be used throughout this book. Photograph courtesy of A McPherson and L Harris.

The structure of a typical antibody molecule.

Antibody molecules are roughly Y-shaped molecules consisting of three equal-sized segments, loosely connected by a flexible tether. Three schematic representations of this structure, determined by X-ray crystallography, are shown in Fig. 3.1. The aim of this section is to explain how this structure is formed, and how it allows antibody molecules to carry out their dual tasks: binding on the one hand to a wide variety of antigens, and on the other, to a limited number of effector molecules and cells. As we shall see, each of these tasks is carried out by a separate part of the molecule; one end is variable between different antibody molecules and is involved in antigen binding, while the other end is conserved and interacts with effector molecules.

All antibodies are constructed in the same way from four polypeptide chains, and the generic term **immunoglobulin (Ig)** is used for all such proteins. Within this general category, however, five classes of immunoglobulins—IgM, IgD, IgG, IgA, and IgE—can be distinguished biochemically as well as functionally, while more subtle differences confined to the variable region account for the specificity of antigen binding. We shall describe the general structural features of immunoglobulin molecules using the IgG molecule as an example.

3-1   IgG antibodies consist of four polypeptide chains.

IgG antibodies are large molecules (with a molecular weight of approximately 150 kDa) composed of two separate polypeptide chains. One, of approximately 50 kDa, is termed the **heavy** or **H chain**, and the other, of 25 kDa, is termed the **light** or **L chain** (Fig. 3.2). The two chains are present in an equimolar ratio, and each intact IgG molecule contains two heavy chains and two light chains [(2 x 50) + (2 x 25) = 150]. The two heavy chains are linked to each other by disulfide bonds and each heavy chain is linked to a light chain by a disulfide bond. In any one immunoglobulin molecule, the two heavy chains and the two light chains are identical.

In all antibodies, there are only two types of light chain, which are termed lambda (λ) and kappa (κ) chains. No functional difference has been found between antibodies having λ or κ light chains. The ratio of the two types of light chain varies from species to species. In mice, the κ to λ ratio is 20:1, whereas in humans it is 2:1, and in cattle it is 1:20. The reason for this variation is unknown. Distortions in this ratio can sometimes be used to detect immune system abnormalities: for example, an excess of λ light chains in a human might indicate the presence of a λ chain-producing B-cell tumor.

By contrast, there are five main **heavy-chain classes** or **isotypes** (and some of these classes have several subtypes), and these determine the functional activity of an antibody molecule. The five functional classes of immunoglobulin are **immunoglobulin M (IgM)**, **immunoglobulin D (IgD)**, **immunoglobulin G (IgG)**, **immunoglobulin A (IgA)**, and **immunoglobulin E (IgE)**, and their heavy chains are denoted by the corresponding lower case Greek letter (μ, δ, γ, α, and ε, respectively). Their distinctive functional properties are conferred by the carboxy-terminal part of the heavy chain, where it is not associated with the light chain. We shall describe the distinct heavy-chain isotypes in more detail later. As the general structural features of all the isotypes are similar, we shall consider IgG, the most abundant isotype in blood plasma, as a typical antibody molecule.

3-2   The heavy and light chains are composed of constant and variable regions.

The amino acid sequences of many immunoglobulin heavy and light chains have been determined and reveal two important features of antibody molecules. First, each chain consists of a series of similar, although not identical, amino acid sequences, each about 110 amino acids in length. The light chain comprises two such sequences, while the heavy chain of the IgG antibody contains four. This suggests that the immunoglobulin chains have evolved by repeated duplication of an ancestral gene corresponding to one folded domain of the protein. As we shall see, these sequences do in fact correspond to separate structural domains in the folded protein (see Fig. 3.1).

The second important feature revealed by sequence comparisons is that the amino-terminal sequences of both the heavy and light chains vary greatly between different antibodies. The variability in sequence is limited to the first 110 amino acids, corresponding to the first domain, while the carboxy-terminal sequences are constant between immunoglobulin chains, either light or heavy, of the same isotype (Fig. 3.3). The variable domains (**V domains**) make up the variable region of the antibody, and the constant domains (**C domains**) make up the constant region.

3-3   The antibody molecule can readily be cleaved into functionally distinct fragments.

The antibody molecule, as we have seen (see Fig. 3.1), comprises three equal-sized globular portions joined by a flexible stretch of polypeptide chain known as the **hinge region** to form a roughly 'Y' shape. Each arm of the Y is formed by the association of a light chain with the amino-terminal half of a heavy chain, while the trunk of the Y is formed by the pairing of the carboxy-terminal halves of the two heavy chains. The association of the heavy and light chains is such that the V_H and V_L domains are paired, as are the C_H1 and C_L domains. The two C_H3 domains pair with each other but the C_H2 domains do not interact; carbohydrate side chains attached to the C_H2 domains lie between the two heavy chains. The two antigen-binding sites of the IgG antibody are formed by the paired V_H and V_L domains at the end of the two arms of the Y (see Fig. 3.1, middle panel).

Proteolytic enzymes (proteases) that cleave polypeptide sequences at particular amino acid sites have been used to dissect the structure of antibody molecules and to determine which parts of the molecule are

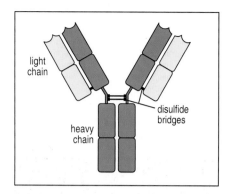

Fig. 3.2 Immunoglobulin molecules are composed of two types of chains: heavy chains and light chains. Each immunoglobulin molecule is made up of two heavy chains (green) and two light chains (yellow) joined by disulfide bridges so that each heavy chain is linked to a light chain and the two heavy chains are linked together.

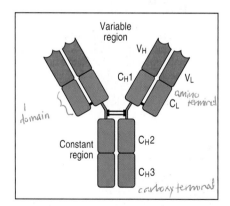

Fig. 3.3 The heavy and light chains of an immunoglobulin can be divided into domains on the basis of sequence similarity. The amino-terminal domain (N-terminus; red) of each chain is variable in sequence when several antibodies are compared; the remaining domains are constant (blue). The two domains of the light chains are termed V_L and C_L. Secreted IgG has four domains in the heavy chain, which are termed V_H, C_H1, C_H2, and C_H3.

responsible for its various functions. Limited digestion with the protease papain cleaves antibody molecules into three fragments (Fig. 3.4). Two fragments are identical and contain the antigen-binding activity, and these are termed the **Fab fragments**, for **F**ragment **a**ntigen **b**inding. The Fab fragments correspond to the arms of the antibody molecule, which contain the complete light chains paired with the V_H and C_H1 domains of the heavy chains. The other fragment contains no antigen-binding activity but was originally observed to crystallize readily, and for this reason was named the **Fc fragment**, for **F**ragment **c**rystall-izable. This fragment corresponds to the paired C_H2 and C_H3 domains and is the part of the antibody molecule that interacts with effector molecules and cells.

The exact pattern of fragments obtained after proteolysis depends upon where the protease cleaves the antibody molecule in relation to the disulfide bonds that link the two heavy chains. These lie in the hinge region between the C_H1 and C_H2 domains, and, as illustrated in Fig. 3.4, papain cleaves the antibody molecule on the amino-terminal side of the disulfide bridges, releasing the two arms of the antibody as separate Fab fragments, while in the Fc fragment the carboxy-terminal halves of the heavy chains remain linked. A second protease, pepsin, cleaves in the same general region of the antibody molecule as papain but on the carboxy-terminal side of the disulfide bridges (see Fig. 3.4), producing a fragment, the $F(ab')_2$ fragment, in which the two arms of the antibody molecule remain linked. In this case the remaining part of the heavy chain is cut into several small fragments. The $F(ab')_2$ fragment has exactly the same

Fig. 3.4 The Y-shaped immunoglobulin molecule can be dissected by partial digestion with proteases. Papain cleaves the immunoglobulin molecule into three pieces, two Fab fragments and one Fc fragment (upper panels). The Fab fragment binds antigens. The Fc fragment is crystall-izable and contains constant regions. Pepsin cleaves an immunoglobulin to yield one $F(ab')_2$ fragment and many small pieces of the Fc fragment, the largest of which is called the pF_c' fragment (lower panels). It is assigned the prime 'F(ab')' because it includes a few more amino acids than Fab, including the cysteine that is necessary for the disulfide bond.

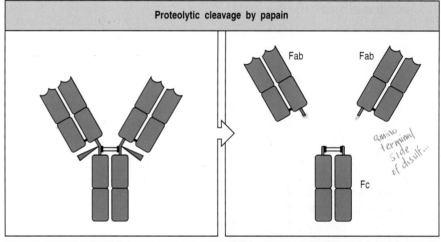

Proteolytic cleavage by papain

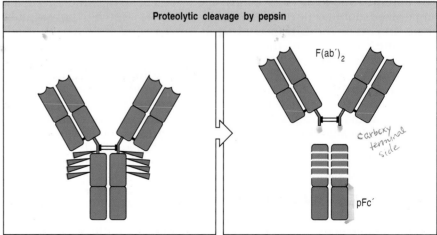

Proteolytic cleavage by pepsin

antigen binding characteristics as the original antibody but is unable to interact with any effector molecules and thus is of potential value in therapeutic applications of antibodies as well as in research into the role of the Fc portion.

Genetic engineering techniques also now permit the construction of a truncated Fab comprising only the variable region of a heavy chain linked by a synthetic 15-residue stretch of peptide to a variable region of a light chain. This is called **single-chain Fv**, named from **Fragment variable**. Fv molecules may become valuable therapeutic agents because of their small size, allowing ready tissue penetration. They may be coupled to protein toxins to yield immunotoxins with potential application, for example, in tumor therapy.

| 3-4 | **The immunoglobulin molecule is flexible, especially at the hinge region.** |

The hinge region that links the Fc and Fab portions of the antibody molecule is, in reality, a flexible tether, allowing independent movement of the two Fab arms, rather than a rigid hinge. For example, electron microscopy of antibody complexes with a bivalent hapten capable of crosslinking two antigen-binding sites demonstrates that the angle between the two Fab arms can vary (Fig. 3.5). Some flexibility is also found at the junction between the V and C domains, allowing bending and rotation of the V domain relative to the C domain—for example, in the crystal structure of the antibody molecule shown in Fig. 3.1 (top panel), not only are the two hinge regions clearly different, but the angle between the V and C domains in each of the two Fab arms is also different. This range of motion has led to the junction between the two domains being

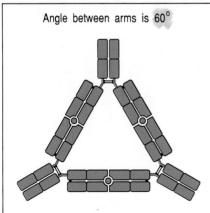

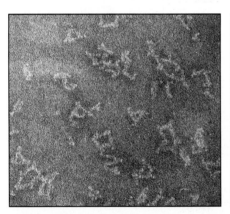

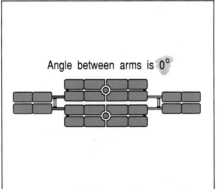

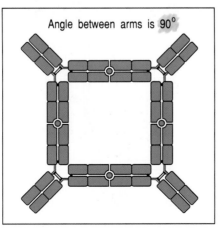

Fig. 3.5 Antibody arms are joined by a flexible hinge. The overall shape of antibodies and the flexibility of the hinge can be seen in the electron micrograph of antibody complexes. A small bifunctional hapten (red ball) that is capable of cross-linking two antigen-binding sites is used to create antigen:antibody complexes. The complexes can be seen to form linear, triangular and square forms, with short projections or spikes. Limited pepsin digestion removes these spikes, which therefore correspond to the Fc portion of the antibody; the F(ab')$_2$ pieces remain crosslinked by antigen. The interpretation of the complexes is shown in the three diagrams. The angle between the arms of the antibody molecule varies from 0° in the antibody dimers to 60° in the triangular forms, and 90° in the square forms, showing that the connections between the arms are flexible. Photograph (x 300 000) courtesy of N M Green.

referred to as a 'molecular ball-and-socket joint'. Such flexibility is required to allow the binding of both arms of the antibody molecule to sites that are different distances apart, for instance with sites on bacterial cell wall polysaccharides. Flexibility of the hinge also permits the interaction of antibodies with the antibody-binding proteins that mediate immune effector mechanisms, as will be described in Chapter 8.

3-5   Each domain of an immunoglobulin molecule has a similar structure.

The discrete globular domains of immunoglobulin chains fall into two distinct structural categories, corresponding to variable and constant domains. The similarities and differences between these two domains can be seen in the diagram of a light chain in Fig. 3.6. Both domains are constructed from two sheets formed by adjacent strands of the polypeptide chain that pack together and which are linked by a disulfide bridge, forming a roughly cylindrical shape. The sheets that form this structure are known as **β sheets** and the structure they form is known as a **β barrel**. β barrels can be formed in many different ways in different proteins: the β barrel that is formed by immunoglobulin chains is known as the **immunoglobulin fold**. In Sections 3-11 and 3-22, we shall see how each domain is encoded by a discrete exon, separated by an intron from the next domain exon.

Fig. 3.6 The structure of immunoglobulin variable and constant domains. The upper panels show schematically the folding pattern of the variable and constant domains of an immunoglobulin light chain. Each domain is a globular structure in which several strands of polypeptide chain come together to form two antiparallel β sheets that are held together by an intrachain disulfide bond between two key cysteine residues. The strands in each sheet are shown in distinct colors in the folded structure but their arrangement can be seen more clearly when the sheets are opened out, as shown in the lower panels. The β strands are lettered sequentially with respect to their occurrence in the amino acid sequence of the domains; the order in each β sheet is characteristic of immunoglobulin domains. The β strands C' and C'' that are found in the variable domains but not in the constant domains are indicated by the shaded background. The characteristic 4-strand plus 3-strand (C-region type domain) or 4-strand plus 5-strand (V-region type domain) are typical immunoglobulin superfamily domain building blocks, found in a whole range of other proteins as well as antibodies.

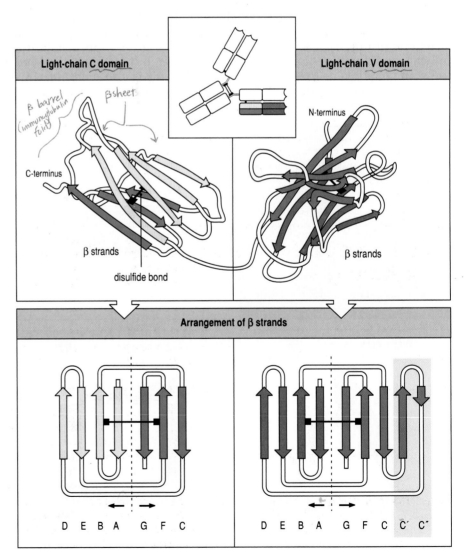

Both the essential similarity of the V and C domains and the critical difference between them are most clearly seen in the bottom panels of Fig. 3.6, where the cylindrical domains are opened out to reveal how the polypeptide chain folds to create each layer. The main difference between the V and C domain structures is that the V domain is larger and has an extra loop of polypeptide chain. We shall see in the next section that the flexible loops of the variable-region domain form the antigen-binding site of the antibody molecule.

Many of the amino acids that are common to all the domains of the heavy and light chains lie in the core of the immunoglobulin fold and are critical to the stability of its structure. For that reason, other proteins having sequences homologous to those of immunoglobulins are believed to have domains with a similar structure. These **immunoglobulin domains** are found in many proteins of the immune and nervous systems, as well as in other proteins thought to be involved in cell–cell recognition.

Summary.

IgG antibodies are made up of four polypeptide chains, comprising two identical light chains and two identical heavy chains and can be thought of as forming a flexible Y-shaped structure. Each of the four chains has a variable region at its amino-terminus, which contributes to the antigen-binding site, and a constant region, which, in the case of the heavy chain, determines isotype and hence the functional properties of the antibody. The light chains are bonded to the heavy chains with disulfide bridges and the variable regions of the heavy and light chains pair to generate two identical antigen-binding sites, which lie at the tips of the arms of the Y. This allows antibody molecules to crosslink antigens. The trunk of the Y, or Fc fragment, is composed of the two carboxy-terminal domains of the two heavy chains. Joining the arms of the Y to the trunk are the flexible hinge regions. The Fc fragment and hinge regions differ in antibodies of different isotypes, thus determining their functional properties. However, the overall plan of all isotypes is similar.

The interaction of the antibody molecule with specific antigen.

In the previous section we described the structure of the antibody molecule and how the variable regions of heavy and light chains fold and pair to form the antigen-binding site. In this section we shall discuss the different ways in which antigens can bind to antibody and shall address the question of how variation in the sequences of the antibody variable domains determines the specificity for antigen.

3-6 | **Localized regions of hypervariable sequence form the antigen-binding site.**

Sequence variability is not distributed evenly throughout the variable regions. The distribution of variable amino acids can be seen clearly using what is termed a **variability** or **Wu and Kabat plot** (Fig. 3.7), where the sequences of many different antibody variable regions are

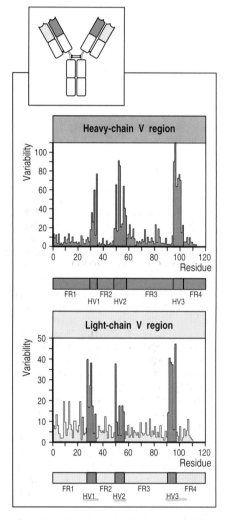

Fig. 3.7 There are discrete regions of hypervariability in variable domains. The figure shows an analysis of a sequence comparison of several dozen heavy- and light-chain variable regions. At each amino acid position the degree of variability is the ratio of the number of different amino acids seen in all of the sequences together to the frequency of the most common amino acid. Three hypervariable regions (HV1, HV2, and HV3) can be seen corresponding to CDR1, CDR2, and CDR3 (red), flanked by less variable framework regions (FR1, FR2, FR3, and FR4, shown in blue or yellow).

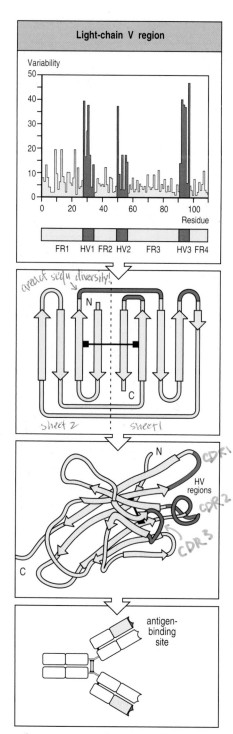

Fig. 3.8 The hypervariable regions lie in discrete loops of the folded structure. When the positions of the hypervariable regions are plotted on the structure of a variable domain, it can be seen that they lie in loops that are brought together in the folded structure. In the antibody molecule, the pairing of the heavy and light chains brings together the hypervariable loops from each chain to create a single hypervariable surface, which forms the antigen-binding site at each tip of the Fab arms.

compared. Three regions of particular variability can be identified, roughly from residues 28 to 35, from 49 to 59, and from 92 to 103. These are designated **hypervariable regions** and are denoted HV1, HV2, and HV3. The most variable part of the domain is in the HV3 region. The rest of the V domain shows less variability and the regions between the hypervariable regions, which are relatively invariant, are termed the **framework regions**. There are four such regions, designated FR1, FR2, FR3, and FR4.

The framework regions form the β sheets that provide the structural framework of the domain, while the hypervariable sequences correspond to three loops at one edge of each sheet that are juxtaposed in the folded protein (Fig. 3.8). Thus, not only is sequence diversity focused on particular parts of the variable regions but it is localized to a particular part of the surface of the molecule. Moreover, when the V_H and V_L domains pair in the antibody molecule, the hypervariable loops from each domain are brought together, creating a single hypervariable site at the tip of the Fab fragment that forms the binding site for antigens, the **antigen-binding site**. As the three hypervariable loops constitute the binding site for antigen and determine specificity by forming a surface complementary to the antigen, they are more commonly termed the **complementarity determining regions**, or **CDRs**, and are denoted **CDR1, CDR2**, and **CDR3**. One consequence of the contribution of CDRs from both V_H and V_L domains to the antigen-binding site is that it is the combination of the heavy and the light chain that determines the final antigen specificity. Thus, one way in which the immune system is able to generate antibodies of different specificities is by generating different combinations of heavy- and light-chain variable regions. This means of producing variability is known as **combinatorial diversity**; we will encounter a second form of combinatorial diversity when we come to consider how the genes encoding the heavy- and light-chain V regions are created from smaller segments of DNA (see Section 3-11).

3-7   Small molecules bind to clefts between the heavy- and light-chain variable domains.

In early investigations of antigen binding, the only available sources of single species of antibody molecules were tumors of antibody-secreting cells, which produce homogeneous antibody molecules. The specificities of the tumor-derived antibodies were unknown, so that large numbers of compounds had to be screened to identify ligands that could be used in the analysis of antigen binding. In general, the substances found to bind to the antibodies were small chemical compounds, or haptens, such as phosphorylcholine or vitamin K1. Structural analysis of antigen:antibody complexes between antibodies and their hapten ligands provided the first direct evidence that the hypervariable regions form the antigen-binding site, and established the structural basis for antigen specificity. Subsequently, with the discovery of monoclonal antibodies (see Section 2-11), it became possible to make large amounts of pure antibody specific for many different sorts of antigens. From these it has been possible to obtain a more general picture of how antibodies react with their antigens, confirming and extending the view of antibody:antigen interactions, derived from the study of haptens.

The surface of the antibody molecule formed by the juxtaposition of the CDRs of the heavy and light chains forms the site to which antigens bind. Clearly, as the sequences of the CDRs will be different in different antibodies, so will the shape of the surface created by these CDRs be different. As a general principle, antibodies bind ligands whose surfaces are complementary to that of the antibody. For small antigens, such as haptens or

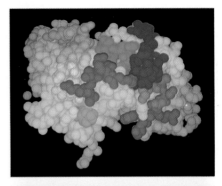

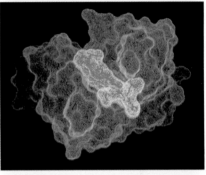

Fig. 3.9　Antigens can bind in pockets or grooves, or on extended surfaces in the binding sites of antibodies. Top panel: space-filling representation of the interaction of a peptide antigen with the complementarity determining regions (CDRs) of a Fab fragment as viewed looking into the antigen-binding site. Seven amino acid residues of the antigen, shown in red, are bound in the antigen-binding pocket. Five of the six CDRs (H1, H2, H3, L1, and L3) interact with the peptide, whereas L2 does not make contact with the peptide. The CDR loops are colored as follows: L1, dark purple; L2, magenta; L3, green; H1, blue; H2, pale purple; H3, yellow. Middle panel: In a complex of an antibody with a peptide from the human immuno-deficiency virus, the peptide (red) binds along a groove formed between the heavy- and light-chain variable domains (green). Bottom panel: in the structure of a complex between hen egg-white lysozyme and the Fab fragment of an antibody to lysozyme, HyHel5, two extended complementary surfaces come into contact, as can be seen from this computer-generated image, where the surface contour of the lysozyme molecule (yellow dots) is superimposed on the antigen-binding site of the antibody. Residues in the antibody that make contact with lysozyme are shown in full (red) while for the rest of the Fab fragment only the peptide backbone is shown (blue). All six CDRs of the antibody are involved in the binding. Photographs courtesy of S Sherriff, I A Wilson, and R L Stanfield.

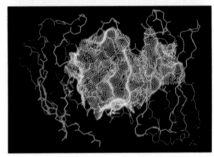

short peptides, the complementary surface may be formed by pockets or grooves lying between the heavy- and light-chain variable domains (Fig. 3.9; top and middle panels). Other antigens, such as protein molecules, can be of the same size or larger than antibodies themselves, and cannot fit into such grooves or pockets. In these cases the interface between the two molecules is often an extended surface involving all of the CDRs and, in some cases, can overlap the framework regions of the antibody (see Fig. 3.9; bottom panel).

3-8 **Antibodies bind to extended sites on the surfaces of native protein antigens.**

The biological function of antibodies is to bind to pathogens and their products and facilitate their removal from the body. Although some of the most important pathogens have polysaccharide coats, in many cases the antigens that provoke an immune response are proteins. For example, protective antibodies against viruses recognize viral coat proteins. In such cases, the antibody binds to the native conformation of the protein and the determinants recognized are therefore areas on the surface of proteins even in very large arrays like a viral capsid. Regions of a molecule that are recognized specifically by antibodies are called **antigenic determinants** or **epitopes**. Such sites on protein surfaces are likely to be composed of amino acids from different parts of the sequence that have been brought together by protein folding. Epitopes of this kind are known as **conformational** or **discontinuous epitopes** since the site is composed of segments of the protein that are discontinuous in the primary sequence but are contiguous in the three-dimensional structure. In contrast, an epitope composed of a single segment of polypeptide chain is termed a **continuous** or **linear epitope**. Although antibodies raised against native proteins usually recognize discontinuous epitopes, some can be found to bind peptide fragments of the protein. Conversely, antibodies raised against peptide fragments of a protein or synthetic peptides corresponding to part of its sequence are occasionally found to bind to the native protein. This makes it possible, in some cases, to use synthetic peptides in vaccines aimed at raising antibodies against an intact protein of a pathogen. We shall discuss the design of such vaccines in Section 13-21.

| 3-9 | **Antigen:antibody interactions involve a variety of forces.** |

The interaction between an antibody and its antigen can be disrupted by high salt concentrations, extremes of pH, detergents, and sometimes by competition by high concentrations of the pure epitope itself. The binding is therefore a reversible non-covalent interaction. The forces, or bonds, involved in these non-covalent interactions are outlined in Fig. 3.10.

The non-covalent forces in antigen:antibody binding can involve electrostatic interactions, either between charged amino acid side chains as in salt bridges, or between electric dipoles as in hydrogen bonds and short-range van der Waals forces. High salt concentrations and extremes of pH disrupt antigen:antibody binding by weakening electrostatic interactions. This principle is employed in purification of antigens by affinity columns of immobilized antibodies or vice versa (see Section 2-7).

Hydrophobic interactions occur when two hydrophobic surfaces come together to exclude water. The strength of hydrophobic interactions is proportional to the surface area that is hidden from water. For some antigens, hydrophobic interactions probably account for most of the binding energy, although this is hard to quantify experimentally.

The contribution of each of these forces to the overall interaction will depend on the specific antibody and antigen involved. A striking difference from other protein–protein interactions is that antibodies possess many aromatic amino acids in their antigen-binding sites; these amino acids participate mainly in van der Waals and hydrophobic interactions, and sometimes hydrogen bonds. Generally speaking the hydrophobic and van der Waals forces operate over very short ranges and serve to pull together two surfaces that are complementary in shape; hills on one surface must fit into valleys on the other for good binding to occur. On the other hand, electrostatic interactions between charged side chains, and hydrogen bonds bridging oxygen and/or nitrogen atoms, accommodate specific features or reactive groups while strengthening the interaction overall. For example, in the complex of hen egg-white lysozyme with the antibody D1.3 (Fig. 3.11), strong hydrogen bonds are formed between the antibody and a particular glutamine in the lysozyme molecule that protrudes between the V_H and V_L domains.

Fig. 3.10 The non-covalent forces that hold together the antigen–antibody complex. Partial charges found in electric dipoles are shown as δ^+ or δ^-. Electrostatic forces diminish as the inverse square of the distance separating the charges, while van der Waal's forces, which are more numerous in most antigen–antibody contacts, fall off as the sixth power of the separation and therefore operate only over very short ranges. Covalent bonds do not occur between antigens and antibodies.

Non-covalent forces	Origin	
Electrostatic forces	Attraction between opposite charges	$-NH_3^{\oplus}$ $^{\ominus}OOC-$
Hydrogen bonds	Hydrogen shared between electronegative atoms (N,O)	$>N\underset{\delta^-}{-}H\underset{\delta^+}{--}\underset{\delta^-}{O}=C<$
Van der Waals forces	Fluctuations in electron clouds around molecules oppositely polarize neighboring atoms	$\delta^+ \rightleftharpoons \delta^-$ $\delta^- \rightleftharpoons \delta^+$
Hydrophobic forces	Hydrophobic groups interact unfavorably with water and tend to pack together to exclude water molecules. The attraction also involves van der Waals forces	H_2O δ^+ δ^- $O<^H_H$ δ^+

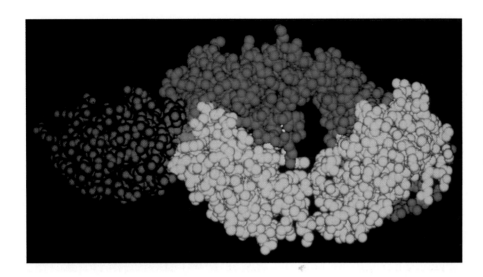

Fig. 3.11 The complex of lysozyme with the antibody D1.3. The interaction of the Fab fragment of D1.3 with hen egg-white lysozyme is shown, with the lysozyme in green, the heavy chain in blue, and the light chain in yellow. A glutamine residue of lysozyme, shown in red, protrudes between the two variable domains of the antigen-binding site and makes hydrogen bonds important to the antigen:antibody binding. Photograph courtesy of R J Poljak.

Lysozymes from partridge and turkey have another amino acid in place of the glutamine and do not bind to the antibody. In the high-affinity complex of hen egg-white lysozyme with another antibody, HyHel5 (see Fig. 3.9 bottom panel), two salt bridges between two basic arginines on the surface of the lysozyme interact with two glutamic acids, one each from the V_H CDR1 and CDR2 loops. Again, lysozymes that lack one of the two arginine residues show a 1000-fold decrease in affinity. Thus, overall surface complementarity, together with specific electrostatic and hydrogen-bonding interactions, appear to determine antibody specificity. Genetic engineering by site-directed mutagenesis can tailor an antibody binding site to its complementary antigenic epitope; this process has its natural counterpart in the maturation to higher affinity by the process of somatic hypermutation as an antibody response progresses, which we discuss later (see Section 3-18).

Summary.

X-ray crystallographic analysis of antigen:antibody complexes has demonstrated that the hypervariable loops of immunoglobulin variable regions determine the specificity of antibodies; in the case of protein antigens, the antibody molecule contacts the antigen over a broad area of its surface that is complementary to the surface recognized on the antigen. Electrostatic interactions, hydrogen bonds, van der Waals forces, and hydrophobic interactions can all contribute to binding. Amino acid side chains in most or all of the hypervariable loops make contact with antigen and determine both the specificity and the affinity of the interaction. Other parts of the variable region play little role in direct contact with the antigen but provide a stable structural framework for the hypervariable loops and help determine their positioning. Antibodies raised against native proteins usually bind to the surface of the protein and make contact with residues that are discontinuous in the primary structure of the molecule; however, they may occasionally bind peptide fragments of the protein, while antibodies raised against peptides derived from a protein can sometimes be used to detect the native protein molecule. Peptides binding to antibodies usually bind in the cleft between the variable regions of the heavy and light chains, where they make specific contact with some, but not necessarily all, of the hypervariable loops. This is also the usual mode of binding carbohydrate antigens and small molecules, or haptens.

The generation of diversity in the humoral immune response.

Virtually any substance can elicit an antibody response. Furthermore, the response even to a simple antigen is diverse, comprising many different antibody molecules each with a unique affinity and fine specificity. The complete collection of antibody specificities available within an individual is known as the **antibody repertoire** and in humans consists of as many as 10^{11} different antibody molecules, and perhaps many more. Before it was possible to examine the immunoglobulin genes directly, there were two main hypotheses for the origin of this diversity. According to one, the **germline theory**, there is a separate gene for each different antibody chain and the antibody repertoire is largely inherited. By contrast, **somatic diversification theories** proposed that a limited number of inherited V-region sequences undergo alteration within B cells during the lifetime of an individual to generate the observed repertoire. The cloning of the genes that encode immunoglobulins showed that the antibody repertoire is, in fact, generated during B cell development by DNA rearrangements that combine and assemble different V-region gene segments from a relatively small group of inherited variable-region sequences at each locus, and that diversity is further enhanced by a process of somatic hypermutation in mature B cells. Thus both theories were partially correct.

3-10   Immunoglobulin genes are rearranged in antibody-producing cells.

The DNA sequences encoding the variable and constant regions of immunoglobulin chains are separated by some considerable distance in the genome in all cells except for lymphocytes of the B lineage, in which rearrangements of the DNA occur early in ontogeny. This was originally discovered 20 years ago in the mouse when it first became possible to study the arrangement of the immunoglobulin genes using restriction enzyme analysis. Chromosomal DNA is first cut with a restriction enzyme, and the DNA fragments containing particular V- and C-region sequences are then identified by hybridization with radiolabeled mRNA probes specific for the relevant V- and C- region sequences. In germline DNA extracted from whole mouse embryos, the V- and C-region sequences are on separate DNA fragments. In DNA from the antibody-producing B cell that was the source of the V- and C-region mRNA probes, however, the probes hybridize to the same DNA fragment, showing that the V- and C-region sequences are adjacent in these cells. A similar experiment using human DNA is shown in Fig. 3.12.

This simple experiment shows that segments of genomic DNA are rearranged in somatic cells of the B lymphocyte lineage. This process of rearrangement is known as **somatic recombination**, to distinguish it from the meiotic recombination that takes place during the production of gametes.

3-11   Complete variable regions are generated by the somatic recombination of separate gene segments.

It is now known that the DNA rearrangements that bring together the DNA encoding the V and C regions of the immunoglobulin chain actually join separate segments of the V-region DNA, one of which is adjacent to the DNA encoding the C region. In the case of the light chain, each variable

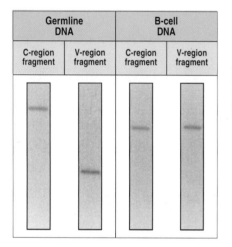

Germline DNA		B-cell DNA	
C-region fragment	V-region fragment	C-region fragment	V-region fragment

Fig. 3.12 Immunoglobulin genes are rearranged in B cells. The two photographs on the left (germline DNA) show agarose gel electrophoresis of a restriction enzyme digest of DNA from peripheral blood granulocytes of a normal person. The locations of immunoglobulin DNA sequences are identified by hybridization with V- and C-region probes. The V and C regions are found in quite separate DNA fragments. They would be the same as this in genuine germline DNA extracted from sperm or ovum. The two photographs on the right (B-cell DNA) are of a similar restriction digest of DNA from peripheral blood lymphocytes from a patient with chronic lymphocytic leukemia (see Chapter 5), in which a particular clone of B cells is greatly expanded. For this reason, one unique rearrangement is visible. In this DNA, the V and C regions are found in the same fragment, which is a different size from either the C-region or the V-region germline fragments. A population of normal B lymphocytes has many thousands of rearranged genes, so they yield a smear of DNA fragment sizes, normally not visible as a crisp band. Photograph courtesy of S Wagner and L Luzzatto.

domain is encoded in two separate DNA segments. The first segment encodes the first 95–101 amino acids of the light chain and is termed a **V gene segment** since it makes up most of the variable domain. The second segment encodes the remainder of the variable domain (up to 13 amino acids) and is termed a **joining** or **J gene segment**.

The process of rearrangement that leads to the production of an immunoglobulin light-chain gene is shown in Fig. 3.13, center panel. The joining of a V and a J gene segment creates a continuous piece of DNA encoding the whole of the light-chain variable region. The J gene segments are separated from the constant region (C) gene segments only by noncoding DNA, and are joined to them by RNA splicing after transcription, not by DNA recombination. In the experiment shown in Fig. 3.12 therefore,

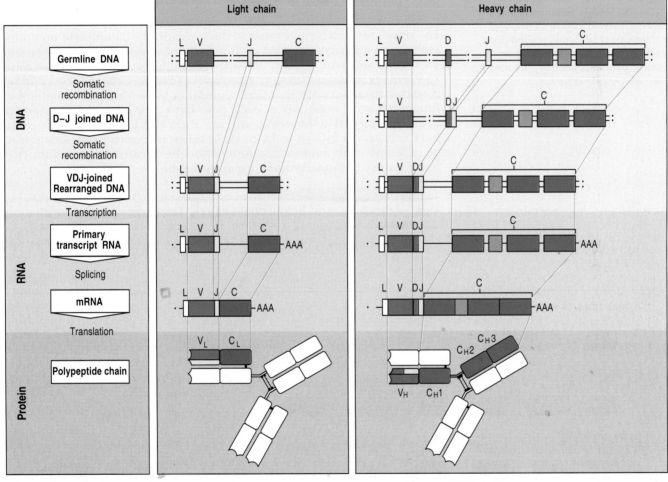

Fig. 3.13 Variable region genes are constructed from gene segments. Light-chain variable region genes are constructed from two segments (center panel). A variable (V) and a joining (J) gene segment in the genomic DNA are joined to form a complete light-chain variable-region gene. The constant region is encoded in a separate exon and is joined to the variable-region gene by RNA splicing of the light-chain message to remove the L to V and the J to C introns. Immunoglobulin chains are extracellular proteins and the V gene segment is preceded by an exon encoding a leader peptide (L), which directs the protein into the cell's secretory pathways and is then cleaved.

Heavy-chain variable regions are constructed from three gene segments (right panel). First the diversity (D) and J gene segments join, then the V gene segment joins to the combined DJ sequence, all at the genomic DNA level. The heavy-chain constant-region sequences are encoded in several exons: note the separate exon encoding the hinge domain (purple). The constant-region exons, together with the leader (L) sequence, are spliced to the variable-domain sequence during processing of the heavy-chain gene RNA transcript. Post-translational alterations remove the L sequence and attach carbohydrate moieties.

Number of segments in human immunoglobulin genes			
Segment	Light chains		Heavy chain
	κ	λ	H
Variable (V)	40	29	51
Diversity (D)	0	0	27
Joining (J)	5	4	6

Fig. 3.14 The numbers of functional gene segments for the variable regions of heavy- and light-chain in human DNA. These numbers are derived from exhaustive cloning and sequencing of DNA from one individual, excluding 44 pseudogenes. Owing to genetic polymorphism, they will not be the same for all humans.

the germline DNA identified by the 'V-region probe' contains the V gene segment, and that identified by the 'C-region probe' actually contains both the J and C gene segments.

The heavy-chain variable regions are encoded in three gene segments. In addition to the V and J gene segments (denoted V_H and J_H to distinguish them from the light-chain gene segments), there is a third gene segment called the **diversity** or **D_H gene segment**, which lies between the V_H and J_H gene segments. The process of recombination that generates a complete heavy-chain variable region is shown in Fig. 3.13 (right panel), and occurs in two separate stages. In the first, a D_H gene segment is joined to a J_H gene segment; then a V_H gene segment rearranges to DJ_H to complete a heavy chain variable-region gene. As with the light chains, RNA splicing joins the assembled variable-region to the constant-region coding sequence found downstream.

3-12   Variable-region gene segments are present in multiple copies.

For simplicity, we have discussed the formation of a complete immunoglobulin variable-region gene as though there were only single copies of each gene segment. In fact, there are multiple copies of all of the gene segments in germline DNA. Their numbers can be estimated by probing restriction enzyme digests of germline DNA: in humans, the numbers of functional gene segments of each type have also been determined by gene cloning and sequencing, and are shown in Fig. 3.14. These numbers can vary between individuals because of insertion or deletion of gene segments by meiotic recombination, or because of mutations that transform a functional gene into a pseudogene.

The functional gene segments are organized into three clusters, one for each of the κ-, λ-, and heavy-chain genes. These clusters are located on different chromosomes and each is organized slightly differently, as shown in Fig. 3.15. For the λ light-chain genes, located on chromosome 22,

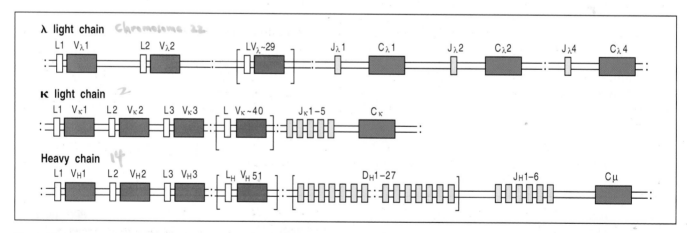

Fig. 3.15 The genomic organization of the heavy- and light-chain gene segments in humans. The upper row shows the gene locus for the λ light chain which has 29 functional V_λ gene segments and four pairs of functional J_λ segments and C_λ genes. The κ locus (middle row) is organized in a similar way, with 40 functional V_κ gene segments accompanied by a cluster of five J_κ segments but with a single C_κ gene. The heavy-chain gene locus (bottom row) has 51 functional V_H gene segments but, in addition, there is a cluster of around 27 D_H segments

lying between the 51 V_H gene segments and the 6 J_H gene segments. The heavy-chain locus also contains a large cluster of C_H genes that will be described in Fig. 3.24. For simplicity we have shown only a single C_H gene in this diagram without illustrating its separate exons, and have omitted pseudogenes. This diagram is not to scale: the total length of the heavy chain cluster is over 2 Megabases, while some of the D segments are only six bases long. L, leader sequence.

there is a cluster of V_λ gene segments, followed by pairs of J_λ gene segments and C_λ genes. In the case of the κ light chain genes, on chromosome 2, the cluster of V_κ gene segments is followed by a cluster of J_κ gene segments, then by a single C_κ gene. Finally, the organization of the heavy chains, on chromosome 14, resembles that of the κ genes, with separate clusters of V_H, D_H, and J_H gene segments and of C_H genes.

The human V gene segments can be grouped into families on the basis of similarity of DNA sequence; both the heavy chain and κ chain V gene segments can be subdivided into seven families whose members are more than 80% homologous, while there are eight families of V_λ gene segments. The families can be further grouped into clans, made up of families that are more similar to each other than to families in other clans. Human V_H gene segments fall into three such clans. All of the V_H gene segments identified from other species also fall into the same three clans, suggesting that all may have evolved by gene duplication from three ancestral V gene segments.

3-13　Rearrangement of V, D, and J gene segments is guided by flanking sequences in DNA.

When the non-coding regions flanking the different heavy and light chain V, D, and J gene segments are compared, conserved sequences are found adjacent to the points at which recombination takes place. The sequences consist of a conserved block of seven nucleotides (the **heptamer** 5′CACAGTG3′), which is always contiguous with the coding sequence, followed by a spacer of roughly 12 or 23 base pairs, followed by a second conserved block of nine nucleotides (the **nonamer** 5′ACAAAAACC3′) (Fig. 3.16). The spacer varies in sequence but its length is conserved and corresponds to one or two turns of the DNA double helix. This would bring the heptamer and nonamer sequences to one side of the DNA helix, where they can be bound by the protein complex that catalyzes recombination. The heptamer-spacer-nonamer is often called a **recombination signal sequence**, RSS.

Recombination occurs only between gene segments located on the same chromosome and the process follows another rule, that recombination can only link a gene segment flanked by a 12mer-spaced recombination signal sequence to one with a 23mer-spaced RSS (**the 12/23 rule**). Thus, for the heavy chain, a D_H gene segment can be joined to a J_H gene segment and a V_H gene segment to a D_H gene segment, but V_H segments cannot be joined to J_H segments directly, as both V and J gene segments are flanked by 23 base pair spacers and the D_H gene segments have 12 base pair spacers on both sides (see Fig. 3.16).

The mechanism of gene segment rearrangement is similar for heavy and light chains, although only one joining event is needed for light-chain genes, whereas two are needed to generate a complete heavy-chain V gene. The commonest mode of rearrangement (Fig. 3.17; left panels) involves the looping-out and deletion of the DNA intervening between two gene segments. The 12mer-spaced and 23mer-spaced recombination signal sequences are brought together by interactions between proteins that specifically recognize the length of spacer between the heptamer and nonamer signals and thus enforce the 12/23 rule for recombination. The two DNA molecules are then broken and re-ligated. The ends of the heptamer sequences are joined precisely in a head-to-head fashion to form a **signal joint** in a circular piece of DNA, which is then lost from the genome when the cell divides. The joining of the V and J gene segments, to form what is called the **coding joint**, is imprecise, and consequently generates much additional variability.

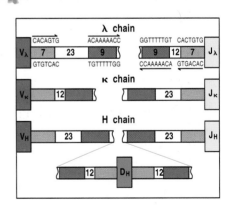

Fig. 3.16 Conserved heptamer and nonamer sequences flank the gene segments encoding the variable regions of heavy (H) and light (λ and κ) chains. The spacing between the heptamer and nonamer sequences is always either approximately 12 or approximately 23 base pairs, and joining almost always involves a 12 base pair and a 23 base pair recombination signal.

Fig. 3.17 Variable-region gene segments are joined by recombination. In every variable region recombination event, the signals flanking the gene segments are brought together to allow recombination to take place. For simplicity, the recombination of light chains is illustrated; for heavy chains, two separate recombination events are required to generate a functional variable region. In many cases, as shown in the left panels, the V and J gene segments have the same transcriptional orientation. Juxtaposition of the recombination signal sequences results in the looping out of the intervening DNA. Heptamers are shown in orange, nonamers in purple and the arrows represent the directions of the recombination heptamer and nonamer signals (see Fig. 3.16), not the direction of V and J transcription. Recombination occurs at the ends of the heptamer sequences, creating a signal joint and releasing the intervening DNA in the form of a closed circle. Subsequently, the joining of the V and J gene segments creates the coding joint. In some cases, as illustrated in the right panels, the V and J gene segments are initially oriented in opposite transcriptional directions. Bringing together the signal sequences in this case requires a more complex looping of the DNA. Joining the ends of the two heptamer sequences now results in the inversion of the intervening DNA. Again, the joining of the V and J gene segments creates a functional variable-region gene.

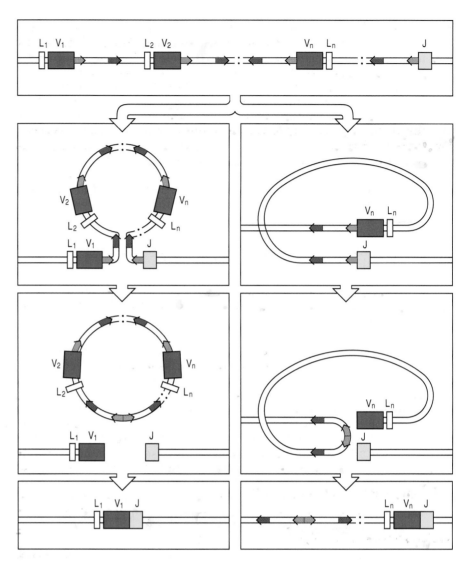

A second mode of recombination can occur between two gene segments that have the opposite transcriptional orientation. This mode of recombination is less common, although such rearrangements account for about half of all V_κ to J_κ joins. The mechanism of recombination is essentially the same but the DNA that lies between the two gene segments meets a different fate (see Fig. 3.17; right panels). When the recombination signals in such cases are brought together and recombination takes place, the intervening DNA is not lost from the chromosome but is retained in an inverted orientation.

3-14   There are four main processes by which antibody diversity is generated.

Antibody diversity is generated in four main ways, three of which are consequences of the process of recombination used to create complete immunoglobulin variable regions, while the fourth is a mutational process that occurs later, acting only on rearranged DNA encoding the variable regions.

First, there are multiple copies of each of the gene segments that make up an immunoglobulin variable region, and different combinations of gene segments can be used in different rearrangement events. This is responsible for a substantial part of the diversity of the heavy- and light-chain variable regions. A second source of combinatorial diversity arises through the pairing of different combinations of heavy- and light-chain variable regions to form the antigen-binding site. With these two ways of generating diversity alone, approximately 2.5×10^6 different antibody molecules could, in theory, be made (see Section 3-15). Third, additional diversity is introduced at the joints between the different gene segments as a result of the recombination process. Finally, **somatic hypermutation** introduces point mutations into rearranged variable region genes and is the only means by which the specificity of an immunoglobulin can be altered after recombination has created functional heavy- and light-chain genes. We will discuss these four mechanisms at greater length in the following sections.

3-15 Inherited gene segments are used in different combinations.

There are multiple copies of the V, D, and J gene segments, each of which is capable of contributing to an immunoglobulin variable region. Many different variable regions can therefore be made by selecting different combinations of these segments. For human κ light chains, there are approximately 40 functional V_κ gene segments and 5 J_κ gene segments, and thus potentially 200 different V_κ regions. For λ light chains there are approximately 29 functional V_λ gene segments and 4 J_λ gene segments, yielding 116 V_λ regions. So in all, 316 different light chains can be made. For the heavy chains of humans, there are 51 functional V_H gene segments, approximately 27 D_H gene segments and 6 J_H gene segments, and thus around 8000 different possible V_H regions ($51 \times 27 \times 6 = 8262$). As both the heavy- and the light-chain variable regions contribute to antibody specificity, each of the 316 different light chains could be combined with each of the 8262 heavy chains to give approximately 2.5×10^6 different antibody specificities. The ability to create many different specificities by making many different combinations of a small number of gene segments ($40 + 5 + 29 + 4 + 51 + 27 + 6 = 162$) is known as combinatorial diversity. For each of these loci, we have given the number of V regions deduced from the number of functional gene segments; the total number of V gene segments is larger but the additional gene segments do not appear in expressed immunoglobulin molecules and are pseudogenes.

In practice, combinatorial diversity is likely to be less than we might expect from the theoretical calculations above. Not all V gene segments are used at the same frequency; some are common, while others are found only rarely. Moreover, not all V_H regions pair successfully with all V_L regions. However, two further processes add greatly to repertoire diversity: imprecise joining of V, D, and J gene segments; and somatic hypermutation.

3-16 Variable addition of nucleotides at the junction between the gene segments encoding the variable region contributes to diversity in the third hypervariable region.

Of the three hypervariable loops in the protein chains of immunoglobulins, two are encoded within the V gene segment DNA. The third falls at the junction between the V gene segments and the J gene segments, and in the heavy chain is partially encoded by the D segment. In both heavy and light chains, the diversity of the third hypervariable region is significantly increased by the addition and deletion of nucleotides at two steps in the formation of the junctions between gene segments. This is known as **junctional diversity**. The added nucleotides are known as **P-nucleotides** and **N-nucleotides** and their addition is schematically illustrated in Fig. 3.18.

Fig. 3.18 Enzymatic steps in the rearrangement of immunoglobulin gene segments. The process is illustrated for a D_H to J_H rearrangement, showing the full sequence of the heptamer signal sequence and the first two nucleotides of the gene segments to be joined; however, the same steps occur in V_H to D_H and in V_L to J_L rearrangements. Rearrangement begins with the action of the RAG-1:RAG-2 complex, which recognizes the recombination signal sequences and cuts one strand of the double-stranded DNA precisely at the end of the heptamer sequences (top panel). The 5' cut end of this DNA strand then reacts with the complementary uncut strand, breaking it to leave a double-stranded break at the end of the heptamer sequence, and forming a hairpin by joining to the cut end of its complementary strand on the other side of the break (second panel). Subsequently, the two heptamer sequences are ligated to form the signal joint, while an endonuclease cleaves the DNA hairpin at a random site (third panel) to yield a single-stranded DNA end (fourth panel). Depending on the site of cleavage, this single-stranded DNA may contain nucleotides that were originally complementary in the double-stranded DNA and which therefore form short DNA palindromes, as indicated by the shaded box in the fourth panel. Such stretches of nucleotides that originate from the complementary strand are known as P-nucleotides. For example, the sequence GA at the end of the D segment shown is complementary to the preceding sequence TC. Where the enzyme terminal deoxynucleotidyl transferase TdT is present, nucleotides are added at random to the ends of the single-stranded segments (fifth panel), indicated by the shaded box surrounding these non-template-encoded or N, nucleotides. The two single-stranded ends then pair (sixth panel). Exonuclease trimming of unpaired nucleotides and repair of the coding joint by DNA synthesis and ligation leaves both the P- and N-nucleotides present in the final coding joint (indicated by shading in the bottom panel). The randomness of insertion of P nucleotides makes an individual P–N region a very valuable unique marker of a B cell clone as it develops, for instance in hypermutation studies (see Fig. 3.19).

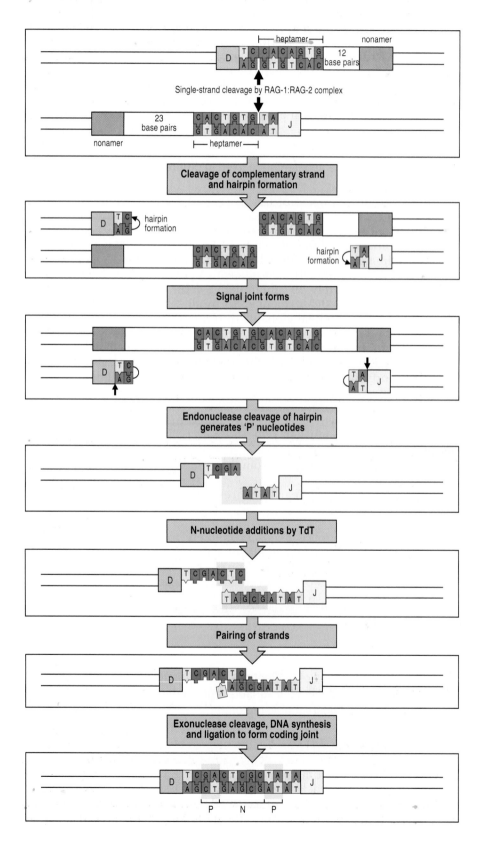

P-nucleotides are so called because they comprise palindromic sequences added to the ends of the gene segments. They are thought to occur in the following way. When the two heptamers of the recombination signal sequence are brought together in the course of DNA rearrangement, the DNA is cleaved precisely between the heptamer and the coding sequence of the gene segments to be joined (see Fig. 3.18, top panel). The two heptamers are then joined to remove the intervening DNA (see Fig. 3.17), but the cleaved ends of the coding segments are not directly ligated to one another. Instead, the cleaved ends are sealed to form hairpins (see Fig. 3.18; second panel) and a single-stranded cleavage subsequently occurs at a random point within the coding sequence so that a single-stranded tail is formed from a few nucleotides of the coding sequence plus the complementary nucleotides from the other DNA strand (see Fig. 3.18; third panel). In most light-chain gene rearrangements, DNA repair enzymes then add the complementary nucleotides to the single-stranded tails and the two double-stranded ends are then rejoined, leaving short palindromic sequences at the joint. In heavy-chain gene rearr-angements and in some human light-chain genes, however, N-nucleotides are first added by a quite different mechanism.

N-nucleotides are so called because they are non-template-encoded. They are added to single-stranded ends of the coding DNA after hairpin cleavage by an enzyme called **terminal deoxynucleotidyl transferase (TdT)**. After the addition of up to 20 nucleotides by this enzyme, the two single strands of N-nucleotides form base pairs over a short region. Repair enzymes then trim off any non-matching bases, synthesize complementary bases to fill in the remaining single-stranded DNA, and ligate them to the P-nucleotides (see Fig. 3.18; last three panels). N-nucleotides are absent from mouse light-chain genes because TdT is expressed only for a short period, during the assembly of the heavy-chain genes, which undergo rearrangement before the light-chain genes are assembled.

Since the total number of nucleotides added by these processes is random, the added nucleotides often disrupt the reading frame of the coding sequences beyond the joint. Such frame shifts will normally lead to a non-functional protein—DNA rearrangements leading to such disruptions are known as **non-productive rearrangements**. As roughly two in every three rearrangements will be non-productive, many B cells never succeed in producing functional immunoglobulin molecules, and junc-tional diversity is therefore achieved only at the expense of considerable wastage. We shall discuss this further when we describe the develop-ment of B cells in Chapter 5. The rearrangement of immunoglobulin genes is tightly regulated in such a way as to ensure that each B cell expresses only one rearranged heavy-chain gene and and one rearranged light-chain gene (see Sections 5-7 and 5-8).

3-17 | **Specialized enzymes are required for somatic recombination of V gene segments.**

The complex of several enzymes which act in concert to effect somatic V-region gene recombination is termed the 'V(D)J recombinase'. This complex comprises mostly the cleavage and repair enzymes pre-sent in all cells and required for the normal maintenance of nuclear DNA in any cell type. The first cleavage step, however, requires an additional specialized heterodimeric endonuclease formed from the products of two genes called *RAG-1* and *RAG-2*, for **recombination-activating genes**. *RAG-1* has sequence similarities to a yeast gene, *HRP-1*, and to bacterial **topoisomerases**, which catalyze the breakage and rejoining of DNA. *RAG-1* and *RAG-2* are normally expressed together only in developing lymphocytes. If they are artificially expressed in cells in culture that do not make antibodies, they can now rearrange introduced unrearranged immunoglobulin gene constructs. Mice with either of the *RAG* gene is knocked out suffer a complete block in primary lymphocyte development at the gene-rearrangement stage (see Section 5-4). A second specialized component of the V(D)J recombinase complex is TdT, discussed in the previous section.

The other components of the recombinase complex are enzymes that normally help repair double-stranded breaks in DNA. They include at least three separate nuclear proteins, one of which is an autoantigen called Ku. Another is the enzyme **DNA-dependent protein kinase**, whose normal role is demonstrated by mutant mice in which it is defective. Such *scid (severe combined immunodeficient)* mice cannot join DNA at the junctions between the gene segments encoding the variable region, and so can make only trivial amounts of immunoglobulin or T- cell receptors.

| 3-18 | Rearranged V genes are further diversified by somatic hypermutation. |

The mechanisms for generating diversity described so far all take place during the rearrangement of gene segments in the initial development of B cells in primary lymphoid organs. There is an additional mechanism that generates diversity throughout the variable region and which operates on B cells in secondary lymphoid organs after functional antibody genes have been assembled. This process, known as **somatic hypermutation**, introduces point mutations into the variable regions of the rearranged heavy- and light-chain genes at a very high rate, giving rise to mutant immunoglobulin molecules on the surface of the B cells (Fig. 3.19). Some of the mutant immunoglobulin molecules bind antigen better than the original surface immunoglobulin, and B cells expressing them are selected, to mature into antibody-secreting cells, giving rise to a phenomenon called **affinity maturation**, which we will discuss in more detail in Chapters 8 and 9.

Somatic hypermutation occurs when B cells respond to antigen. The immunoglobulin constant-region genes, and other genes expressed in the B cells, are not affected, whereas all rearranged variable region genes are mutated even if they are the result of non-productive rearrangements and are not expressed. The pattern of nucleotide base changes in non-productive variable-region genes illustrates the result of somatic hypermutation without selection for enhanced binding to antigen. The base changes are distributed widely through the V region, but not completely randomly: there are certain 'hotspots' of mutation that indicate a preference for characteristic short motifs of four to five nucleotides, and perhaps also certain ill-defined secondary structural features. The pattern of base changes in the expressed variable-region genes is different. The net result of selection for enhanced binding to antigen is that base changes that alter amino acid sequences are clustered in the CDR1 and CDR2 regions, while silent mutations which preserve amino acid sequence and do not alter structure are scattered throughout the framework regions.

Most of the diversity of antibodies in an adult individual derives from somatic alterations acquired during the lifetime of the individual. The combination of heritable and acquired components of diversity that we have described operates in several mammalian immune systems. Other species achieve a mix of inherited and acquired diversity by different means: birds do not employ somatic recombination or hypermutation to create diversity, but create their repertoires by gene conversion from germline pseudogenes. Overall, it would appear that there is

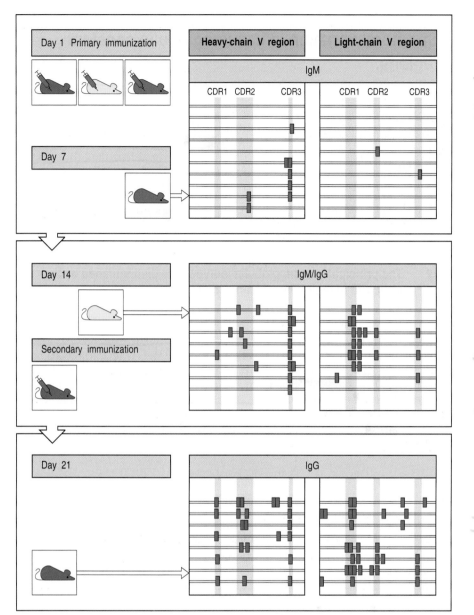

Fig. 3.19 Somatic hypermutation introduces diversity into expressed immunoglobulin genes. This figure illustrates an experiment in which somatic hypermutation in immunoglobulin variable regions was demonstrated by sequencing of heavy- and light-chain variable regions of immunoglobulins specific for the same antigen at different times after immunization. Three groups of mice were immunized, in this case with a small hapten, oxazolone, for which the majority of antibodies produced use a single V_H and V_L. B cells were taken from the first group of animals and oxazolone-specific hybridomas were produced from them 7 days after immunization. The hybridomas secreted predominantly IgM antibodies and showed little sequence variation in the V regions. Amino acid positions that differ from the prototypic variable region sequences are shown as bars on the lines representing the sequences. At day 7 most of the differences lie in the junctional regions, that is, in CDR3. After a further 7 days the oxazolone-specific antibodies from the second group of mice were analyzed. At this time, both IgG and IgM antibodies were present and several sequence changes were found affecting all six CDRs. A third group of mice were given a secondary immunization and were analyzed after a further 7 days. In this last group most of the antibodies were of the IgG type and all showed extensive changes in the V regions. Both productive and silent changes were seen throughout the variable region but productive changes were concentrated in CDRs.

strong selective pressure to generate sufficient diversity in the immune system to protect the organism from common pathogens, and that several different mechanisms can be co-opted towards this end.

Summary.

Diversity in antibody molecules is achieved by several means. Many variable-region gene segments are present in the genome of an individual, and thus provide a heritable source of diversity. Additional diversity results from the formation of a complete variable-region gene by the random recombination of separate V, D, and J gene segments. Variability of the junctions between segments is increased by the insertion of random numbers of P- and N- nucleotides. The association of different light- and heavy-chain variable regions to form the antigen-binding site subsequently contributes further diversity. Finally, after an antibody has been expressed, the coding sequences of its variable regions are modified by somatic hypermutation upon stimulation of the B cell by antigen. The combination of all these sources of diversity creates a vast repertoire of antibody specificities from a relatively limited number of genes.

Structural variation in immunoglobulin constant regions.

So far we have focused on the structural versatility of the variable region of the antibody molecule, discussing only the general structural features of the constant region as illustrated by IgG, the most abundant type of antibody in plasma. We now turn to the structural features that distinguish the heavy-chain constant regions of antibodies of the five major isotypes and confer on them their specialized functional properties. A given variable region may be expressed with any of the different constant regions, through a mechanism known as **isotype switching** and involving further DNA rearrangements.

| 3-19 | **The principal immunoglobulin isotypes are distinguished by the structure of their heavy-chain constant regions.** |

The five main isotypes of immunoglobulin are IgM, IgD, IgG, IgE, and IgA. IgG antibodies can be subdivided further into four subclasses in humans (IgG1, IgG2, IgG3, and IgG4) and in mice (IgG1, IgG2a, IgG2b, and IgG3), while IgA antibodies are found as two subclasses (IgA1 and IgA2) in humans. The heavy chains that define these isotypes are designated by the lower-case Greek letters μ, δ, γ, ε, and α, as shown in Fig. 3.20, which also lists the major physical properties of the different human isotypes. IgM forms pentamers in serum, which accounts for its high molecular weight.

Fig. 3.20 The properties of the human immunoglobulin isotypes. IgM is so called because of its size: although monomeric, IgM is only 190 KDa, it normally forms pentamers, known as **macroglobulin** (hence the M), of very large molecular weight (see Fig. 3.22). IgA dimerizes to give a molecular weight of around 390 KDa in secretions. IgE has been called **'reaginic' antibody** to denote its association with immediate-type hypersensitivity. When fixed to tissue mast cells IgE has a much longer half-life than in plasma (shown here). The activation of the alternative pathway of complement by IgA1 does not result from the Fc but its Fab portion.

	Immunoglobulin								
	IgG1	IgG2	IgG3	IgG4	IgM	IgA1	IgA2	IgD	IgE
Heavy chain	γ_1	γ_2	γ_3	γ_4	μ	α_1	α_2	δ	ε
Molecular weight (kDa)	146	146	165	146	970	160	160	184	188
Serum level (mean adult mg ml⁻¹)	9	3	1	0.5	1.5	3.0	0.5	0.03	5x10⁻⁵
Half-life in serum (days)	21	20	7	21	10	6	6	3	2
Classical pathway of complement activation	++	+	+++	–	+++	–	–	–	–
Alternative pathway of complement activation	–	–	–	–	–	+	–	–	–
Placental transfer		+		+					
Binding to macrophages and other phagocytes	+	–	+	–	–	–	–	–	+
High-affinity binding to mast cells and basophils	–	–	–	–	–	–	–	–	+++
Reactivity with staphylococcal Protein A	+	+	–/+	+	–	–	–	–	–

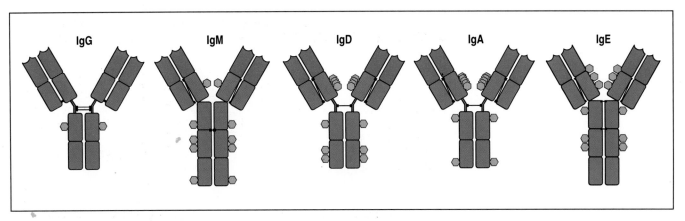

Fig. 3.21 The structural organization of the main human immunoglobulin isotype monomers. In particular, note the differences in the numbers and location of the disulfide bonds linking the chains. Both IgM and IgE lack a hinge region but each contains one extra C-terminal heavy-chain domain. The isotypes also differ in the distribution of N-linked carbohydrate groups, as shown in turquoise.

Sequence differences between immunoglobulin heavy chains cause the various isotypes to differ in several characteristic respects. These include the number and location of interchain disulfide bonds, the number of attached oligosaccharide moieties, the number of constant domains, and the length of the hinge region (Fig. 3.21). IgM and IgE heavy chains contain an extra constant-region domain that replaces the hinge region found in γ, δ, and α chains. The absence of the hinge region does not imply that the IgM and IgE molecules lack flexibility; electron micrographs of IgM molecules binding to ligands show that the Fab arms can bend relative to the Fc portion. However, such a difference in structure may have functional consequences that are not yet characterized.

3-20 | IgM and IgA can form polymers.

Although all immunoglobulin molecules are constructed from a basic unit of two heavy and two light chains, both IgM and IgA can form multimers (Fig. 3.22). IgM molecules are found as pentamers, and occasionally hexamers in serum, while IgA in mucous secretions, but not in plasma, is mainly found as a dimer (see Fig. 3.22). An additional separate 15 kDa polypeptide chain called the J chain (this should not be confused with the J gene segment, see Section 3-11) promotes polymerization by linking carboxy-terminal cysteines, which are found only in the secreted forms of the M and A chains (see Section 3-24). In the case of IgA, polymerization is required for transport through epithelia, as we discuss further in Chapter 8.

The polymerization of immunoglobulin molecules is thought to be important in antibody binding to repetitive epitopes. The dissociation rate of one individual epitope from one individual binding site influences the strength of binding, or **affinity**, of that site: the lower the dissociation rate, the higher the affinity (see Section 2-12). An antibody molecule has two or more identical antigen-binding sites, and if it attaches to two or more repeating epitopes on a single target antigen, it will only dissociate when all sites are empty. The dissociation rate of the whole antibody from the whole antigen will therefore be much slower than the rate for the individual binding sites, giving a

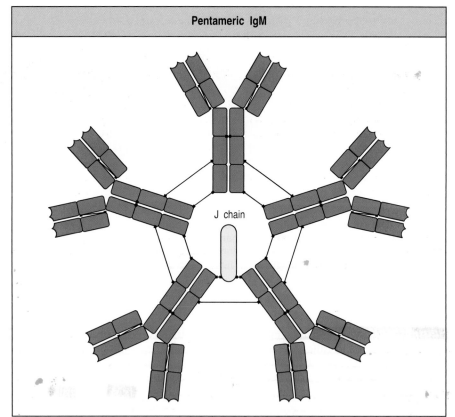

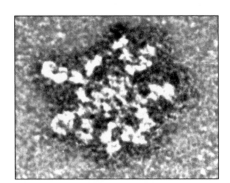

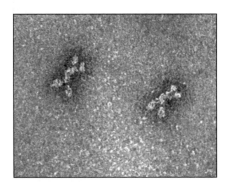

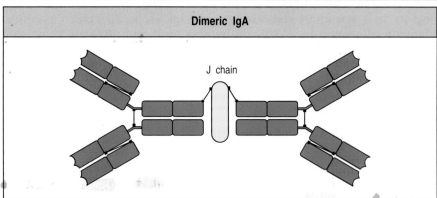

Fig. 3.22   The IgM and IgA molecules can form multimers. IgM and IgA are usually synthesized as multimers in association with an additional polypeptide chain, the J chain. In pentameric IgM, the monomers are crosslinked by disulfide bonds to each other and to the J chain. The top left panel shows an electron micrograph of an IgM pentamer, showing the arrangement of the monomers in a flat disc. IgM can also form hexamers that lack a J chain but are more efficient in complement activation. In dimeric IgA, the monomers have disulfide bonds to the J chain and not to each other. The bottom left panel shows an electron micrograph of dimeric IgA. Photographs (x 900 000) courtesy of K H Roux and J M Schiff.

greater effective binding strength, or **avidity**. This consideration is particularly relevant for pentameric IgM, which has 10 antigen-binding sites. IgM antibodies frequently recognize repetitive epitopes such as those expressed by bacterial cell wall polysaccharides, but the binding of individual sites is often of low affinity because IgM is made early in immune responses, before affinity maturation. Multi-site binding makes up for this, dramatically improving the overall functional binding strength.

3-21 | Immunoglobulin constant regions confer functional specialization.

The secreted immunoglobulins protect the body in a variety of ways, as we have outlined briefly here and shall discuss further in Chapter 8. In some cases it is enough for the immunoglobulin to bind antigen. For instance, by binding tightly to a toxin or virus, an antibody can prevent it from recognizing its receptor on a host cell. The variable regions on their own are sufficient for this. The constant region is essential, however, for recruiting the help of other cells and molecules to destroy and dispose of pathogens, and confers functionally distinct properties on each of the various isotypes. It has three main effector functions.

First, the Fc portions of IgG1 and IgG3 antibodies are recognized by Fc receptors expressed on the surface of phagocytic cells such as macrophages and neutrophils, which can thereby bind and engulf pathogens coated with antibodies of these isotypes. The Fc portion of IgE is recognized by Fc receptors on mast cells in tissues, and their blood-borne relatives, basophils, which respond by releasing inflammatory mediators.

Second, the Fc portions of antigen-antibody complexes can bind to complement (see Fig. 1.22) and initiate the complement cascade, which helps to recruit and activate phagocytes and which can also directly destroy pathogens (see Chapter 8). Complement is activated by IgM and IgG, which initiate the cascade by binding to a protein called C1q through a region of charged residues on the side of C_H3 in IgM, and to IgG at a similar region of the C_H2 domain. C1q binding is affected by the glycosylation of the C_H2 domain, and shows a range of preference for the different subtypes of IgG antibodies. The C1q molecule has six Fc-binding sites of which at least two must be occupied before the complement cascade is activated. The pentameric IgM molecule has five targets for C1q on its Fc tails and is therefore very efficient at stimulating complement: just one molecule of the pentamer is sufficient to activate the cascade. For activation by IgG, the requirement for occupation of more than one binding site means that at least two antigen-bound IgG molecules must be closely adjacent in order for activation to occur.

The third important effector function of the Fc portion is to deliver antibodies to places they would not reach without active transport. These include the mucous secretions and also tears and milk (IgA), and the fetal blood circulation by transfer from the pregnant mother (some IgG subclasses). Again, this system uses Fc receptors, this time on the transporting cells of the appropriate epithelia or the placenta. The remnants of the Fc receptor used to transport IgA remain attached to it as secretory piece.

The role of the Fc portion in these effector functions can be demonstrated by studying enzymatically treated immunoglobulins that have had one or other domain of the Fc cleaved off (see Section 3-3). Genetic engineering by site-directed mutagenesis permits detailed mapping of the exact amino-acid residues within the Fc that are needed. Many kinds of microorganisms appear to have responded to the destructive potential of the Fc portion by manufacturing proteins that either bind to it, or proteolytically cleave it, and so prevent the Fc piece from working. Examples of these are protein A and protein G made by *Staphylococcus* spp. (Fig. 3.23), and protein D of *Haemophilus* spp. Researchers can exploit these to help to map the Fc, and as immunological reagents (see Section 2-9).

Fig. 3.23 Protein A of *Staphylococcus aureus* bound to a fragment of the Fc regions of IgG. A fragment of the Fc portion of a single IgG heavy chain is complexed with a fragment of the immunoglobulin-binding protein, Protein A, from *S. aureus*. The Fc fragment has two domains, C_H2 and C_H3, shown in purple. A carbohydrate chain is attached to an asparagine residue in the C_H2 domain: all the atoms are shown and the surface is outlined in green. The fragment of Protein A (white) is bound between the two domains of the Fc fragment. The amino acids that bind to the complement component C1q (red) lie in the C_H2 domain. Photograph courtesy of C Thorpe.

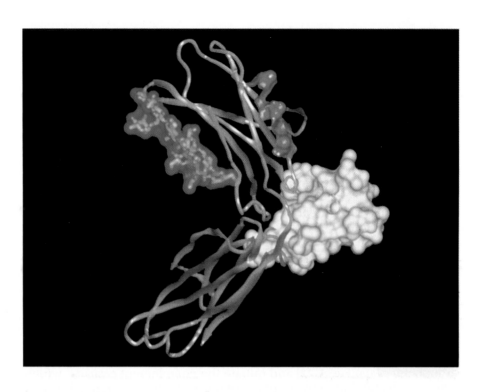

3-22   The same V_H region can associate with different C_H regions in the course of an immune response.

The variable-region genes expressed by any given B cell are determined during its early differentiation in the bone marrow and, although they may subsequently be modified by somatic hypermutation, no further V-segment recombination occurs. All the progeny of that B cell will therefore express the same assembled V genes. By contrast, the C-region genes expressed in a B-cell change in its progeny as they mature and proliferate in the course of an immune response. Every B cell begins by expressing IgM, and the first antibody produced in an immune response is always IgM. Later in the immune response, however, the same assembled V region may be expressed in IgG, IgA, or IgE. This change is known as the **isotype switch** and is stimulated in the course of an immune response by cytokines released by T cells. How cytokines influence B-cell responses will be discussed in detail in Chapter 8. Here we are concerned with the molecular basis of the isotype switch.

The immunoglobulin constant-region genes form a large cluster spanning about 200 kb to the 3' side of the J_H gene segments (Fig. 3.24): each

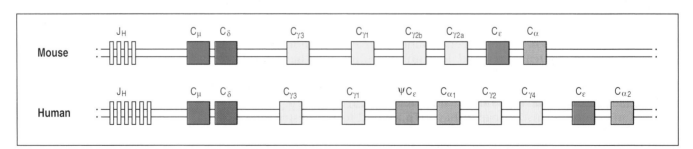

Fig. 3.24   The organization of the immunoglobulin heavy-chain constant-region genes in mice and humans (not to scale). In humans, the cluster shows evidence of evolutionary duplication of a unit consisting of two γ genes, an ε, and an α gene. One of the ε genes has become inactivated and is now a pseudogene (ψ), hence only one subtype of IgE is expressed. For simplicity, other pseudogenes are not illustrated, and the exon details within each C gene are not shown.

constant-region gene is split into separate exons corresponding to the separate domains of the folded protein. The constant-region exons encoding the μ chain lie closest to the J_H gene segments, and therefore closest to the assembled V gene after DNA rearrangement and, in the absence of isotype switching, a complete μ heavy-chain transcript is produced from the rearranged gene. Any J_H gene segments remaining between the assembled V gene and the C_μ gene are removed during RNA processing to generate the mature mRNA. μ heavy chains are therefore the first to be expressed, and IgM is the first immunoglobulin isotype to be produced after maturation of a B cell.

Immediately 3′ to the μ gene lies the δ gene encoding the constant region of the IgD heavy chain. IgD is co-expressed with IgM on almost all B cells, although this isotype is secreted in only small amounts and its function is unknown. Indeed, mice in which the delta exons have been deleted by homologous recombination appear to have essentially normal immune systems. The possibility that changes in the ratio of surface IgD to IgM may be associated with unresponsiveness or with memory in B cells will be discussed in Chapter 5. B cells expressing IgM and IgD have not undergone isotype switching, which, as we shall see shortly, entails an irreversible change in the DNA. Instead, these cells produce a long primary transcript that is processed to yield two distinct mRNA molecules. In one of these, the V_H segments are linked to the C_μ exons to yield a μ heavy chain mRNA, and in the other, the V_H segments are linked to the C_δ exons (Fig. 3.25).

Switching to other isotypes occurs only after B cells have been stimulated by antigen, through a specialized mechanism guided by a stretch of repetitive DNA known as a **switch region** lying in the intron between the rearranged VDJ_H sequence and the μ gene, and at an equivalent site upstream of the C genes encoding each of the other heavy-chain isotypes, with the exception of the δ gene (Fig. 3.26, top panel). The μ switch region (S_μ) consists of about 150 repeats of the sequence $[(GAGCT)_n(GGGGGT)]$, where n is usually three but can be as many as seven. The sequences of the other switch regions (S_γ, S_α, and S_ϵ) differ in detail but all contain repeats of the GAGCT and GGGGGT sequences.

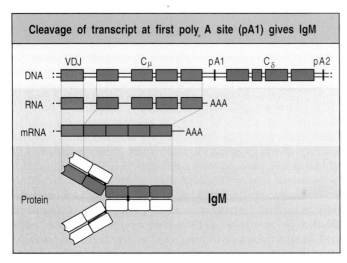

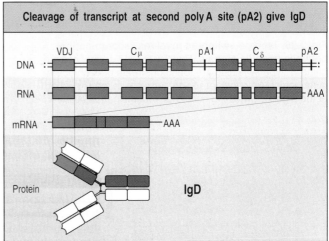

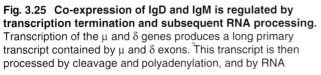

Fig. 3.25 Co-expression of IgD and IgM is regulated by transcription termination and subsequent RNA processing. Transcription of the μ and δ genes produces a long primary transcript contained by μ and δ exons. This transcript is then processed by cleavage and polyadenylation, and by RNA splicing. Cleavage and polyadenylation at the μ site (pA1) and subsequent processing yields a messenger RNA encoding a μ heavy chain (left panel). Cleavage at δ site (pA2) leads to a different pattern of splicing that yeilds a δ mRNA (right panel).

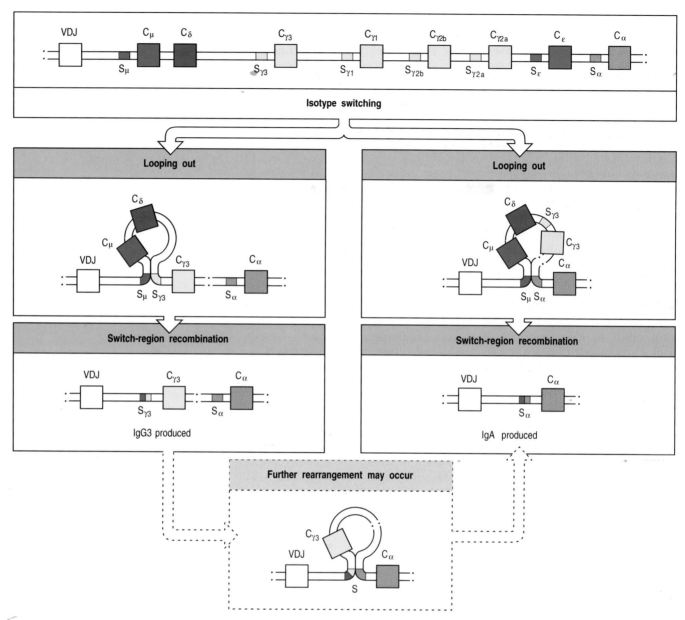

Fig. 3.26 Isotype switching involves recombination between specific signals. Repetitive DNA sequences that guide isotype switching are found upstream of each of the immunoglobulin constant-region genes, with the exception of the δ gene. Switching occurs by recombination between these repetitive sequences, or switch signals, with deletion of the intervening DNA. The initial switching event takes place from the μ switch region; switching to other isotypes can take place subsequently from the recombinant switch region formed after μ switching. S, switch region.

When a B cell switches from co-expression of IgM and IgD to express IgG, DNA recombination occurs between S_μ and S_γ, the C_μ and C_δ coding regions are deleted, and gamma heavy-chain transcripts are made from the recombined gene (illustrated for switching to γ3 in Fig. 3.26, left panels). Some of the progeny of this IgG-producing cell may subsequently undergo a further switching event to produce a different isotype, for example IgA, as shown in the bottom panel of Fig. 3.26. Alternatively, as shown in the right panels of Fig. 3.26, the switch recombination may occur between S_μ and one of the switch regions downstream of the γ genes so that the cell switches from IgM to IgA or IgE (illustrated for IgA only).

All switch recombination events produce genes that can encode a functional protein because the switch sequences lie in introns and therefore cannot cause frame shifts.

Switch recombination is unlike variable-gene segment recombination in several different ways. First, all isotype switch recombination is productive; second, it uses different recombination signal sequences and enzymes; third, it happens after antigen stimulation and not during B-cell development in the bone marrow (see Chapter 5); and fourth, the switching process is not random but is regulated by T cells, as discussed in Chapter 8.

3-23 | Various differences between immunoglobulins can be detected by antibodies.

When an immunoglobulin is used as an antigen, it will be treated like any other foreign protein and will elicit an antibody response. Anti-immunoglobulin antibodies can be made that recognize the amino acids that characterize the isotype of the injected antibody (see Section 2-9). Such anti-isotypic antibodies recognize all immunoglobulins of the same isotype in all members of the species from which the injected antibody came.

It is also possible to raise antibodies that recognize differences in antibodies from members of the same species that are due to genetic variation or **polymorphism**. Such allelic variants are called **allotypes** and represent polymorphic differences at the loci encoding heavy- and light-chain constant regions. In contrast to anti-isotypic antibodies, anti-allotypic antibodies will recognize immunoglobulins of a particular isotype only in some members of a species. Finally, as individual antibodies differ in their variable regions, one can raise antibodies against unique sequence variants, which are called **idiotypes**.

A schematic picture of the differences between idiotypes, allotypes, and isotypes is shown in Fig. 3.27. Historically, the main features of immuno-globulins were defined using isotypic and allotypic markers. The independent segregation of allotypic markers revealed the existence of separate heavy-chain, κ, and λ chain genes. Rabbits, which are unique in having heavy-chain variable-region allotypes, provided the earliest evidence that the variable and constant regions were encoded by distinct gene segments. The finding that variable-region allotypes could be associated with different isotypes of immunoglobulin confounded the dogma that one gene encoded one polypeptide chain and presaged the discovery of somatic recombination.

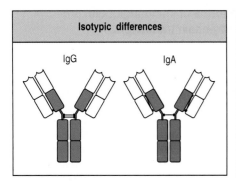
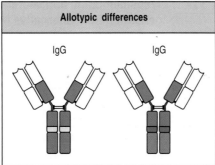
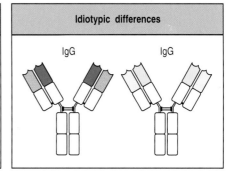

Fig. 3.27 Amino acid variation in immunoglobulin chains can be recognized by other immunoglobulins. Differences between constant-region genes are called isotypes, those between two alleles of the same constant genes are called allotypes, and amino acid changes specific to a particular rearranged V_H and V_L gene are called idiotypes.

Summary.

The isotypes of immunoglobulins are defined by their heavy-chain constant regions, each isotype being encoded by a separate constant-region gene. The heavy-chain constant-region genes lie in a cluster 3' to the variable-region genes. A productively rearranged variable-region gene is initially expressed in μ and δ heavy chains, but the same variable-region gene can subsequently be associated with any one of the other isotypes by the process of isotype switching in which the DNA is rearranged to place the variable region 5' to different constant-region genes. Unlike VDJ recombination, isotype switching occurs only in specifically activated B cells and is always productive. The immunological functions of the various isotypes differ; thus isotype switching varies the response to the same antigen at different times or under different conditions.

The B-cell antigen receptor and B-cell activation.

Antibodies were originally discovered in their secreted form as proteins that appeared in the plasma following immunization or infection. However, before antibody can be produced, immunoglobulin encoded by exactly the same rearranged heavy- and light-chain genes must function as the cell-surface antigen receptor for the B cell. We shall use the terms **cell-surface immunoglobulin**, **B-cell antigen receptor** or simply **B-cell receptor** interchangeably in this book. Antigen binding to these transmembrane immunoglobulin molecules initiates B-cell activation, leading to the clonal expansion of the B cell and the differentiation of its progeny into antibody-secreting plasma cells. Although some antigens can activate B cells just by binding surface immunoglobulin, B-cell responses to most antigens require specialized interactions with other cells that provide additional signals. These cell–cell interactions will be discussed in detail in Chapters 7 and 8. In the following sections, we shall be concerned chiefly with the mechanism whereby B cells switch from the production of membrane immunoglobulin to the secreted molecule, and with the complex of associated chains that enables the surface immunoglobulin to signal to the interior of the cell upon antigen binding.

3-24   Transmembrane and secreted forms of immunoglobulin are generated from alternative heavy-chain transcripts.

Antibodies of all heavy-chain isotypes can be produced either in secreted form or as a membrane-bound receptor. The membrane forms of all isotypes are monomers: IgM and IgA only polymerize when secreted.

In its membrane-bound form, the immunoglobulin molecule has a hydrophobic transmembrane domain of about 25 amino acid residues, which anchors it to the surface of the B lymphocyte; this domain is absent from the secreted form. The two different carboxy termini of the transmembrane and secreted forms of immunoglobulin heavy chains are encoded in separate exons and the production of both membrane and secreted versions of the heavy chain is achieved by similar mechanisms to those that allow the co-expression of IgM and IgD (Fig. 3.28). The last exon of

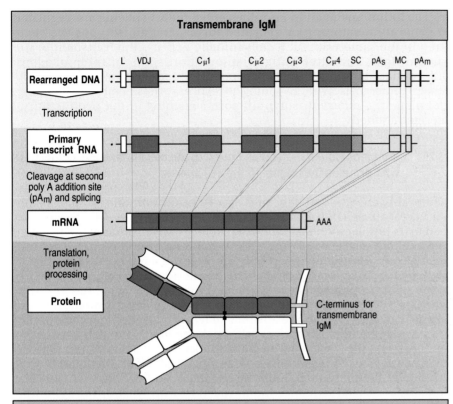

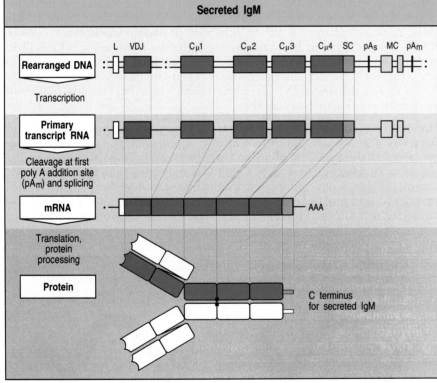

Fig. 3.28 Transmembrane and secreted forms of immunoglobulins are derived from the same gene by alternative RNA processing. Each immunoglobulin gene has two exons (MC; yellow) that encode the transmembrane region and cytoplasmic tail of the transmembrane form and an SC sequence (orange) encoding the carboxy terminus of the secreted form. In the case of IgD, the SC sequence is present on a separate exon but, for the other isotypes, including IgM shown here, the SC sequences are contiguous with the last constant-domain exon. The events that dictate whether an immunoglobulin RNA will encode a secreted or transmembrane immunoglobulin occur during the processing of the initial transcript. Each immunoglobulin gene has two potential polyadenylation sites (shown as pA_s and pA_m). In the upper panel, the transcript is cleaved and polyadenylated at the second site (pA_m). Splicing between a site located between the $C\mu4$ and the SC sequences, and a second site at the 5' end of the MC axons, results in the removal of SC sequences adn the joining of $C\mu4$ to MC sequences, to generate the transmembrane form of immunoglobulin. In the lower panel, the primary transcript is cleaved and polyadenylated at the first site (pA_s) thus eliminating the transmembrane exons and giving rise to the secreted immunoglobulin molecule.

the constant-region gene contains the sequence encoding the transmembrane region of the heavy chain. If the primary transcript includes all exons, the sequence encoding the carboxy-terminal of the secreted form is removed during RNA processing and the cell-surface form of immunoglobulin is produced. If transcription is terminated before the last exon, only the secreted molecule can be produced. Both

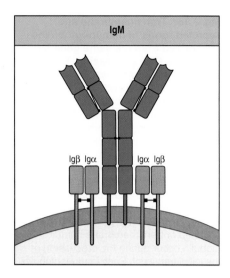

Fig. 3.29 Transmembrane immuno-globulins are found in a complex with two other proteins, Igα and Igβ. Igα and Igβ are disulfide-linked but the exact stoichiometry is unknown, nor is it known which chain binds to the heavy chain. The ratio of two Igα and Igβ chains to each immunoglobulin molecule as shown here is a guess. Igα varies in its glycosylation depending on which heavy chain it associates with.

transcription termination and differential mRNA splicing are regulated to generate membrane or secreted forms, and all isotypes are regulated in the same way. All B cells initially express the transmembrane form of IgM, and after antigen stimulation some of their progeny differentiate into plasma cells producing the secreted form of IgM, while others undergo isotype switching to express transmembrane immuno-globulins of a different isotype before switching to the production of secreted antibody.

3-25   Immunoglobulin molecules bound to the cell surface are associated with proteins that signal to the cell interior.

When antigen binds to the membrane-bound immunoglobulin at the surface of a B cell, it initiates a cascade of events in the cell interior that lead to its proliferation and ultimately to the differentiation of the progeny into antibody-secreting plasma cells. Membrane-bound immunoglobulin itself has a cytoplasmic tail of only about three amino acids, too few to play any part in signal transduction to the interior of the cell. Transmission of the signal depends instead on at least two other chains, **Igα** and **Igβ**, which are closely associated with immunoglobulin in the membranes of B cells (Fig. 3.29), and in the absence of Igα and Igβ, no immunoglobulin is expressed on the cell surface, although the heavy and light chains are synthesized and remain in an intracellular compartment. Igα and Igβ have extracellular single-domain immunoglobulin folds that bind noncovalently to the immunoglobulin heavy chain, and cytoplasmic tails that contain specialized sequence motifs called **immunoreceptor tyrosine activation motifs** (**ITAMs**), which are found in the cytoplasmic domains of several immune system signaling molecules, including those of the T-cell receptor complex. When they are phosphorylated on tyrosine, ITAMs are recognized by cytoplasmic signaling molecules, which bind to them and are thereby activated. These in turn activate a variety of other intracellular signaling molecules. Tyrosine phosphorylation of the ITAMs is thus the first step in an intracellular signaling cascade triggered by antigen binding to the receptor.

The essential role of the antigen in triggering the signaling cascade is to crosslink the surface immunoglobulin molecules and thereby cause clustering of the signaling complex, bringing receptor-associated tyrosine kinase molecules together with the ITAMs they phosphorylate (Fig. 3.30). Natural antigens with multiple repeating epitopes therefore trigger B cells effectively, and most of what we know about the mechanism of signaling through the B-cell receptor has been learned from experiments *in vitro*

Fig. 3.30   Antigen binding to surface immunoglobulin causes aggregation of the receptor complex, allowing receptor-associated kinases to phosphorylate ITAMs. The receptor-associated kinases, which include Blk, Fyn and Lyn, phosphorylate two tyrosine's in the ITAMs and the doubly phosphorylated ITAM is then recognized by the cytoplasmic kinase Syk.

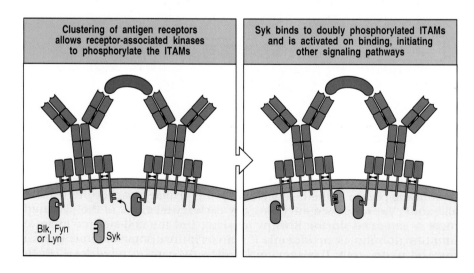

in which the effects of such antigens are mimicked by anti-immuno-globulin antibodies, which are used to cause the aggregation of the receptor molecules in the membrane.

Three **tyrosine kinases** have been found in association with the receptor complex of activated B cells: **Fyn**, **Blk**, and **Lyn**. On receptor aggregation they are thought to phosphorylate two tyrosine residues in the ITAMs of the cytoplasmic tails of Igβ. The doubly phosphorylated ITAM is then recognized by another tyrosine kinase, called **Syk**, which binds to the phosphorylated ITAM and is thereby activated. Syk then activates, in turn, a cascade of intracellular signaling molecules.

As the activated receptor-associated kinases tend to phosphorylate themselves as well as one another, once activation is initiated the activating signal is quickly amplified. It is therefore important that signaling through the antigen receptor is not initiated accidentally. It is thus not surprising that the kinases that trigger the intracellular signaling cascade are subject to negative controls. One of these operates directly on the receptor-associated kinases. They are activated by phosphorylation at one site but are inhibited by phosphorylation at another. Their activation therefore requires dephosphorylation at the inhibitory site, as well as phosphorylation at the activating site. Dephosphorylation of the inhibitory site is mediated by a membrane protein called **CD45**, which is found on all white blood cells and is therefore also known as the **leukocyte common antigen**. CD45 has a tyrosine-specific phosphatase on its cytoplasmic tail and contributes to the activation of lymphocytes by removing the inhibitory phosphates from the receptor- associated kinases.

A second phosphatase, SHP, is responsible for switching off the activated tyrosine kinases, thereby limiting the response of the activated cell. SHP is a cytoplasmic phosphatase that acts by removing the activating phosphate groups. In mutant mice lacking this enzyme, the lymphocytes respond to much lower levels of antigen than they do in normal mice and, because of the abnormal proliferation of both lymphocytes and other white blood cells, they develop autoimmune disease of which they die within a few weeks of birth.

The downstream targets of the activated receptor-associated kinases are outlined in Fig. 3.31. One of the most important is the enzyme **phospholipase C-γ**, which cleaves the membrane phospholipid phosphatidylinositol-4,5-bisphosphate (PIP_2) into two signaling molecules: **inositol trisphosphate**, which releases calcium ions from intracellular stores; and **diacylglycerol**, an activator of protein kinase C, which phosphorylates a further group of downstream targets.

The cascade of intracellular reactions that follows the activation of the receptor-associated kinases leads ultimately to changes in gene expression, which result in the proliferation and differentiation of the B cell. We shall see in Chapter 4 that a very similar signaling cascade links antigen recognition to changes in gene expression in T cells.

3-26 | Activation of B cells normally requires other membrane complexes in addition to the antigen receptor complex.

Crosslinking of surface immunoglobulin is often insufficient on its own to activate B cells, and most antigens do not have repeating epitopes and are not capable of crosslinking surface immunoglobulin. The initiation of most B-cell responses therefore requires other signals. The most important of these are the signals delivered by a specialized subset of T cells, the **helper T cells**, which recognize antigen on the surface

Fig. 3.31 Crosslinking of cell-surface immunoglobulin molecules initiates an intracellular signaling cascade. Antigens that bind and crosslink surface immunoglobulin molecules activate the Src-family protein tyrosine kinases Blk, Fyn, and Lyn, which become associated with the receptor complex. The CD45 phosphatase, which can remove a specific inhibitory phosphate from these kinases, is probably also involved. Activation of the receptor-associated kinases results in a signaling cascade involving several reaction pathways. First, the receptor-associated kinases phosphorylate the ITAMs in the receptor complex, which then bind and activate Syk. Syk then initiates the phosphorylation of phospholipase C-γ, which cleaves the membrane phospholipid phosphatidyl-inositol-4,5-bisphosphate (PIP$_2$) into inositol trisphosphate and diacylglycerol. Inositol trisphosphate releases calcium ions from intracellular stores, and calcium influx through a membrane channel is also stimulated, increasing intracellular calcium concentrations, while diacyglycerol activates the serine/threonine protein kinase C. Finally, the GTP-binding protein Ras is activated, and in turn activates an associated protein kinase, Raf, which in turn activates protein kinases that phosphorylate gene transcription regulatory proteins. This model does not account for all observations, and is likely to be incomplete.

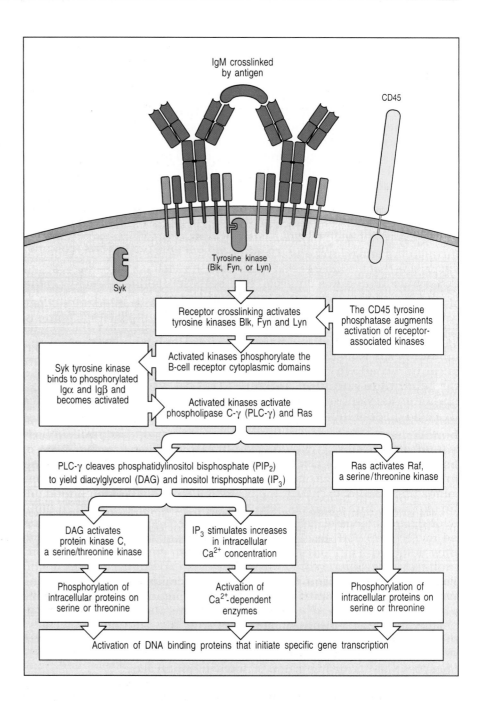

of B cells and are thereby stimulated to deliver activating signals to them. We discuss these interactions in detail in Chapter 8. Other signals are delivered by macrophages and by activated components of the complement system, which we also discuss in Chapter 8. At present, our understanding of the interplay between the different cell surface molecules that contribute to B-cell activation is very incomplete, and what we know of their intracellular signaling pathways depends almost entirely on experiments with artificial ligands *in vitro*. A central part is played, however, by a complex of cell-surface molecules called the **CD19/CR2/TAPA-1 complex** (Fig. 3.32).

CD19 is a molecule expressed on all B cells from an early stage in B-cell ontogeny. It is implicated in B-cell activation by three lines of evidence. First, anti-CD19 antibodies help activate B cells *in vitro*; second, knock-out mice lacking CD19 make deficient B-cell responses to many antigens;

and third, CD19 amplifies the intracellular effects of signaling through the B-cell antigen receptor complex. Moreover, CR2 (CD21), with which CD19 is associated in the cell membrane, is a receptor for components of complement that are known to be important in inducing efficient B-cell responses, and ligation of CR2 induces phosphorylation of CD19 by the receptor-associated kinases. The third component of the complex, TAPA-1 (CD81) plays an unknown part in this process.

On tyrosine phosphorylation, CD19 binds phosphatidylinositol 3-kinase (PI 3-kinase) and a multifunctional intracellular signaling molecule called vav. These then become activated and amplify the signaling cascade generated through the B-cell receptor complex. These combined signals have many effects. Not only do they initiate the proliferation and thereby the clonal expansion of the B cell, they also induce the expression of surface molecules necessary for interactions with T cells and other cell types, and increase the expression of molecules essential in enabling B cells to display antigen on their surface in a form that can be recognized by the appropriate T cell. The ability of specialized cells to present antigen appropriately to T cells is critical to the initiation of almost all adaptive immune responses, and the machinery of antigen presentation is the first topic we address in Chapter 4.

Summary.

Immunoglobulin exists both as a serum protein and on the surface of all B cells where it acts as the receptor for antigen. The transmembrane and secreted forms of immunoglobulin produced by one B cell share the same antibody specificity and the difference between the two forms results from alternative heavy-chain termination of transcription and subsequent RNA processing. Thus, one principle of the clonal selection hypothesis, that the antigen specificity of the secreted antibody should be identical to that of the cellular antigen receptor, is upheld. Expression of transmembrane immunoglobulins at the cell surface and signal transduction by immunoglobulins on antigen binding require the association of the heavy chains with two other membrane proteins, Igα and Igβ, to form a complex in the cell membrane. Crosslinking of the complex by antigen is required to activate enzymes within the cell that initiate a series of biochemical processes leading to the activation of several different protein kinases and raised intracellular calcium ion concentrations. Antigens that do not strongly crosslink surface immunoglobulin molecules cannot activate B cells in the absence of helper T cells or signals from other sources. Activated complement components provide one such signal, acting by binding complement receptors that form a complex with other molecules in the B-cell membrane and thereby amplifying the effect of the antigen.

Summary to Chapter 3.

This chapter has provided an overview of the antibody molecule. In Chapter 1 we introduced the clonal selection hypothesis and suggested that the principles of clonal selection provide a framework for understanding the immune system. The clonal selection hypothesis requires that there be a broad repertoire of antibody specificities and that these specificities be distributed clonally. The organization of the antibody molecule and of the genes encoding the antibody molecule allows diversity to be generated within the antigen-binding site. Moreover, the mechanisms that create this diversity ensure that the specificity of each receptor is unique to the B cell in which it occurs, and hence is distributed

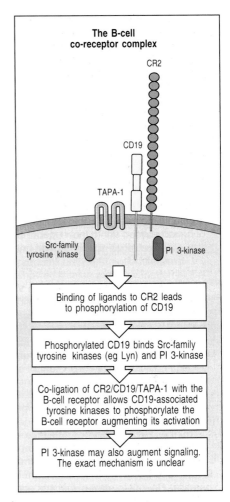

Fig. 3.32 The B-cell antigen receptor is modulated by a co-receptor complex of at least three cell-surface molecules, CD19, TAPA-1, and CR2. Binding of ligands to the CR2 component of the co-receptor results in the phosphorylation of tyrosine residues in the cytoplasmic domain of CD19, possibly because of their close proximity to the antigen-receptor complex. Co-ligation of the B-cell receptor with the co-receptor brings the Igα bound Lyn in close proximity to the CD19 cytoplasmic domain which it phosphorylates. The phosphorylated CD19 can then bind vav and one or more of the many isoforms of phosphatidyl-inositol 3-kinase, and this may augment signaling. The exact role of phosphatidylinositol 3-kinase is unclear. Vav can activate the GDP/GTP exchange that leads to ras activation (see Fig. 3.31).

clonally. A second principle of the clonal selection hypothesis requires that the effector antibody molecules secreted by a B cell have the same specificity as the cellular receptor. Alternative transcription termination and then splicing of heavy-chain RNA transcripts, varying the carboxy-terminal sequences of the heavy chains, ensures that the antigen specificity remains the same for both transmembrane and secreted immunoglobulins. Different heavy-chain constant-region genes determine the different effector functions of distinct antibody isotypes. Moving an active heavy-chain variable-region gene to a new expression site adjacent to various constant-region genes switches the isotype and ensures that the same antigen specificity is retained in antibodies of different functional properties. The transmembrane form of immunoglobulin exists in association with at least two other proteins, forming a complex that functions as an antigen receptor able to signal to the interior of the cell that antigen has bound. This can activate B cells when the receptors are crosslinked by multivalent antigens in the presence of growth factors but a second signal is required for other antigens and this is provided by signaling molecules expressed by helper T cells.

General references.

Ager, A., Callard, R., Ezine, S., Gerard, C., and Lopez-Botet, M.: **Immune receptor supplement.** *Immunol. Today.* 1996, **17**.

Carayannopoulos, L., and Capra, J.D. *Immunoglobulins: structure and function,* in: Paul W.E., ed. *Fundamental Immunology.* (3rd ed.) New York, Raven Press, 1993.

Casali, P., and Silberstein, L.E.S.eds.: **Immunoglobulin gene expression in development and disease.** *Ann. N. Y. Acad. Sci.* 1995, **764**.

Davies, D.R., and Chacko, S.: **Antibody structure.** *Acc. Chem. Res.* 1993, **26**:421-427.

DeFranco, A.L., Blum, J.H., Stevens, T.L., Law, D.A., Chan, V.W.F., Foy, S.P., Datta, S.K., and Matsuuchi, L.: **Structure and function of the B-cell antigen receptor.** *Chem. Immunol.* 1994, **59**:156-172.

Fearon, D.T., and Carter, R.H.: **The CD19/CR2/TAPA-1 complex of B lymphocytes—linking natural to acquired immunity.** *Ann. Rev. Immunol.* 1995, **13**:127-149.

Hames, B.D., and Glover, D.M. *Molecular Immunology,* in *Frontiers in molecular biology* (2nd ed.). Oxford, IRL Press, 1996.

Honjo, T., and Alt, F.W., eds. *Immunoglobulin Genes* (2nd ed.). London, Academic Press, 1995.

Max, E.E.: *Immunoglobulins: molecular genetics* in: Paul W.E., ed. *Fundamental Immunology* (3rd ed.). New York, Raven Press, 1993.

Poljak, R.J.: **Structure of antibodies and their complexes with antigens.** *Mol. Immunol.* 1991, **28**:1341-1345.

Reth, M.: **The B-cell antigen receptor complex and co-receptors.** *Immunol. Today* 1995, **16**:310-313.

Schatz, D.G., Oettinger, M.A., and Schlissel, M.S.: **V(D)J recombination—molecular biology and regulation.** *Ann. Rev. Immunol.* 1992, **10**:359-383.

Stavnezer, J.: **Antibody class switching.** *Adv. Immunol.* 1996, **61**:79-146.

Wagner, S.D., and Neuberger, M.S.: **Somatic hypermutation of immunoglobulin genes.** *Ann. Rev. Immunol.* 1996, **14**:441-457.

Section references.

3-1   IgG antibodies consist of four polypeptide chains.

Edelman, G.M.: **Antibody structure and molecular immunology.** *Scand. J. Immunol.* 1991, **34**:4-22.

Harris, L.J., Larson, S.B., Hasel, K.W., Day, J., Greenwood, A., and McPherson, A.: **The 3-dimensional structure of an intact monoclonal antibody for canine lymphoma.** *Nature* 1992, **360**:369-372.

3-2   The heavy and light chains are composed of constant and variable regions.

Han, W.H., Mou, J.X., Sheng, J., Yang, J., and Shao, Z.F.: **Cryo-atomic force microscopy—a new approach for biological imaging at high resolution.** *Biochem.* 1995, **34**:8215-8220.

3-3   The antibody molecule can readily be cleaved into functionally distinct fragments.

Porter, R.R.: **Structural studies of immunoglobulins.** *Scand. J. Immunol.* 1991, **34**:382-389.

Yamaguchi, Y., Kim, H., Kato, K., Masuda, K., Shimada, I., and Arata, Y.: **Proteolytic fragmentation with high specificity of mouse IgG—mapping of proteolytic cleavage sites in the hinge region.** *J. Immunol. Methods* 1995, **181**:259-267

3-4   The immunoglobulin molecule is flexible, especially at the hinge region.

Gerstein, M., Lesk, A.M., and Chothia, C.: **Structural mechanisms for domain movements in proteins.** *Biochem.* 1994, **33**:6739-6749.

Kim, J.K., Tsen, M.F., Ghetie, V., and Ward, E.S.: **Evidence that the hinge region plays a role in maintaining serum levels of the murine IgG1 molecule.** *Mol. Immunol.* 1995, **32**:467-475.

3-5 Each domain of an immunoglobulin molecule has a similar structure.

Barclay, A.N., Brown, M.H., Law, S.K., McKnight, A.J., Tomlinson, M.G., and van der Merwe, P.A., eds. *The Leukocyte Antigen Factsbook*, (2nd ed.). London, Academic Press, 1997 in press.

Hsu, E., and Steiner, L.A.: **Primary structure of immunoglobulin through evolution.** *Curr. Opin. Struct. Biol.* 1992, **2**:422-430.

3-6 Localized regions of hypervariable sequence form the antigen-binding site.

Chitarra, V., Alzari, P.M., Bentley, G.A., Bhat, T.N., Eisele, J.L., Houdusse, A., Lescar, J., Souchon, H., and Poljak, R.J.: **3-dimensional structure of a heteroclitic antigen-antibody cross reaction complex.** *Proc. Nat. Acad. Sci.* 1993, **90**:7711-7715.

Gilliland, L.K., Norris, N.A., Marquardt, H., Tsu, T.T., Hayden, M.S., Neubauer, M.G., Yelton, D.E., Mittler, R.S., and Ledbetter, J.A.: **Rapid and reliable cloning of antibody variable regions and generation of recombinant single-chain antibody fragments.** *Tissue Antigens* 1996, **47**:1-20.

3-7 Small molecules bind to clefts between the heavy- and light-chain variable domains.

Padlan, E.A.: **Anatomy of the antibody molecule.** *Mol. Immunol.* 1994, **31**:169-217.

3-8 Antibodies bind to extended sites on the surfaces of native protein antigens.

Davies, D.R., and Cohen, G.H.: **Interactions of protein antigens with antibodies.** *Proc. Nat. Acad. Sci.* 1996, **93**:7-12.

Stanfield, R.L., Takimoto-Kamimura, M., Rini, J.M., Profy, A.T., and Wilson, I.A.: **Major antigen-induced domain rearrangements in an antibody.** *Structure* 1993, **1**:83-93.

Stanfield, R.L., and Wilson, I.A.: **Protein-peptide interactions.** *Curr. Opin. Struct. Biol.* 1995, **5**:103-113.

Wilson, I.A., and Stanfield, R.L.: **Antibody-antigen interactions—new structures and new conformational changes.** *Curr. Opin. Struct. Biol.* 1994, **4**:857-867.

3-9 Antigen:antibody interactions involve a variety of forces.

Braden, B.C., and Poljak, R.J.: **Structural features of the reactions between antibodies and protein antigens.** *Faseb J.* 1995, **9**:9-16.

Mariuzza, R.A., Poljak, R.J., and Schwarz, F.P.: **The energetics of antigen-antibody binding.** *Res. Immunol.* 1994, **145**:70-72.

3-10 Immunoglobulin genes are rearranged in antibody-producing cells.

Tonegawa, S.: **Somatic generation of immune diversity.** *Scand. J. Immunol.* 1993, **38**:305-317.

Waldmann, T.A.: **The arrangement of immunoglobulin and T-cell receptor genes in human lymphoproliferative disorders.** *Adv. Immunol.* 1987, **40**:247-321.

3-11 Complete variable regions are generated by the somatic recombination of separate gene segments

Feeney, A.J., and Riblet, R.: **D(ST4)—a new, and probably the last, functional D(H) gene in the BALB/c mouse.** *Immunogen.* 1993, **37**:217-221.

Lansford, R., Okada, A., Chen, J., Oltz, E.M., Blackwell, T.K., Alt, F.W., and Rathbun, G.: *Mechanism and control of immunoglobulin gene rearrangement*, in *Molecular Immunology* (2nd ed.). Oxford, IRL Press, 1995.

3-12 Variable-region gene segments are present in multiple copies.

Cook, G.P., and Tomlinson, I.M.: **The human immunoglobulin V-H repertoire.** *Immunol. Today* 1995, **16**:237-242.

Kofler, R., Geley, S., Kofler, H., and Helmberg, A.: **Mouse variable-region gene families—complexity, polymorphism, and use in nonautoimmune responses.** *Immunol. Rev.* 1992, **128**:5-21.

Matsuda, F., and Honjo, T.: **Organization of the human immunoglobulin heavy-chain locus.** *Adv. Immunol.* 1996, **62**:1-29.

3-13 Rearrangement of V, D, and J gene segments is guided by flanking sequences in DNA.

Lieber, M.: **Immunoglobulin diversity—rearranging by cutting and repairing.** *Curr. Biol.* 1996, **6**:134-136.

Steen, S.B., Gomelsky, L., and Roth, D.B.: **The 12/23-rule is enforced at the cleavage step of V(D)J recombination** *in vivo. Genes to Cells* 1996, **1**:543-553.

3-14 There are four main processes by which antibody diversity is generated.

Fanning, L.J., Connor, A.M., and Wu, G.E.: **Development of the immunoglobulin repertoire.** *Clin. Immunol. and Immunopath.* 1996, **79**:1-14.

Stewart, A.K., and Schwartz, R.S.: **Immunoglobulin V Regions and the B cell.** *Blood* 1994, **83**:1717-1730.

3-15 Inherited gene segments are used in different combinations.

Lee, A., Desravines, S., and Hsu, E.: *IgH diversity in an individual with only one million B lymphocytes.* *Develop. Immunol.* 1993, **3**:211-222.

Radic, M.Z., and Weigert, M.: **Genetic and structural evidence for antigen selection of anti-DNA antibodies.** *Ann. Rev. Immunol.* 1994, **12**:487-520.

Winter, G., Griffiths, A.D., Hawkins, R.E., and Hoogenboom, H.R.: **Making antibodies by phage display technology.** *Ann. Rev. Immunol.* 1994, **12**:433-455.

3-16 Variable addition of nucleotides at the junction between the gene segments encoding the variable region contributes to diversity in the third hypervariable region

Gauss, G.H., and Lieber, M.R.: **Mechanistic constraints on diversity in human V(D)J recombination.** *Mol. Cell. Biol.* 1996, **16**:258-269.

Lewis, S.M.: **The mechanism of V(D)J joining—lessons from molecular, immunological, and comparative analyses.** *Adv. Immunol.* 1994, **56**:27-150.

3-17   Specialized enzymes are required for somatic recombination of V gene segments.

Blunt, T., Finnie, N.J., Taccioli, G.E., Smith, G.C.M., Demengeot, J., Gottlieb, T.M., Mizuta, R., Varghese, A.J., Alt, F.W., Jeggo, P.A., and Jackson, S.P.: **Defective DNA-dependent protein kinase activity is linked to V(D)J recombination and DNA-repair defects associated with the murine *scid* mutation**. *Cell* 1995, **80**:813-823

Jeggo, P.A., Taccioli, G.E., and Jackson, S.P.: **Ménage-à-Trois—double-strand break repair, V(D)J recombination, and DNA-PK**. *Bioessays* 1995, **17**:949-957.

Lin, W.C., and Desiderio, S.: **V(D)J recombination and the cell-cycle**. *Immunol. Today* 1995, **16**:279-289.

Li, Z.Y., Otevrel, T., Gao, Y.J., Cheng, H.L., Seed, B., Stamato, T.D., Taccioli, G.E., and Alt, F.W.: **The XRCC4 gene encodes a novel protein involved in DNA double-strand break repair and V(D)J recombination**. *Cell* 1995, **83**:1079-1089.

Zhu, C.M., Bogue, M.A., Lim, D.S., Hasty, P., and Roth, D.B.: **Ku86-deficient mice exhibit severe combined immunodeficiency and defective processing of V(D)J recombination intermediates**. *Cell* 1996, **86**:379-389.

3-18   Rearranged V genes are further diversified by somatic hypermutation.

Milstein, C.: **From the structure of antibodies to the diversification of the immune response**. *Scand. J. Immunol.* 1993, **37**:386-397.

Neuberger, M.S., and Milstein, C.: **Somatic hypermutation**. *Curr. Opin. Immunol.* 1995, **7**:248-254.

Peters, A., and Storb, U.: **Somatic hypermutation of immunoglobulin genes is linked to transcription initiation**. *Immunity* 1996, **4**:57-65.

Storb, U.: **The molecular basis of somatic hypermutation of immunoglobulin genes**. *Curr. Opin. Immunol.* 1996, **8**:206-214.

Tomlinson, I.M., Walter, G., Jones, P.T., Dear, P.H., Sonnhammer, E.L.L., and Winter, G.: **The imprint of somatic hypermutation on the repertoire of human germline V genes**. *J. Mol. Biol.* 1996, **256**:813-817.

3-19   The principal immunoglobulin isotypes are distinguished by the structure of their heavy-chain constant regions.

Davies, D.R., and Metzger, H.: **Structural basis of antibody function**. *Ann. Rev. Immunol.* 1983, **1**:87-117.

Jefferis, R., Lund, J., and Goodall, M.: **Recognition sites on human IgG for Fcγ receptors—the role of glycosylation**. *Immunol. Letters* 1995, **44**:111-117.

Kabat, E.A. *Structural concepts in immunology and immunochemistry* (2nd ed.). New York, Holt, Rinehart, Winston. 1976.

3-20   IgM and IgA can form polymers.

Hendrickson, B.A., Conner, D.A., Ladd, D.J., Kendall, D., Casanova, J.E., Corthesy, B., Max, E.E., Neutra, M.R., Seidman, C.E., and Seidman, J.G.: **Altered hepatic transport of IgA in mice lacking the J chain**. *J. Exp. Med.* 1995, **182**:1905-1911.

Niles, M.J., Matsuuchi, L., and Koshland, M.E.: **Polymer IgM assembly and secretion in lymphoid and nonlymphoid cell-lines—evidence that J chain is required for pentamer IgM synthesis**. *Proc. Nat. Acad. Sci.* 1995, **92**:2884-2888.

3-21   Immunoglobulin constant regions confer functional specialization.

Helm, B.A., Sayers, I., Higginbottom, A., Machado, D.C., Ling, Y., Ahmad, K., Padlan, E.A., and Wilson, A.P.M.: **Identification of the high affinity receptor binding region in human IgE**. *J. Biol. Chem.* 1996, **271**:7494-7500.

Jefferis, R., Lund, J., and Goodall, M.: **Recognition sites on human IgG for Fcγ receptors—the role of glycosylation**. *Immunol. Letters* 1995, **44**:111-117.

3-22   The same V_H region can associate with different C_H regions in the course of an immune response.

Stavnezer, J.: **Immunoglobulin class switching**. *Curr. Opin. Immunol.* 1996, **8**:199-205.

3-23   Various differences between immunoglobulins can be detected by antibodies.

Fields, B.A., Goldbaum, F.A., Ysern, X., Poljak, R.J., and Mariuzza, R.A.: **Molecular basis of antigen mimicry by an anti idiotope**. *Nature* 1995, **374**:739-742.

3-24   Transmembrane and secreted forms of immunoglobulin are generated from alternative heavy-chain transcripts.

Caldwell, J., McElhone, P., Brokaw, J., Anker, R., and Pollok, B.A.: **Coexpression of full length and truncated Igμ chains in human B lymphocytes results from alternative splicing of a single primary RNA transcript**. *J. Immunol.* 1991, **146**:4344-4351.

Lyczak, J.B., Zhang, K., Saxon, A., and Morrison, S.L.: **Expression of novel secreted isoforms of human IgE proteins**. *J. Biol. Chem.* 1996, **271**:3428-3436.

3-25   Immunoglobulin molecules bound to the cell surface are associated with proteins that signal to the cell interior.

Bolen, J.B.: **Protein tyrosine kinases in the initiation of antigen receptor signaling**. *Curr. Opin. Immunol.* 1995, **7**:306-311.

DeFranco, A.L.: **Transmembrane signaling by antigen receptors of B lymphocytes and T lymphocytes**. *Curr. Opin. Cell Biol.* 1995, **7**:163-175.

Gold, M.R., and DeFranco, A.L.: **Biochemistry of B lymphocyte activation**. *Adv. Immunol.* 1994, **55**:221-295.

Pleiman, C.M., Dambrosio, D., and Cambier, J.C.: **The B cell antigen receptor complex—structure and signal-transduction**. *Immunol. Today* 1994, **15**:393-399.

3-26   Activation of B cells normally requires other membrane complexes in addition to the antigen receptor complex.

DeFranco, A.L.: **B cell co-receptors—the two-headed antigen**. *Curr. Biol.* 1996, **6**:548-550.

Dempsey, P.W., Allison, M.E.D., Akkaraju, S., Goodnow, C.C., and Fearon, D.T.: **C3d of complement as a molecular adjuvant—bridging innate and acquired immunity**. *Science* 1996, **271**:348-350.

Doody, G.M., Dempsey, P.W., and Fearon, D.T.: **Activation of B lymphocytes—integrating signals from CD19, CD22 and FcγRIIb1**. *Curr. Opin. Immunol.* 1996, **8**:378-382.

Engel, P., Zhou, L.J., Ord, D.C., Sato, S., Koller, B., and Tedder, T.F.: **Abnormal B-lymphocyte development, activation, and differentiation in mice that lack or overexpress the CD19 signal transduction molecule**. *Immunity* 1995, **3**:39-50.

Antigen Recognition by T Lymphocytes

In an adaptive immune response, antigen is recognized by two distinct sets of highly variable receptor molecules—the immunoglobulins that serve as antigen receptors on B cells, and the antigen-specific receptors of T cells. As we saw in Chapter 3, immunoglobulins are secreted as antibodies by activated B cells, and bind pathogens or their toxic products in the extracellular spaces of the body. Binding by antibody neutralizes viruses, and marks pathogens for destruction by phagocytes and complement; these mechanisms will be discussed in Chapter 8. T cells, by contrast, recognize only antigens that are displayed on cell surfaces. These antigens may derive from pathogens, such as viruses or intracellular bacteria, that replicate within cells; or from pathogens or their products that cells internalize by endocytosis from the extracellular fluid.

T cells can detect the presence of intracellular pathogens because infected cells display on their surface peptide fragments derived from the pathogens' proteins. These foreign peptides are delivered to the cell surface by specialized host-cell glycoproteins encoded in a large cluster of genes that were first identified by their potent effects on the immune response to transplanted tissues. For that reason, the gene complex was termed the **major histocompatibility complex** (**MHC**), and the peptide-binding glycoproteins are still called **MHC molecules**. The recognition of antigen as a small peptide fragment bound to an MHC molecule and displayed at the cell surface is one of the most distinctive features of T cells, and will be the central focus of this chapter.

We shall begin by discussing the mechanisms of antigen processing and presentation, whereby protein antigens are degraded into peptides inside cells and the peptides are then carried to the cell surface stably bound to MHC molecules. We shall see that there are two different classes of MHC molecules, known as MHC class I and MHC class II, that deliver peptides from different cellular compartments to the surface of the infected cell. Peptides bound to MHC class I molecules are recognized by CD8 T cells, and those bound to MHC class II molecules are recognized by CD4 T cells. The two functional subsets of T cells are thereby activated to initiate the destruction of pathogens resident in these two different cellular compartments. CD4 T cells may also activate B cells that have internalized specific antigen, and thus stimulate the production of antibodies to extracellular pathogens and their products.

In the second part of this chapter, we shall see that there are several genes for each class of MHC molecule, that is, the MHC is polygenic. Each of these genes has many alleles, that is, the MHC is also highly polymorphic. Indeed, the most remarkable feature of MHC genes is their genetic variability. MHC polymorphism has a profound effect on antigen recognition by T cells, and the combination of polygeny and polymorphism greatly extends the range of peptides that can be presented to T cells by one individual.

Finally, we will describe the **T-cell receptors** themselves. As might be expected from their function as highly variable antigen-recognition structures, T-cell receptors are closely related to antibody molecules in structure and, like immunoglobulins, are encoded in V, D, and J gene segments, which rearrange to form a complete variable-region exon. T-cell receptors are complexes of proteins very similar to B-cell receptors; they signal the cell when they bind antigen, using analogous biochemical pathways. There are, however, important differences between T-cell receptors and immunoglobulins, which reflect the unique features of antigen recognition by the T-cell receptor.

The generation of T-cell ligands.

The actions of T cells depend on their ability to recognize cells that are harboring pathogens or that have internalized pathogens or their products. T cells do this by recognizing peptide fragments of pathogen-derived proteins in the form of complexes of peptide and MHC molecules on the surface of these cells. In this section, we shall see how the structure and intracellular transport of the two classes of MHC molecules enables them to bind to a wide range of peptides derived from pathogens and their antigens present in the cytosol or in the vesicular compartment of cells, and to present them for recognition by the appropriate functional type of T cell.

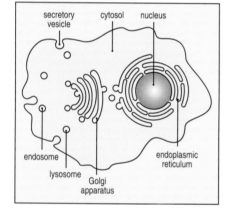

Fig. 4.1 There are two major compartments within cells, separated by membranes. The first is the cytosol, which is contiguous with the nucleus via the nuclear pores in the nuclear membrane. The second is the vesicular system, which comprises the endoplasmic reticulum, Golgi apparatus, endosomes, lysosomes, and other intracellular vesicles. The vesicular system can be thought of as contiguous with the extracellular fluid, as secretory vesicles bud off from the endoplasmic reticulum and are transported via the Golgi membranes to move vesicular contents out of the cell, while endosomes take up extracellular material into the vesicular system. All cell-surface proteins, including the MHC class I and MHC class II molecules, are synthesized on ribosomes attached to the cytoplasmic face of the endoplasmic reticulum and co-translationally transported into the lumen, where they are modified and folded.

4-1 | **T cells with different functions recognize peptides produced in two distinct intracellular compartments.**

Infectious agents can replicate in either of two distinct intracellular compartments (Fig. 4.1). Viruses and certain bacteria replicate in the cytosol or in the contiguous nuclear compartment (Fig. 4.2, left panel) while many pathogenic bacteria and some eukaryotic parasites replicate in the endosomes and lysosomes that form part of the vesicular system (see Fig. 4.2, center panel). The immune system has different strategies for eliminating infections from these two sites. Cells infected with viruses or with bacteria that live in the cytosol are eliminated by cytotoxic T cells; these T cells are distinguished by the cell-surface molecule **CD8**. The function of CD8 T cells is to kill infected cells; this is an important means of eliminating sources of new viral particles and cytosolic bacteria and thus freeing the host of infection.

Pathogens and their products in the vesicular compartments of cells are detected by a different class of T cell, distinguished by surface expression of the molecule **CD4**. CD4 T cells are specialized to activate other cells and fall into two functional classes: T_H1 cells (sometimes known as inflammatory T cells), which activate macrophages to kill the intravesicular bacteria they harbor, and T_H2 cells or helper T cells, which activate B cells to make antibody. Microbial antigens may enter the vesicular compartment in either of two ways. Some bacteria, including the mycobacteria that cause tuberculosis and leprosy, invade macrophages and flourish in intracellular vesicles. Other bacteria, which normally

Cytosolic pathogens	Intravesicular pathogens	Extracellular pathogens and toxins
	macrophage	B cell

	Cytosolic pathogens	Intravesicular pathogens	Extracellular pathogens and toxins
Degraded in	Cytoplasm	Acidified vesicles	Acidified vesicles
Peptides bind to	MHC class I	MHC class II	MHC class II
Presented to	CD8 T cells	CD4 T cells	CD4 T cells
Effect on presenting cell	Cell death	Activation to kill intravesicular bacteria and parasites	Activation of B cells to secrete Ig to eliminate extracellular bacteria/toxins

Fig. 4.2 Pathogens and their products can be found in either the cytoplasmic or the vesicular compartment of cells. Left panel: all viruses and some bacteria replicate in the cytosolic compartment. Their antigens are presented by MHC class I molecules to CD8 T cells. Center panel: other bacteria and some parasites are engulfed into endosomes, usually by phagocytic cells such as macrophages, and are able to proliferate within the vesicles themselves. Their antigens are presented by MHC class II molecules to CD4 T cells. Right panel: proteins derived from extracellular pathogens may enter the vesicular system of cells by binding to surface molecules followed by endocytosis. This is illustrated for proteins bound by surface immunoglobulin of B cells, which thereby present antigens to CD4 helper T cells, which they stimulate to produce soluble antibody. (The endoplasmic reticulum and Golgi apparatus have been omitted for simplicity.) Other types of cells may also internalize antigens in this way and be able to activate T cells.

proliferate outside cells, secrete toxins and other proteins, and these and bacterial degradation products can be internalized by cells by endocytosis, indeed they enter intracellular vesicles in that way. In particular, B cells take up and internalize specific antigen by receptor-mediated endocytosis of antigen bound to their surface immunoglobulin receptor (see Fig. 4.2, right panel).

To produce an appropriate response to infectious microorganisms, T cells need to be able to distinguish between foreign material coming from the cytosolic and vesicular compartments. This is achieved through delivery of peptides to the cell surface from each of these intracellular compartments by a different class of MHC molecule. MHC class I molecules deliver peptides originating in the cytosol to the cell surface, where the peptide:MHC complex is recognized by CD8 T cells. MHC class II molecules deliver peptides originating in the vesicular system to the cell surface, where they are recognized by CD4 T cells (see Fig. 4.2).

Since the generation of peptides from an intact antigen involves modification of the native protein, it is commonly referred to as **antigen processing**, while the display of the peptide at the cell surface by the MHC molecule is referred to as **antigen presentation**. In the sections that follow, we shall see how the two classes of MHC molecules differ in structure and how they bind selectively to peptides generated in different intracellular sites and deliver them to the cell surface. Later, when we discuss the recognition of MHC molecules by the T-cell receptor, we will also see how the molecules CD4 and CD8, which characterize the two major subsets of T cells, help in the differential recognition of MHC class I and MHC class II molecules by the T-cell receptor.

4-2   **The two classes of MHC molecule have a distinct subunit structure but a similar three-dimensional structure.**

The **MHC class I** and **MHC class II** molecules are cell-surface glycoproteins closely related in overall structure and function, although they have different subunit structures. MHC class I structure is outlined

Fig. 4.3 The structure of an MHC class I molecule, determined by X-ray crystallography. Panel a shows a computer graphic representation of a human MHC class I molecule, HLA-A2, which has been cleaved from the cell surface by the enzyme papain. Panel b shows a ribbon diagram of that structure. Shown schematically in panel d, the MHC class I molecule is a heterodimer of a membrane-spanning α chain (43 000 Da), non-covalently associated with β2-microglobulin (12 000 Da), which does not span the membrane. The α chain folds into three domains, α1, α2, and α3. The α3 domain and β2-microglobulin show similarities in amino acid sequence to immunoglobulin constant domains and have a similar folded structure, while the α1 and α2 domains fold together into a single structure consisting of two segmented α helices lying on a sheet of eight antiparallel β-strands. The folding of the α1 and α2 domains creates a long cleft or groove, which is the site at which peptide antigens bind to the MHC molecules. The transmembrane region and the short stretch of peptide that connects the external domains to the cell surface are not seen in panels a and b as they have been removed by the papain digestion. As can be seen in panel c, looking down on the molecule from above, the sides of the cleft are formed from the inner faces of the two α helices, while the β-pleated sheet formed by the pairing of the α1 and α2 domains creates the floor of the cleft. We shall use the schematic representation in panel d throughout this text. Photograph courtesy of C Thorpe.

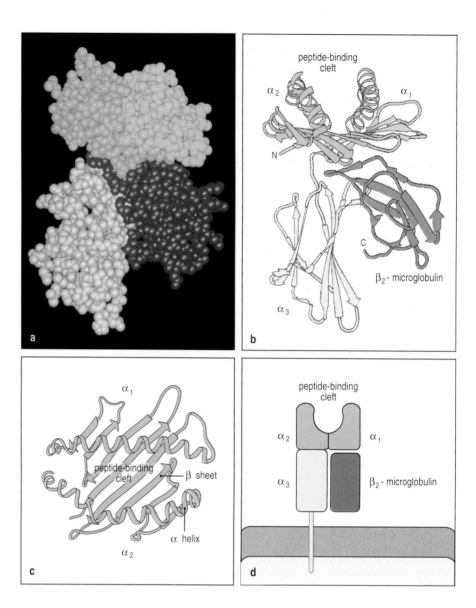

in Fig. 4.3. MHC class I molecules consist of two polypeptide chains, an α or heavy chain encoded in the MHC, and a smaller non-covalently associated chain, β2-microglobulin, which is not encoded in the MHC. Only the class I α chain spans the membrane. The molecule has four domains, three formed from the MHC-encoded α chain, and one contributed by β2-microglobulin. The α3 domain and β2-microglobulin have a folded structure that closely resembles that of an immunoglobulin domain (see Section 3-5). The most remarkable feature of MHC molecules is the structure of the α1 and α2 domains, which pair to generate a cleft on the surface of the molecule that is the site of peptide binding.

MHC class II molecules consist of a non-covalent complex of two chains, α and β, both of which span the membrane (Fig. 4.4). The crystal structure of the MHC class II molecule shows that it is folded very much like the MHC class I molecule. The major differences lie at the ends of the peptide-binding cleft, which are more open in MHC class II molecules. The main consequence of this is that the ends of a peptide bound to an MHC class I molecule are substantially buried within the molecule, while the ends of peptides bound to MHC class II molecules are not.

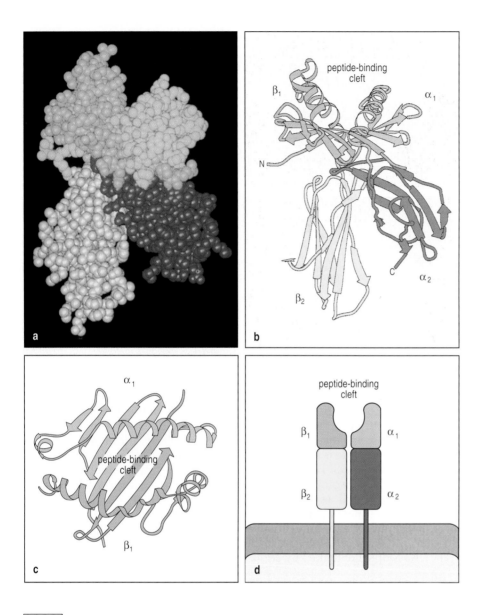

Fig. 4.4   MHC class II molecules resemble MHC class I molecules in structure. The MHC class II molecule is composed of two transmembrane glycoprotein chains, α (34 000 Da) and β (29 000 Da), as shown schematically in panel d. Each chain has two domains, and the two chains together form a compact four-domain structure similar to that of the class I molecule (compare with panel d of Fig. 4.3). Panel a shows a computer graphic representation of the MHC class II molecule, in this case, the human protein HLA-DR1; panel b shows the equivalent ribbon diagram. The α_2 and β_2 domains, like the α_3 and β_2-microglobulin domains of the MHC class I molecule, have amino acid sequence and structural similarities to immunoglobulin constant domains; in the MHC class II molecule, the two domains forming the peptide-binding cleft are contributed by different chains, and are therefore not joined by a covalent bond (see panels c and d). Another important difference, not apparent in this diagram, is that the peptide-binding groove of the MHC class II molecule is open at both ends. Photograph courtesy of C Thorpe.

4-3	**T cells recognize a complex of a peptide fragment bound to an MHC molecule.**

The recognition of protein antigens by B-cell receptors and their secreted counterpart, antibody molecules, involves direct binding to the native protein structure. It can be shown by X-ray crystallography that, typically, antibodies bind to the protein surface, contacting amino acids that are discontinuous in the primary structure but are brought together in the folded protein. As T cells do not secrete their receptors, it has been difficult to obtain purified receptors in sufficient quantity to allow a detailed physical and structural analysis. The use of protein engineering techniques to produce soluble T-cell receptors should soon make it possible to obtain a description of T-cell receptor:MHC:peptide interactions comparable with that of antibody:antigen interactions. Until such data are available, the features of antigen recognition by T cells have to be deduced from the functional assays described in Chapter 2. T cells always respond to contiguous short amino acid sequences in proteins that are often buried in their native structure. The peptides that stimulate T cells are recognized only when bound to the appropriate MHC molecule. This has been shown conclusively by stimulating T cells with purified peptide:MHC complexes. Purified peptide: MHC complexes have been characterized

Fig. 4.5 MHC molecules bind peptides tightly within the cleft. The original crystal structure of an MHC class I molecule contained a mixture of naturally occurring peptide antigens and details of the peptide:MHC interaction could not be discerned. When MHC molecules are crystallized with a single synthetic peptide antigen bound to their cleft, the details of peptide binding are revealed. In MHC class I molecules (panel a) the peptide is bound in an elongated conformation with both ends tightly bound at either end of the cleft. In the case of MHC class II molecules (panel b), the peptide is also bound in an elongated conformation but the ends of the peptide are not tightly bound and the peptide extends beyond the cleft. The upper surface of the peptide:MHC complex is recognized by T cells, and is composed of residues of the MHC molecule (shown in white for MHC class I molecules in panel c and for MHC class II molecules in panel d) and of the peptide (shown in red in panels c and d). Photographs courtesy of C Thorpe.

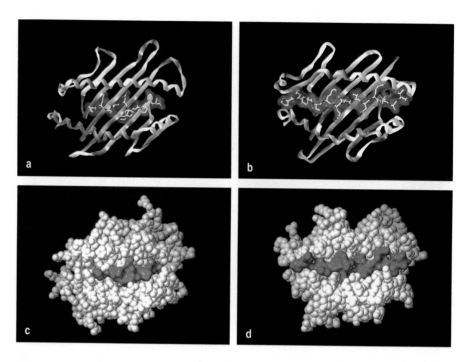

structurally (Fig. 4.5); the peptide binds to the cleft on the outer face of the MHC molecule so that, viewed from above as a T-cell receptor would see the complex, the peptide occupies the center of this face of the molecule. In an MHC class I molecule, the bound peptide is surrounded by the two α helices from the α_1 and α_2 domains. Similarly, in the MHC class II molecule, the peptide is held between the α helices of the α_1 and β_1 domains. Assuming that a T-cell receptor interacts with this ligand much as an antibody does with a protein, then ~700–900 Å^2 of surface area will be in contact with the T-cell receptor, with the periphery of the binding site consisting of contacts with the MHC molecule and the center of contacts with the peptide fragment of antigen. As we shall see in the last part of this chapter, the most variable part of the T-cell receptor is made up of the central CDR3 loops that make key contacts with the peptide.

4-4 | Peptides are stably bound to MHC molecules through invariant and variable contacts.

Cells make only a few distinct MHC molecules but an individual may be infected by a wide variety of different pathogens whose proteins will not necessarily have peptide sequences in common. If T cells are to be alerted to all possible intracellular infections, therefore, the MHC molecules on each cell must be able to bind stably to many different peptides. This behavior is quite distinct from that of peptide-binding receptors, such as those for peptide hormones, which bind only a single peptide with great specificity. Rather, it resembles the binding of some proteases where, although the binding site encompasses some six amino acids, only a single amino acid of the substrate determines its ability to bind. The crystal structures of peptide:MHC complexes have helped to show how a single binding site can bind peptides with high affinity, while retaining the ability to bind a wide variety of different peptides. We shall first discuss the peptide-binding properties of MHC class I molecules, whose structure was solved before that of MHC class II molecules. Unlike other peptide-binding proteins, MHC molecules bind peptide ligands as an integral part of the MHC molecular structure, and MHC molecules are unstable when peptides are not bound. This stable binding is important because otherwise, peptide exchanges occurring at the cell surface would prevent peptide:MHC complexes being reliable indicators of infection or of specific antigen uptake. As a result of this stability, when MHC class I molecules are purified from cells, their bound peptides co-purify with them, and this has enabled the peptides bound by specific MHC class I molecules to be analyzed. For this purpose, the peptides are eluted from the MHC class I molecules by denaturing the complex in acid to release the bound peptides, which can then be purified and sequenced. Pure synthetic versions of these peptides can also be co-crystallized with previously empty MHC class I molecules and the structure of the complex determined, revealing details of the contacts between the MHC molecule and the peptide. From an analysis of the sequences of peptides bound to specific MHC molecules, and a structural analysis of the peptide:MHC complex, a detailed picture of the binding interactions has been built up.

Peptides that bind to MHC class I molecules are usually eight to ten amino acids long. The binding of the peptide is stabilized at its two ends by contacts between atoms in the free amino and carboxy termini, and invariant sites in the peptide-binding groove of all MHC class I molecules. The terminal amino group of the peptide makes contact with an invariant site at one end of the peptide-binding groove, and the terminal carboxyl group binds to an invariant site at the other end of the groove. These contacts are thought to be the main stabilizing contacts for peptide:MHC class I complexes since synthetic peptide analogs lacking terminal amino and carboxyl groups fail to stabilize MHC class I molecules. The peptide lies in an elongated conformation along the groove; variations in peptide length appear to be accommodated, in most cases, by a kinking in the peptide backbone. However, a single case where the peptide is able to extend out of the groove at the carboxy terminus suggests that some length variation may also be accommodated in this way.

These interactions provide broad peptide:MHC binding specificity. MHC molecules are highly polymorphic at certain sites in the peptide-binding cleft, however, and interactions between the polymorphic amino acids and side chains on the peptide mean that different allelic variants of MHC molecules preferentially bind different peptides. Peptides binding to a given allelic variant of an MHC molecule have been shown to have the same or very similar amino acid residues at two or three specific positions along the peptide sequence.

The amino acid side chains at these positions insert into pockets in the MHC molecule that are lined by the polymorphic amino acids. Since the binding of these side chains anchors the peptide to the MHC molecule, the peptide residues involved have been called **anchor residues**. Most peptides that bind to MHC class I molecules have an anchor residue at the carboxy terminus, and this residue is almost always hydrophobic (Fig. 4.6). Changing any anchor residue can prevent the peptide from binding, and conversely, most synthetic peptides of correct length that contain these anchor residues will bind the appropriate MHC class I molecule, in most cases irrespective of the sequence of the peptide at other positions. These features of peptide binding allow MHC class I molecules to bind a wide variety of different peptides of suitable length. Moreover, because the peptides can kink in the middle where they protrude above the groove and contact the T-cell receptor, the anchor residues are not always at precisely the same position in the linear sequence of peptides that bind to a given MHC class I molecule.

Although only a few residues of the peptide may protrude above the peptide-binding cleft and be available for recognition by the T-cell receptor, T cells are clearly able to discriminate efficiently between different peptide:MHC complexes. From a comparison of the structures of different peptides bound by the same MHC class I molecule, it is clear that even for peptides of the same length, the conformation of the peptide

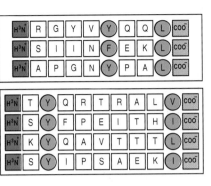

Fig. 4.6 Peptides bind to MHC molecules through structurally related anchor residues. Peptides eluted from two different MHC class I molecules are shown. The anchor residues (green) differ for peptides binding different MHC molecules but are similar for all peptides binding to the same MHC molecule. The upper and lower panels show peptides that bind to two different MHC class I molecules respectively. The anchor residues binding a particular MHC molecule need not be identical but are always related (for example, phenylalanine (F) and tyrosine (Y) are both aromatic amino acids, whereas valine (V), leucine (L) and isoleucine (I) are all hydrophobic amino acids). Peptides also bind to MHC class I molecules through their amino (blue) and carboxy termini (red).

backbone can vary, depending on its sequence. Finally, when different peptides are bound by the same MHC class I molecule, there can be small changes in the conformation of the MHC class I molecule itself, which could also influence the binding of the T-cell receptor.

| 4-5 | **The length of the peptides bound by MHC class II molecules is not constrained.** |

Peptide binding to MHC class II molecules has also been analyzed by elution of bound peptides and by X-ray crystallography, and is different in several ways from peptide binding to MHC class I molecules. Peptides that bind to MHC class II molecules are at least 13 amino acids in length and can be much longer. The clusters of residues that in MHC class I molecules bind the two ends of a peptide are not found in MHC class II molecules and the ends of the peptide are not bound. Instead, the peptide lies in an extended conformation along the MHC class II peptide-binding groove. It is held in this groove both by peptide side chains that protrude into shallow and deep pockets lined by residues that vary between MHC class II molecules, and by binding of the peptide backbone with side chains of conserved MHC class II residues that line all MHC class II peptide-binding grooves. Although there are fewer crystal structures of MHC class II-bound peptides than of MHC class I, the available data show that amino acid side chains at residues 1, 4, 6, and 9 of a minimal MHC class II-bound peptide are held in these binding pockets.

These pockets are more permissive than those of the MHC class I molecule, making it more difficult to detect a peptide-binding motif for MHC class II molecules (Fig. 4.7). Nevertheless, it is usually possible to detect a pattern of binding with different alleles of MHC class II molecules, and to associate

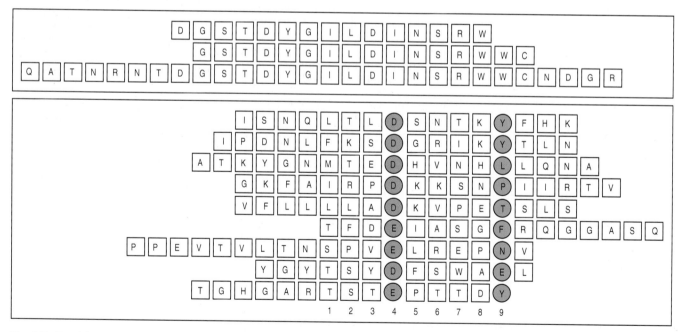

Fig. 4.7 Peptides that bind MHC class II molecules are variable in length and their anchor residues lie at various distances from the ends of the peptide. The sequences of a set of peptides that bind to the mouse MHC class II A^k allele are shown in the upper panel. All contain the same core sequence but differ in length. In the lower panel, different peptides binding to the human MHC class II allele HLA-DR3 are shown. The lengths of these peptides can vary, and so by convention the first anchor residue is denoted as residue 1, or P1. Note that all of the peptides share a negatively charged residue [aspartic acid (D) or glutamic acid (E)] in the fourth, or P4 position (blue) and tend to have a hydrophobic residue [eg tyrosine (Y), leucine (L), proline (P), phenylalanine (F)] in the P9 position (green).

this binding motif with the amino acids that make up the groove of the MHC class II allele. By binding the peptide backbone and allowing the bound peptide to emerge from both ends of the binding groove, there is in principle, no upper limit on the length of peptides binding to MHC class II molecules. However, it appears that longer peptides bound to MHC class II molecules are trimmed by peptidases to peptides of 13–17 amino acids in most cases. As for MHC class I molecules, MHC class II molecules that lack bound peptide are unstable but the critical stabilizing interactions that the peptide makes with the MHC class II molecule are not yet known.

| 4-6 | **The two classes of MHC molecules are expressed differentially on cells.** |

MHC class I and MHC class II molecules have a distinct distribution among cells that reflects directly the different effector functions of the T cells that recognize them (Fig. 4.8). MHC class I molecules, as we saw in Section 4-1, present peptides from pathogens in the cytosol, commonly viruses, to CD8 cytotoxic T cells, which are specialized to kill any cell that they specifically recognize. As viruses can infect any nucleated cell, almost all such cells express MHC class I molecules, although the level of constitutive expression varies from one cell type to the next (see Fig. 4.8). Cells of the immune system express abundant MHC class I on their surface, while liver cells (hepatocytes) express relatively low levels.

Tissue	MHC class I	MHC class II
Lymphoid tissues		
T cells	+++	+*
B cells	+++	+++
Macrophages	+++	++
Other antigen-presenting cells (eg Langerhans' cells)	+++	+++
Epithelial cells of the thymus	+	+++
Other nucleated cells		
Neutrophils	+++	−
Hepatocytes	+	−
Kidney	+	−
Brain	+	−†
Non-nucleated cells		
Red blood cells	−	−

Fig. 4.8 The expression of MHC molecules differs between tissues. MHC class I molecules are expressed on all nucleated cells, although they are most highly expressed in hematopoietic cells. MHC class II molecules are normally only expressed by a subset of hematopoietic cells and by thymic stromal cells, although they may be expressed by other cell types on exposure to the inflammatory cytokine interferon-γ.
* In humans, activated T cells express MHC class II molecules, while in mice, all T cells are MHC class II-negative.
† In the brain, most cell types are MHC class II-negative but microglia, which are related to macrophages, are MHC class II-positive.

As might be expected, the level of MHC molecule expression influences T-cell activation; cells that express few MHC class I molecules may not be easily killed by cytotoxic T cells. Non-nucleated cells, such as mammalian red blood cells, express little or no MHC class I, and thus the interior of red blood cells is a site in which an infection can go undetected by cytotoxic T cells. As red blood cells cannot support viral replication, this is of no great consequence for viral infection but it may be the absence of MHC class I that allows the *Plasmodium* species that cause malaria to live in this privileged site.

The main function of CD4 T cells, by contrast, is to activate other effector cells of the immune system. Thus MHC class II molecules are normally found on B lymphocytes and macrophages—cells that participate in immune responses—but not on other tissue cells (see Fig. 4.8). When helper T cells recognize peptides bound to MHC class II molecules on B cells, they stimulate the B cells to produce antibody. Likewise, T_H1 cells recognizing peptides bound to MHC class II molecules on macrophages activate these cells to destroy the pathogens in their vesicles. We shall see in Chapter 7 that MHC class II molecules are also expressed on specialized antigen-presenting cells in lymphoid tissues where naive T cells encounter antigen and are first activated. Expression of both MHC class I and MHC class II molecules is regulated by cytokines, in particular interferons, released in the course of immune responses. Interferon-γ, for example, can induce the expression of MHC class II molecules on certain cell types that do not normally express them, with important consequences for autoimmunity. Interferons also play a central part in the antigen-presenting function of MHC class I molecules, not only by up-regulating the expression of the MHC class I molecules themselves but also by inducing the expression of key components of the intracellular machinery, which is required to enable peptides to be loaded onto these molecules. It is to this machinery that we now turn.

4-7 Peptides that bind to MHC class I molecules are actively transported from the cytosol to the endoplasmic reticulum.

Typically, the antigen fragments that bind to MHC class I molecules for presentation to CD8 T cells are derived from viruses that take over the cell's biosynthetic mechanisms to make their own proteins. All proteins are made in the cytosol. Proteins destined for the cell surface, including both classes of MHC molecule, are translocated during their synthesis from the cytosol into the lumen of the endoplasmic reticulum, where they must fold correctly before they can be transported to the cell surface. Since the peptide-binding site of the MHC class I molecule is formed in the lumen of the endoplasmic reticulum and never exposed to the cytosol, how are peptides derived from viral proteins in the cytosol able to bind to MHC class I molecules for delivery to the cell surface?

The answer to this question was suggested first by the behavior of mutant cells with a defect in antigen presentation by MHC class I molecules. Although both chains of MHC class I molecules are synthesized normally in these cells, the MHC class I proteins are expressed only at very low levels on the cell surface. The defect in these cells can be corrected by the addition of synthetic peptides, suggesting both that the mutation affects the supply of peptides to MHC class I molecules and that peptide is required for their normal cell-surface expression. This was the first indication that MHC molecules are unstable in the absence of bound peptide.

Analysis of the affected DNA in the mutant cells showed that two genes encoding members of the ATP-binding cassette, or ABC, family of proteins are mutant or absent in these cells. These two genes map within the MHC itself (see Section 4-14). ATP-binding cassette proteins are associated with membranes in many cells, including bacterial cells, where they mediate ATP-dependent transport, whether of ions, sugars, amino acids, or peptides, across membranes. The two ATP-binding cassette proteins deleted in the mutant cells are associated with the endoplasmic reticulum membrane. They are encoded in the MHC and are inducible by interferon. Transfection of the mutant cells with both genes restores presentation of cytosolic peptides by the cell's MHC class I molecules. These proteins are now called **Transporters associated with Antigen Processing-1** and **-2** (**TAP-1** and **TAP-2**). The two TAP proteins form a heterodimer (Fig. 4.9) and mutations in either TAP gene can prevent antigen presentation by MHC class I molecules.

In assays *in vitro* using microsomal vesicles that mimic the endoplasmic reticulum, vesicles from normal cells will internalize peptides, which then bind to MHC class I molecules already present in the microsomal lumen. Vesicles from TAP-1 or TAP-2 mutant cells do not transport peptides. Peptide transport into the normal microsomes requires ATP hydrolysis, proving that the TAP-1:TAP-2 complex is an ATP-dependent peptide transporter that selectively loads peptides into the lumen of the endoplasmic reticulum. Such experiments have also shown that the TAP transporter has some specificity for the peptides it will transport. The TAP-1:TAP-2 transporter prefers peptides of eight or more amino acids with hydrophobic or basic residues at the carboxy terminus, the exact features of peptides that bind MHC class I molecules. In the rat, there are two allelic variants of the TAP-2 transporter that differ in their capacity to transport peptides. One variant (TAP-2^a) transports peptides with either basic or hydrophobic carboxy-terminal residues, while the other (TAP-2^u) transports only those peptides with hydrophobic carboxy-terminal residues. Genetic variation in the TAP proteins can thus affect the repertoire of peptides available for binding by MHC class I molecules; hence the original description of the TAP-2 locus in the rat as the class I modifier, or *cim* locus.

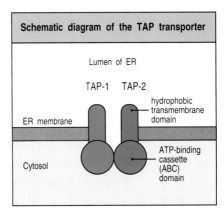

Fig. 4.9 The TAP-1 and TAP-2 transporter molecules form a heterodimer in the endoplasmic reticulum membrane. All protein molecules that belong to the ATP-binding cassette (ABC) transporter family have four domains, two complex transmembrane domains which each have multiple transmembrane regions, and two ATP-binding domains. Both TAP-1 and TAP-2 encode one hydrophobic and one ATP-binding domain and assemble into a heterodimer to form a four-domain transporter. On the basis of similarities between the TAP molecules and other members of the ABC-transporter family, it is believed that the ATP-binding domains lie within the cytoplasm of the cell, while the hydrophobic domains project through the membrane into the lumen of the endoplasmic reticulum (ER).

| 4-8 | **Newly synthesized MHC class I molecules are retained in the endoplasmic reticulum by binding a TAP-1 associated protein until they bind peptide.** |

The discovery of the TAP-1:TAP-2 heterodimer explained how peptides get from the cytosol to the lumen of the endoplasmic reticulum, and the ability of TAP-1 and TAP-2 genes to restore antigen presentation in mutant cells suggested that peptide binding is necessary for the cell-surface expression of newly synthesized MHC class I molecules. This is because, without bound peptide, the MHC class I molecule is unstable and newly synthesized MHC class I molecules are held in the endoplasmic reticulum in a partially folded state until they bind peptide. This explains why cells with mutations in TAP-1 or TAP-2 fail to express MHC class I molecules at the cell surface.

In humans, newly synthesized MHC class I α chains rapidly bind an 88 kDa membrane-bound protein known as **calnexin**, which retains the MHC class I molecule in a partially folded state in the endoplasmic reticulum. Calnexin also associates with partially folded T-cell receptors, immunoglobulins, and MHC class II molecules, and so has a central role in the assembly of many molecules important in immunology. When β$_2$-microglobulin binds to the α chain, the α:β$_2$-microglobulin heterodimer dissociates from calnexin and now binds to a complex of proteins, one of which, calreticulin, is similar to calnexin and probably carries out a similar chaperone function. A second component of the complex is the

TAP-1 associated protein **tapasin**, which binds to the TAP-1 subunit of the transporter, allowing the partially folded α:β₂-microglobulin heterodimer to await the transport of a suitable peptide from the cytosol. Finally, the binding of a peptide to the partially folded heterodimer releases it from TAP and allows the now fully folded MHC class I molecule to leave the endoplasmic reticulum and be transported to the cell surface (Fig. 4.10). Most of the peptides transported by TAP will not bind to the MHC molecules in that cell and are cleared out of the endoplasmic reticulum rapidly; there is evidence that they are transported back into the cytosol by an ATP-dependent transport mechanism distinct from the TAP transporter. It is not yet clear whether the TAP transporter plays a direct role in loading MHC class I molecules with peptide or whether binding to the TAP transporter merely allows the MHC class I molecule to scan the transported peptides before they diffuse through the lumen of the endoplasmic reticulum and are transported back into the cytosol.

In cells with mutant TAP genes, the MHC class I molecules are unstable and appear to be degraded within the endoplasmic reticulum, indicating that it is the binding of peptide to the MHC class I molecule that allows it to complete its folding and to be transported onwards from the endoplasmic reticulum. Even in normal cells, MHC class I molecules are retained in the endoplasmic reticulum for some time, suggesting that MHC class I molecules are usually present in excess of peptide. This is very important for the function of MHC class I molecules because they must be immediately available to transport viral peptides to the cell surface at any time the cell becomes infected. In uninfected cells, peptides derived from self proteins fill the peptide-binding cleft of mature MHC class I molecules present at the cell surface. When a cell is infected by a

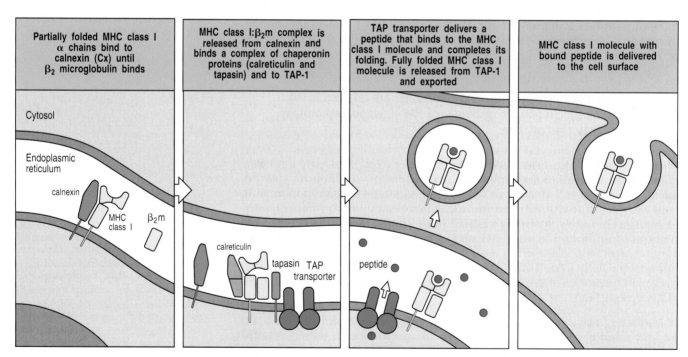

Fig. 4.10 MHC class I molecules do not leave the endoplasmic reticulum unless they bind peptides. Peptides generated by degradation of proteins in the cytoplasm are transported into the lumen of the endoplasmic reticulum. MHC class I α chains assemble in the endoplasmic reticulum with a membrane-bound protein, calnexin (Cx). When this complex binds β₂-microglobulin (β₂m) it is released from calnexin and the partially folded MHC class I molecule then binds to the TAP-1 subunit of the TAP transporter by interacting with one molecule of the TAP-associated protein tapasin, and a chaperonin, calreticulin. It is retained in the endoplasmic reticulum until released by binding of a peptide, completing the folding of the MHC class I molecule. The peptide:MHC complex is then transported through the Golgi complex to the cell surface.

virus, the presence of excess MHC class I molecules in the endoplasmic reticulum allows the rapid presentation at the cell surface of peptides derived from the pathogen.

Since the presentation of viral peptides by MHC class I molecules signals CD8 T cells to kill the infected cell, some viruses have evolved mechanisms to evade recognition by interfering with this pathway. The herpes simplex virus, for example, prevents transport of viral peptides into the endoplasmic reticulum by producing a protein that binds to and inhibits the TAP transporter. A second mechanism is that used by adenoviruses, which encode a protein that binds to MHC class I molecules and retains them in the endoplasmic reticulum, again preventing the appearance at the cell surface of MHC class I molecules loaded with viral peptides. The advantage to a virus of blocking recognition of infected cells is so great that it would not be surprising if other steps in the formation of peptide:MHC complexes, for example the association of the MHC class I:chaperone complex with the TAP transporter, were found to be inhibited by some viruses.

4-9   Peptides of cytosolic proteins are generated in the cytosol prior to transport into the endoplasmic reticulum.

Proteins in cells are continuously being degraded and replaced with newly synthesized proteins. A major part in cytosolic protein degradation is played by a large, multicatalytic protease complex of 28 subunits, each between 20 and 30 kDa, called the **proteasome** (Fig. 4.11). Various lines of evidence implicate the proteasome in the production of peptide ligands for MHC class I molecules. For example, the proteasome takes part in the ubiquitin-dependent degradation pathway for cytosolic proteins; experimentally tagging proteins with ubiquitin also results in the more efficient presentation of their peptides by MHC class I molecules. Moreover, inhibitors of the proteolytic activity of the proteasome also inhibit antigen presentation by MHC class I molecules. Whether the proteasome is the only cytosolic protease capable of generating peptides for transport into the endoplasmic reticulum is not known.

Two subunits of the proteasome, called LMP2 and LMP7, are encoded within the MHC near the TAP-1 and TAP-2 genes (see Section 4-14) and their expression is induced by interferon, like that of the MHC class I and TAP molecules. LMP2 and LMP7 substitute for two constitutive subunits of the proteasome, which they displace in cells in which they are expressed. A third subunit, MECL-1, which is not encoded within the MHC, is also induced by interferon treatment and also displaces a constitutive proteasome subunit. These three inducible subunits and their constitutive counterparts are thought to be active proteases. The replacement of the constitutive components by their interferon-inducible counterparts seems to change the activity of the proteasome; in interferon-treated cells, there is increased cleavage of polypeptides after hydrophobic and basic residues, and reduced cleavage after acidic residues. This produces peptides with carboxy-terminal residues that are preferred anchor residues for peptide binding to most MHC class I molecules and are also the preferred structures for transport by TAP.

If the peptides that bind to MHC class I molecules are produced in the cytosol, how can MHC class I molecules present peptide fragments of membrane or secreted proteins, which are normally translocated into the lumen of the endoplasmic reticulum during their synthesis? Probably a small fraction of such proteins fail to be translocated correctly into the endoplasmic reticulum and, instead, remain within the cytosol where they are degraded into peptides. Certain amino-terminal amino acids that protect cell-surface and secreted proteins from degradation in

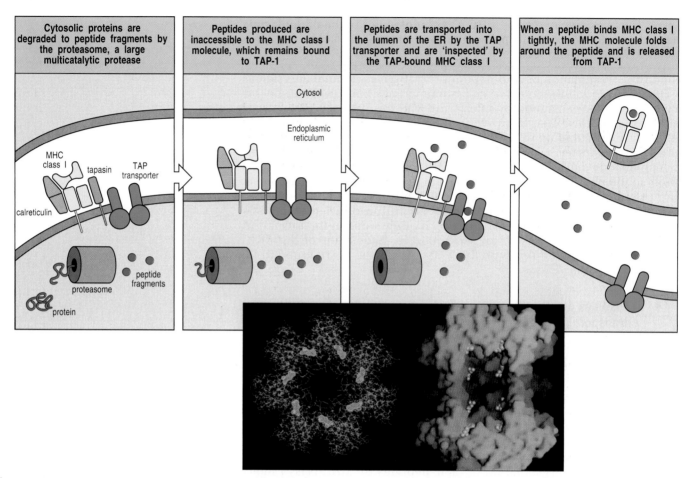

| Cytosolic proteins are degraded to peptide fragments by the proteasome, a large multicatalytic protease | Peptides produced are inaccessible to the MHC class I molecule, which remains bound to TAP-1 | Peptides are transported into the lumen of the ER by the TAP transporter and are 'inspected' by the TAP-bound MHC class I | When a peptide binds MHC class I tightly, the MHC molecule folds around the peptide and is released from TAP-1 |

Fig. 4.11 Degradation and transport of antigens that bind MHC class I molecules. The source of peptides for MHC class I molecules is the degradation of proteins in the cytosol. The digestion of cytosolic proteins is carried out by a large protease complex, the proteasome. The proteasome contains 28 subunits arranged, as shown in cross-section in panel a and in longitudinal section in panel b, to form a cylindrical structure composed of four rings, each of seven subunits. It is not known exactly how the mammalian proteasome degrades cytosolic proteins. It has six active proteolytic sites, which correspond to the N-terminal threonine residues of three of the seven β subunits, and are found in the center of the cylinder. Thus, it is likely that proteins have to unfold and pass through the center of the cylindrical structure as shown here for degradation to occur. Peptide fragments generated by the proteasome are transported into the lumen of the endoplasmic reticulum (ER) by the TAP transporter. There, the peptides bind to the complex of the partially folded MHC molecule, liberating the MHC class I molecule from the TAP/tapasin complex, thus allowing the peptide:MHC complex to be delivered to the cell surface. Photographs of bacterial proteasome structure (x 667 000) courtesy of W Baumeister.

the endoplasmic reticulum are associated with rapid degradation in the cytosol (and vice versa); thus, any misdirected cell-surface or secreted proteins that end up in the cytosol will be targeted for rapid degradation, providing a source of peptides that can be transported across the endoplasmic reticulum membrane to interact with MHC class I molecules. This mechanism may explain, for example, how viral envelope glycoproteins produce peptides that are presented by MHC class I molecules.

4-10   **Peptides presented by MHC class II molecules are generated in acidified intracellular vesicles.**

Whereas viruses and some bacteria replicate in the cytosol, several classes of pathogens, including *Leishmania* spp. and the mycobacteria that cause leprosy and tuberculosis, replicate in intracellular vesicles in macrophages. As they reside in membrane-enclosed vesicles, the proteins of these pathogens are not accessible to proteasomes. Instead, proteins in these sites are degraded by vesicular proteases into peptide fragments that bind to MHC class II molecules for delivery to the cell surface (Fig. 4.12) where they are recognized by CD4 T cells. CD4 T cells also recognize peptide fragments derived from extracellular pathogens and proteins that are internalized into similar intracellular vesicles.

Most of what we know about the processing of proteins in vesicles has come from experiments in which simple proteins are fed to macrophages; in this way processing of added antigen can be quantified. Proteins that bind to surface immunoglobulin on B cells and are internalized by B-cell receptor-mediated endocytosis are processed by the same pathway. Internalized protein antigens that enter cells through endocytosis become enclosed in vesicles known as endosomes that become increasingly acidic as they progress into the interior of the cell. The vesicles of the endosomal pathway contain proteases, known as acid proteases, which are activated at low pH, and eventually degrade proteins contained in the vesicles.

Drugs, such as chloroquine, that raise the pH of vesicles, inhibit the presentation of antigens that enter the cell in this way, suggesting that acid proteases are responsible for the processing of internalized antigen. Among these acid proteases are cathepsins B and D, and cathepsin L, which is the most active enzyme in this family of related proteases. Antigen processing can be mimicked to some extent by digestion of proteins with these enzymes *in vitro* at acid pH. Proteins of pathogens growing in intracellular vesicles are also handled by this pathway of antigen processing.

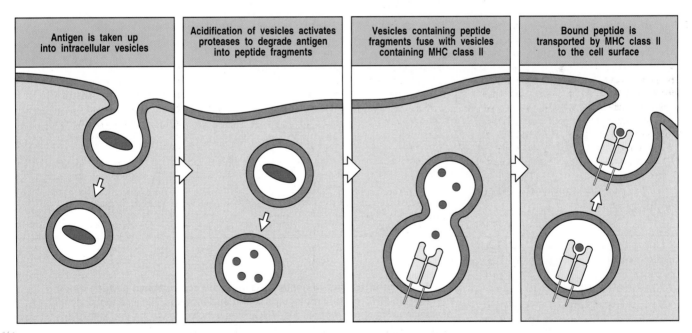

Antigen is taken up into intracellular vesicles

Acidification of vesicles activates proteases to degrade antigen into peptide fragments

Vesicles containing peptide fragments fuse with vesicles containing MHC class II

Bound peptide is transported by MHC class II to the cell surface

Fig. 4.12 Antigens that bind to MHC class II molecules are degraded in acidified endosomes. In some cases, the source of the peptides may be bacteria or parasites that have invaded the cell to replicate in intracellular vesicles. In other cases, as illustrated here, microorganisms or foreign proteins may be engulfed by phagocytic cells and routed to lysosomes for degradation, or endocytosed by other professional antigen-presenting cells. En route to the lysosomes, the pH of the vesicles (endosomes) containing the engulfed pathogens progressively decreases, activating proteases that reside within the endosome to degrade the engulfed material. At some point on their pathway to the cell surface, newly synthesized MHC class II molecules pass through such acidified endosomes and bind peptide fragments of the pathogens, transporting the peptides to the cell surface.

4-11   The invariant chain directs newly synthesized MHC class II molecules to acidified intracellular vesicles.

The function of MHC class II molecules is to present peptides generated in the intracellular vesicles of B cells, macrophages, and other antigen-presenting cells to CD4 T cells. However, the biosynthetic pathway for MHC class II molecules, like that of other cell-surface glycoproteins, starts with their translocation into the endoplasmic reticulum, and they must therefore be prevented from binding prematurely to peptides transported into the endoplasmic reticulum lumen by the TAP transporter, or to the cell's own newly synthesized polypeptides. As the endoplasmic reticulum is richly endowed with unfolded and partially folded polypeptide chains, a general mechanism is needed to prevent their binding in the open-ended MHC class II peptide-binding groove.

Binding is prevented by the assembly of newly synthesized MHC class II molecules with a protein known as the MHC class II-associated **invariant chain (Ii)**. The invariant chain forms trimers, with each subunit binding non-covalently to a class II α:β heterodimer (Fig. 4.13; for convenience, we show the MHC class II:invariant chain complex as only a single α:β:Ii complex). Ii binds to the MHC class II molecule with part of its polypeptide chain lying within the peptide-binding groove (see Fig. 4.13, lower left panel), thus blocking the groove and preventing the binding

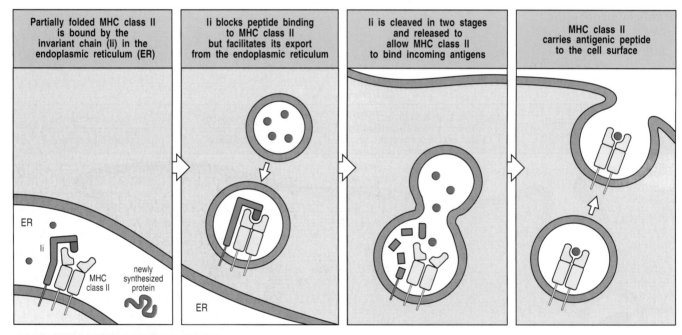

| Partially folded MHC class II is bound by the invariant chain (Ii) in the endoplasmic reticulum (ER) | Ii blocks peptide binding to MHC class II but facilitates its export from the endoplasmic reticulum | Ii is cleaved in two stages and released to allow MHC class II to bind incoming antigens | MHC class II carries antigenic peptide to the cell surface |

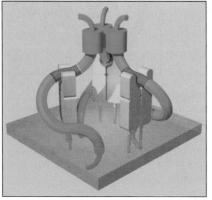

Fig. 4.13 The MHC class II-associated invariant chain delays peptide binding and targets MHC class II molecules to the endosomes. The invariant chain (Ii) assembles with newly synthesized MHC class II molecules in the endoplasmic reticulum where it prevents the MHC class II molecule from binding intracellular peptides and partially folded proteins present in the lumen. The invariant chain directs export of MHC Class II molecules through the Golgi apparatus to acidified endosomes containing peptides of resident bacteria or engulfed extracellular proteins. Here the invariant chain is cleaved in stages, and the MHC class II molecule binds antigenic peptide and is transported to the cell surface. A model for the trimeric invariant chain bound to αβ heterodimers is shown in the lower left. The CLIP portion is shown in red, the rest of the invariant chain in green, and the α:β MHC class II heterodimer in yellow. Model structure courtesy of P Cresswell.

of either peptides or partially folded proteins. While this complex is being assembled in the endoplasmic reticulum, its component parts are associated with calnexin. Only when assembly is completed to produce a nine-chain complex is it released from calnexin for transport onward from the endoplasmic reticulum. In this nine-chain complex, the MHC class II molecule cannot bind peptides or unfolded proteins, so that peptides present in the endoplasmic reticulum are not usually presented by MHC class II molecules. Moreover, in the absence of invariant chains there is evidence that many MHC class II molecules are retained in the endoplasmic reticulum as complexes with misfolded proteins.

The invariant chain has a second function, which is to target delivery of the MHC class II molecules from the endoplasmic reticulum to an appropriate low pH endosomal compartment. The complex of MHC class II α:β heterodimers with invariant chain is retained for 2–4 hours in this compartment. During this time, the invariant chain is cleaved by proteases such as cathepsin L in several steps (see Fig. 4.13). The initial cleavage events generate a truncated form of the invariant chain that remains bound to the MHC class II molecule and retains it within the proteolytic compartment. A subsequent cleavage releases the MHC class II molecule, bound to a short fragment of Ii, called **CLIP** (for **class II-associated invariant-chain peptide**). MHC class II molecules that have CLIP associated with them still cannot bind other peptides, and CLIP must either dissociate or be displaced to allow peptides to bind and be delivered to the cell surface.

The intracellular location at which invariant chain is cleaved and MHC class II molecules encounter peptides is not clearly defined. Most newly synthesized MHC class II molecules are brought towards the cell surface in vesicles, which at some point fuse with incoming endosomes. However, there is also evidence that some MHC class II:Ii complexes are first transported to the cell surface and then re-internalized into endosomes. In either case, MHC class II:Ii complexes enter the endosomal pathway and are there exposed to an acidic, proteolytic environment in which the invariant chain is cleaved and pathogens and their proteins are broken down into peptides available to bind to the MHC class II molecule. Electron microscopy studies using antibodies tagged with gold particles suggest that this may occur in a specialized vesicular compartment, called the **MIIC** (**MHC class II compartment**), late in the endosomal pathway (Fig. 4.14).

The MIIC does not appear to be a simple vesicular compartment. There are at least two types of MIIC characterized by different morphologies; one type has several concentric membranes and is called a multilaminar vesicle, while the other contains multiple discrete vesicles and hence is called a multivesicular body. Within the multilaminar MIIC, the invariant chain appears to be uncleaved, while within the multivesicular MIIC only the CLIP fragment remains associated with MHC class II molecules. It is not known at present whether the invariant chain is cleaved within a single vesicle that matures from a multilaminar form to a multivesicular form, or whether the Ii:MHC class II complex moves from one type of vesicle to another.

As with MHC class I molecules, MHC class II molecules in uninfected cells bind peptides derived from self proteins. MHC class II molecules that do not bind peptide after dissociation from the invariant chain are unstable, leading to aggregation and rapid degradation at the acidic pH of the endosomal compartment. It is therefore not surprising that peptides derived from MHC class II molecules themselves form a large proportion of the peptides presented by MHC class II

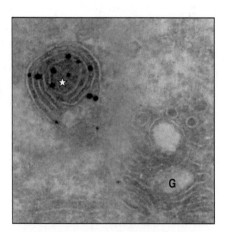

Fig. 4.14 Electron micrograph showing a multivesicular body(☆) containing internalized proteins and MHC class II molecules. MHC class II molecules and the invariant chain are labeled with different sized gold particles, the larger particles showing the presence of MHC class II molecules, and the smaller particles the invariant chain. G, Golgi apparatus. Photograph courtesy of F Sanderson.

molecules in normal cells. This suggests that, as for MHC class I molecules, excess MHC class II molecules are generated. Thus, when a cell is infected by mycobacteria or other pathogens that proliferate in cellular vesicles, when a phagocyte engulfs a pathogen, or a B cell binds antigen to its immunoglobulin receptor, the peptides generated from them find plentiful empty MHC class II molecules to bind.

4-12 | A specialized MHC class II-like molecule catalyzes loading of MHC class II molecules with endogenously processed peptides.

Just as mutant cell lines first led to an appreciation of the role of the TAP transporters in peptide loading on MHC class I molecules, observations on mutant human B-cell lines revealed an unsuspected component of the vesicular antigen-processing pathway. MHC class II molecules in these mutant cell lines assemble correctly with the invariant chain and seem to follow the normal vesicular route, but fail to bind peptides derived from internalized proteins, and often arrive at the cell surface with the CLIP peptide still bound. These CLIP-associated MHC class II molecules are unstable and dissociate in the ionic detergent sodium dodecylsulfate at room temperature.

The defect in these mutant cells lies in a MHC class II-like molecule, called **HLA-DM** in humans (H-2M in mice), which is encoded near the TAP and LMP genes in the class II region of the MHC (see Fig. 4.16). The HLA-DM locus encodes an α chain and a β chain that closely resemble those of other MHC class II molecules, although, unlike other class II molecules, HLA-DM does not appear to require peptide for stabilization. The DM molecule is not expressed at the cell surface but rather is found predominantly in the MIIC compartment. When HLA-DR:CLIP complexes from HLA-DM deficient cells are mixed with DM, the CLIP fragment is released. If antigenic peptides are also added, CLIP is released and the stability of the HLA-DR molecule is restored. This suggests that the HLA-DM molecule directs the release of the CLIP fragment and the subsequent loading of peptides onto MHC class II molecules (Fig. 4.15). DM molecules stabilize HLA-DR molecules when added in sub-stoichiometric amounts together with peptide, indicating that they act catalytically. There is also evidence that DM molecules stabilize empty MHC class II molecules by binding to them, further increasing the yield of stable peptide:MHC class II complexes.

The role of the DM molecule in facilitating the binding of peptides to MHC class II molecules appears to parallel the role of the TAP molecules in facilitating the binding of peptides to MHC class I molecules. Thus it seems likely that both classes of MHC molecule interact inefficiently with peptides free in solution and that a specialized mechanism to deliver peptides efficiently has co-evolved with the MHC molecules themselves.

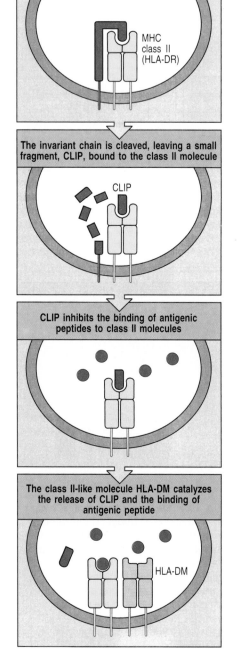

Class II molecules are transported to the MIIC in association with the invariant chain

MHC class II (HLA-DR)

The invariant chain is cleaved, leaving a small fragment, CLIP, bound to the class II molecule

CLIP

CLIP inhibits the binding of antigenic peptides to class II molecules

The class II-like molecule HLA-DM catalyzes the release of CLIP and the binding of antigenic peptide

HLA-DM

Fig. 4.15 HLA-DM facilitates the loading of antigenic peptides onto MHC class II molecules. The invariant chain directs the α:β:li complex to a specialized endosomal compartment (MIIC). Here the invariant chain is cleaved (first panel) and a small fragment, called the class II-associated invariant chain peptide, or CLIP, remains bound to the MHC class II molecule, in this example HLA-DR (second panel). Under normal circumstances the CLIP peptide is replaced by antigenic peptides but, in the absence of HLA-DM, this does not occur (third panel). HLA-DM binds to MHC class II molecules and, although the exact mechanism is not yet defined, is able to catalyze the release of the CLIP fragment and the binding of other peptides (fourth panel).

| 4-13 | **The characteristics of peptide binding by MHC molecules allow effective antigen presentation at the cell surface.** |

To enable MHC molecules to perform their essential function of signaling intracellular infection, it is important that the peptide:MHC complex should be stable at the cell surface. If the complex were to dissociate too readily, the pathogen in the infected cell could escape detection. Conversely, MHC molecules on uninfected cells could pick up peptides released by MHC molecules on infected cells and falsely signal to cytotoxic T cells that a healthy cell is infected, triggering its unwarranted destruction. The stable binding of peptide by MHC molecules makes both these undesirable outcomes unlikely.

It can be seen from the peptide:MHC complexes shown earlier in Fig. 4.5 that the peptide is actually enclosed within the three-dimensional structure of the MHC molecule. Moreover, it can be shown that peptide:MHC complexes expressed on live cells are lost at the same rate as the MHC molecule itself, indicating that the binding of peptide is essentially irreversible. This stability of binding permits even rare peptides to be transported efficiently to the cell surface by MHC molecules, and allows long-term display of these complexes on the surface of the infected cell, thus fulfilling the first of the requirements for effective antigen presentation.

The second criterion for effective antigen presentation is that if dissociation of a peptide from an MHC molecule should occur, new peptides would not be able to bind to the now empty peptide-binding groove. In fact, removal of the peptide from a purified MHC class I molecule requires denaturation of the molecule. When peptide dissociates at the cell surface, the MHC class I molecule changes conformation, the β_2-microglobulin moiety dissociates, and the α chain is internalized and rapidly degraded. Thus, although some MHC class I molecules are able to rebind peptide, most empty MHC class I molecules are quickly lost from the cell surface.

At neutral pH, empty MHC class II molecules are more stable than empty MHC class I molecules, yet empty MHC class II molecules are also removed from the cell surface. Peptide loss from MHC class II molecules is most likely when the molecules are recycled through acidified intracellular vesicles. At the acidic pH of these endocytic vesicles, MHC class II molecules are able to bind peptides that are present in the vesicles but those that fail to do so aggregate and are rapidly degraded. Thus, loss of peptide again leads to the rapid loss of the empty MHC molecule. This feature of peptide binding is important in the antigen presentation function of MHC molecules as it helps to prevent the MHC molecules on a cell surface from acquiring peptides from the surrounding extracellular fluid. This ensures that T cells act selectively on infected cells that efficiently display foreign peptides bound to MHC molecules on their surfaces, while sparing surrounding healthy cells.

| | **Summary.** |

The most distinctive feature of antigen recognition by T cells is the form of the ligand recognized by the T-cell receptor. This comprises a peptide derived from the foreign antigen bound to an MHC molecule. MHC molecules are cell-surface glycoproteins whose non-cytoplasmic face has a peptide-binding groove that can bind a wide variety of different peptides. The MHC molecule binds the peptide in an intracellular location and delivers it to the cell surface, where the combined ligand can be recognized by a T cell. There are two classes of MHC molecule, MHC class I and MHC class II, which deliver peptides from proteins degraded in different intracellular sites. MHC class II molecules, which present peptides to CD4 T cells, bind peptides from proteins that are degraded in acidified intracellular vesicles. Typically, a macrophage infected with mycobacteria, or a B cell that has bound and internalized a specific protein antigen, will present peptides from these foreign proteins, bound to MHC class II molecules, to CD4 T cells, which then activate the macrophage or B cell. MHC class I molecules, which present peptides to CD8 T cells, bind peptides from proteins degraded in the cytosol. Typically, foreign peptides presented by MHC class I molecules come from viral proteins, and the CD8 T cell kills the infected cell upon recognizing the foreign peptide:MHC class I complex on the cell surface. Thus, the two classes of MHC molecule deliver peptides from different cellular compartments to the cell surface where they are recognized by T cells mediating distinct and appropriate effector functions.

The major histocompatibility complex of genes: organization and polymorphism.

The function of the MHC molecules is to bind peptide fragments derived from pathogens and display them on the cell surface for recognition by the appropriate T cells. The consequences of such presentation are almost always deleterious to the pathogen; virus-infected cells are killed, macrophages are activated to kill bacteria in intracellular vesicles, and B cells are activated to produce antibody molecules capable of eliminating or neutralizing extracellular pathogens. Thus, there is strong selective pressure in favor of any pathogen that can mutate its structural genes to escape presentation by an MHC molecule.

Two separate properties of the MHC make it difficult for pathogens to evade immune responses in this way: first, the MHC is **polygenic**—there are several MHC class I and MHC class II genes, encoding proteins with different ranges of peptide-binding specificities; second, the MHC is highly **polymorphic**—there are multiple alleles of each gene. The MHC genes are, in fact, the most polymorphic genes known. In this section, we shall describe the organization of the genes in the MHC and discuss how the allelic variation in MHC molecules arises. We shall also see how the effect of polygeny and polymorphism on the range of peptides bound contributes to the ability of the immune system to respond to a multitude of different and rapidly evolving pathogens.

4-14   The proteins involved in antigen processing and presentation are encoded by genes in the major histocompatibility complex.

The major histocompatibility complex extends over 2–3 centimorgans of DNA, or about 4×10^6 base pairs, and contains more than 100 genes in humans. The genes encoding the α chains of MHC class I molecules and the α and β chains of MHC class II molecules are linked within the complex; the genes for β_2-microglobulin and the invariant chain lie on separate chromosomes. Fig. 4.15 shows the general organization of these genes in the MHC of humans and of the mouse. The particular combination of MHC alleles found on an individual chromosome is known as an **MHC haplotype**.

In humans, there are three class I α-chain genes, called HLA-A, -B, and -C. There are also three pairs of MHC class II α- and β-chain genes, called HLA-DR, -DP, and -DQ. However, in many haplotypes, the HLA-DR cluster

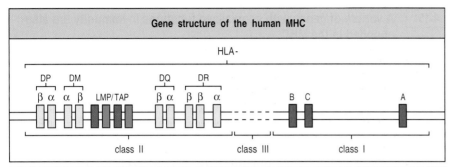

Gene structure of the human MHC

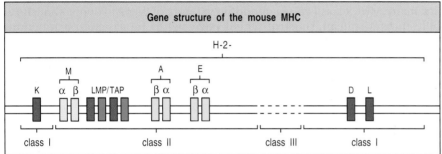

Gene structure of the mouse MHC

Fig. 4.16 The genetic organization of the major histocompatibility complex (MHC) in humans and the mouse. The organization of the principal MHC genes is shown for both human (where the MHC is called HLA and is on chromosome 6) and mouse (where the MHC is called H-2 and is on chromosome 17). The organization of the MHC genes is similar in both species. There are separate regions of MHC class I and MHC class II genes, although in the mouse an MHC class I gene appears to have translocated relative to the human MHC so that, in mice, the class I region is split in two. In both species there are three main class I genes, which are called HLA-A, -B, and -C in humans and H-2K,D, and L in the mouse. The gene for β_2-microglobulin, although it encodes part of the MHC class I molecule, is located on a different chromosome—15 in humans and 2 in the mouse. The genes for the TAP-1:TAP-2 peptide transporter, the LMP genes that encode proteasome subunits, and the DMA and DMB genes (encoding DMα and DMβ chains) are also in the MHC class II region. The so-called class III genes encode various other proteins with functions in immunity (see Fig. 4.17).

contains an extra β-chain gene whose product can pair with the DRα chain. This means that the three sets of genes give rise to four types of MHC class II molecule. All the MHC class I and class II molecules are capable of presenting antigens to T cells and, as each protein binds a different range of peptides, the presence of several loci means that any one individual is equipped to present a much broader range of different peptides than if only one MHC protein of each class were expressed at the cell surface.

The two TAP genes lie in the MHC class II region, in close association with the LMP genes that encode components of the proteasome. The genetic linkage of the MHC class I molecules, which deliver cytosolic peptides to the cell surface with the TAP and proteasome genes, which encode the molecules that generate these peptides in the cytosol and transport them into the endoplasmic reticulum, suggests that the entire major histocompatibility complex has been selected during evolution for antigen processing and presentation.

Moreover, when cells are treated with the cytokines interferon-α, -β or -γ, transcription of MHC class I α chain, β_2-microglobulin, and the MHC-linked proteasome and TAP genes are all markedly increased. Interferon-γ is produced early in viral infections as part of the innate immune response, as described in more detail in Chapter 9, and this effect of interferon-γ, which increases the ability of cells to process viral proteins and present the resulting peptides at the cell surface, can help to activate T cells and initiate the later phases of the immune response. The coordinated regulation of the genes encoding these components may be facilitated by the linkage of many of them in the MHC.

The DM genes, whose function is to catalyze peptide binding to MHC class II molecules, are clearly related to the class II genes. They are coordinately regulated with the genes encoding other MHC class II molecules and the invariant chain; expression of all of them is induced by interferon-γ (but not by interferon-α or -β), which induces the production of a transcriptional activator known as **MHC class II transactivator (CIITA)**. The absence of CIITA in patients with the bare lymphocyte syndrome causes severe immunodeficiency as described later, in Chapter 10.

4-15   **A variety of genes with specialized functions in immunity are also encoded in the MHC.**

While the most important known function of the gene products of the MHC is the processing and presentation of antigens to T cells, many other genes map within this region and, although some of these are known to have other roles in the immune system, many have yet to be characterized functionally. Fig. 4.17 shows the detailed organization of the human MHC.

In addition to the highly polymorphic MHC class I and class II genes, there are many MHC class I genes encoding variants of these proteins that show little polymorphism, most of which have yet to be assigned a function. These genes are linked to the class I region of the MHC and the exact number of genes varies greatly between species and even between members of the same species. These genes have been termed **MHC class IB** genes, and like MHC class I genes, they encode β2-microglobulin-associated

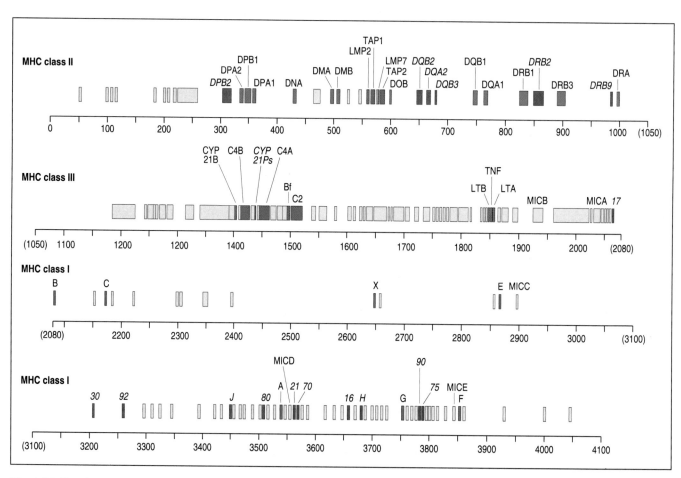

Fig. 4.17 Detailed map of the human MHC region. The organization of the class I, class II, and class III regions of the MHC are shown, with approximate genetic distances given in thousands of base pairs (kb). Most of the genes in the class I and class II region are mentioned in the text; the additional genes indicated in the class I region (for example HLA-E, -F, -G, -H, -J, and -X) are class I-like genes, encoding class IB molecules, while the additional class II genes are pseudogenes. The genes shown in the class III region encode the complement proteins C4 (there are two C4 genes, shown as C4A and C4B), C2 and Factor B (shown as Bf) as well as genes that encode the cytokines tumor necrosis factor (TNF) -α and -β. Closely linked to the C4 genes are the genes encoding 21-hydroxylase (shown as CYP 21A and CYP 21B), an enzyme involved in steroid synthesis. Deficiencies in 21-hydroxylase cause congenital adrenal hyperplasia and salt-wasting syndrome. Many other genes (unmarked boxes) are also present in this part of the genome. It is not known if these have any role in the immune system.

cell-surface molecules. Their expression on cells is variable, both in the amount expressed at the cell surface and in the tissue distribution.

In mice, one of these molecules, H2-M3, can present peptides with N-formylated amino-termini, which is of interest since all prokaryotes initiate protein synthesis with N-formylmethionine. Cells infected with cytosolic bacteria can be killed by CD8 T cells that recognize N-formylated bacterial peptides bound to this MHC class IB molecule. Whether an equivalent class IB molecule exists in humans is not known.

The large number of MHC class IB genes (50 or more in the mouse) means that many different class IB molecules can exist in a single animal. These may, like the protein that presents N-formylmethionyl peptides, have specialized roles in antigen presentation. Some class IB genes appear to be under a different regulatory control from the classical MHC class I genes and are induced in response to cellular stress (such as heat shock). These MHC class IB genes may play a part in innate immunity, or in the induction of immune responses in circumstances where interferons are not produced.

Other MHC class IB genes may function to inhibit cell killing by NK cells, a role apparently played by several class I MHC molecules, and one we will discuss in more detail in Chapter 9. Such a role has been suggested for the MHC class I molecule HLA-G, which is expressed on fetal-derived placental cells that migrate into the uterine wall. These cells express no classical MHC class I molecules and cannot be recognized by CD8 T cells but, unlike other cells lacking classical MHC class I molecules, they are not killed by NK cells. The combination of the lack of classical MHC class I molecules and the expression of HLA-G may protect the fetus from attack by either CD8 T cells or NK cells.

In addition to the DM molecule discussed in Section 4-12, another non-polymorphic MHC class II-like molecule is encoded within the MHC class II region. The DO molecule is formed from the pairing of the DNα and DOβ chains; these genes appear to be expressed only in the thymus and on B cells. The role of the DO gene products in the immune system is unknown.

Of the other genes that map within the MHC, some have products such as the complement components C2, Factor B and C4 or the cytokines tumor necrosis factor-α and tumor necrosis factor-β (lymphotoxin), that have important functions in immunity. These have been termed MHC class III genes, and are shown in Fig. 4.17. The functions of these genes will be discussed in Chapters 8 and 9.

Some MHC class I-like genes map outside the MHC region. One family of such genes, called CD1, also functions in antigen presentation to T cells, although it does not present peptide antigens. In cells infected with mycobacteria, the CD1 molecule is able to bind and present the mycobacterial membrane components mycolic acid and lipoarabinomannan. Whether CD1 molecules can also present peptide antigens remains to be determined.

As we shall see in Chapter 12, many studies have established associations between susceptibility to certain diseases and particular allelic variants of genes in the MHC. While most of these diseases are known, or suspected to have an immune etiology, this is not true of all of them, and it is important to remember that there are many genes lying within the MHC that have no known or suspected immunological function. One of these is the enzyme 21-hydroxylase, deficiencies of which cause congenital adrenal hyperplasia and, in severe cases, salt-wasting syndrome. Disease associations mapping to the MHC must therefore be interpreted with caution, in the light of a detailed understanding of its genetic structure and the functions of its individual genes. Much remains to be learned about the latter and about the significance of all the genetic variation localized within the MHC. For instance, the C4 genes are highly polymorphic, and this genetic variability may have adaptive significance in resistance to disease, as in the case of the MHC class I and class II proteins, to which we now turn.

4-16 | The protein products of MHC class I and class II genes are highly polymorphic.

Since there are three genes encoding MHC class I molecules and four possible sets of MHC class II molecules, every individual will express at least three different MHC class I proteins and four MHC class II proteins on his or her cells. In fact, the number of different MHC proteins expressed on the cells of most individuals is greater because of the extreme polymorphism of the MHC and the co-dominant expression of MHC genes.

The term **polymorphism** comes from the Greek *poly*, meaning many, and *morph*, meaning shape or structure. As used here, it means variation at a single genetic locus and its product within a species; the individual variant genes are termed **alleles**. There are more than 100 alleles of some MHC class I and class II loci (Fig. 4.18), each allele being present at a relatively high frequency in the population. For these reasons, the chance that the corresponding MHC locus on both chromosomes of an individual will encode the same allele is small; most individuals will be **heterozygous** at these loci. The products of both alleles are expressed on the same cell, so expression is said to be co-dominant, and both function in presenting antigens to T cells (Fig. 4.19). The extensive polymorphism at each locus has the potential to double the number of distinct MHC molecules expressed in an individual and thereby increases the diversity already available through polygeny, the existence of multiple functionally equivalent loci (Fig. 4.20).

Thus, with three MHC class I genes and four potential sets of MHC class II genes on each chromosome, a typical human will express six different

Fig. 4.18 Human MHC genes are highly polymorphic. With the notable exception of the DRα locus, which is monomorphic, each locus has many alleles. The number of different alleles is shown in this figure by the height of the bars and is obtained from studies mainly of Caucasoid populations. In other populations, such as Amerindian or Oriental populations, new alleles are found, so that the total diversity in these loci is greater than represented here. In fact, it is impossible to determine the total amount of variability at these loci without detailed worldwide studies.

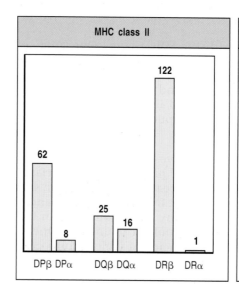
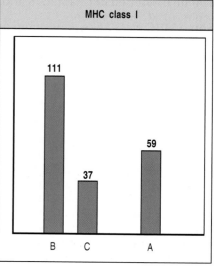

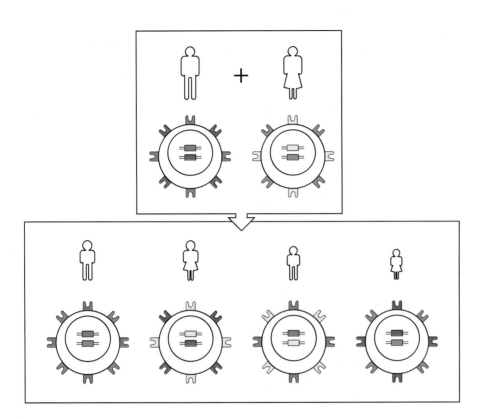

Fig. 4.19 Expression of MHC alleles is co-dominant. The MHC is so polymorphic that most individuals are likely to be heterozygous at each locus. Alleles are expressed from both MHC haplotypes in any one individual, and the products of all alleles are found on all expressing cells. In any mating, there are four possible combinations of haplotypes that can be found in the offspring; thus siblings are also likely to differ in the MHC alleles they express, there being one chance in four that an individual will share both haplotypes with a sibling. One consequence of this is the difficulty in finding suitable donors for tissue transplantation.

MHC class I molecules and eight different MHC class II molecules on his or her cells. For the MHC class II genes, the number of different products may be increased still further by the combination of α and β chains from different chromosomes (so that two α chains and two β chains can give rise to four different products). In mice, it has been shown that not all combinations of α and β chains can pair to form stable dimers and so, in practice, the exact number of different MHC class II molecules expressed will depend on which alleles are present on each chromosome.

All MHC products are polymorphic to a greater or lesser extent, with the exception of the DRα chain and its homolog Eα in the mouse. These chains do not vary in sequence between different individuals and are said to be **monomorphic**. This might indicate a functional constraint that prevents variation in the DRα and Eα proteins but no such special function has yet been found. Many mice, both domestic and wild, have a mutation in the Eα gene that prevents synthesis of the Eα protein, and thus lack cell-surface E molecules; so if E molecules have a special function it is unlikely to be an essential one. All other MHC class I and class II genes are polymorphic.

Fig. 4.20 Polymorphism and polygeny contribute to the diversity of MHC molecules expressed by an individual. The MHC genes are highly polymorphic, so that each individual is likely to be heterozygous, that is, to express two different allelic MHC molecules from each locus. However, no matter how polymorphic the genes, no individual can express more than two alleles of a given gene. The duplication of the MHC genes, leading to polygeny, overcomes this limitation. Polymorphism and polygeny combine to produce the diversity in MHC molecules seen both within an individual, and in the population at large.

Polymorphism

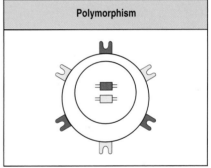

Polygeny

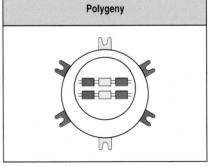

Polymorphism and polygeny

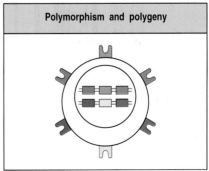

| 4-17 | MHC polymorphism affects antigen recognition indirectly by controlling peptide binding. |

The products of individual MHC alleles can differ from one another by up to 20 amino acids, making each allele quite distinct. Most of these differences are localized to exposed surfaces of the outer domain of the molecule, and to the peptide-binding groove in particular (Fig. 4.21). The polymorphic residues that line the peptide-binding groove determine the peptide-binding properties of the different MHC molecules.

We have seen that peptides bind to MHC class I molecules through specific anchor residues (see Section 4-4), which are peptide amino-acid side chains bound in pockets lining the peptide-binding groove. Polymorphism in MHC class I molecules affects the amino acids lining these pockets and thus their binding specificity. In consequence, the anchor residues of peptides that bind to each allelic variant are different. The set of anchor residues that allows binding to a given MHC class I molecule is called a **sequence motif**. These sequence motifs make it possible to identify peptides within a protein that can potentially bind the appropriate MHC molecule, which may be very important in designing peptide vaccines (see Chapter 13). Different allelic variants of MHC class II molecules also bind different peptides but the more open structure of the MHC class II peptide-binding groove, and the greater length of the peptides bound in it, allow greater flexibility in peptide binding. It is therefore more difficult to predict which peptides will bind to MHC class II molecules.

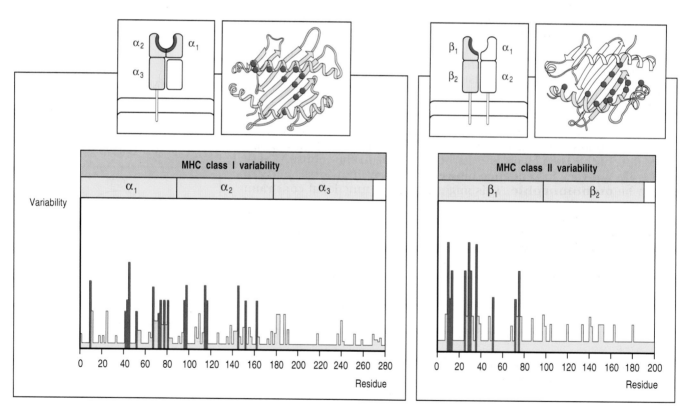

Fig. 4.21 Allelic variation occurs at specific sites within the MHC molecules. Variability plots of the MHC molecules show that the variation arising from polymorphism in the MHC molecules is restricted to the amino-terminal domains (α_1 and α_2 domains of class I and predominantly the β_1 domain of MHC class II molecules), the domains that form the peptide-binding cleft. Moreover, allelic variability is clustered in specific sites within the amino-terminal domains, lying in positions that line the peptide-binding cleft, either on the floor of the groove or directed inwards from the walls.

As different MHC molecules bind different peptides, the T cells responding to a given protein antigen presented by several different MHC molecules will usually have to recognize different peptides. In rare cases, a protein will have no peptides with a suitable motif for binding to any of the MHC molecules expressed on the cells of an individual. When this happens, the individual fails to respond to the antigen. Such failures in responsiveness to simple antigens were first reported in inbred animals, where they were called **immune response (Ir) gene defects**, long before the function of MHC molecules was understood. These defects could be mapped to genes within the MHC and were the first clue to the antigen-presenting function of MHC molecules; however, it was only much later that the Ir genes were shown to encode MHC class II molecules. Ir gene defects are common in inbred strains of mice because the mice are homozygous for all their MHC genes and thus express only one allelic variant from each gene locus. Ordinarily, the polymorphism of MHC molecules guarantees a sufficient number of different MHC molecules in a single individual to make this type of non-responsiveness unlikely, even to relatively simple antigens such as small toxins. This has obvious importance for host defense.

4-18 MHC polymorphism directly affects antigen recognition by T cells.

Ir gene defects were identified in experimental animals (guinea pigs and subsequently mice) through the failure to mount an immune response to specific foreign antigens. Initially, the only evidence linking the defect to the MHC was genetic—mice of one MHC genotype could make antibody in response to a particular antigen, while mice of a different MHC genotype, but otherwise genetically identical, could not. MHC molecules were somehow controlling the ability of the immune system to detect or respond to specific antigens but it was not clear at that time that direct recognition of MHC molecules was involved.

This emerged from later experiments. The immune responses affected by the Ir genes were known to be dependent upon T cells, and this led to a series of experiments aimed at ascertaining how MHC polymorphism might control the responses of T cells. The earliest of these experiments showed that T cells could be activated only by macrophages or B cells that shared MHC alleles with the mouse in which the T cells originated; this provided the first evidence that T cells recognize MHC molecules themselves. The clearest example of this recognition, however, came from studies of virus-specific cytotoxic T cells for which Peter Doherty and Rolf Zinkernagel won the Nobel Prize in 1996.

When mice are infected with a virus, they generate cytotoxic T cells that kill self cells infected with the virus, while sparing uninfected cells or cells infected with unrelated viruses. The cytotoxic T cells are thus virus-specific. A particularly striking outcome of these experiments, however, was that the specificity of the cytotoxic T cells was also affected by allelic polymorphism in MHC molecules: cytotoxic T cells induced by viral infection in mice of MHC genotype a (MHC^a) would kill any MHC^a cell infected with that virus but would not kill cells of MHC genotype b, or c, and so on, even if they were infected with the same virus. Since the MHC genotype restricts the antigen specificity of T cells, this effect is called **MHC restriction**. Together with the earlier studies on both B cells and macrophages, this showed that MHC restriction is a critical feature of antigen recognition by all functional classes of T cells.

Since different MHC molecules bind different peptides, MHC restriction in responses to viruses and other complex antigens could be explained solely on this indirect basis. However, it can be seen from Fig. 4.21 that some of the polymorphic amino acids on MHC molecules are located on the α helices flanking the peptide-binding cleft in such a way that they

Fig. 4.22 T-cell recognition of antigens is MHC-restricted. The antigen-specific receptor of T cells (TCR) recognizes a complex of antigenic peptide and MHC. One consequence of this is that a T cell specific for peptide x and a particular MHC allele, MHC^a (left panel), will not recognize the complex of peptide x with a different MHC allele, MHC^b (center panel), or the complex of antigen y with MHC^a (right panel). The co-recognition of peptide and MHC molecule is known as MHC restriction because the MHC molecule is said to restrict the ability of the T cell to recognize antigen. This restriction may result either from direct contact between MHC molecule and T-cell receptor, or be an indirect effect of MHC polymorphism on the peptides that bind or on their bound conformation.

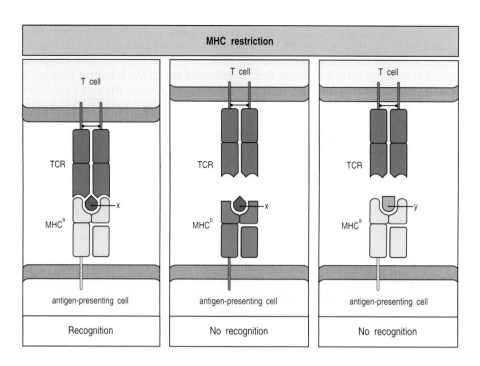

would be exposed on the outer surface of the peptide:MHC complex. It is therefore not surprising that, when T cells are tested for their ability to recognize the same peptide bound to different MHC molecules, they readily distinguish peptide-bound MHC^a from the same peptide bound to MHC^b. Thus, specificity in a T-cell receptor is defined both by the peptide and by the MHC molecule binding it (Fig. 4.22). This restricted recognition is sometimes caused by differences in the conformation of the bound peptide imposed by the different MHC molecules and sometimes by the conformational changes that occur in the MHC molecule on binding different peptides, rather than by direct recognition of polymorphic amino acids on the MHC molecule itself. However, it can be shown by other means that direct contact of the T-cell receptor with polymorphic residues on the MHC molecule affects antigen recognition, and thus MHC restriction in antigen recognition reflects the combined effect of differences in peptide binding, and of direct contact between the MHC molecule and the T-cell receptor.

The discovery of MHC restriction, in revealing the physiological function of the MHC molecules, also led to the explanation of the otherwise puzzling phenomenon of non-self MHC recognition in graft rejection, to which we shall turn briefly before discussing other implications of MHC polymorphism.

4-19   Non-self MHC molecules are recognized by 1–10% of T cells.

Transplanted tissues or organs from donors bearing MHC molecules that differ from those of the recipient are reliably rejected. Tissue grafts can be rejected on the basis of MHC molecules that differ by as little as one amino acid. This rapid and very potent cell-mediated immune response results from the presence of large numbers of T cells in any individual that are specifically reactive to particular non-self or **allogeneic** MHC molecules. Studies on T-cell responses to allogeneic MHC molecules using the mixed lymphocyte reaction (see Section 2-24) have shown that roughly 1–10% of all T cells in an individual will respond to stimulation by cells from any allogeneic individual. This type of T-cell response is called **alloreactivity** because it represents recognition of allelic polymorphism on allogeneic MHC molecules.

Foreign peptide: self-MHC binding	Peptide-dominant binding	MHC-dominant binding
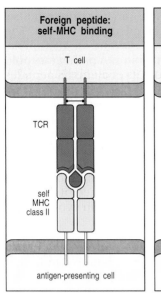	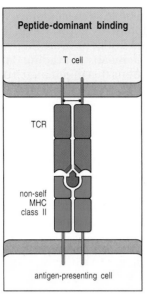	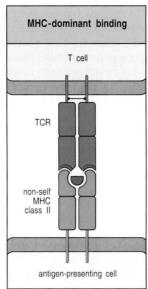

Fig. 4.23 Two modes of cross-reactive recognition that may explain allo-reactivity. A T cell that is specific for one peptide:MHC combination (left panel) may cross-react with peptides presented by other (allogeneic) MHC molecules. This may come about in either of two ways: most commonly, the peptides bound to the allogeneic MHC molecule fit well to the T-cell receptor (TCR), allowing binding even though there is not a good fit with the MHC molecule (center panel); alternatively, but less often, the allogeneic MHC molecule may provide a better fit to the T-cell receptor, giving a tight binding that is independent of the peptide bound to the MHC molecule (right panel).

Before the role of the MHC molecules in antigen presentation was understood, it was a mystery why so many T cells should recognize non-self MHC molecules, as there is no reason why the immune system should have evolved a defense against tissue transplants. It is now thought that this alloreactivity reflects cross-reactivity of T-cell receptors normally specific for a variety of foreign peptides bound by self MHC molecules. This cross-reactivity results, in part, because the spectrum of peptides bound by non-self MHC molecules on the transplanted tissues differ from those bound by the host's own MHC molecules, and the host's T cells are not tolerant to these new peptide:MHC complexes.

Given a T-cell receptor that is normally specific for a self MHC molecule binding a foreign peptide (Fig. 4.23, left panel), there are two ways in which it may bind to non-self MHC molecules. In some cases, the peptide bound by the non-self MHC molecule interacts strongly with the T-cell receptor, and the T-cells bearing this receptor are stimulated to respond. This type of cross-reactive recognition is known as peptide-dominant binding (see Fig. 4.23, center panel). In a second type of cross-reactive recognition, known as MHC-dominant binding, alloreactive T cells respond because of direct binding of the T-cell receptor to distinctive features of the non-self MHC molecule (see Fig. 4.23, right panel). In these cases, the recognition is independent of the type of peptide bound; T-cell receptor binding to unique features of the non-self MHC molecule generates a strong signal because of the high concentration of the non-self MHC molecule on the surface of the presenting cell. Both these mechanisms contribute to the high frequency of T cells responding to the non-self MHC molecules on the transplanted tissue, which clearly reflects the commitment of the T-cell receptor to the recognition of MHC molecules in general.

4-20 | MHC polymorphism extends the range of antigens to which the immune system can respond.

Most polymorphic genes encode proteins that vary by only one or a few amino acids. As we have seen, the different allelic variants of MHC proteins differ by up to 20 amino acids. The extensive polymorphism of the MHC proteins has almost certainly evolved to outflank the evasive strategies of pathogens.

Pathogens have several possible strategies for avoiding an immune response, either by evading detection or by suppressing the ensuing response. The requirement that pathogen antigens must be presented by an MHC molecule provides two possible means of evading detection. A pathogen could escape detection by mutations that eliminated from its proteins all peptides able to bind MHC molecules. An example of this type of strategy can be seen in regions of South East China and in Papua New Guinea, where about 60% of individuals in these small isolated populations carry the HLA-A11 allele. Many isolates of the Epstein-Barr virus obtained in these populations have mutated a dominant epitope presented by HLA-A11, so that the mutant peptides no longer bind to HLA-A11 and cannot be recognized by HLA-A11-restricted T cells. This strategy is plainly much more difficult to follow if there are many different MHC molecules, and the presence of different loci encoding functionally related proteins may have been an evolutionary adaptation by hosts to this strategy by pathogens.

In large outbred populations, polymorphism at each locus can potentially double the number of different MHC molecules expressed by an individual, as most individuals will be heterozygotes. Polymorphism has the additional advantage that different individuals in a population will differ in the combinations of MHC molecules they express and will therefore present different sets of peptides from each pathogen. This makes it unlikely that all individuals in a population will be equally susceptible to a given pathogen and its spread will therefore be limited. That exposure to pathogens over an evolutionary timescale can select for expression of particular MHC alleles is strongly indicated by the strong association of the HLA-B53 allele with recovery from a potentially lethal form of malaria; this allele is very common in individuals from West Africa where malaria is endemic.

Similar arguments apply to a second possibility for evading recognition. If pathogens could develop mechanisms to block the presentation of their peptides by MHC molecules, they could avoid the adaptive immune response. Adenoviruses encode a protein that binds to MHC class I molecules in the endoplasmic reticulum and prevents their transport to the cell surface, thus preventing recognition of viral peptides by CD8 cytotoxic T cells. This MHC-binding protein must interact with a polymorphic region of the MHC class I molecule, as some alleles are retained in the endoplasmic reticulum while others are not. Increasing the variety of MHC molecules expressed therefore reduces the likelihood that a pathogen will be able to block presentation by all of them, and so completely evade an immune response.

These arguments raise a question: if having three MHC class I loci offers an advantage that is amplified by allelic variation, why are there not far more MHC class I loci? A full answer to this question must await a discussion of the mechanisms by which the repertoire of T-cell receptors is selected in the thymus, which will be the topic of Chapter 6. Briefly, the probable explanation is that each time a distinct MHC molecule is added to the MHC repertoire, all T cells that can recognize self peptides bound to that molecule must be removed in order to maintain self tolerance. It seems that the number of MHC loci present in humans and mice is about optimal to balance out the advantages of presenting an increased range of foreign peptides and the disadvantages of increased presentation of self peptides and the loss of T cells that accompanies it.

4-21   Multiple genetic processes generate MHC polymorphism.

MHC polymorphism appears to have been selected strongly by evolutionary pressures. However, for selection to work efficiently in slowly reproducing organisms like humans, there must also be powerful mechanisms that

Fig. 4.24 Gene conversion can create new allelic variants by transferring sequences from one MHC gene to another. Sequences can be transferred from one gene to a similar gene by a process known as gene conversion. In this process, which can occur between two alleles or, as shown here, between two closely related genes generated by gene duplication during evolution, the two genes are apposed during meiosis. This can occur as a consequence of the misalignment of the two chromosomes when there are many copies of similar genes arrayed in tandem—somewhat like buttoning in the wrong buttonhole. The DNA sequence from one chromosome can then be copied to the other, giving rise to a new gene sequence. In this way several nucleotide changes can be inserted all at once into a gene and can cause several amino acid changes between the new gene and the original gene. The process of gene conversion has occurred many times in the evolution of MHC alleles.

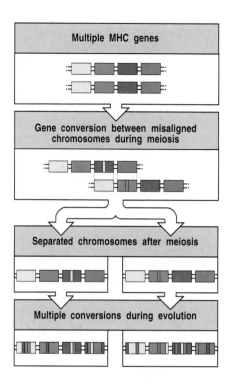

generate variability in MHC alleles on which selection can act. The generation of polymorphism in MHC molecules is an evolutionary problem not readily analyzed in the laboratory; however, it is clear that several genetic mechanisms contribute to the generation of new alleles. Some new alleles are the result of point mutations but many arise from combining sequences from different alleles either by genetic recombination or by **gene conversion**, in which one sequence is replaced, in part, by another from a homologous gene (Fig. 4.24).

Evidence for gene conversion comes from studies of the sequences of different MHC alleles, which reveal that some changes involve clusters of several amino acids in the MHC molecule and require multiple nucleotide changes in a contiguous stretch of the gene. Even more significantly, the same sequences are found within other MHC genes on the same chromosome, a prerequisite for gene conversion. Recombination between alleles at the same locus may, however, have been more important than gene conversion in generating MHC polymorphism. A comparison of sequences of MHC alleles shows that many different alleles could represent recombination events between a set of hypothetical ancestral alleles. If one postulates a small number of ancestral alleles, most present-day alleles could have been generated by one or more recombination events (Fig. 4.25).

The effects of selective pressure in favor of polymorphism can be seen clearly in the pattern of point mutations in the MHC genes. Point mutations can be classified as replacement substitutions, which change an amino acid, or silent substitutions, which simply change the codon but leave the amino acid the same. Replacement substitutions occur within the MHC at a higher frequency relative to silent substitutions than would be expected, providing evidence that polymorphism has been actively selected for in the evolution of the MHC.

Summary.

The major histocompatibility complex (MHC) of genes consists of a linked set of genetic loci encoding many of the proteins involved in antigen presentation to T cells, most notably the MHC glycoproteins that present peptides to the T-cell receptor. The outstanding feature of MHC genes is their extensive polymorphism. This polymorphism is of critical importance in antigen recognition by T cells. A T cell recognizes antigen as a peptide bound by a particular allelic variant of an MHC molecule,

Position of polymorphic regions in one domain of MHC structure

Strain 1

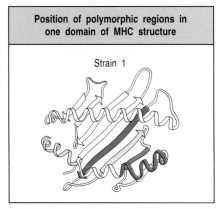

Position of polymorphic regions in one domain of MHC structure

Strain 8

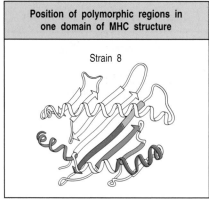

Polymorphic regions in alleles from closely related strains

Strain 1

Strain 2

Strain 3

Strain 4

Polymorphic regions in alleles from distantly related strains

Strain 5

Strain 6

Strain 7

Strain 8

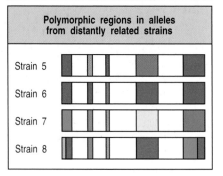

Fig. 4.25 Recombination can create new alleles by reassorting discrete polymorphic regions. Recombination differs from gene conversion in that the DNA segments are exchanged between different chromosomes rather than, as in gene conversion, being copied so that one sequence replaces sequences in another gene. Analysis of many MHC allele sequences has shown that the swapping of segments of DNA has occurred many times in the evolution of MHC alleles. The variable parts of MHC domains correspond to segments of the structure, such as β strands or parts of the α helix, as shown in the upper two panels. Closely related strains of mice have MHC genes where only one or two segments have been swapped between alleles (third panel), while more distantly related strains show a patchwork effect that results from the accumulation of many such recombination events (fourth panel).

and will not recognize the same peptide bound to other MHC molecules. This behavior of T cells is called MHC restriction. Most MHC alleles differ from one another by multiple amino acid substitutions, and these differences are focused on the peptide-binding site and adjacent regions that make direct contact with the T-cell receptor. At least three properties of MHC molecules are affected by MHC polymorphism: the range of peptides bound; the conformation of the bound peptide; and the interaction of the MHC molecule directly with the T-cell receptor. Thus the highly polymorphic nature of the MHC has functional consequences, and the evolutionary selection for this polymorphism suggests that it is critical to the role of the MHC molecules in the immune response. Powerful genetic mechanisms generate the variation that is seen among MHC alleles, and an argument can be made that selective pressure to maintain a wide variety of MHC molecules in the population comes from infectious agents.

The T-cell receptor complex.

The mechanisms by which a diverse set of B-cell antigen receptors is generated through recombination of a limited set of gene segments are so powerful that it is not surprising that the antigen receptor of T cells is generated by the same mechanism. The T-cell antigen receptor resembles a membrane-bound Fab fragment of immunoglobulin and, like the surface immunoglobulin of B cells (see Section 3-25), is associated on the cell surface with a complex of invariant proteins that are required for signal transduction. In this section, we shall describe the structure of the T-cell receptor proteins and the organization of the T-cell receptor genes. We shall also see how, despite their overall similarity, T-cell receptors differ from immunoglobulins in important ways, and how the MHC-binding co-receptor molecules CD4 and CD8 contribute to antigen recognition.

4-22   The T-cell receptor resembles a membrane-associated Fab fragment of immunoglobulin.

T-cell receptors were first identified using monoclonal antibodies specific for individual cloned T-cell lines (see Section 2-20) that could specifically inhibit antigen recognition. These **clonotypic** antibodies were then used to show that each T cell bears about 30 000 antigen receptor molecules

Fig. 4.26 The T-cell receptor resembles a membrane-bound Fab fragment. The Fab fragment of antibody molecules is a disulfide-linked heterodimer, each chain of which contains one immunoglobulin constant domain and one variable domain; the juxtaposition of the variable domains forms the antigen-binding site (see Chapter 3). The T-cell receptor is also a disulfide-linked heterodimer, with each chain containing an immunoglobulin constant-like domain and an immunoglobulin variable-like domain. Finally, as in the Fab fragment, the juxtaposition of the variable regions forms the antigen-recognition site.

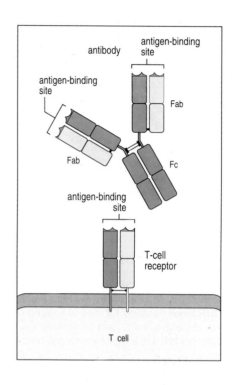

on its surface, each receptor consisting of two different polypeptide chains, termed the **T-cell receptor α and β chains**, bound to one another by a disulfide bond in a structure that is very similar to the Fab fragment of an immunoglobulin molecule (Fig. 4.26). These α:β heterodimers account for antigen recognition by all the functional classes of T cells we have described so far. There is an alternative type of T-cell receptor made up of different polypeptides designated γ and δ but its discovery was unexpected and its functional significance is not yet clear, as we shall see later (see Section 4-31).

Although the use of clonotypic antibodies enabled some characteristic features of the **α:β T-cell receptor** to be determined, most of what we now know about its structure and function came from studies of cloned DNA encoding the receptor chains. The genes encoding the T-cell receptor α and β chains were first identified as cDNAs that were isolated on the basis of their expression in T cells but not B cells. As T and B cells are closely related, there are relatively few such cDNAs. Those encoding the T-cell receptor were sought on the basis of two criteria. First, it was expected that they would be encoded by gene segments that had undergone rearrangement only in T cells. The second criterion was sequence homology to immunoglobulin. Using these approaches, the first cDNAs encoding T-cell receptor α and β chains were identified. Preliminary peptide fragmentation studies of T-cell receptors isolated using clonotypic antibodies indicated that, like antibodies, they contain variable and constant peptides. However, it was the predicted amino-acid sequence from T-cell receptor cDNAs that demonstrated clearly that both chains of the T-cell receptor have an amino-terminal variable region with homology to an immunoglobulin V domain, a constant region with homology to an immunoglobulin C domain, and a short hinge region with a cysteine residue that forms the interchain disulfide bond (Fig. 4.27). Each chain spans the lipid bilayer by a hydrophobic transmembrane domain whose notable feature is the presence of positively charged amino acids. The presence of such charged residues in transmembrane domains is unusual and would normally tend to destabilize them. We will see later that these charged residues play an important part in the interaction of the T-cell receptor chains with oppositely charged polypeptides known as CD3 γ, δ, and ε, which are homologous to the Igα and Igβ proteins of the B-cell receptor. Finally, each chain ends with a short cytoplasmic domain.

Fig. 4.27 Structure of the T-cell receptor. The T-cell receptor heterodimer is composed of two transmembrane glycoprotein chains, α and β. The external portion of each chain consists of two domains, resembling immunoglobulin variable and constant domains, respectively. Both chains have carbohydrate side chains attached to each domain. A short segment, analogous to an immunoglobulin hinge region, connects the immunoglobulin-like domains to the membrane and contains the cysteine that forms the interchain disulfide bond. The transmembrane helices of both chains are unusual in containing positively charged (basic) residues within the hydrophobic transmembrane segment. The α chains carry two such residues, while the β chains have one.

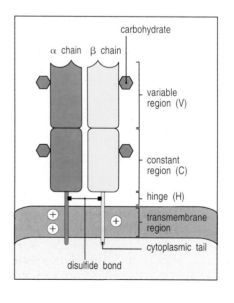

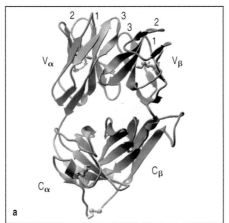 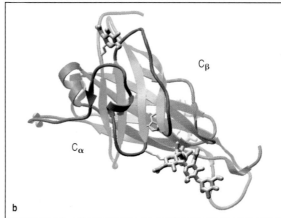 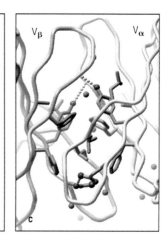

Fig. 4.28 The crystal structure of an α:β T-cell receptor resolved at 2.5 Å. In all panels the α chain is shown in purple and the β chain in blue. In panel a, the T-cell receptor is viewed as it would sit on a cell surface with the MHC:peptide binding CDR loops (labelled 1,2, and 3) arrayed across its relatively flat top. In panel b, the C_α and C_β domains are shown. The C_α domain does not fold into a typical immunoglobulin-like domain, one face of the domain being mainly composed of irregular strands of polypeptide rather than β sheet. In panel c, the V_α:V_β interface is shown. The number of residues forming this interface is small enough to accomodate conformational changes upon ligand binding, although there is as yet no evidence that such changes occur. Photographs courtesy of I A Wilson.

The V-like domains comprise V-, D- and J-like elements in the β chain and V- and J-like elements in the α chain. It is these close similarities of T-cell receptor chains to the heavy and light immunoglobulin chains that lead to the conclusion that T-cell receptor proteins must closely resemble a Fab fragment of immunoglobulin. The structure of the T-cell receptor heterodimer has been determined directly. As expected, it folds in much the same way as an antibody Fab fragment (Fig. 4.28). However, there are also distinct differences. The CDR loops align relatively closely with those of antibody molecules (see Fig. 4.28, left panel) but there is some displacement relative to those of the antibody molecule. Second, the packing of the C domains is distinctive, which produces a different angle in the bend between the V_β and C_β, assisted by carbohydrate packing in the structure (see Fig. 4.28, center panel). Third, there are relatively fewer contacts between the two V domains than in antibody molecules, perhaps explaining the difficulty initially encountered in preparing such crystals (see Fig. 4.28, right panel). It remains to be seen whether this structure is shared by all T-cell receptors, and what the effect is of ligand binding on the overall structure.

T-cell receptors differ from B-cell receptors in that the T-cell receptor is monovalent, while immunoglobulin is bivalent, and in that the T-cell receptor is never secreted, while immunoglobulin is adapted to be secreted upon B-cell activation (see Fig. 3.33).

4-23   The T-cell receptor genes resemble immunoglobulin genes.

The organization of the gene segments encoding T-cell receptor α and β chains (Fig. 4.29) is generally homologous to that of the immunoglobulin gene segments (see Sections 3-11 and 3-12 for comparison). The α chains, like immunoglobulin light chains, are assembled from V and J gene segments, although the T-cell receptor α-chain genes have many more J gene segments. 61 J_α gene segments are distributed over about 80 kb of DNA, while immunoglobulin light-chain genes have only five J gene segments. We shall see later that this has important consequences for the recognition of antigen by the T-cell receptor. The β-chain genes, like those of immunoglobulin heavy chains, have D gene segments in addition to V and J gene segments.

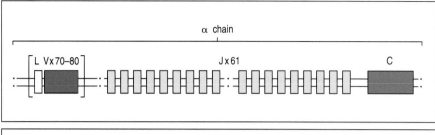

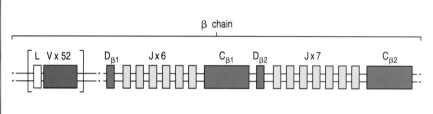

Fig. 4.29 The organization of the mouse T-cell receptor α- and β-chain genes. The arrangement of the gene segments resembles that of the immunoglobulins with separate variable (V), diversity (D), joining (J) and constant (C) gene segments. The α-chain gene consists of 70–80 variable segments, each containing an exon encoding a variable region (V) preceded by an exon encoding the leader sequence (L) that targets the protein to the endoplasmic reticulum for transport to the cell surface. How many of these are functional is not known exactly. A cluster of about 60 J gene segments is located a considerable distance from the V gene segments. The J gene segments are followed by a single constant-domain gene, which contains separate exons for the constant and hinge domains and a single exon encoding the transmembrane and cytoplasmic regions. The β-chain gene has a different organization with a cluster of about 50 functional V gene segments located distantly from two separate clusters each containing a single D gene segment, together with six or seven J gene segments and a single constant region gene. Each β-chain constant gene has separate exons encoding the constant, hinge, trans-membrane, and cytoplasmic regions. The α-chain locus is interrupted between the J and V segments by another TCR locus—the δ-chain locus (not shown here; see Fig. 4.37).

Like immunoglobulin genes in B cells, the T-cell receptor gene segments rearrange during development to form complete V-domain exons (Fig. 4.30). The process of T-cell receptor gene rearrangement takes place in the thymus and is dealt with in detail in Chapter 6, where selection of the T-cell repertoire is also discussed. Essentially, however, the mechanics of gene rearrangement are similar for B and T cells. The T-cell receptor gene segments are flanked by heptamer and nonamer recombination signal sequences homologous to those found in immunoglobulin genes (see Section 3-16) and are recognized by the same enzymes: defects in three distinct genes that control gene segment rearrangement affect T- and B-cell receptor genes equally, and animals with these genetic defects lack functional lymphocytes altogether.

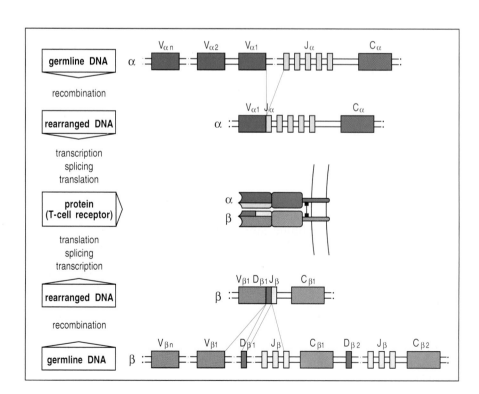

Fig. 4.30 T-cell receptor α- and β-chain gene rearrangement and expression. The T-cell receptor α- and β-chain genes are composed of discrete segments that are joined by somatic recombination during development of the T cell. Functional α- and β-chain genes are generated by the somatic recombination of gene segments in the same way that complete immunoglobulin genes are created. For the α chain, a V_α gene segment rearranges to a J_α gene segment to create a functional exon. Transcription and splicing of the VJ_α exon to C_α generates the mRNA that is translated to yield the T-cell receptor α-chain protein. For the β chains, like the immunoglobulin heavy chains (see Chapter 3), the variable domain is encoded in three gene segments, V_β, D_β, and J_β. Rearrangement of these gene segments generates a functional exon that is transcribed, spliced to join VDJ_β to C_β and the resulting mRNA translated to yield the T-cell receptor β-chain protein. The α and β chains pair soon after their biosynthesis to yield the α:β T-cell receptor heterodimer. Not all J gene segments are shown.

A further shared feature of immunoglobulin and T-cell receptor gene rearrangement is the presence of P- and N-nucleotides in the junctions between the V, D, and J gene segments of the β chain, although in T cells P- and N-nucleotides are also added between the V and J gene segments of all α chains, while V to J gene segment joints in immunoglobulin light-chain genes are only modified in some instances.

The main differences between the immunoglobulin genes and those encoding the T-cell receptor reflect the fact that all the effector functions of B cells depend upon secreted antibodies whose distinct constant-region isotypes trigger distinct effector mechanisms. The effector functions of T cells, on the other hand, depend upon cell–cell contact and are not mediated directly by the T-cell receptor, which serves only for antigen recognition. Thus, the constant-region genes of the T-cell receptor are much simpler than those of antibodies: there is only one C_α gene and, although there are two C_β genes, there is no known functional distinction between their products. The T-cell receptor constant-region genes encode only transmembrane polypeptides: there are no exons encoding an alternative secreted form.

4-24   T-cell receptor diversity is focused in CDR3.

The extent and pattern of diversity of T-cell receptors and immunoglobulins reflects the distinct nature of their ligands. While antibodies must conform to the surfaces of an almost infinite variety of different antigens, the ligand for the T-cell receptor is always an MHC molecule; the T-cell receptors therefore have a relatively invariant shape, with most of the variability focused on the bound antigenic peptide occupying the center of the surface in contact with the receptor.

The three-dimensional structure of a complete T-cell receptor looks much like that of an antibody molecule. In an antibody, the center of the antigen-binding site is formed by the third complementarity determining regions (CDR3) of the heavy and light chains. The structurally equivalent loops of the T-cell receptor α and β chains, to which the D and J gene segments contribute, also form the center of the antigen-binding site on T-cell receptors, while the periphery of the site consists of the equivalent of the CDR1 and CDR2 loops, which are encoded within the germline V gene segments for the α and β chains (see Fig. 4.28). T-cell receptor genes have roughly the same number of V gene segments as immunoglobulins, but only immunoglobulins show extensive diversification of expressed rearranged variable-region genes by somatic hypermutation. Thus, diversity in the periphery of the antigen-binding site of an antibody molecule comprising the CDR1 and CDR2 loops will be far greater than it is in a T-cell receptor.

Thus, comparing the origins of diversity in T-cell receptors and immunoglobulins (Fig. 4.31) bears out the prediction above. It can be seen that most of the variability in T-cell receptors occurs within the junctional region encoded by D-, J-, and N-nucleotides. This region encodes the CDR3 loops in immunoglobulins and T-cell receptors that form the center of the antigen-binding site. Thus, the center of the T-cell receptor will be highly variable, while the periphery will be subject to relatively little variation. So, when one superimposes the proposed structure of a T-cell receptor on its ligand, the most variable part of the receptor lies over the most variable part of the ligand, the bound foreign peptide. The periphery of the receptor, formed mainly from the CDR1 and CDR2 loops of the α and β variable domains, will contact the periphery of the ligand, comprising mainly amino acids contributed by the α helices of the two outer MHC domains. Exactly how the T-cell receptor is oriented with respect to the peptide:MHC complex, and whether the orientation

Element	Immunoglobulin		$\alpha\beta$ receptors	
	H	$\kappa+\lambda$	β	α
Variable segments (V)	51	69	52	~70
Diversity segments (D)	~30	0	2	0
D segments read in 3 frames	rarely	–	often	–
Joining segments (J)	5	5	13	61
Joints with N and P nucleotides	2	(1)	2	1
Number of V gene pairs	3519		3640	
Junctional diversity	~10^{13}		~10^{13}	
Total diversity	~10^{16}		~10^{16}	

Fig. 4.31 The numbers of human T-cell receptor gene segments and the sources of T-cell receptor diversity compared with those of immunoglobulin. The number of κ-chain joints with N and P regions is shown in brackets as only about half of human κ chains contain N and P regions.

is the same for different T-cell receptors, will remain unknown until the structure of a number of ternary T-cell receptor:MHC:peptide complexes is determined, but recent experiments suggest that the T-cell receptor α chain is oriented over the α_1 domains of the MHC class I or class II molecule while the β chain is oriented over the α_2 or β_1 domain.

4-25 **Somatic hypermutation is not a major mechanism for generating diversity in T-cell receptors.**

When we discussed the generation of antibody diversity in Section 3-14, we saw that somatic hypermutation increases the diversity of all three complementarity determining regions of both immunoglobulin chains. As a general principle, somatic hypermutation does not occur in T-cell receptor genes, so that variability of the CDR1 and CDR2 regions is limited to that of the germline V gene segments. Somatic mutation has been reported for the α and β chain V regions expressed by T cells isolated from germinal centers but it is not known whether these mutated α and β chains contribute to a cell-surface T-cell receptor and so generate an altered specificity. At present, therefore, it appears as though the bulk of diversity in T-cell receptors is generated during rearrangement and is consequently focused on the CDR3 regions.

Why T-cell and B-cell receptors differ in their ability to undergo somatic hypermutation is not clear but several explanations can be suggested on the basis of the functional differences between T and B cells. Since the central role of T cells is to stimulate both humoral and cellular immune responses, it is crucially important that T cells do not react with self proteins. T cells that recognize self antigens are rigorously purged during development (see Chapter 6) and the absence of somatic hypermutation helps to ensure that somatic mutants recognizing self proteins do not arise later in the course of immune responses. This constraint does not apply with the same force to B-cell receptors, as B cells usually require T-cell help in order to secrete antibodies. A B cell whose receptor mutates to become self reactive would, under normal circumstances, fail to make antibody for lack of self-reactive T cells to provide this help (see Section 3-26).

An additional argument might be that T cells already interact with a self component, namely the MHC molecule that makes up part of the ligand for the receptor, and thus might be unusually prone to developing self-recognition capability through somatic hypermutation. In this case, the converse argument can also be made: because T-cell receptors must be able to recognize self MHC molecules as part of their ligand, it is important to avoid somatic mutation that might result in the loss of recognition and consequent loss of any ability to respond. However, the strongest argument for this difference between immunoglobulins and T-cell receptors is the simple one that somatic hypermutation is an adaptive specialization for B cells alone, because they must make very high-affinity antibodies in order to capture toxin molecules in the extracellular fluids. We shall see in Chapter 8 that they do this through somatic hypermutation followed by selection for antigen binding.

4-26   Many T cells respond to superantigens.

Not all antigens that bind to MHC class II molecules are presented as peptides in the peptide-binding groove. A few fall into a distinct class known as **superantigens**, which have a distinctive mode of binding that enables them to stimulate very large numbers of T cells, often with disastrous consequences. Superantigens are produced by many different pathogens, including bacteria, mycoplasmas, and viruses, and bind directly to MHC molecules without being processed previously; indeed, fragmentation of a superantigen destroys its biological activity. Instead of binding in the groove of the MHC molecule, superantigens bind to the outer surface of both the MHC class II molecule and the Vβ region of the T-cell receptor (Fig. 4.32). Thus, the α chain V region and the DJ junction of the β chain of the T-cell receptor have little effect on superantigen recognition, which is determined largely by the V gene segment of the β chain gene. Each superantigen can bind one or a few of the different products of Vβ gene segments, of which there are 20–50 in mice and humans, so a superantigen can stimulate 2–20% of all T cells.

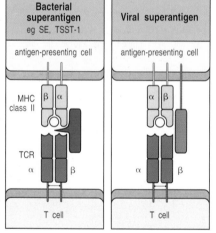

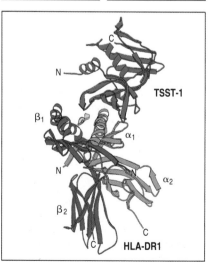

Fig. 4.32 Superantigens bind directly to T-cell receptors (TCR) and to MHC molecules. Superantigens interact with MHC class II molecules and T-cell receptors in a way that is quite distinct from the way that normal peptide antigens bind. Superantigens can bind independently to MHC class II molecules and to T-cell receptors, binding to the Vβ domain of the T-cell receptor, away from the complementarity determining regions, and to the outer faces of the MHC class II molecule, outside the peptide-binding site. Two distinct classes of superantigens have been described so far. Bacterial superantigens, like staphlyococcal enterotoxins (SEs) or the toxic shock syndrome toxin (TSST-1), are soluble proteins secreted by bacteria. The so-called endogenous viral superantigens are proteins expressed by some viruses that infect mammalian cells and integrate into the DNA of their host. The best characterized viral superantigens are membrane proteins produced by endogenous viruses of mice, especially the murine mammary tumor virus, MMTV. The crystal structures of complexes of MHC class II molecules with staphylococcal enterotoxin B (SEB) and with TSST-1 have been determined (that of the HLA-DR1:TSST-1 complex is shown in the lower panel) and show clearly that the superantigen binds to the α chain of the MHC class II molecule. In the case of the TSST-1 superantigen, peptides bound by the class II molecule and parts of the β chain may also contact the superantigen and influence its binding. The viral superantigen MMTV-7 has a CLIP-like peptide and appears to compete with the MHC class II invariant chain for binding to MHC class II molecules. Each of these superantigens contacts a separate site on the T-cell receptor Vβ domain. Complex structure courtesy of J Kim.

This mode of stimulation does not prime an adaptive immune response specific for the pathogen. Instead, it causes massive production of cytokines by CD4 T cells, the predominant responding population of T cells. These cytokines have two effects on the host—systemic toxicity and suppression of the adaptive immune response. Both of these effects contribute to microbial pathogenicity. Among the bacterial superantigens are the **staphylococcal enterotoxins (SEs)**, which cause common food poisoning, and the **toxic shock syndrome toxin-1 (TSST-1)**.

The role of viral superantigens is less clear. Endogenous viral superantigens are very common in mice and we shall see in Chapter 6 that the study of these superantigens has played a critical role in elucidating one of the major mechanisms of self tolerance. In humans, the T-cell response to rabies virus and the Epstein-Barr virus indicate the existence of superantigens encoded by these viruses; however, the genes encoding these superantigens have not yet been identified.

4-27 | The T-cell receptor associates with the invariant proteins of the CD3 complex.

Neither chain of the T-cell receptor heterodimer has a large cytoplasmic domain that might serve to signal the cell that the T-cell receptor has bound its peptide:MHC ligand. Instead, that function is carried out by a complex of three types of proteins known as the **CD3 complex**, which is stably associated with the T-cell receptor on the cell surface (Fig. 4.33). The three proteins are known as CD3γ, CD3δ, and CD3ε and are encoded by linked genes. In addition, a fourth molecule known as the ζ chain and encoded by an unlinked gene is associated with the receptor. CD3γ, CD3δ, and CD3ε have extracellular domains that bear weak amino acid homology to immunoglobulin domains and small cytoplasmic domains. Their transmembrane domains are characterized by an acidic (negatively charged) residue appropriately placed to form a salt bridge with the basic (positively charged) amino acids in the transmembrane region of the T-cell receptor. The ζ chain is a disulfide-linked dimer, very little of which extends outside the cell, the bulk of the polypeptide chain lying in the cytoplasm. The cytoplasmic domains of all the CD3 proteins contain sequences called **immunoreceptor tyrosine-based activation motifs (ITAMs)** (see Section 3-25) that allow them to associate with cytosolic **protein tyrosine kinases** following receptor stimulation and thereby signal to the interior of the cell. The cytoplasmic domains of the ζ chain and the CD3ε chain are particularly important for signaling through tyrosine kinases.

The genes encoding CD3γ, δ, and ε are closely linked in the genome, and their expression is coordinately regulated. The CD3 proteins are also required for the cell-surface expression of the T-cell receptor, although this regulation is at the level of assembly of the complex, and not of transcription. Individuals deficient in expression of particular CD3 chains (in one case the γ chain and in another the ε chain) show significantly reduced levels of T-cell receptor at the T-cell surface and suffer from immunodeficiency. In mice, mutant cells lacking any one of the γ, δ, or ε chains of the CD3 complex fail to express any of the chains at the cell surface. Sequences lying within the plasma membrane, which contain the acidic residues of the CD3γ, δ, or ε chains respectively (see Fig. 4.33), seem to be required for the complex to assemble and be transported to the cell surface. Mutant cells lacking ζ chains express much reduced levels of the T-cell receptor at the cell surface, suggesting that the ζ chain plays an important, but not essential, role in transport.

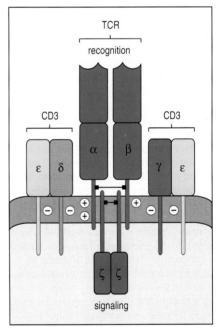

Fig. 4.33 The outline structure of the T-cell receptor (TCR):CD3 complex. The receptor for antigens on the surface of T cells is composed of eight polypeptide chains. Two are the disulfide-bonded chains of the T-cell receptor heterodimer that recognizes antigen (TCR). Four other chains, collectively called CD3, associate with the TCR heterodimer and transport it to the cell surface. These CD3 chains, along with a homodimer of ζ chains, signal to the interior of the cell that antigen binding has occurred.

4-28 The co-receptor molecules CD4 and CD8 cooperate with the T-cell receptor in antigen recognition.

We have seen that T cells fall into two major classes that differ in the class of MHC molecule they recognize, have different effector functions, and are distinguished by the cell-surface proteins CD4 and CD8. CD4 and CD8 were known for some time as markers for different functional sets of T cells before it became clear that they play an important part in the differential recognition of MHC class II and MHC class I molecules. It is now known that CD4 binds to invariant parts of the MHC class II molecule and CD8 to invariant parts of the MHC class I molecule. During antigen recognition, CD4 and CD8 molecules associate on the T-cell surface with components of the T-cell receptor. For this reason, they are called **co-receptors**.

CD4 is a single-chain molecule composed of four immunoglobulin-like domains (Fig. 4.34). The first two domains (D1 and D2) of the CD4 molecule are packed tightly together to form a rigid rod some 60Å long, which is believed to be joined by a flexible hinge to a similar rod formed by the third and fourth domains (D3 and D4). The cytoplasmic domain interacts strongly with a cytoplasmic tyrosine kinase called Lck, which enables the CD4 molecule to participate in signal transduction. CD4 binds MHC class II molecules through a region that lies mainly on a lateral face of the first domain (D1), although it is thought that residues in the second domain may also be involved. CD4 binding to MHC class II is weak on its own and it is not clear whether such binding is able to transmit a signal to the interior of the T cell. As CD4 binds to a site on the β_2 domain of the MHC class II molecule that is well away from the site where the T-cell receptor binds (Fig. 4.35), the CD4 molecule and the T-cell receptor can bind the same peptide:MHC class II complex. As they bind independently to the peptide:MHC class II complex, they come together only during antigen recognition when they act synergistically in signaling. The presence of CD4 results in a marked increase in the sensitivity of a T cell to antigen presented by MHC class II molecules, lowering by 100-fold the dose of antigen required for activation, as discussed in the next section.

Fig. 4.34 The outline structures of the CD4 and CD8 co-receptor molecules. The CD4 molecule exists as a monomer (panel a) and contains four immunoglobulin-like domains. The crystal structure of the first two domains of human CD4 has been obtained and is shown in panel b. The amino-terminal domain, D1, in white, is similar in structure to an immunoglobulin variable domain. The second domain, D2, in purple, although it is clearly related to immunoglobulin domains, is different from both V and C domains and has been termed a C2 domain. The first two domains of CD4 form a rigid rod-like structure that is linked to the two carboxy-terminal domains by a flexible link. The binding site for MHC class II molecules is thought to involve both the D1 and D2 domains of CD4. The CD8 molecule is a heterodimer of an α and a β chain that are covalently associated by a disulfide bond (panel a). The two chains of the dimer have very similar structures, each having a single domain resembling an immunoglobulin variable domain and a stretch of peptide believed to be in a relatively extended conformation that links the variable region-like domain to the cell membrane. The structure shown in panel c is that of a homodimer of CD8 α chains, which both resembles and functions like the α:β heterodimer. Photographs courtesy of C Thorpe.

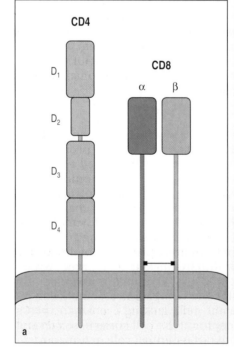

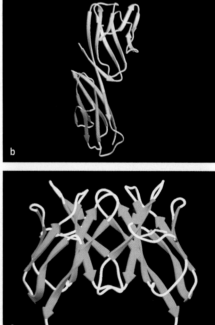

Fig. 4.35 The binding sites for CD8 and CD4 on MHC class I and class II molecules lie in the immunoglobulin-like domains. The binding sites for CD8 and CD4 on the MHC class I and class II molecules respectively lie in the immunoglobulin-like domains nearest to the membrane, distant from the peptide-binding cleft. CD8 binds to a site, shown surfaced in green in panel a, at the base of the α_3 domain of the MHC class I molecule. The α chain of the class I molecule is shown in white while the β_2-microglobulin is shown in purple. CD4 binds to a site on the β_2 domain of a MHC class II molecule, which as shown in panel b, is also at the base of the domain and distant from the peptide-binding site. The α chain of the class II molecule is shown in purple while the β chain is in white. Photographs courtesy of C Thorpe.

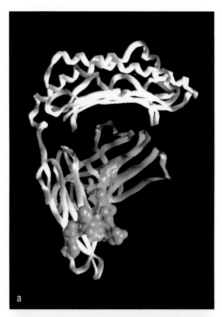

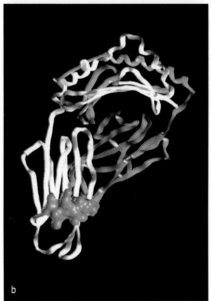

Although CD4 and CD8 both function as co-receptors, their structures are quite distinct. The CD8 molecule is a disulfide-linked heterodimer comprising α and β chains, each containing a single immunoglobulin-like domain linked to the membrane by a segment of polypeptide chain that is believed to have an extended conformation (see Fig. 4.34). It is not known whether a single domain of the CD8 molecule contacts MHC class I proteins or whether the binding site is formed by the interaction of the CD8α and CD8β chains, although it is known that CD8α homo-dimers can also bind MHC class I molecules. CD8 binds weakly on its own to the α_3 domain of MHC class I molecules (see Fig. 4.35), allowing it to bind simultaneously with the T-cell receptor to specific peptide:MHC class I complexes. CD8 also binds Lck with its cytoplasmic tail and increases the sensitivity of T cells bearing the CD8 co-receptor to antigen presented by MHC class I molecules by about 100-fold. Thus, the two co-receptor proteins have similar functions, although their structures are only distantly related.

4-29 | Antigen recognition activates protein tyrosine kinases in the T cell.

Signaling through the antigen-specific T-cell receptor requires aggregation of the receptors by the array of peptide:MHC complexes on the target cell, just as stimulation of B cells requires crosslinking of surface immuno-globulin. Optimal signaling through T-cell receptors occurs only on clustering of the T-cell receptor with the co-receptors CD4 or CD8, just as CD19 co-aggregation with immunoglobulin is required for optimal B-cell signaling (see Section 3-26). Receptor aggregation activates the cell by bringing tyrosine kinases associated with the cytoplasmic domains of the co-receptors together with their targets on the cytoplasmic domains of the CD3 receptor complex and initiating a cascade of signaling reactions leading ultimately to the activation of genes required for cell prolifera-tion and differentiation, or for the effector activities of the T cell. We shall focus here on the intracellular signaling events triggered by antigen binding to receptors on effector T cells.

The initial events in signaling are believed to depend upon two tyrosine kinases—Lck, which is constitutively associated with the cytoplasmic domain of the co-receptor molecules CD4 and CD8, and Fyn, a cytoplasmic tyrosine kinase that binds to the cytoplasmic domains of the CD3ζ and CD3ε chains upon receptor aggregation. Both Fyn and Lck phosphory-late sites on the CD3ζ and ε chains that can then bind a second cytosolic tyrosine kinase, ζ-associated protein-70, or ZAP-70, which is closely related to the B-cell tyrosine kinase Syk. The second and pivotal step in the signaling cascade is the phosphorylation by Fyn and Lck of ZAP-70. This activates ZAP-70 and triggers all subsequent signaling events (Fig. 4.36): individuals lacking ZAP-70 have T cells that mature normally but do not respond to signaling through their antigen receptors.

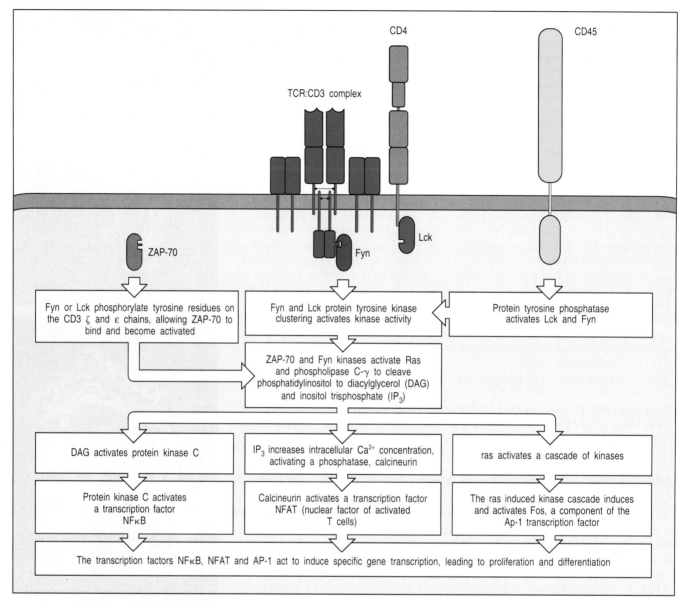

Fig. 4.36 Binding of antigen to the T-cell receptor initiates a series of biochemical changes within the T cell. Protein tyrosine phosphorylation plays an important part in the activation of T cells, and both the T-cell receptor complex and the co-receptor (in this example the CD4 molecule) are associated with cytoplasmic tyrosine kinases. Further, the CD45 molecule, a T-cell surface protein known to be required for activation of T cells, has protein tyrosine phosphatase activity in its cytoplasmic domain. In T cells studied in culture, it is thought that ligand binding to the T-cell receptor and the co-receptor brings together CD4, the T-cell receptor:CD3 complex, and CD45, thus allowing the CD45 tyrosine phosphatase to remove inhibitory phosphate groups and thereby activate the Lck and Fyn tyrosine kinases associated with the co-receptor and T-cell receptor:CD3 complex, respectively. The events occurring after the activation of these tyrosine kinases are not known in detail. One effect is to phosphorylate the ζ chain, which then binds and induces the activation of a cytosolic tyrosine kinase called ζ-associated protein-70 (ZAP-70). In freshly isolated T cells, ZAP-70 is constitutively bound to the ζ chain and so the role of the Lck kinase appears to be simply to activate the bound ZAP-70. Activation of ZAP-70 leads to three important signaling pathways, two of which are initiated by the activation of phospholipase C-γ, which cleaves the phospholipid, phosphatidylinositol-4,5-bisphosphate (PIP$_2$), to yield diacylglycerol (DAG) and inositol trisphosphate (IP$_3$). DAG acts within the cell to activate a protein serine/threonine kinase, protein kinase C, which in turn leads to the activation of the transcription factor NFκB. Meanwhile, IP$_3$ acts to release calcium ions (Ca^{2+}) from intracellular stores. In addition, a calcium-specific ion channel is opened in the T-cell membrane to allow the influx of Ca^{2+} from extracellular sources. The elevated concentration of Ca^{2+} activates a cytoplasmic phosphatase NFAT. However, full NFAT activity also requires a member of the AP-1 family of transcription factors; these are dimers of members of the Fos and Jun families of transcription regulators. A third signaling pathway initiated by activated ZAP-70, the activation of Ras and the subsequent activation of a cascade of kinases, culminates in the activation of Fos and hence of the AP-1 transcription factors. The combination of the NFκB, NFAT and AP-1 transcription factors acts upon the T-cell chromosomes, initiating new gene transcription that results in the differentiation, proliferation and effector actions of T cells, which will be discussed in more detail in Chapter 7.

Co-aggregation of the T-cell receptor and the co-receptor molecules is essential for normal signaling. About 100 specific peptide:MHC complexes are required on a target cell to trigger a T cell expressing the appropriate co-receptor. In the absence of the co-receptor, 10 000 identical complexes (about 10% of all the MHC molecules on a cell) would be required.

Most of what we know about signaling through the T-cell receptor derives from observations of cultured T-cell lines. In T cells isolated directly from the lymph nodes or the thymus, ZAP-70 is already bound to the phosphorylated ζ chains but is not yet activated. It therefore seems likely that most circulating T cells have already undergone the first step required for their activation, and subsequent encounter with antigen, by bringing the antigen receptor together with CD4 or CD8, then initiates the second step, in which Lck activates ZAP-70.

How T cells are held poised part way along their activation pathway is not clear; however, it is known that an additional regulatory element is provided by a tyrosine phosphatase called CD45. CD45 is a trans-membrane molecule that is believed to activate the tyrosine kinases associated with the receptor and co-receptor molecules by removing inhibitory phosphate groups. T cells that lack CD45 are defective in signaling through the T-cell receptor. CD45 is thought to associate physically with the T-cell receptor complex but the mechanism of association is not known. How far the activation of a T cell progresses may depend upon the balance of many kinase and phosphatase activities.

Once ZAP-70 is activated, it in turn initiates three separate signaling pathways. One of these is mediated by the activation of Ras, a GTP-binding protein of 21 kDa which is a ubiquitous intracellular signaling molecule. Ras subsequently triggers a cascade of protein kinases that ultimately induce the transcription and activation of members of a family of gene regulatory proteins called Fos. Fos proteins pair with members of a second family, called Jun, to produce a transcriptional activator called AP-1 which plays a part in gene regulation in many cell types. AP-1 can act alone to induce new gene transcription and its activation is important in many proliferative responses. In T-cell activation, however, it also acts in association with a T-cell specific factor, NFAT.

NFAT is one of a small family of molecules present in an inactive form in the cytoplasm of T cells before they are activated. On activation, NFAT is translocated to the nucleus within minutes of receptor stimulation. This is achieved through the second of the three pathways initiated by ZAP-70. ZAP-70 first activates the enzyme phospholipase C-γ to produce inositol trisphosphate (IP$_3$), which releases Ca^{2+} from intracellular stores. In addition, a channel specific for Ca^{2+} is opened in the T-cell membrane, allowing entry of Ca^{2+} from the surrounding extracellular fluid. The elevated concentration of cytosolic Ca^{2+} activates a cytoplasmic protein phosphatase, **calcineurin**, which removes a phosphate group from the cytoplasmic NFAT proteins. This allows NFAT proteins to enter the nucleus and bind to AP-1 to create the active NFAT transcription factor. While the AP-1 transcription factor is active in many cell types, cytoplasmic NFAT and hence the NFAT transcription factor itself, are restricted to T cells. For that reason blockade of the signaling pathway that leads to NFAT is an important means of specifically inhibiting T-cell responses. Signal transduction in T cells is potently inhibited by two drugs called **cyclosporin A** and **FK506** (see Chapter 13). These drugs are used widely to prevent graft rejection, which they do by inhibiting the activation of alloreactive T cells. Cyclosporin A and FK506 both inhibit calcineurin and hence prevent the formation of active NFAT.

A third signaling pathway is initiated by the diacylglycerol produced by activation of phospholipase C-γ, which activates protein kinase C. Protein kinase C is, in turn, able to activate a variety of enzymes within the cell, and plays an essential role in the induction of the transcription factor NFκB. Together with AP-1 and NFAT, NFκB induces new gene expression, leading to cell proliferation and the subsequent effector function (see Chapter 7).

The signaling events described here occur in fully differentiated effector T cells and lead to the release of effector molecules by the activated T cell—these may be cytotoxins released by CD8 cytotoxic T cells, or cytokines released by CD4 T cells. The mechanisms of release of effector molecules by fully differentiated T cells will be discussed in detail in Chapter 7. The same signals are also crucial earlier in the development of T cells, both for the proper differentiation of T cells during their development in the thymus and for maturation to effector status on first encounter with antigen. However, in these latter settings other signals are also required, as discussed in Chapters 6 and 7.

| 4-30 | **Certain peptides generate partial signals for activation or inhibit T-cell responses.** |

So far, we have assumed that any peptide:MHC complex that is recognized by a T-cell receptor will activate the T cell. However, some experiments originally designed to explore the structural basis for antigen recognition by T cells showed unexpectedly that recognition does not necessarily lead to activation. Rather, some peptide:MHC complexes that do not themselves activate a given T cell can actually inhibit its response to the peptide:MHC complex that it normally recognizes. These peptides are usually called **antagonist peptides**, or **altered peptide ligands**.

In these experiments, variants of a known peptide ligand were made in which the changes were thought to affect amino acids that contact the T-cell receptor but not those that bind to the MHC molecule. Some of these peptides could not stimulate responses in the appropriate T cells, while others (called **partial agonist peptides**) elicited partial responses. More surprisingly, some peptides rendered the T cells unresponsive to stimulation with agonist peptides, whether presented to the T-cell receptor on the same antigen-presenting cell or, even more strikingly, when exposed to the activating peptide at a later time.

The extent to which agonist and partial agonist peptides influence physiological immune responses is not known, although they may contribute to some persistent viral infections. For example, mutant peptides of epitopes on cells infected with human immunodeficiency virus can inhibit activation of CD8 T cells at a 1:100 ratio of antagonist to agonist; it is possible that this allows the infected cells to survive in the presence of virus-specific cytotoxic cells. Differential signaling by variants of agonist peptides may also be important for the development of T cells in the thymus, where the immature cells are selected for their potential to recognize foreign peptide antigens in the context of self MHC molecules. This process, which we shall discuss in detail in Chapter 6, would seem to require immature T cells to be signaled by a self-peptide:self-MHC complex that is related to but not identical to the foreign peptide:self-MHC complex that the mature T cell will recognize.

The basis for the incomplete activating signal delivered by antagonist peptides is also unknown but it has been shown that recognition of these ligands fails to activate the ZAP-70 tyrosine kinase. Why this occurs is not known. The affinity of the T-cell receptor for the antagonist peptide:MHC complex is lower than that for the activating complex and the T-cell receptor may dissociate too quickly from its ligand for a full activating signal to be delivered. An alternative possibility is that conformational changes in the T-cell receptor contribute to signaling and that antagonist peptides fail to trigger these conformational changes.

4-31 Some T cells bear an alternative form of T-cell receptor with γ and δ chains.

At the time of the discovery of the T-cell receptor α:β heterodimer, all known specific immune responses could be accounted for by the action of T cells bearing these polypeptides. Thus, it was a real surprise when, during the search for genes encoding T-cell receptors, a third T cell-specific cDNA was discovered that also encoded a protein with homology to immunoglobulin and whose gene rearranged in T lymphocytes. As this gene clearly did not encode either the α or the β chain of the T-cell receptor, it was termed T-cell receptor γ. The γ polypeptide is found on the cell surface associated with a second polypeptide, the T-cell receptor δ chain. The **γ:δ heterodimer**, like the homologous α:β heterodimer, is also associated with a CD3 complex on the cell surface and the γ:δ T-cell receptor chains should not be confused with the CD3 γ and δ chains.

The organization of the γ and δ genes (Fig. 4.37) resembles that of the α and β genes, although there are some important differences. The gene complex encoding the δ chain is found entirely within the T-cell receptor α-chain gene complex between the Vα and the Jα gene segments. As a result, any rearrangement of the α-chain genes inactivates the genes encoding δ chains. There are many fewer V gene segments at the γ and δ loci than at either the T-cell receptor α or β gene loci or for any of the immunoglobulin loci. Increased junctional variability in the δ chains may compensate for the small number of possible variable regions and has the effect of focusing almost all of the variability in the γ:δ receptor in the junctional region. As we have seen, the amino acids encoded by the junctional regions lie at the center of the T-cell receptor binding site.

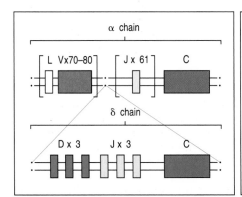

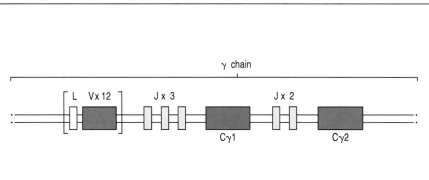

Fig. 4.37   The organization of the T-cell receptor γ and δ chain genes of the human. The γ and δ genes, like the α and β T-cell receptor genes, have discrete V, D, J, and C gene segments. Uniquely, the gene encoding the δ chain is located entirely within the gene encoding the α chain, lying between the cluster of Vα gene segments and the cluster of Jα gene segments. There are three Dδ gene segments, three Jδ gene segments, and a single constant region gene. The Vδ gene segments are interspersed among the Vα gene segments; it is not known exactly how many Vδ gene segments there are but there are at least four. The human γ chain resembles the β chains, with two constant-region gene segments each with its own J gene segments. The mouse γ genes (not shown) have a more complex organization and there are three functional clusters of γ genes, each containing V and J gene segments and a constant region gene. Rearrangement of the γ and δ genes proceeds as for the other T-cell receptor genes, with the exception that during δ-chain rearrangement both D segments can be used in the same gene. Use of two D segments greatly increases the variability, mainly because extra N-region nucleotides can be added at the junction between the two D gene segments as well as at the VD and DJ junctions.

T cells bearing γ:δ receptors are a distinct lineage of cells of unknown function. The ligands for these receptors are also unknown, although some γ:δ T cells can recognize products of certain class IB genes (see Section 4-14), while others appear to be able to recognize antigen directly, much as antibodies do, without the requirement for presentation by an MHC molecule or processing of the antigen. Detailed analysis of the rearranged variable regions of γ:δ T-cell receptors show that they resemble variable regions of antibody molecules more than they resemble the variable regions of α:β T-cell receptors. In peripheral lymphoid tissues, only a very small percentage (generally 1–5%) of CD3-positive cells express γ:δ receptors. However, in epithelial tissues, especially in the epidermis and small intestine of the mouse, most T cells express γ:δ receptors. The receptors of these epithelial γ:δ T cells show extremely restricted variability. We shall return to the possible functional significance of these findings in Chapter 9.

Summary.

T-cell receptors are structurally similar to immunoglobulins and are encoded by homologous genes. Diversity is distributed differently in T-cell receptors, which have roughly the same number of V gene segments but more J and D gene segments and more powerful mechanisms for diversification of junctions between gene segments. Moreover, functional T-cell receptors are not known to diversify their V genes after rearrangement through somatic hypermutation. This leads to a T-cell receptor structure where the highest diversity is in the central part of the receptor, which contacts the bound peptide fragment of the ligand. The cell-surface T-cell receptor resembles in many ways the cell-surface form of immunoglobulins. Both are associated in the cell membrane with a complex of invariant proteins that are required for transport of the receptors to the cell surface and for signal transduction. Both receptors must not only bind antigen but also become clustered or crosslinked in order to trigger the cell. The co-receptor molecules, CD4 and CD8, bind MHC class II and MHC class I molecules respectively, and act synergistically with the T-cell receptor in signaling, resulting in about a 100-fold increase in the sensitivity of T cells to antigen. The biochemical events that follow from antigen binding to the T-cell receptor share many features with other signaling systems, in which cell growth or cell activation is regulated by the binding of growth factors or hormones.

Summary to Chapter 4.

The T-cell receptor is very similar to immunoglobulins, both in structure and in the way in which variability is introduced into the antigen-binding site. However, there are also important differences between T-cell receptors and immunoglobulins that are related to the nature of the antigens recognized by T cells. The mechanism of generation of diversity in T-cell receptors focuses the diversity into the CDR3 loops of T-cell receptor variable regions, which lie in the center of the antigen-binding site. This pattern of diversity reflects the recognition of antigen by the T-cell receptor, specific for foreign peptide antigen bound to an MHC molecule on the target cell surface. There are two classes of MHC molecule: MHC class I molecules, which bind peptides derived from proteins synthesized and degraded in the cytosol; and MHC class II molecules, which bind peptides derived from proteins degraded in cellular vesicles. There are several genes for each class of MHC molecule, arranged in a cluster in the major histocompatibility complex (MHC), together with genes involved in the degradation of protein antigens into peptides and their transport to the cell surface bound to MHC molecules. Since the genes for the MHC class I and class II molecules are highly polymorphic, each cell expresses several different MHC class I and class II proteins, and is thus able to bind many different peptide antigens. The binding site for the peptide on an MHC molecule lies in a cleft between two α helices; thus the T-cell receptor recognizes a ligand that has a region of high variability (the peptide antigen) lying between regions of lesser variability (the α helices of the MHC). The distribution of variability in the T-cell receptor thus correlates with the distribution of variability in the ligand it must recognize. Moreover, T cells manifest MHC-restricted antigen recognition, such that a given T cell is specific for one peptide bound to one MHC molecule. Unlike immunoglobulins, T-cell receptors are not known to use somatic hypermutation as a means of increasing receptor variability. Thus, T-cell receptors can only recognize a limited range of ligands.

General references.

Klein, J.: *Natural History of the Major Histocompatibility Complex.* New York: J. Wiley & Sons; 1986.

Bodmer, J.G., Marsh, S.G.E., Albert, E.D., Bodmer, W.F., DuPont, B., Erlich, H.A., Mach, B., Mayr, W.R., Parham, P., Saszuki, T., et al.: **Nomenclature for factors of the HLA system, 1991**. *Tissue Antigens* 1992, **39**:161-173.

Moller, G. (ed): **Origin of major histocompatibility complex diversity.** *Immunol. Rev.* 1995, **143**:5-292.

Germain, R.N.: **MHC-dependent antigen processing and peptide presentation: Providing ligands for T lymphocyte activation.** *Cell* 1994, **76**:287-299.

Section references.

4-1 | T cells with different functions recognize peptides produced in two distinct intracellular compartments.

Morrison, L.A., Lukacher, A.E., Braciale, V.L., Fan, D.P., and Braciale, T.J.: **Differences in antigen presentation to MHC class I- and class II-restricted influenza virus-specific cytolytic T-lymphocyte clones.** *J. Exp. Med.* 1986, **163**:903.

Song, R. and Harding C.V.: **Roles of proteasomes, transporter for antigen presentation (TAP), and** β_2 **-microglobulin in the processing of bacterial or particulate antigens via an alternate class I MHC processing pathway.** *J. Immunol.* 1996, **156**:4182-4190.

4-2 | The two classes of MHC molecule have a distinct subunit structure but a similar three-dimensional structure.

Fremont, D.H., Hendrickson, W.A., Marrack, P. and Kappler, J.: **Structures of an MHC class II molecule with covalently bound single peptides.** *Science* 1996, **272**:1001-1004.

Madden, D.R.: **The three-dimensional structure of peptide-MHC complexes.** *Ann. Rev. Immunol.* 1995, **13**:587-622.

4-3 | T cells recognize a complex of a peptide fragment bound to an MHC molecule.

Fremont, D.H., Rees, W.A., Kozono, H.: **Biophysical studies of T cell receptors and their ligands.** *Curr. Opin. Immunol.* 1996, **8**:93-100.

4-4 | Peptides are stably bound to MHC molecules through invariant and variable contacts.

Madden, D.R., Gorga, J.C., Strominger, J.L. and Wiley, D.C.: **The three-dimensional structure of HLA-B27 at 2.1Å resolution suggests a general mechanism for tight peptide binding to MHC.** *Cell* 1992, **70**:1035-1048.

Fremont, D.H., Matsumura, M., Stura, E.A., Peterson, P.A. & Wilson, I.: **Crystal structures of two viral peptides in complex with murine MHC class 1 H-2K[b].** *Science* 1992, **257**:919-927.

4-5 | The length of the peptides bound by MHC class II molecules is not constrained.

Rammensee, H.G.: **Chemistry of peptides associated with MHC class I and class II molecules.** *Curr. Opin. Immunol.* 1995, **7**:85-96.

Rudensky, A,Y., Preston-Hurlburt, P., Hong, S-C., Barlow, A., Janeway Jr, C.A.: **Sequence analysis of peptides bound to MHC class II molecules.** *Nature* 1991, **353**:622.

4-6 | The two classes of MHC molecule are expressed differentially on cells.

Steimle, V., Siegrist, C.A., Mottet, A., Lisowska-Grospierre, B.and Mach, B.: **Regulation of MHC class II expression by interferon-γ mediated by the transactivator gene CIITA.** *Science* 1994, **265**:106-109.

4-7 | Peptides that bind to MHC class I molecules are actively transported from cytosol to the endoplasmic reticulum.

Shepherd, J.C., Schumacher, T.N.M., Ashton-Rickardt, P.G., Imaeda, S., Ploegh, H.L., Janeway, C.A. Jr., and Tonegawa, S.: **TAP1-dependent peptide translocation** *in vitro* **is ATP-dependent and peptide-selective.** *Cell* 1993, **74**:577-584.

Townsend, A., Ohlen, C., Foster, L., Bastin, J., Lunggren, H.-G., and Karre, K.: **A mutant cell in which association of class I heavy and light chains is induced by viral peptides.** *Cold Spring Harbor Symp. Quant. Biol.* 1989, **54**:299-308.

4-8   Newly synthesized MHC class I molecules are retained in the endoplasmic reticulum by binding a TAP-1 associated protein until they bind peptide.

Van Kaer, L., Ashton-Rickardt, P.G., Eichelberger, M., Gaczynska, M., Nagashima, K., Rock, K.L., Goldberg, A.L., Doherty, P.C., Tonegawa, S.: **Altered peptides and viral specific T cell responses in LMP2 mutant mice.** *Immunity* 1994, **1**:533-541.

Shastri, N.: **Needles in haystacks: identifying specific peptide antigens for T-cells.** *Curr. Opin. Immunol.* 1996, **8**:271-277.

Williams, D.B., Watts, T.H.: **Molecular chaperones in antigen presentation.** *Curr. Opin. Immunol.* 1995, **7**:77-84.

4-9   Peptides of cytosolic proteins are generated in the cytosol prior to transport into the endoplasmic reticulum.

Lehner, P.J., Cresswell, P.: **Processing and delivery of peptides presented by MHC class I molecules.** *Curr. Opin. Immunol.* 1996, **8**:59-67.

York, I.A., Rock, K.L.: **Antigen processing and presentation by the class-I major histocompatibility complex.** *Ann. Rev. Immunol.* 1996, **14**:369-396.

Howard, J.C.: **Supply and transport of peptides presented by class I MHC molecules.** *Curr. Opin. Immunol.* 1995, **7**:69-76.

4-10   Peptides presented by MHC class II molecules are generated in acidified intracellular vesicles.

Cresswell, P.: **Assembly, transport, and function of MHC class II molecules.** *Ann. Rev. Immunol.* 1994, **12**:259-293.

Germain, R,N., Castellino, F., Han, R.E., Sousa, C.R., Romagnoli, P., Sadegh Nasseri, S., Zhong, G.M.: **Processing and presentation of endocytically acquired protein antigens by MHC class I and class II molecules.** *Immunol. Rev.* 1996, **151**:5-30.

Lanzavecchia, A.: **Mechanisms of antigen uptake for presentation.** *Curr. Opin. Immunol.* 1996, **8**:348-354.

4-11   The invariant chain directs newly synthesized MHC class II molecules to acidified intracellular vesicles.

Amigorena, S., Drake, J.R., Webster, P., Mellman, I.: **Transient accumulation of new class II MHC molecules in a novel endocytic compartment in B lymphocytes.** *Nature* 1994, **369**:113-120.

Cresswell, P., Denzin, L.K.: **HLA-DM induces CLIP dissociation from MHC class II α:β dimers and facilitates peptide loading.** *Cell* 1995, **82**:155-165.

Sant, A.J., Miller, J.: **MHC class II antigen processing: Biology of invariant chain.** *Curr. Opin. Immunol.* 1994, **6**:57-63.

4-12   A specialized MHC class II-like molecule catalyzes loading of MHC class II molecules with endogenously processed peptides.

Busch, R., Mellins, E.D.: **Developing and shedding inhibitions: How MHC class II molecules reach maturity.** *Curr. Opin. Immunol.* 1996, **8**:51-58.

Morris, P., Shaman, J., Attaya, M., Amaya, M., Goodman, S., Bergman, C., Monaco, J., Mellins, E.: **An Essential Role for HLA-DM in Antigen Presentation by Class II Major Histocompatibility Molecules.** *Nature* 1994, **368**:551.

Denzin, L.K., Cresswell, P.: **HLA-DM Induces CLIP Dissociation from MHC Class II α:β Dimers and Facilitates Peptide Loading.** *Cell* 1995, **82**:155-165.

Sloan, V. S., Cameron, P., Porter, G., Gammon, M., Amaya, M., Mellins, E. , Zaller, D.M.: **Mediation by HLA-DM of Dissociation of Peptides from HLA-DR.** *Nature* 1995, **375**:802.

4-13   The characteristics of peptide binding by MHC molecules allow effective antigen presentation at the cell surface.

Lanzavecchia, A., Reid, P.A., and Watts, C.: **Irreversible association of peptides with class II MHC molecules in living cells.** *Nature* 1992, **357**:249-252.

4-14   The proteins involved in antigen processing and presentation are encoded by genes in the major histocompatibility complex.

Trowsdale, J., Campbell, R.D.: **Complexity in the major histocompatibility complex.** *Eur. J. Immunogen.* 1992, **19**:45-55.

Trowsdale, J.: **'Both man and bird and beast': Comparative organization of MHC genes.** *Immunogenetics* 1995, **41**:1-17.

4-15   A variety of genes with specialized functions in immunity are also encoded in the MHC.

Blumberg, R.S., Gerdes, D., Chott, A., Porcelli, S.A., Balk, S.P.: **Structure and function of the CD1 family of MHC-like cell surface proteins.** *Immunol. Rev.* 1995 **147**:5-29.

Porcelli, S.A., Morita, C.T., Modlin, R.L.: **T cell recognition of non-peptide antigens.** *Curr. Opin. Immunol.* 1996, **8**:510-516.

Campbell, R.D., Trowsdale, J.: **Map of the human MHC.** *Immunol. Today* 1995, **14**:349-352.

4-16   The protein products of MHC class I and class II genes are highly polymorphic.

Klein, J., Satta, Y., O'Huigin, C.: **The molecular descent of the major histocompatibility complex.** *Ann. Rev. Immunol.* 1993, **11**:269-295.

Parham, P., Adams, E.J., Arnett, K.L.: **The origins of HLA-ABC polymorphism.** *Immunol.Rev.* 1995, **143**:141-180.

4-17   MHC polymorphism affects antigen recognition indirectly by controlling peptide binding.

Babbitt, B., Allen, P.M., Matsueda, G., Haber, P., Unuanue, E.R.: **Binding of immunogenic peptides to Ia histocompatibility molecules.** *Nature* 1985, **317**:359.

Hammer, J.: **New methods to predict MHC-binding sequences within protein antigens.** *Curr. Opin. Immunol.* 1995, **7**:263-269.

4-18   MHC polymorphism directly affects antigen recognition by T cells.

Zinkernagel, R.M., and Doherty, P.C.: **Restriction of *in vivo* T-cell mediated cytotoxicity in lymphocytic choriomeningitis within a syngeneic or semiallogeneic system.** *Nature* 1974, **248**:701-702.

Rosenthal, A.S., and Shevach, E.M.: **Function of macrophages in antigen recognition by guinea pig T lymphocytes. I. Requirement for histocompatible macrophages and lymphocytes.** *J. Exp. Med.* 1973, **138**:1194.

Katz, D.H., Hamaoka, T., Dorf, M.E., Maurer, P.H., and Benacerraf, B.: **Cell interactions between histoincompatible T and B lymphocytes. IV. Involvement of immune response (Ir) gene control of lymphocyte interaction controlled by the gene**. *J. Exp. Med.* 1973, **138**:734.

4-19 Non-self MHC molecules are recognized by 1-10% of T cells.

Kaye, J., and Janeway, C.A. Jr.: **The Fab fragment of a directly activating monoclonal antibody that precipitates a disulfide-linked heterodimer from a helper T-cell clone blocks activation by either allogeneic Ia or antigen and self-Ia**. *J. Exp. Med.* 1984, **159**:1397-1412.

4-20 MHC polymorphism extends the range of antigens to which the immune system can respond.

Hill, A.V., Elvin, J., Willis, A.C., Aidoo, M., Allsopp, C.E.M., Gotch, F.M., Gao, X.M., Takiguchi, M., Greenwood, B.M., Townsend, A.R.M., McMichael, A.J., Whittle, H.C.: **Molecular analysis of the association of B53 and resistance to severe malaria**. *Nature* 1992, **360**:434-440.

Potts, W.K., Slev, P.R.: **Pathogen-based models favouring MHC genetic diversity**. *Immunol. Rev.* 1995, **143**:181-197.

Franco, A., Ferrari, C., Sette, A., Chisari, F.V.: **Viral mutations, TCR antagonism and escape from the immune response**. *Curr. Opin. Immunol.* 1995, **7**:524-531

4-21 Multiple genetic processes generate MHC polymorphism.

Andersson, L., Mikko, S.: **Generation of MHC class II diversity by intra- and intergenic recombination**. *Immunol. Rev.* 1995, **143**:5-12.

4-22 The T-cell receptor resembles a membrane-associated Fab fragment of immunoglobulin.

Bentley, G.A., Mariuzza, R.A.: **The structure of the T cell antigen receptor**. *Ann. Rev. Immunol.* 1996, **14**:563-590.

Garcia, K.C., Degano, M., Stanfield, R.L., Brunmark, A., Jackson,M.L., Peterson, P.A., Teyton, L., Wilson, I.A.: **An α:β T cell receptor structure at 2.5Å and its orientation in the TCR-MHC complex**. *Science* 1996, **274**:209-219.

Sant Angelo, D.B., Waterbury, G., Preston-Hurlburt, P., Yoon, S.T., Medzhitov, R., Hong, S.C. and Janeway, C.A.Jr.: **The specificity and orientation of a TCR to its peptide-MHC class II ligands**. *Immunity* 1996, **4**:367-376.

4-23 The T-cell receptor genes resemble immunoglobulin genes.

Rowen, L., Koop, B.F. and Hood, L.: **The complete 685-kilobase DNA sequence of the human β T cell receptor locus**. *Science* 1996, **272**:1755-1762.

4-24 T-cell receptor diversity is focused in CDR3.

Davis, M.M. and Bjorkman, P.J.: **T-cell antigen receptor genes and T cell recognition**. *Nature 1988,* **334**:395-402.

4-25 Somatic hypermutation is not a major mechanism of generating diversity in T-cell receptors.

Zheng, B., Xue, W., and Kelsoe, G.: **Locus-specific somatic hypermutation in germinal centre T cells**. *Nature* 1994, **372**:556-559.

4-26 Many T cells respond to superantigens.

Hong, S.C., Waterbury, G. and Janeway, C.A.Jr.: **Different Superantigens interact with distinct sites in the Vβ domain of a single T cell receptor**. *J. Exp. Med.* 1996, **183**:1437-1446.

Webb, S.R., Gascoigne, N.R.J.: **T Cell activation by superantigens**. *Curr. Opin. Immunol.* 1994, **6**:467-475.

McDonald, H.R., Acha-Orbea, H.: **Superantigens of mouse mammary tumor virus**. *Ann. Rev. Immunol.* 1995, **13**:459-486.

4-27 The T-cell receptor associates with the invariant proteins of the CD3 complex.

Malissen, B., Malissen, M.: **Functions of TCR and preTCR subunits: Lessons from gene ablation**. *Curr. Opin. Immunol.* 1996, **8**:394-401.

4-28 The co-receptor molecules CD4 and CD8 cooperate with the T-cell receptor in antigen recognition.

Janeway, C.A. Jr.: **The T-cell receptor as a multicomponent signaling machine: CD4/CD8 coreceptors and CD45 in T-cell activation**. *Ann. Rev. Immunol.* 1992, **10**:645-674.

4-29 Antigen recognition activates protein tyrosine kinases in the T cell.

Cantrell, D.: **T cell antigen receptor signal transduction pathways**. *Ann. Rev. Immunol.* 1996, **14**:259-274.

Plas, P.R., Johnson, R., Pingel, J.T., Matthews, R.J., Dalton, M., Roy, G., Chan, A.C. and Thomas, M.L.: **Direct regulation of ZAP-70 by SHP-1 in T cell antigen receptor signaling**. *Science* 1996, **272**: 1173-1176.

Samelson, L.E., Patel, M.D., Weissman, A.M., Harford, J.B., and Klausner, R.D.: **Antigen activation of murine T cells induces tyrosine phosphorylation of a polypeptide associated with the T-cell antigen receptor**. *Cell* 1986, **46**:1083.

Irving, B.A., and Weiss, A.: **The cytoplasmic domain of the T cell receptor chain is sufficient to couple to receptor-associated signal-transduction pathways**. *Cell* 1991, **64**:891.

4-30 Certain peptides generate partial signals for activation or inhibit T-cell responses.

Jameson, S.C., Carbone, F.R., Bevan, M.J.: **Clone-specific T-cell receptor antagonists of major histocompatibility complex class I-restricted cytotoxic T cells**. *J. Exp. Med.* 1993, **177**:1541-1550.

Sloan-Lancaster, J., Allen, P.M.: **Altered peptide ligand-induced partial T-cell activation: Molecular mechanisms and roles in T-cell biology**. *Ann. Rev. Immunol.* 1996, **14**:1-27.

4-31 Some T cells bear an alternative form of T-cell receptor with γ and δ chains.

Chien, Y., Jores, R., Crowley, P.: **Recognition by γ/δ T cells**. *Ann. Rev. Immunol.* 1996, **14**:511-532.

PART III

THE DEVELOPMENT OF LYMPHOCYTE REPERTOIRES

The Development of B Lymphocytes

5

In order that an individual may make antibodies against the wide range of pathogens encountered during a lifetime, B lymphocytes expressing a diverse repertoire of immunoglobulins must be generated continually. Each B cell expresses immunoglobulin of a single antigen specificity, which is determined early in its differentiation, when the genes encoding the immunoglobulin heavy and light chains are assembled from gene segments. In humans and mice, immunoglobulin diversity is largely generated by this process of gene rearrangement, which begins in the fetal liver and continues throughout life in the bone marrow, albeit at a diminishing rate. As we saw in Chapter 3, many thousands of rearrangements are possible for both heavy- and light-chain genes; ongoing gene rearrangement in developing B cells is therefore continually providing a new population of immature B cells bearing a highly diverse repertoire of surface immunoglobulin molecules that act as specific receptors for antigen.

The expression of antigen receptors on the surface of a B lymphocyte marks a watershed in its development. The B cell can now detect ligands in its environment and potentially self-reactive cells must therefore be eliminated before further maturation is allowed. The stimulation of B cells at this stage of their development by molecules binding to surface immunoglobulin leads to loss or inactivation of the B cell, and in this way tolerance is established to ubiquitous self antigens. The cells that survive to form part of the long-lived pool of mature peripheral B cells are only a small fraction of those generated in the bone marrow. Nonetheless, these cells express a large repertoire of receptors capable of responding to a virtually unlimited variety of non-self structures. This repertoire provides the raw material on which clonal selection acts in an adaptive immune response.

In this chapter, we shall define the different stages of B-cell development in the bone marrow of mice and humans, and see how the unselected B-cell receptor repertoire is generated, before discussing what is known of the mechanisms by which tolerance can be ensured once a B cell expresses a complete immunoglobulin molecule at the cell surface. The development of B cells can be divided into four broad phases (Fig. 5.1). We shall follow the fate of newly generated B cells as they leave the bone marrow and circulate through the lymphoid tissues, although the final stages in the life history of a B cell, in which an encounter with foreign antigen activates it to become an antibody-producing plasma cell, will be discussed in Chapter 8. In this chapter we also consider a second population of B cells that develop by a different pathway, and look at how B-cell tumors can capture features of the different stages in normal B-cell development.

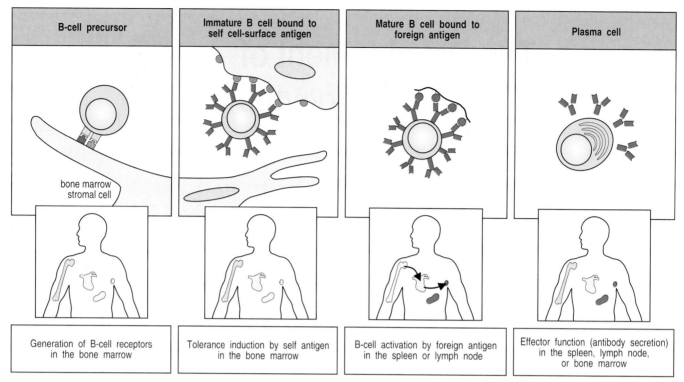

B-cell precursor	Immature B cell bound to self cell-surface antigen	Mature B cell bound to foreign antigen	Plasma cell
bone marrow stromal cell			
Generation of B-cell receptors in the bone marrow	Tolerance induction by self antigen in the bone marrow	B-cell activation by foreign antigen in the spleen or lymph node	Effector function (antibody secretion) in the spleen, lymph node, or bone marrow

Fig. 5.1 The development of B cells can be divided into four broad phases. First panel: B cells develop from progenitor cells in the bone marrow and rearrange their immunoglobulin genes to produce a receptor with unique antigen specificity. As this receptor cannot be expressed until gene rearrangement is completed, the process cannot be driven by specific antigen. It is, however, dependent on interactions with bone marrow stromal cells. Second panel: immature B cells expressing surface IgM can interact with antigens in their environment; those that are stimulated by antigen at this stage are either deleted or inactivated. Third panel: B cells not reactive to self antigens can mature to express IgD as well as IgM and survive after emerging into the periphery, where they may be activated by encounter with foreign antigen in a secondary lymphoid organ. Fourth panel: the activation of a mature B cell leads to its proliferation and differentiation into the last phase of B-lineage development, the antibody-secreting plasma cell, which may remain in the lymphoid organ or migrate to the bone marrow.

Generation of B cells.

The successive stages of B-cell differentiation in mice and humans are marked by successive steps in the rearrangement and expression of the immunoglobulin genes, as well as by changes in the expression of cell-surface and intracellular molecules. This developmental program begins to generate B cells in the fetal liver and continues after birth in the bone marrow. In this section we look at the steps leading to the production of mature B cells expressing surface immunoglobulin (see Fig. 5.1, first and second panels). B-cell development must also be regulated so that each mature B cell produces only one heavy chain and one light chain, and thus bears receptors of a single specificity. We shall see that this entails two series of gene rearrangements, each of which is terminated when a protein product is made successfully, and whose success determines whether further development can occur.

5-1   B-cell development proceeds through several stages.

The stages in primary B-cell development are defined by the sequential rearrangement and expression of heavy- and light-chain immunoglobulin genes (Fig. 5.2). The earliest B-lineage cells are known as **pro-B cells**,

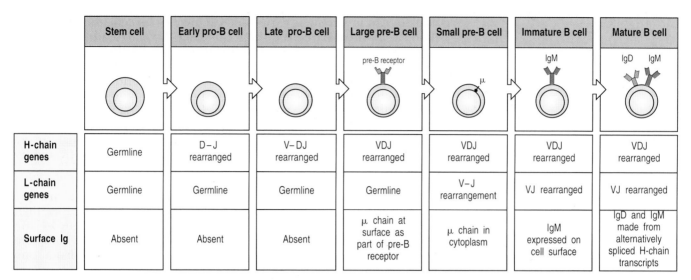

	Stem cell	Early pro-B cell	Late pro-B cell	Large pre-B cell	Small pre-B cell	Immature B cell	Mature B cell
H-chain genes	Germline	D–J rearranged	V–DJ rearranged	VDJ rearranged	VDJ rearranged	VDJ rearranged	VDJ rearranged
L-chain genes	Germline	Germline	Germline	Germline	V–J rearrangement	VJ rearranged	VJ rearranged
Surface Ig	Absent	Absent	Absent	μ chain at surface as part of pre-B receptor	μ chain in cytoplasm	IgM expressed on cell surface	IgD and IgM made from alternatively spliced H-chain transcripts

Fig. 5.2 The development of a B-lineage cell proceeds through several stages marked by the rearrangement and expression of the immunoglobulin genes. The stem cell has not yet begun to rearrange its immunoglobulin genes; they are said to be in the germline configuration as found in all non-lymphoid cells. The heavy-chain locus (H-chain genes) rearranges first. Rearrangements of D_H gene segments to J_H gene segments occur in early pro-B cells, generating late pro-B cells in which a V_H gene segment becomes joined to the rearranged DJ_H. A successful VDJ_H rearrangement leads to the expression of an intact immunoglobulin heavy chain at the cell surface as part of the pre-B receptor. Once this occurs the cell is defined as a large pre-B cell, which, like the progenitor B cells, is large and actively dividing. Large pre-B cells then cease dividing to become small resting pre-B cells in which the μ heavy chain is found inside the cell, and in which the light-chain genes (L-chain genes) can be rearranged. Upon successfully assembling a light-chain gene, the cell becomes an immature B cell that expresses light chains and μ heavy chains as surface IgM molecules. Mature B cells are marked by the additional appearance of IgD on the cell surface.

as they are progenitor cells with limited self-renewal capacity. They are derived from pluripotential hematopoietic cells and are identified by the appearance of cell-surface proteins characteristic of early B-lineage cells. Rearrangement of heavy-chain immunoglobulin gene segments takes place in these pro-B cells; D_H to J_H joining at the **early pro-B cell** stage is followed by V_H to DJ_H joining at the **late pro-B cell** stage. Productive VDJ_H joining leads to expression of an intact μ chain, which is the hallmark of the next main stage of development, the **pre-B cell** stage. The μ chain in **large pre-B cells** is expressed transiently at the cell-surface in combination with a surrogate light chain as part of a **pre-B cell receptor** and this permits the cell to divide further before giving rise to **small pre-B cells**.

The pre-B cell receptor consists of a productively rearranged μ heavy chain, the surrogate light chains VpreB and λ5, and the Igα and Igβ signal transduction units (Fig. 5.3), and is discussed further in Section 5-7. This receptor is expressed at the cell surface, and its expression is required for further development. In mice lacking the μ chain, B-cell development does not progress through this stage and such mice are completely deficient in B cells. Upon encountering its ligand, which is as yet unknown, this receptor launches the large pre-B cell into the cell cycle, leading to significant expansion of all pre-B cells with in-frame VDJ_H joins. It also signals for heavy-chain rearrangement to cease, thus ensuring that each cell ends up with only a single rearranged heavy-chain gene on its surface.

The proliferating large pre-B cell eventually gives rise to non-dividing small pre-B cells in which the μ heavy chain is found intracellularly, the pre-B cell receptor is no longer displayed, and in which light-chain gene rearrangements proceed. Once a light-chain gene is assembled and a

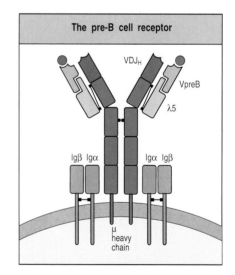

Fig. 5.3 The pre-B cell receptor. This protein complex is expressed on the surface of large pre-B cells. It is thought to resemble an immunoglobulin molecule and consist of two rearranged μ heavy chains together with a surrogate light chain consisting of VpreB and λ5, and to be complexed with the signal transduction molecules Igα and Igβ. The ligand for this receptor is unknown.

complete IgM molecule is expressed on the cell surface, the cell is now defined as an **immature B cell**. At this stage the cell is subject to selection for self-tolerance and its ability to survive in the periphery, as described in the next part of this chapter. All the preceding stages of development take place in the bone marrow, independent of antigen; as the surviving B cells now emerge into the periphery, they undergo further differentiation to become **mature B cells** expressing immunoglobulin D in addition to immunoglobulin M. These cells, also called **naive B cells** until they encounter their specific antigen, now recirculate through secondary lymphoid tissues where they may encounter and be activated by foreign antigen.

The expression of the immunoglobulin heavy and light chains are key milestones in this differentiation pathway. These events do more than simply delineate stages of the pathway; as we shall see in Section 5-7, the surface expression first of an intact heavy chain, and later a complete immunoglobulin molecule, actively regulates progression from one stage to the next.

Other markers of early B-cell development are the changes seen in cell-surface molecules (see Fig. 5.23), growth factor dependence, cell size, and location within the bone marrow. Antibodies to stage-specific cell-surface markers are particularly useful to clinicians who wish to identify lymphoproliferative diseases (see Section 5-17) and immunodeficiencies affecting B-cell development, while researchers can use such antibodies to separate subpopulations of cells from each stage in order to study them further (see Section 2-17). Evidence for the order of steps in B-cell development can be derived by studying the further development of such sorted populations, and by analyzing spontaneously occurring or genetically engineered mutants in which B-cell development is blocked. Such developmental blocks are associated with defects in a variety of cellular proteins including recombination enzymes, signaling molecules, and transcription factors, all of which play an important role in B-cell development, as we shall see.

5-2   The bone marrow provides an essential microenvironment for early B-cell development.

Immature B cells are initially generated in the fetal liver and later, exclusively in the bone marrow. B-cell development is dependent upon the non-lymphoid stromal cells found in these sites: stem cells removed from the bone marrow and grown in culture fail to differentiate into B cells unless fetal liver or bone marrow stromal cells are also present. The stroma, whose name derives from the Greek word for a mattress, thus provides a necessary support for B-cell development. The contribution of the stromal cells is twofold. First, they form specific adhesion contacts with the developing B-lineage cells by interactions between cell adhesion molecules (CAMs) and their ligands. Second, they provide growth factors, for instance the membrane-bound stem cell factor (SCF) which is recognized by the surface receptor Kit on early B-lineage cells, and the secreted cytokine interleukin-7, which is recognized by late pro-B and pre-B cells (Fig. 5.4). In addition, a small cytokine known as PBSF/SDF-1, which is produced constitutively by bone marrow stromal cells, plays an important role in early stages of B-cell development, as shown by the failure of B-cell development in mice lacking the gene for this cytokine. Other adhesion molecules and growth factors produced by stromal cells may have a role in B-cell development; this is an active area of research and a full understanding of the factors that regulate B-cell differentiation has yet to be achieved.

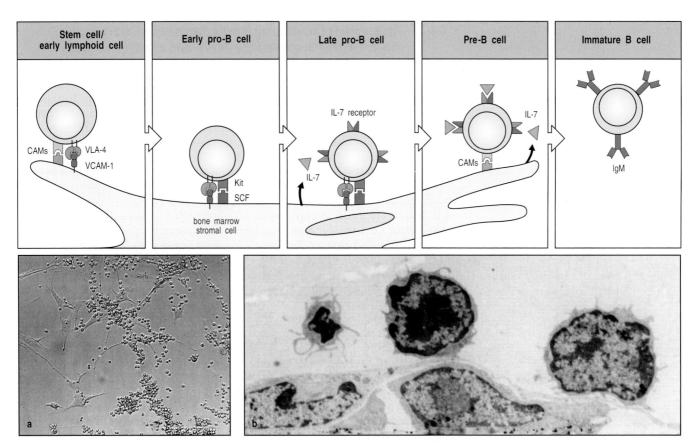

Fig. 5.4 **The early stages of B-cell development are dependent on bone marrow stromal cells.** Top panels: lymphoid progenitor cells and early pro-B cells bind to VCAM-1 on stromal cells through the integrin VLA-4; there are also interactions through other cell adhesion molecules (CAMs). This promotes the binding of their surface Kit receptor tyrosine kinase to stem-cell factor (SCF) on the stromal cell, activating the kinase and inducing proliferation of the B cell. Later stages require interleukin-7 (IL-7) for their growth and maturation. Panel a: light micrograph showing small round cells, which are the B-lymphoid progenitors in intimate contact with cultured stromal cells, which have extended processes fastening them to the plastic dish on which they are grown. Panel b: a high magnification electron micrograph, where two lymphoid cells are seen adhering to a flattened stromal cell. Photographs courtesy of A Rolink (a); P Kincade and P L Witte (b).

As B-lineage cells mature, they migrate in contact with stromal cells within the marrow. The earliest stem cells lie in a region called the subendosteum, which is adjacent to the bone surface. As maturation proceeds, B-lineage cells move towards the central axis of the marrow cavity (Fig. 5.5). Later stages of maturation become less dependent on contact with stromal cells. Final development from immature B cells into mature B cells can occur either in the bone marrow or in secondary lymphoid organs such as the spleen.

Fig. 5.5 **B-lineage cells move within the bone marrow towards its central axis as they mature.** This transverse section of a rat femur was photographed using ultraviolet illumination to identify fluorescent cells stained for terminal deoxynucleotidyl transferase (TdT), which marks the pro-B stage (see Fig. 5.8). Immature pro-B cells expressing TdT are concentrated near the endosteum (the inner bone surface), as seen towards the upper right quadrant of the picture. As development proceeds, cells lose TdT and pass towards the axis of the marrow cavity (lower left), where they wait in sinuses ready for export. Photograph courtesy of D Opstelten and M Hermans.

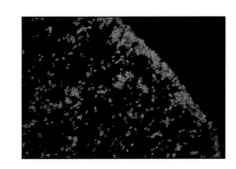

5-3
The survival of developing B cells depends on the productive, sequential rearrangement of a heavy- and a light-chain gene.

A large number of developing B cells are lost because they fail to rearrange their immunoglobulin gene segments productively to form one functional heavy-chain gene and one functional light-chain gene. This failure is caused by imprecise joining of the gene segments, which in turn is a consequence of the way diversity is created at the junctions during gene rearrangement (see Section 3-16). The imprecise joining mechanism means that it is a matter of chance whether V gene segments and J gene segments are assembled in a way that preserves their correct reading frames; each time a V gene segment undergoes rearrangement to a J or a DJ gene segment there is a roughly two-in-three chance of generating an out-of-frame sequence downstream from the join. The points at which non-productive rearrangements may lead to cell loss as B cells sequentially rearrange their immunoglobulin genes are shown in Fig. 5.6. As we shall see, far fewer cells are lost as a consequence of failing to make productive light-chain gene rearrangements than are lost at the stage of heavy-chain gene rearrangements, because the opportunity for successive rearrangement attempts is much greater in the case of the light-chain genes.

Immunoglobulin heavy-chain gene rearrangement begins with a D_H gene segment joining to a J_H gene segment. D_H to J_H rearrangements occur in early pro-B cells, and often occur on both chromosomes of the diploid set before the cell, now classified as a late pro-B cell, proceeds to rearrange a V_H gene to join a DJ_H complex. Most $D–J_H$ joins in humans are potentially

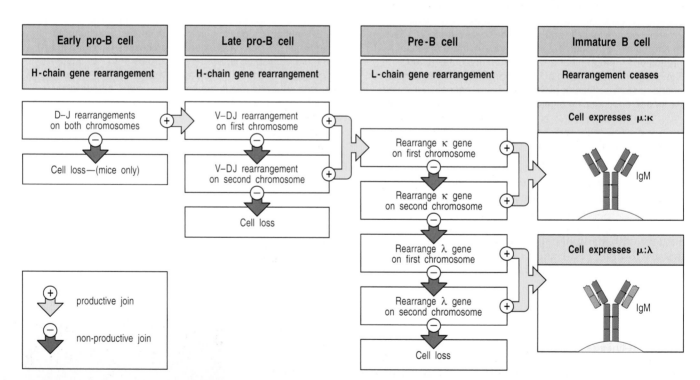

Fig. 5.6 Steps in immunoglobulin gene rearrangement leading to the expression of cell-surface immunoglobulin. The developmental program usually rearranges first heavy-chain genes and then light-chain genes. Cells are allowed to progress to the next stage when a productive rearrangement has been achieved in a prior stage. Each rearrangement has about a

one-in-three chance of being successful, but if the first attempt is non-productive, development is suspended and there is a chance for one or more further attempts. The scope for repeated rearrangements is greater in the case of the light-chain genes (see Fig. 5.7), so that fewer cells are lost between the pre-B and immature B-cell stages than in the pro-B to pre-B transition.

useful, as almost all human D gene segments can be translated in all three reading frames. In mice, however, most D gene segments can only be used productively in one of the three possible reading frames, and some DJ_H joins abort further development because they give rise to a truncated heavy chain which can be expressed at the cell surface but cannot form a functional pre-B cell receptor (see Section 5-7). Thus, in mice, some developing B cells are lost at this stage, while a significant proportion of the cells that proceed carry DJ_H rearrangements that are out-of-frame and unable to give rise to productive V_H–DJ_H rearrangements.

V_H to DJ_H rearrangement occurs first on only one chromosome, and the chances of this rearrangement generating a joint that puts the V gene in-frame with downstream sequences is, in humans, one-in-three. Taking into account the possibility of rearranging one of the considerable number of V_H pseudogenes, the probability of generating a productive V_H–DJ_H rearrangement on the first attempt will be something less than one-in-three. A successful first rearrangement means that intact μ chains are produced and the cell progresses to become a pre-B cell. In at least two out of three cases, however, the first rearrangement will be non-productive, and rearrangement will continue on the other chromosome, again with a chance of less than one-in-three of being productive. Overall this gives a rough estimate of the chance of generating a pre-B cell of something less than $\frac{1}{3} + (\frac{1}{3} \times \frac{2}{3}) = 0.55$, and in mice, for the reasons explained already, the probability of success will be lower. The pro-B cells in which both rearrangements are non-productive are unable to receive a survival signal. Some of these cells may be rescued by a secondary rearrangement, which replaces their V gene segment sequences with another V_H gene (we shall discuss this mechanism further in Section 5-11), but most appear to be lost from the lineage and this is therefore the fate of a considerable proportion of pro-B cells.

The large pre-B cells, in which a successful heavy-chain gene rearrangement has just occurred, are dividing actively. In the mouse they divide five or six times, thus undergoing approximately 30- to 60-fold expansion before becoming resting, small pre-B cells. These divisions are thought to occur after successful rearrangement of a heavy-chain gene and the transient expression of a μ heavy chain at the cell surface as part of the pre-B receptor (see Fig. 5.2). A large pre-B cell with a particular rearranged heavy-chain gene can therefore give rise to many progeny, each of which can make different light-chain gene rearrangements upon reaching the small pre-B cell stage.

In the mouse and human B-cell lineages, κ-gene segments tend to rearrange before λ-gene segments. This was first deduced from the observation that λ-chain-secreting myeloma cells generally have both their κ- and λ-genes rearranged, but only their κ-genes are rearranged if they are κ producers. This order is occasionally reversed, however, and λ-chain gene rearrangement does not absolutely require the prior rearrangement of the κ genes. Whatever the order, rearrangement only occurs at one locus at a time in each individual cell; B cells never make simultaneous rearrangements of both their κ and λ genes.

As in the case of the heavy-chain genes, light-chain gene rearrangements also take place on only one chromosome at a time. Unlike the heavy-chain genes, however, there is scope for repeated rearrangements of unused V and J gene segments (Fig. 5.7). Several successive attempts at productive rearrangement of a light-chain gene can therefore be made on one chromosome before initiating any rearrangements on the second chromosome. Each V–J join has a one-in-three chance of assembling a productive light-chain gene and the chances of eventually generating an intact light chain are greatly increased by the potential for multiple success-ive rearrangement events on each chromosome and at each of the two

Fig. 5.7   Non-productive light-chain gene rearrangements may be rescued by further gene rearrangement. The organization of the light-chain genes in mice and humans offers many opportunities for rescue of pre-B cells that initially make an out of frame light-chain gene rearrangement. Light-chain rescue is illustrated for the mouse κ locus, where it has been demonstrated experimentally. If the first rearrangement is non-productive, a 5′ V_κ gene segment can recombine with a 3′ J_κ gene segment to remove the out of frame join and replace it. In principle, this can happen up to four times on each chromosome, since there are four functional J_κ segments in the mouse (the fifth is a pseudogene). In humans, there are five functional J_κ segments. If all rearrangements of κ-chain genes fail to yield a productive light-chain join, λ-chain gene rearrangement may succeed (not shown). The λ light-chain genes are arranged in four sets of V, J, and C gene segments (see Fig. 3.15); although one of these is a pseudogene, this organization nonetheless can allow several λ light-chain gene rearrangements to occur on each chromosome. Thus, there is a very high probability of productive light-chain gene rearrangement in developing B cells and most pre-B cells successfully complete their differentiation to immature B cells. Similar repeated rearrangements for the heavy chain locus are much less likely because there exists no spare downstream DJ_H joints to which a new V_H could join and the 12-23 rule prevents V_H rearranging directly to J_H.

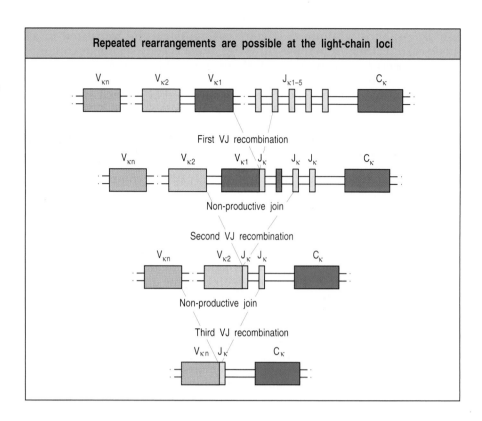

Repeated rearrangements are possible at the light-chain loci

First VJ recombination

Non-productive join

Second VJ recombination

Non-productive join

Third VJ recombination

light-chain loci. As a result of the redundancy in light-chain genes, most B-cell precursors that reach the pre-B cell stage succeed in generating progeny that bear intact IgM molecules and can be classified as immature cells; the success rate is about 85% in mice. Overall, the proportion of B-lineage cells that survive the process of primary receptor diversification should theoretically be no more than 0.85 x 0.55 = 0.47, and may be considerably less if pseudogenes are taken into account.

5-4   The expression of proteins regulating immunoglobulin gene rearrangement and function is developmentally programmed.

While the sequential steps in immunoglobulin gene rearrangement and immunoglobulin chain production provide defining markers for the different stages in B-cell differentiation, a variety of other proteins contribute to this process. Fig. 5.8 lists some of these, and shows how their expression is regulated through the different stages of B-cell development.

Immunoglobulin gene rearrangement is itself dependent on expression of the recombination activation genes **RAG-1** and **RAG-2** (see Section 3-17). The enzymes encoded by these genes also mediate rearrangement of the T-cell receptor genes and they are active in very early stages of lymphoid development, before the B- and T-cell lineages have diverged. In both these lineages there is a later temporary suppression of *RAG* gene expression after the first successful rearrangement event. In the B-cell lineage, *RAG* transcripts are in the large cycling pre-B cells that express an intact immunoglobulin heavy chain as part of the pre-B cell receptor at the cell surface. They accumulate again as these cells divide further but RAG-2 protein and RAG activity is only seen again when the

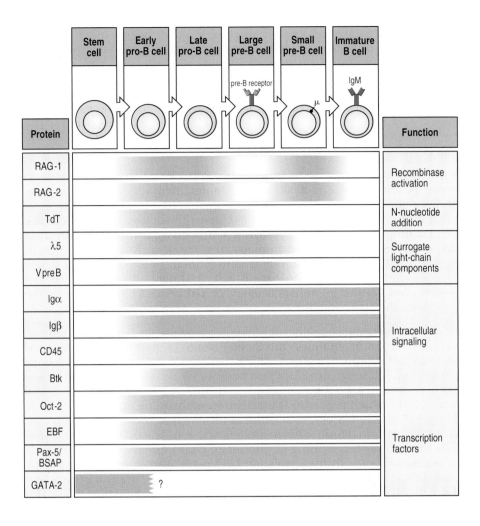

Fig. 5.8 The expression of several important cellular proteins changes during B-cell development. The proteins listed here are a selection of those known to be associated with early B-lineage development, and have been included because of their proven importance in the developmental sequence, largely on the basis of studies in mice. Their individual contributions to B-cell development are discussed in the text, with the exception of the Octamer Transcription Factor, Oct-2, which binds the octamer ATGCAAAT found in the heavy-chain promoter and elsewhere, and GATA-2, which is one example of the many transcription factors that are active in several hematopoietic lineages. CD45 refers to the high molecular weight isoform of the phosphotyrosine phosphatase expressing the A, B, and C exons, which is restricted to the B-cell lineage and is known as B220 in mice. The *pax-5* gene product known as B-lineage specific activator protein (BSAP) is involved in regulating the expression of several of the other proteins listed. The tight temporal regulation of the expression of these proteins, and of the immunoglobulin genes themselves, would be expected to impose a strict sequence on the events of B-cell differentiation.

cells cease cycling and become small pre-B cells—the stage at which light-chain gene rearrangement occurs. *RAG* gene expression ceases again when a complete immunoglobulin molecule is expressed at the cell surface and the cell becomes an immature B cell.

Another enzyme, **terminal deoxynucleotidyl transferase (TdT)**, contributes to the diversity of both B- and T-cell antigen-receptor repertoires by adding N-nucleotides at the rearrangement joints. As with the *RAG* genes, TdT is expressed in early lymphoid progenitors but, unlike the RAG-1/RAG-2 enzyme, it is not essential to the rearrangement process; indeed, at the time that the peripheral immune system is first being supplied with T and B lymphocytes, TdT is not expressed at all. It ceases to be expressed at the pre-B cell stage in adult mice when heavy-chain gene rearrangement is complete and light-chain gene rearrangement has commenced. This timing explains why N-nucleotides are found in the V–D and D–J joints of heavy-chain genes and in about half of human V–J joints of light-chain genes. Mice have N-nucleotides only rarely in their light-chain joints, showing that they switch off TdT earlier.

Proteins required for the cell-surface expression of the immunoglobulin chains are also essential for B-cell development. These include the Igα (CD79a) and Igβ (CD79b) components of the B-cell and pre-B cell antigen receptor, which transduce signals from these receptors by interacting with intracellular tyrosine kinases through their cytoplasmic tails. Igα and Igβ are expressed from the pro-B cell stage until death of the cell or its terminal differentiation into an antibody-secreting plasma cell.

For reasons that are not known, mice lacking Igβ have a block in B-cell development at the pro-B cell stage before VDJ$_H$ rearrangements are complete. Formation of the pre-B receptor complex also requires λ5 and VpreB, which together make up a surrogate light chain that combines with the product of newly rearranged heavy-chain gene. The pre-B receptor complex appears only briefly at the cell surface, perhaps because λ5 and VpreB cease to be expressed as soon as this occurs. The cell-surface expression of the pre-B receptor is an important checkpoint in B-cell development and will be discussed further in Section 5-7.

A third category of proteins included in Fig. 5.8 are signal-transduction proteins with a role in B-cell development. Bruton's tyrosine kinase, Btk, is a good example of a signaling molecule that has received intense scrutiny because mutations in the *Btk* gene cause a profound B-lineage specific immune deficiency, **Bruton's X-linked agammaglobulinemia (XLA)** (see Section 10-7). In humans, the block in B-cell development caused by *XLA* locus mutations is almost total, interrupting the transition from pre-B cell to immature B cell. A similar, though less severe defect called X-linked immunodeficiency, or **xid**, arises from mutations in the corresponding gene in mice.

Finally, several gene regulatory proteins are essential for B-cell development, as shown by deficiencies of the B-cell lineage in genetically engineered mutants lacking these proteins. At least 10 transcription factors necessary for normal B-lineage development have been described, and there are likely to be others. One essential transcription factor is the early B-cell factor, EBF, which regulates transcription of the gene for Igα. Another is the *pax-5* gene product, one isoform of which is the B-lineage specific activator protein (BSAP). This protein is active in late pro-B cells and permits the proper functioning of the heavy chain enhancer; it also binds to regulatory sites in the genes for λ5, VpreB, and other B-cell specific proteins. It seems likely that these regulatory proteins and others like them together direct the developmental program of B-lineage cells. The gene-regulatory proteins involved in the tissue-specific transcriptional regulation of immunoglobulin genes are likely to be particularly important in regulating the order of events in gene rearrangement, to which we now turn.

| 5-5 | **Immunoglobulin gene rearrangement is closely co-ordinated with gene transcription.** |

The **V(D)J recombinase** system (see Section 3-17) operates in both B- and T-lineage cells and employs the same core enzymes, which recognize the same conserved recombination signal sequences in both immunoglobulin and T-cell receptor genes. Yet productive rearrangements of T-cell receptor genes do not occur in B-lineage cells, and although T cells show some DJ$_H$ rearrangements in their immunoglobulin genes, these may occur before the two lineages diverge, and VDJ$_H$ rearrangements are not seen. The close temporal co-ordination between the initiation of rearrangement and transcription of the segments that are to be joined suggests that this may be achieved by controlling gene rearrangement using gene-regulatory proteins specific to T or B cells.

Before a gene rearrangement occurs, there is a low level of transcription from the separate immunoglobulin gene segments that are to be joined at that step. This transcription is initiated at a promoter located upstream of each V gene segment, and at another upstream of the J and C gene segments. The activity of these promoters is controlled by the binding of gene-regulatory proteins to tissue-specific enhancers which, in the case of heavy-chain genes and the κ light-chain genes, lie in the intron between the J gene segments and the C-region exons and also 3' to the C exons (Fig. 5.9). Mice mutated in either of the κ enhancers show reduced but not completely abolished rearrangement of their κ gene segments, supporting the idea that specific DNA-binding proteins contribute to the initiation of gene rearrangement events.

One model proposes that gene-regulatory proteins control the accessibility of the immunoglobulin gene chromatin to the recombination enzymes. For example, B-lineage specific proteins such as BSAP that bind to the immunoglobulin enhancers could make the chromatin in the region accessible, not only to transcriptional activation but also to the enzymes that mediate somatic recombination. The gene-regulatory proteins might also act in a more direct way. Some enhancer-binding proteins may activate transcription by interacting with the basal transcription machinery bound to the promoter, a mechanism that would involve 'looping-out' the intervening DNA and which might, in itself, promote access to the recombination signal sequences included in the loop.

In principle, therefore, master genes that encode gene-regulatory proteins can execute a developmental program of lineage- and stage-specific activation that could account for the ordered control of immunoglobulin

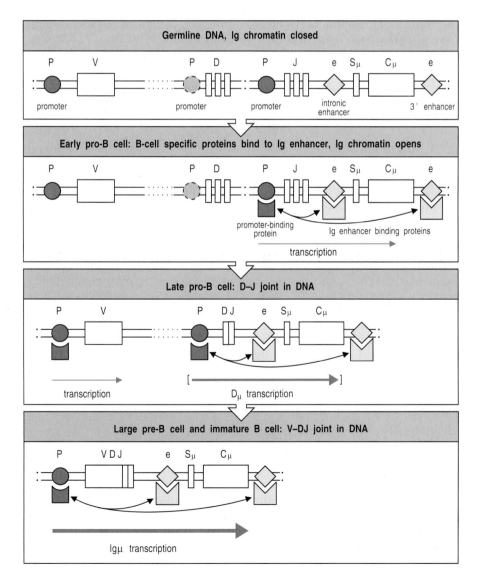

Fig. 5.9 Proteins binding to promoter and enhancer elements contribute to the sequence of gene rearrangement and regulate the level of RNA transcription. First panel: in germline DNA, stem cells, and non-lymphoid cells, the chromatin containing the immunoglobulin genes is in a closed conformation. Second panel: in the early pro-B cell, specific proteins bind to the Ig enhancer elements (e); for the heavy chain, these are in the J–C intron and 3' to the C exons. The DNA is now in an open conformation, and low-level transcription from promoters (P) upstream of the J gene segments is seen. Third panel: the rearrangement D to J_H that follows the initiation of transcription of the J gene segments activates a low level of transcription from promoters located upstream of the D gene segments. For some D–J_H joins in the mouse this may result in the expression of a truncated heavy-chain (D_μ) at levels sufficient to abort further development but, in most cases, it is followed by initiation of low-level transcription of an upstream V_H gene segment. Fourth panel: subsequent rearrangement of a V gene segment brings its promoter under the influence of the heavy-chain enhancers, leading to enhanced production of a μ heavy-chain mRNA in large pre-B cells and their progeny. S_μ represents the switch signal sequence for isotype switching (see Section 3-22).

gene rearrangement and expression. More exact descriptions of this control must await better fundamental knowledge of the stepwise activation of the regulatory genes themselves and of how DNA-binding protein complexes assemble and function.

5-6   Gene rearrangement alters the activity of the immunoglobulin gene promoters.

Immunoglobulin gene rearrangement dramatically increases the transcriptional activity of the rearranged gene segments. Before rearrangement, the heavy-chain J and C gene segments are transcribed at a low level from the weak promoter upstream of the J gene segments and transcription of V_H gene segments is variably activated (see Fig. 5.9, top three panels). Once rearrangement has occurred, the promoter upstream of the V gene segment is brought nearer to the enhancers, with the result that, in mature B cells, the rearranged gene is transcribed at a much higher rate (see Fig. 5.9, bottom panel). Thus, gene rearrangement can be viewed as a powerful mechanism for regulating gene expression, as well as for generating receptor diversity. Several cases of gene rearrangement bringing genes under the control of a new promoter are known from prokaryotes and single-celled eukaryotes but, in vertebrates, only the immunoglobulin and T-cell receptor genes are known to use gene rearrangement to regulate gene expression.

5-7   Cell-surface expression of the products of rearranged immunoglobulin genes act as checkpoints of B-cell development.

Each fully differentiated B cell has only one successfully rearranged heavy-chain gene and one successfully rearranged light-chain gene. The increased transcription of successfully rearranged immunoglobulin genes and the resulting rapid appearance of their protein products play an important part in ensuring this outcome. This is shown dramatically by introducing an already rearranged immunoglobulin heavy-chain gene into the germline of a mouse; virtually all B cells in this transgenic mouse will express the product of the rearranged transgene and, in these B cells, rearrangement of the endogenous heavy-chain genes is suppressed. The endogenous light-chain genes rearrange normally, however, thus generating a variety of complete immunoglobulin molecules. A similar though less efficient suppression of endogenous light-chain gene rearrangement occurs in mice transgenic for a rearranged light-chain gene. Transgenic mice carrying both a rearranged heavy-chain and a rearranged light-chain gene make B cells in which rearrangements of all endogenous immunoglobulin genes are overwhelmingly suppressed. These mice therefore express a B-cell repertoire with the single dominant specificity conferred by the transgenes, and have been very valuable in studies of self-tolerance, as we shall see in Section 5-10.

In contrast to the effects of transgenes expressing complete immunoglobulin chains, a heavy-chain transgene lacking the transmembrane exon fails to suppress the rearrangement of endogenous heavy-chain genes. This is because membrane insertion and cell-surface expression of the heavy chain is needed for the suppression to occur. As we have seen, the heavy chain is expressed briefly at the cell surface as part of the pre-B receptor as soon as it is made. This appearance depends on an association between the heavy chain and two proteins made in pro-B cells, which pair non-covalently to form a **surrogate light chain** (Fig. 5.10). One of these proteins is called **λ5** because of its close similarity to the known C_λ light-chain domains, while the other, called **VpreB**, resembles a V domain but bears an extra N-terminal protein sequence. Together, λ5, VpreB, the μ heavy chain, and the attendant constant Igα and Igβ chains form a cell-surface complex that resembles a complete cell-surface immunoglobulin receptor. This cell-surface complex is called the **pre-B cell receptor** (see Fig. 5.3).

The pre-B cell receptor complex is only expressed transiently, perhaps because production of λ5 stops as soon as it is formed. Nevertheless, it mediates an important checkpoint in B-cell development. In mice lacking λ5, or possessing mutant heavy-chain genes that cannot produce transmembrane heavy chains, the pre-B cell receptor cannot be formed and development is blocked after heavy-chain gene rearrangement. Such mice have rearrangements of the heavy-chain genes on both chromosomes in all cells, and two productive VDJ_H rearrangements therefore

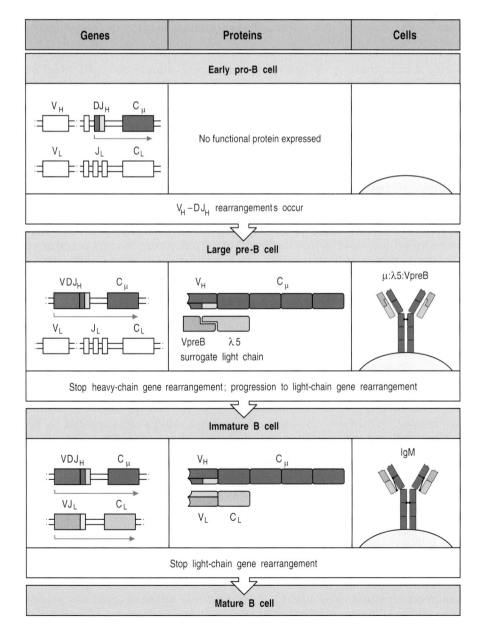

Fig. 5.10 Productively rearranged immunoglobulin genes encode proteins that are expressed immediately at the surface of the cell. First panel: in early pro-B cells, no functional μ protein is expressed. Second panel: as soon as a productive heavy-chain gene rearrangement has taken place, μ chains are expressed at the surface of the cell in an immunoglobulin-like complex with two chains, λ5 and VpreB, which together make up a surrogate light chain. Signaling via this immunoglobulin-like molecule suppresses heavy-chain gene rearrangement and drives the transition to the large pre-B cell stage by inducing proliferation. The progeny of large pre-B cells stop dividing to become small pre-B cells in which light-chain gene rearrangements commence. Third panel: successful light-chain gene rearrangement results in the production of a light chain that binds the μ chain to form a complete IgM molecule at the cell surface. Assembly of the IgM molecules is thought to trigger the cessation of light-chain gene rearrangement.

occur in about 10% of cells. In normal mice, the appearance of the pre-B cell receptor coincides with inactivation of the RAG-2 protein by phosphorylation, and degradation of *RAG-1* and *RAG-2* mRNA, suggesting that this is the mechanism by which further rearrangement is suppressed. Expression of the pre-B cell receptor at the cell surface is also associated with cell enlargement followed by a burst of proliferation. Such cells then undergo the transition to small resting pre-B cells, in which the RAG-1/RAG-2 enzyme is again active, and light-chain genes are rearranged. The pre-B cell receptor therefore appears to signal to the cell that a complete μ heavy-chain gene has been formed, that further rearrangements at this locus should be suppressed, and that development to the next stage can proceed.

The feedback loop mediating the suppression of further rearrangements may occasionally be prematurely activated in mice as a result of certain DJ$_H$ rearrangements which lead to the expression of a truncated heavy chain able to interact with the λ5-VpreB pair. The formation of this incomplete version of the pre-B cell receptor, which is known as a D$_μ$ protein (see Fig. 5.9), shuts down further heavy-chain gene rearrangement. It does not, however, deliver a signal that leads to further maturation, and in the absence of complete heavy chains, further development of the pro-B cell is aborted.

Once a light-chain gene has been rearranged successfully, its product combines with the heavy chain to form intact IgM (see Fig. 5.10), which is expressed at the cell surface in a complex with Igα and Igβ. It is not yet clear how the cell senses that a functional immunoglobulin receptor has been expressed in the absence of its specific antigen. Nevertheless, at this point further light-chain gene rearrangement ceases, and it appears that this checkpoint, like that mediated by the pre-B cell receptor, requires a signal from the receptor to suppress any further light-chain gene rearrangement and to trigger the maturation of the B cell. A role for Igα in signaling at both these checkpoints is indicated by the reduction in B-lineage cells in mice expressing Igα with a truncated cytoplasmic domain. In these mice the population of immature B cells in the marrow is reduced four-fold, while the number of peripheral B cells is reduced 100-fold, showing that an ability to signal through Igα is particularly important in dictating survival once a complete immunoglobulin molecule is expressed.

5-8   The immunoglobulin gene rearrangement program leads to monospecificity of individual B cells.

We saw in Chapter 1 that individual B cells must produce only one specificity of antibody to ensure that all the antibodies secreted by an activated B cell are specific for the antigen that originally triggered its proliferation. This prevents the secretion of antibodies of other specificities that could be wasteful or even harmful. We can now see that the regulated program of immunoglobulin gene rearrangement guarantees monospecificity, and how this, in turn, explains the phenomena of allelic and isotypic exclusion). Allelic exclusion signifies the expression of a gene from only one of the two parental chromosomes in each individual cell (Fig. 5.11) and occurs for both the heavy- and light-chain genes. Isotypic exclusion in immunoglobulin occurs only in the case of the light chains, which are produced from only one of the four light-chain loci in each individual cell. The phenomenon of allelic exclusion was first discovered 30 years ago, when it provided one of the original key pieces of experimental support for the clonal selection theory for lymphocytes.

Allelic exclusion appears to operate without substantial allelic preference, as the alleles at each locus are generally expressed in roughly equal frequencies; chance probably therefore determines which allele rearranges first. However, for isotype exclusion the situation is different, and the ratios of κ-expressing versus λ-expressing mature B cells vary from extreme to extreme in different species; in mice and rats it is 95:5, in humans typically 65:35, and in cats it is the opposite of mice. These ratios correlate with the kinetics and efficiency of rearrangements measured in a population of developing B cells and indicate that the relative probability of initiating a gene rearrangement at each of these loci must vary from species to species. The measurement of κ:λ ratios in mature lymphocyte populations is useful in clinical diagnostics, as an aberrant κ:λ ratio indicates the dominance of one clone and the presence of a lymphoproliferative disorder, which may be malignant (see Section 5-17).

Once a complete immunoglobulin molecule is generated, the monospecific B cell, now called an **immature B cell**, is exposed to selection by antigens in its environment. Before immature B cells leave the bone marrow and populate the peripheral lymphoid tissues, where they can be stimulated to make antibody, those that are stimulated by self antigens must be removed or inactivated to ensure self tolerance. We shall describe some mechanisms of ensuring B-cell tolerance in subsequent sections of this chapter, and also in Chapter 12, while the activation of B cells in the periphery will be discussed in Chapter 8. First, however, we look at the fate of the new B cells generated in the bone marrow as they first emerge into the periphery.

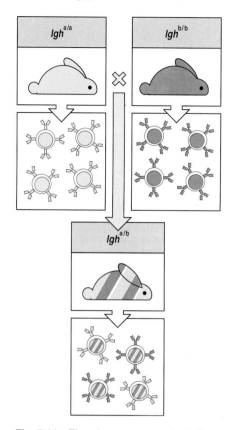

Fig. 5.11 The phenomenon of allelic exclusion in single B cells. Most species have genetic polymorphisms of the constant regions of their immunoglobulin heavy- and light-chain genes known as allotypes. In rabbits, for example, all of the B cells in an individual homozygous for the *a* allele of the immunoglobulin heavy chain (*Igh*) will express immunoglobulin of type *a*, while in an individual homozygous for the *b* allele, all the B cells make immunoglobulin of type *b*. In a heterozygous animal, carrying both *a* and *b* alleles, allelic exclusion can be shown by staining the surface of B cells with anti-allotype antibodies (see Section 3-23) coupled to two different dyes. Each individual B cell stains either one color or the other but not both. Most often, equal frequencies of the B cells bearing each allele are made but sometimes there is a bias. The expression of only one of the parental alleles in any one B cell reflects productive rearrangement of only one of the two parental chromosomes carrying the Igh locus. For light chains, isotype exclusion is seen as well as allelic exclusion, and only one allele from one of the two light-chain loci is expressed in each individual cell.

5-9 Lymphoid follicles are thought to provide a second essential environment for B cells.

After B cells leave the bone marrow, they recirculate around the body, passing from the blood into the secondary lymphoid organs—the spleen, lymph nodes and mucosal-associated lymphoid tissues (see Chapter 1)—and returning from these organs to the blood via the lymphatic system, or directly in the case of the spleen. Within the secondary lymphoid organs, the B cells are localized in discrete clusters, called **follicles**, comprised primarily of B cells and a specialized stromal cell, **the follicular dendritic cell**. Mature resting B lymphocytes appear to need signals from follicles, possibly from the follicular dendritic cells, to survive and continue to recirculate. This has been deduced from experiments that trace the fate of transgenic B cells expressing surface immunoglobulin of a single known specificity. When these B lymphocytes are transfused intravenously into recipients in which a space has been cleared for them, for example by irradiation, they survive. If they are introduced into a recipient with normal lymphocyte numbers, however, most are excluded from the follicles by other B cells and die. It therefore seems that the microenvironment of the lymphoid follicle provides signals essential for the survival of B cells, although the identity of these signals and their source still remain to be determined. B cells that succeed in migrating into a follicle receive a survival signal, then move on into the efferent lymphatics and back into the blood. Their continued survival depends, however, on further recirculation through the follicles of secondary lymphoid tissue.

New B cells continue to be produced by the bone marrow throughout life, yet the number of follicles is limited; exclusion from these follicles may explain why the majority of newly generated B cells that emerge from the bone marrow die in the periphery after only a few days. Thus the life of a B cell can be viewed as a continuing Darwinian struggle in which B cells compete with each other for access to lymphoid follicles.

The competition for follicular signals could explain the normal regulation of the size of the mature B lymphocyte pool in the body. As we shall see, this competition may also play an important part in the elimination of some self-reactive B cells.

Summary.

B cells are generated throughout life in the specialized environment of the bone marrow, and may require a second environment, the lymphoid follicle to maintain their existence as mature recirculating B cells. As B cells differentiate from primitive stem cells, they proceed through stages that are marked by the sequential rearrangement of immunoglobulin gene segments to generate a diverse repertoire of antigen receptors. This developmental program also involves changes in the expression of other cellular proteins and is directed by transcription factors. It is characterized by two important checkpoints; as each intact immunoglobulin chain is generated by somatic gene rearrangement, it signals the developing cell to cease rearrangement of the set of gene segments specifying that chain and to progress to the next developmental step. However, if successive rearrangements fail to generate first a heavy-chain that can form a pre-B cell receptor, and then a light-chain which can be expressed as part of a complete immunoglobulin molecule at the cell surface, the developing B cell fails to progress and dies. The end-product of this process is a B cell with surface immunoglobulin of a single specificity. At this stage in its development, the B cell is ready for selective events driven by antigen binding to these cell-surface receptors.

Selection of B cells.

If an antigen binds specifically to the newly expressed surface IgM of an immature B lymphocyte, the cell is eliminated or inactivated. Thus, those B cells that recognize self molecules while still immature are prevented from developing further and from secreting antibodies that bind self cells or tissues. This results in a B-cell receptor repertoire tolerant of the self molecules encountered up to this stage. We shall see that the form of presentation of a self molecule, for instance whether membrane-bound or soluble, and its abundance, make a vital difference to whether it leads to tolerance. The immature B cell may die, survive for a short time but become non-functional, or edit its receptors to a new specificity. Only after this screening for potential autoreactivity do the B cells migrate to the peripheral lymphoid tissues, completing their maturation. Here, they may encounter other self molecules that were not available to immature B cells. There are also a variety of supplementary mechanisms that render mature self-reactive B cells unresponsive to self antigens, which are described in Chapter 12.

5-10   **Immature B cells can be eliminated or inactivated by contact with self antigens.**

The immature B cells generated in the bone marrow express only surface IgM. The completion of B-cell development involves emigration from the bone marrow and the alternative splicing of heavy-chain transcripts to generate mature B cells expressing surface IgM and IgD (see Fig. 3.25). A proportion of newly generated immature B cells fail to make this transition, however, and one reason for this is the elimination of potentially self-reactive cells.

Immature B cells expressing only IgM are eliminated or inactivated if they bind to abundant multivalent ligands. This can be demonstrated by using anti-μ chain antibodies to crosslink the surface IgM of immature B cells, mimicking the effect of multivalent antigens; such treatment results in the inactivation or death of all immature B cells. This distinguishes immature B cells from mature B cells, which are normally activated by multivalent antigens (see Section 8-10). Thus, immature B cells bearing self-reactive receptors must be eliminated during the few days before this transition in reactivity occurs.

Experiments with transgenic mice have shown that two different mechanisms ensure tolerance to self antigens encountered by immature B cells. One of them operates in the case of multivalent antigens, for example multiple copies of an MHC molecule on a cell surface; the other operates when the antigens are of low valence, for example small soluble proteins (Fig. 5.12). The effect of encounter with a multivalent antigen was tested in mice transgenic for both chains of an antibody specific for H-2K^b MHC class I molecules; in such mice, for the reasons discussed earlier, all B cells that develop bear the anti-MHC antibody as surface IgM. If the transgenic mouse does not express H-2K^b, normal numbers of B cells develop, all bearing transgene-encoded anti-H-2K^b receptors. However, in mice bearing both H-2K^b and the immunoglobulin transgenes, B-cell development is blocked: normal numbers of pre-B cells are found but B cells expressing the anti-H-2K^b antibody as surface IgM never develop; instead most of these immature B cells die in the bone marrow by apoptosis. This antigen-induced loss from the B-cell population is known as **clonal deletion** (see Fig. 5.12, left panels). Similar results have been obtained in mice doubly transgenic for an antibody

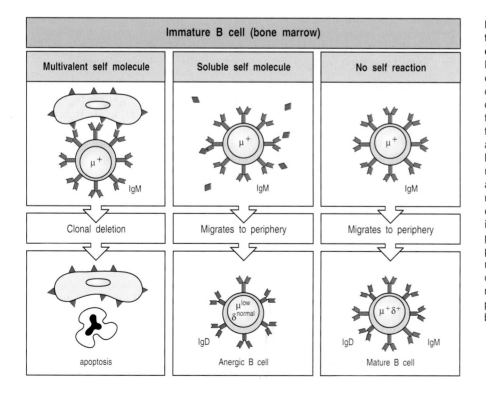

Immature B cell (bone marrow)

Multivalent self molecule	Soluble self molecule	No self reaction
μ$^+$ IgM	μ$^+$ IgM	μ$^+$ IgM
Clonal deletion	Migrates to periphery	Migrates to periphery
apoptosis	μ^{low} δ^{normal} IgD — Anergic B cell	μ$^+$δ$^+$ IgD IgM — Mature B cell

Fig. 5.12 Binding to self molecules in the bone marrow can lead to the deletion or inactivation of immature B cells. Left panels: when developing B cells express receptors that recognize ubiquitous cell-surface molecules, such as MHC class I molecules, they are deleted from the repertoire. These B cells are believed to undergo programmed cell death or apoptosis. Center panels: immature B cells that bind soluble self antigens are rendered unresponsive or anergic to the antigen and bear little surface IgM. They migrate to the periphery where they express IgD but remain anergic, and if in competition with other B cells in the periphery, they are rapidly lost. Right panels: only immature B cells that do not encounter antigen at this early stage of development mature normally, and migrate from the bone marrow to the peripheral lymphoid tissues as B cells bearing both IgM and IgD on their surface.

and for its ligand expressed as a cell-surface molecule. Clonal deletion has also been shown to occur when potentially self-reactive B cells encounter a multivalent antigen on first emerging into the periphery. This was demonstrated in mice transgenic for anti-H-2K^b receptors and for H-2K^b expressed under the control of a liver promoter so that it is made only in liver cells; in these mice, immature H-2K^b-specific B cells are found in the bone marrow but no mature peripheral B cells are seen.

In contrast, when soluble antigen binds an immature B cell, the cell is inactivated but not killed. Thus, when hen egg lysozyme (HEL) is expressed in soluble form (from a transgene) in mice that are also transgenic for high-affinity anti-HEL antibody, the HEL-specific B cells mature but are unable to respond to antigen. The non-responsive cells retain their IgM within the cell and transport little to the surface. In addition, they develop a partial block in signal transduction so that, despite normal levels of HEL-binding surface IgD, the cells cannot be stimulated by crosslinking this receptor. It appears that this blockade in signal transduction lies prior to the phosphorylation of the Igα and Igβ associated with the B-cell receptor (see Section 3-25), although its exact nature is not yet known. This state of non-reactivity is called **anergy**, and such B cells are defined as **anergic** (see Fig. 5.12, center panels).

An extension of these experiments shows that anergy is induced in a similar way in mature B cells that encounter and bind an abundant soluble antigen. The HEL transgene is placed under the control of an inducible promoter that can be regulated by changes in the diet of the mouse. It is thus possible to vary the stage of development at which the lysozyme is produced and thereby study its effects on B cells at different stages of maturation. Such experiments have demonstrated that inactivation occurs whether the B cells are chronically or acutely exposed to the soluble antigen, and is independent of the developmental stage of the B cell at the time of the encounter.

In a normal animal, in which the B cells binding soluble antigen are in a minority, they are detained in the T-cell areas of the secondary lymphoid tissue and excluded from the primary lymphoid follicles. Since anergic B cells cannot be activated by T cells, and T-cell help will not in any case be available for self antigens to which the T cells themselves are tolerant, these antigen-binding B cells will not be activated to secrete antibody. Instead they are rapidly lost, thus ensuring that the long-lived pool of peripheral B cells is purged of such potentially self-reactive cells.

Peripheral antigens that are not present in the tissues through which naive B cells circulate, will not be able to purge newly generated B cells as they emerge, and cells expressing receptors specific for such antigens may therefore survive. However, in the event of such a cell contacting these self antigens, it will usually be held in check and then eliminated because of its dependence on T cells, as explained in the preceding paragraph and in Section 12-24.

5-11   Some potentially self-reactive B cells may be rescued by further immunoglobulin gene rearrangement.

In the discussion of success rates of rearrangement (see Section 5-3), we saw that a rearrangement attempt on a given chromosome may be repeated. While this may normally occur after an unproductive rearrangement (see Fig. 5.7), it has also been shown to rescue immature self-reactive B cells, by deleting a rearrangement that encodes an autoreactive receptor and replacing it with the product of a further rearrangement event. These **receptor editing** phenomena have been demonstrated in mice bearing site-directed transgenes for autoantibody heavy and light chains. Unlike ordinary transgenic mice, whose transgenes may be integrated anywhere in the genome, the site-directed transgenes are placed in their normal site within the immunoglobulin V and J gene segment loci by a method explained in Section 2-37. In this way, the transgene imitates a primary rearrangement and is surrounded by unused endogenous gene segments. In mice that express the antigen recognized by the transgene-encoded receptor, the few peripheral B cells that emerge are not self-reactive (Fig. 5.13) because they have used these surrounding gene segments for further rearrangements that delete the autoreactive transgene.

At a light-chain locus, the conventional recombination signal sequences that flank these unused gene segments can be used for a further rearrangement, just as is thought to occur after a non-productive rearrangement, as illustrated for κ in Fig. 5.7. At the heavy-chain locus, however, receptor editing requires the use of embedded recombination signal sequences in a recombination event that displaces the V gene segment sequence from the autoreactive rearrangement and replaces it with a new V gene segment (Fig. 5.14). These recombination signal sequences are found in highly conserved regions at the 3′ end of most V_H gene segments and they may also be used in replacing non-productive rearrangements at the heavy-chain locus, although this has yet to be demonstrated. So far, receptor editing has only been demonstrated in mice transgenic for rearranged immunoglobulin genes; however, rare immature B cells with active RAG-1 and RAG-2 have been found in the bone marrow of normal mice—these may represent self-reactive B cells undergoing further receptor gene rearrangement. This process only occurs while B cells are still immature, before they have left the bone marrow.

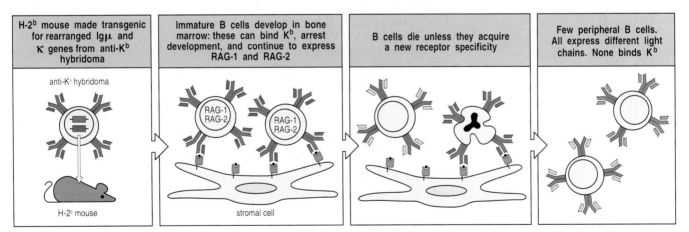

Fig. 5.13 Replacement of light chains by receptor editing can rescue some self-reactive B cells from elimination by changing their antigen specificity. If an H-2^d mouse is made transgenic for the heavy- and light-chain genes of an immunoglobulin specific for the MHC class I molecule, H-2K^b, normal numbers of B cells develop. They all express the transgenes and are specific for H-2K^b (not shown). First panel: if the same rearranged immunoglobulin genes are introduced into an H-2K^b mouse, which expresses the H-2K^b molecule on its tissues, the developing B cells express the immunoglobulin at a very early stage and can bind to the H-2K^b molecule in the bone marrow. Second panel: binding to H-2K^b in the bone marrow appears to signal the B cells to arrest their development and continue to express RAG-1 and RAG-2. Third panel: this enables some B cells to make further light-chain gene rearrangements which generate new receptor specificities (yellow). Most of the B cells do not make new rearrangements and are deleted. Fourth panel: if a B cell makes a new receptor which does not bind self antigens in the bone marrow, it can mature and enter the peripheral circulation. Thus, in the transgenic H-2K^b mice, there are many fewer peripheral B cells than normal and none expresses the transgenic light chain.

Fig. 5.14 Immunoglobulin heavy-chain gene rearrangements may be rescued by further rearrangements that make use of recombination signal sequences found at the 3′ end of V_H gene segments. The first recombination event that takes place at the heavy-chain locus excises all unused D_H segments so that further rearrangements using conventional recombination signal sequences flanking unused gene segments are not possible. Instead, recombination signal sequences that are embedded in the 3′ end of most V_H coding regions can be used to displace the autoreactive V from the first VDJ join with a different V_H coding region.

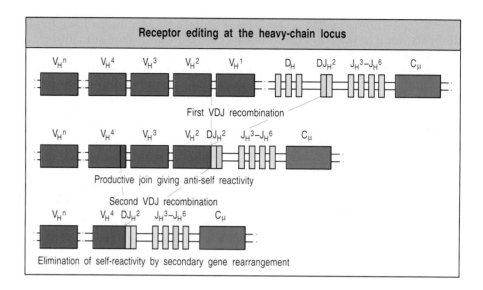

Receptor editing at the heavy-chain locus

First VDJ recombination

Productive join giving anti-self reactivity

Second VDJ recombination

Elimination of self-reactivity by secondary gene rearrangement

---

5-12   In some species, most immunoglobulin gene diversification occurs after gene rearrangement.

In humans and mice, all stages of B-cell development and immunoglobulin gene rearrangement occur in the bone marrow, and much receptor diversity is generated during rearrangement (see Section 3-14). In some other species, B cells develop in a different fashion. In birds, rabbits, and sheep, there is little or no **germline diversity** in the V, D, and J gene segments that form the initial B-cell receptors, and the rearranged variable region sequences are identical or similar in all immature B cells. These B cells then migrate to a specialized microenvironment, the best known of which is the bursa of Fabricius in chickens. Here, surface immunoglobulin-positive B cells proliferate rapidly, and their already rearranged receptor genes undergo further diversification (Fig. 5.15). In birds and rabbits, this occurs by a process of **gene conversion**, in which an unused V gene segment exchanges short sequences with the expressed rearranged variable-region gene. In sheep, diversification is the result of somatic hypermutation, which occurs in a novel organ known as the ileal Peyer's patch.

It is possible that the B-cell receptor first generated in these animals is specific for a ligand expressed by cells in the bursa of Fabricius or its equivalent, and that recognition of this ligand by the invariant B-cell receptor drives the intense B-cell proliferation found at such sites. According to this model, the cells can only stop proliferating and emerge from the bursa as mature B cells when their receptors have diversified to such an extent that they no longer recognize this self ligand (see Fig. 5.15).

It is not known why this alternative strategy of diversifying an initially homogeneous pool of receptors exists in these species. The phenomenon is in some respects analogous to the receptor editing that occurs in mice when immature B cells bind self antigens (see Section 5-11). It may turn out to be a general rule that lymphocyte repertoires are selected both positively and negatively by the signals they receive from self ligands as they mature. We shall see in Chapter 6 that the interaction of receptors on newly formed lymphocytes with self molecules in a specialized microenvironment is crucial for the development of the other major lymphocyte subset—the T cells. This positive selection in the T-cell lineage might be seen as a parallel to the proposed recognition of self ligands in the B-cell lineage, but this is very controversial.

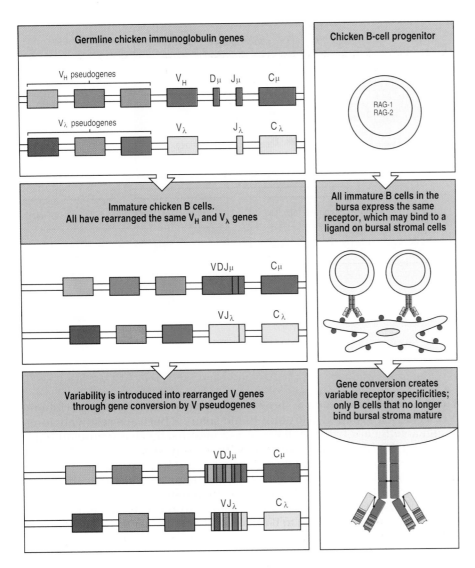

Germline chicken immunoglobulin genes

V_H pseudogenes V_H D_μ J_μ C_μ

V_λ pseudogenes V_λ J_λ C_λ

Immature chicken B cells. All have rearranged the same V_H and V_λ genes

VDJ_μ C_μ

VJ_λ C_λ

Variability is introduced into rearranged V genes through gene conversion by V pseudogenes

VDJ_μ C_μ

VJ_λ C_λ

Chicken B-cell progenitor

RAG-1
RAG-2

All immature B cells in the bursa express the same receptor, which may bind to a ligand on bursal stromal cells

Gene conversion creates variable receptor specificities; only B cells that no longer bind bursal stroma mature

Fig. 5.15 Binding to a self ligand may drive the diversification of chicken immunoglobulins. In chickens, all B cells express the same surface immunoglobulin initially; there is only one active V(D) and J gene segment for both the chicken heavy- and light-chain genes (top left panel), and gene rearrangement can produce only a single receptor specificity. Immature B cells expressing this receptor migrate to the bursa of Fabricius, where the receptor is thought to bind to a self cell-surface molecule, inducing proliferation (middle panels). Gene-conversion events introduce sequences from adjacent V pseudogenes into the expressed gene, creating diversity in the receptors. In this scheme, only when a B cell loses reactivity to the bursal antigen does it cease to proliferate and emigrate to the periphery (bottom panels).

5-13 **B cells are produced continuously but only some contribute to a relatively stable peripheral pool.**

Our knowledge of the dynamics of B-cell populations comes from labeling experiments in the bone marrow of normal young adult mice. Here, about 35 million large pre-B cells enter mitosis each day. However, only 10–15 million new mature B lymphocytes emerge as the end-products of primary development in the bone marrow. The loss of more than half of the initial pre-B cells must be caused by their failure to make a productive light-chain gene rearrangement and to the deletion of self-reactive B cells while still in the bone marrow. The daily output of 10–20 million B cells is roughly 5–10% of the total B lymphocyte population in the steady-state peripheral pool, although the size of this pool is not easy to measure. Fig. 5.16 shows the possible fates of mature B cells entering the periphery. The stream of new mature B cells must compensate for the death of an equal number of peripheral B cells. These deaths are chiefly in the short-lived peripheral B-cell population, which has a turn-over time of less than a week. Many B cells have a short life span once they leave the bone marrow and enter the peripheral B-cell pool, perhaps because they are excluded from the lymphoid follicles (see Section 5-9).

Fig. 5.16 Proposed population dynamics of conventional B cells.
B cells are produced as receptor-positive cells in the bone marrow. Most autoreactive B cells are removed at this stage. Upon maturation, B cells migrate to the periphery, where they enter the recirculating pool. There appear to be two classes of B cell, long-lived B cells and short-lived B cells. It is estimated that 10–20 million mature B cells are produced by the bone marrow and exported each day in a mouse and an equal number are lost from the periphery. Most of the turnover of short-lived B cells may result from B cells that fail to enter lymphoid follicles. However, about half of all mature B cells are long-lived. Memory B cells, which have been activated previously by antigen and T cells, have a long life, sustained by autocrine production of nerve growth factor. The short-lived B cells are recently formed B cells by definition.

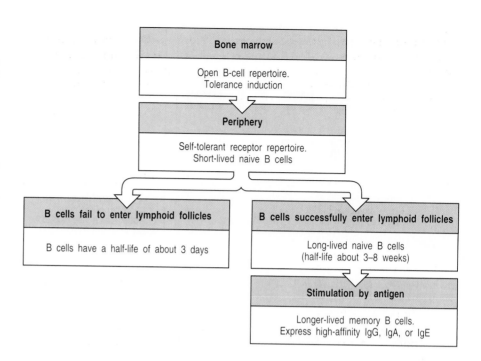

The labeling studies in mice show that the remaining, long-lived peripheral B cells have a broad distribution of life spans. There are relatively long-lived naive B cells with a half-life of 1–2 months; these are thought to be sustained by signals received each time they pass through follicles. There are also non-dividing B cells that are very long-lived. These include the memory B cells that differentiate from mature B cells after their first encounter with antigen. Memory B cells persist for extended periods after antigenic stimulation, and also appear to require intermittent follicular signals; we shall return to B-cell memory in Chapter 9. The production and loss of new B cells ensures that different receptors are produced continuously to meet new antigenic challenges, while the persistence of the progeny of cells that have been activated ensures that those cells proven to recognize pathogens are retained to combat reinfection.

Summary.

Experiments using transgene-encoded receptors have demonstrated three different mechanisms which prevent potentially self-reactive B cells from developing to the stage at which encounter with antigen can trigger a primary immune reponse. B cells specific for ubiquitous multivalent ligands such as self MHC molecules are eliminated soon after their antigen receptor is first expressed, in a process known as clonal deletion. A small proportion of self-reactive immature B cells may escape this fate, however, by replacing their receptors with new receptors that are no longer autoreactive. This occurs by a process of further gene rearrangements and is known as receptor editing. B cells binding soluble self antigens can be rendered anergic as immature or mature B cells, and although they are exported from the bone marrow, they are excluded from lymphoid follicles, and do not survive for long in the periphery. Thus, the mature peripheral B-cell repertoire is a selected subset of the immature B-cell repertoire. Indeed, only a small proportion of newly made immature B cells survive to form a part of the long-lived peripheral B-cell pool, which indicates that this selection is extensive, although how much of it is ligand mediated and governed by receptor specificity remains unclear. A very different strategy of generating a diverse peripheral B-cell repertoire is seen in some mammals and in birds. In these species, immature B cells expressing only a few limited gene rearrangements migrate to specialized organs where their receptors are diversified either by gene conversion or by somatic hypermutation. This may be a ligand-driven process whose end-products are selected for a loss of reactivity to self.

B-cell heterogeneity.

The B cells in peripheral lymphoid tissues are heterogeneous; different populations are found in different locations and are distinguished by the different cell-surface molecules they express. Part of this heterogeneity results from B-cell maturation in the periphery in response to antigenic stimulation: naive recirculating B cells are clearly distinct from the B lymphoblasts actively responding to antigen, whereas the very long-lived memory B lymphocytes can be distinguished from naive B cells by the expression of isotypes other than IgM and IgD, as well as by other cell-surface changes. There is also a population of B cells that may arise from distinct stem cells early in an animal's development and which renews itself by continuing division in the peripheral lymphoid tissues of adult animals. These cells are known as B-1 B cells to distinguish them from the conventional B-2 B cells whose development we have described in the first part of this chapter, and they appear to represent a distinct developmental lineage of B cells.

In the remaining part of this chapter, we describe these populations of B cells and some malignant tumors of B-lineage cells that reflect their distinctiveness. Since tumors of B cells are a source of large numbers of cells that can be identified by their identical immunoglobulin gene rearrangements, they have proven invaluable for studying B-cell development, homing behavior, and function. Tumors of fully differentiated antibody-secreting plasma cells provided the means for understanding the genetic basis of antibody diversity and isotype switching; tumors of less differentiated B-lineage cells have illustrated the steps through which B-cell development proceeds. Some tumors representing B cells at early stages of development retain the ability to rearrange their immunoglobulin genes, and much of what we know about gene rearrangement has come from studying these B-cell tumor lines. Malignant tumors of B cells have also shed light on the normal processes by which B-cell growth is controlled, as we shall see in the last part of this chapter.

5-14　B cells bearing surface CD5 express a distinctive repertoire of receptors.

Not all B cells conform to the developmental pathway we have described in previous sections. A significant subset of B cells in mice and humans, and the major population in rabbits, arises early in ontogeny and has a distinctive receptor repertoire and functional properties (Fig. 5.17). These B cells were first identified by surface expression of the protein CD5 and are also characterized by displaying surface IgM with little or no IgD even when mature. These unconventional B-lineage cells are termed **B-1 B cells**, because their development precedes that of the conventional B cells, sometimes termed **B-2 B cells**. They are also known as **CD5 B cells**, although CD5 itself cannot be essential for their function since cells that have similar traits develop normally in mice lacking the CD5 gene, and in rats B-1 B cells do not display CD5.

Fig. 5.17 A comparison of the properties of B-1 B cells and conventional or B-2 B cells.

Fig. 5.17 A comparison of the properties of B-1 B cells and conventional or B-2 B cells. B-1 B cells may develop in unusual sites in the fetus, such as the omentum, in addition to the liver, and are only produced by the bone marrow for a short time around the time of birth. An autonomous pool of these cells then establishes itself outside the marrow. The limited diversity of the B-1 cell repertoire, and their propensity to produce low-affinity autoreactive antibodies, suggest that they mediate a more primitive, less adaptive immune response than the conventional or B-2 B cells. Although the surface molecule CD5 was extremely useful in first identifying B-1 B cells, it now seems that it is not essential to B-1 B-cell development or function; the developmental relationship, if any, between B-1 B cells that are CD5-positive and B-1 B cells that do not carry CD5 is not clear.

Property	B-1 B cells	Conventional B-2 B cells
When first produced	Fetus	After birth
Mode of renewal	Self-renewing	Replaced from bone marrow
Production of immunoglobulin	High	Low
Specificity	Degenerate	Precise
Isotypes secreted	IgM >> IgG	IgG > IgM
Somatic hypermutation	Low–none	High
Response to carbohydrate antigen	Yes	Maybe
Response to protein antigen	Maybe	Yes

Currently little is known about the function of B-1 B cells. Although relatively sparse in lymph nodes or spleen, they are the predominant B-cell population in the peritoneal and pleural cavities. B-1 B cells make little contribution to the adaptive immune responses to protein antigens but contribute strongly to some antibody responses against carbohydrate antigens, as we shall see in Chapter 8. Moreover in mice, a large proportion of serum IgM in normal non-immune animals derives from B-1 B cells. These distinguishing features may reflect the different developmental origin of B-1 B cells and the distinct repertoire of their receptors.

B-1 B cells arise early in ontogeny. In mice, they derive from an immature stem cell that is most active in the prenatal period (Fig. 5.18). In the B-1 B cells, the immunoglobulin heavy-chain gene rearrangements are dominated by those using V_H gene segments that lie closest to the D gene segments in the germline. As TdT is not active in the prenatal period, these early heavy-chain gene rearrangements are accompanied by few, if any, N-nucleotide insertions. The VDJ junctions expressed by B-1 B cells are thus less diverse than those of conventional B-2 B cells. The recognition

Fig. 5.18 Stem cells at different stages of development give rise to distinct B-cell populations. Stem cells in fetal mice give rise to progenitors that have little or no terminal deoxynucleotidyl transferase (TdT), which in turn give rise to B-1 B cells. These cells have fewer N-nucleotides in their V(D)J junctions and are self-renewing. Adult bone marrow stem cells give rise only to conventional B cells that have high junctional diversity and a range of life spans; they are not self-renewing and are replaced continuously by new cells generated in the bone marrow.

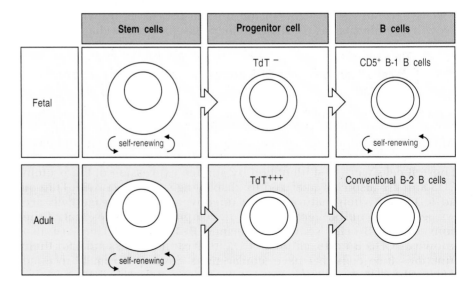

properties of the receptors on B-1 B cells also differ from those of conventional B-2 B cells. B-1 B-cell receptors and the antibodies these cells produce tend to bind numerous different ligands at relatively low affinity, a property known as **polyspecificity**, with a preference for binding common bacterial polysaccharides. Indeed, the V gene segments that encode B-1 B-cell receptors may have evolved by natural selection to recognize common bacterial antigens, allowing them to contribute to early phases of immunity, which will be discussed in detail in Chapter 9.

B-1 B cells that develop postnatally use a more diverse repertoire of V genes and their rearranged immunoglobulin genes have abundant N-nucleotides. As mice develop, however, the bone marrow stem cells seem to undergo a developmental change such that only B-2 B cells are produced (see Fig. 5.18). In adult animals, the population of B-1 B cells is maintained by continued division in peripheral sites, a process that requires interleukin-10. B-1 B cells are also of interest to clinicians, as they are the origin of the common B-cell tumor in the disease chronic lymphocytic leukemia (CLL). CLL cells often display CD5, which is a useful diagnostic clue.

There are some striking similarities between the development of B-1 B cells and that of the second lineage of T cells, the γ:δ T cells. As we shall see in Chapter 6, γ:δ T cells expressing a limited repertoire of receptors with no N-region additions dominate T-cell production early in ontogeny whereas later γ:δ T cells are generated with more diverse receptors and their production is secondary to that of the major lineage of α:β T cells.

| 5-15 | **B cells at different developmental stages are found in different anatomical sites.** |

B cells are not sessile. They change their location as they mature in the bone marrow and upon reaching maturity, they leave the bone marrow to migrate through the B-cell rich areas of peripheral lymphoid tissues, such as the follicles of lymph nodes and spleen. Those mature B cells that survive form part of the recirculating lymphocyte pool, perpetually passing from the blood into primary lymphoid follicles and back into the blood (Fig. 5.19). Many B cells are found in the gut-associated lymphoid tissues, which have high B- to T-cell ratios. These include the very large gut-associated lymphoid follicles known as Peyer's patches, the appendix and the tonsils, all of which provide specialized sites where B cells can become committed to synthesizing IgA.

Fig. 5.19 The distribution of conventional B cells within lymphoid organs. B-lineage cells are found in bone marrow, blood, lymphoid organs, and lymph. In adult mammals, B cells develop in the bone marrow, migrate via the blood to the secondary lymphoid organs, where they leave the circulation and enter the cortex of the lymphoid organ. In the absence of antigen, they migrate through primary follicles and return to the circulation, via the lymphatic vessels, which join the blood via the thoracic duct. In the presence of appropriately presented antigen, B cells are activated by helper T cells to form primary foci of proliferating cells from which the B cells then migrate to form the germinal center within a follicle (see also Fig. 8.10). Germinal centers are sites of rapid B-cell proliferation and differentiation in which the rapidly dividing B cells are known as lymphoblasts. Some of these cells then migrate to the medullary cords of the lymph node, or to the bone marrow, where they complete their differentiation into antibody-secreting plasma cells. A few weeks after it forms, the germinal center reaction has died down to leave a residual follicle called a secondary lymphoid follicle. We have illustrated a lymph node here: the other major peripheral lymphoid tissues are the spleen and Peyer's patches of the gut.

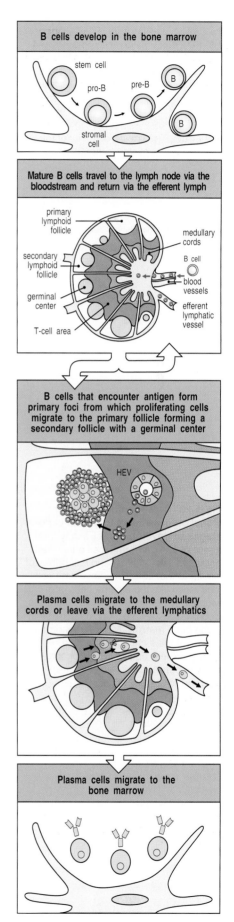

If B cells encounter antigen on entering the lymphoid tissue, they are detained in the T-cell areas and may be activated to proliferate by appropriate helper T cells. Some of these activated B cells differentiate into antibody-secreting plasma cells, while others migrate to a nearby lymphoid follicle where they establish **germinal centers** (see Fig. 5.19). Here, the activated B cells undergo intense proliferation that is accompanied by somatic hypermutation of their rearranged variable-region genes and the further maturation of cells bearing receptors with a higher affinity for the stimulating antigen (see Section 3-18 and Chapter 8). As some of the progeny B cells develop into antibody-secreting plasma cells they migrate again; plasma cells are found predominantly in the medullary cords of lymph nodes, in red pulp in the spleen, and in the bone marrow. The bone marrow can be an important site of IgG antibody production. In hyperimmune animals producing IgG antibody in response to repeated immunization with antigen, up to 90% of the antibody can be derived from plasma cells in the bone marrow. However, in the case of IgA responses, which mostly develop in the gut-associated lymphoid tissue, the lamina propria of the mucosa is the destination of the antibody-producing cells.

5-16   B-cell tumors often occupy the same site as their normal counterparts.

Tumors retain many of the characteristics of the cell type from which they arose, especially when the tumor is relatively differentiated and slow-growing. This is clearly illustrated in the case of B-cell tumors. Tumors corresponding to essentially all stages of B-cell development have been found in humans, from the earliest stages to the myelomas that represent malignant outgrowths of plasma cells (Fig. 5.20). Furthermore, each

Fig. 5.20 B-cell tumors represent clonal outgrowths of B cells at various stages of development. Each type of tumor cell has a normal cell equivalent, homes to similar sites, and has behavior similar to that cell. Thus, myeloma cells look much like the plasma cells from which they derive, they secrete immunoglobulin, and they are found predominantly in the bone marrow. Many lymphomas and myelomas may go through a preliminary less aggressive lymphoproliferative phase, and some mild lymphoproliferations appear to be benign.

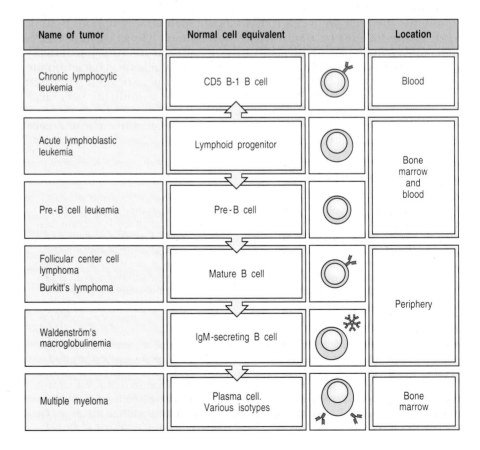

Name of tumor	Normal cell equivalent		Location
Chronic lymphocytic leukemia	CD5 B-1 B cell		Blood
Acute lymphoblastic leukemia	Lymphoid progenitor		Bone marrow and blood
Pre-B cell leukemia	Pre-B cell		
Follicular center cell lymphoma Burkitt's lymphoma	Mature B cell		Periphery
Waldenström's macroglobulinemia	IgM-secreting B cell		
Multiple myeloma	Plasma cell. Various isotypes		Bone marrow

type of tumor retains its characteristic homing properties. Thus, a tumor that resembles mature, naive B cells homes to follicles in lymph nodes and spleen, giving rise to a follicular center cell lymphoma, while a tumor of a plasma cell usually disperses to many different sites in bone marrow, from which comes the clinical name of multiple myeloma (tumor of bone marrow). These similarities mean that it is possible to use tumor cells, which are available in large quantities, to study the cell-surface molecules and signaling pathways responsible for homing behavior.

5-17   Malignant B cells frequently carry chromosomal translocations that join immunoglobulin loci to genes regulating cell growth.

The general conclusion that a tumor represents the clonal outgrowth of a single transformed cell is very clearly illustrated by tumors of B-lineage cells. All the cells in a B-cell tumor have the identical immunoglobulin gene rearrangement, decisively documenting their origin from one cell. This is useful for clinical diagnosis, as tumor cells can be detected by sensitive assays for these homogeneous rearrangements (Fig. 5.21; see also Fig. 3.12). Only on rare occasions are biclonal tumors with two patterns of rearrangement found.

The unregulated growth that is the most striking characteristic of tumor cells is caused by mutations that release the cell from the normal restraints on its growth. In B-cell tumors, the disruption of normal growth controls is often associated with an aberrant immunoglobulin gene rearrangement, which joins one of its immunoglobulin loci to a gene on another chromosome. This genetic fusion with another chromosome is known as a translocation, and in B-cell tumors such translocations are found to disrupt the expression and function of genes important for controlling cell growth. Cellular genes that cause cancer when their function or expression is disrupted are termed **proto-oncogenes**. Many of them were first discovered as a result of studying RNA tumor viruses that could transform cells directly. The viral genes responsible for this were named **oncogenes**, and it was later found that they were derived from normal cellular genes that perform key roles in the control of cell growth, division, and differentiation.

The translocations between immunoglobulin loci and proto-oncogenes give rise to chromosomal abnormalities that are visible microscopically in metaphase. These abnormalities are characteristic of tumors of different types, and reflect the involvement of a particular proto-oncogene in each tumor type. Characteristic translocations, involving the T-cell receptor loci, are also seen in T-cell tumors. Immunoglobulin and T-cell receptor loci are sites in which double-stranded DNA breaks occur during normal gene rearrangement, so it is not surprising that they are especially prone to be sites of chromosomal translocation in T and B cells.

The analysis of chromosomal abnormalities has revealed much about the regulation of B-cell growth and the disruption of growth control in tumor cells. In Burkitt's lymphoma cells, the *myc* proto-oncogene on chromosome 8 is recombined with an immunoglobulin locus by translocations that involve either chromosome 14 (heavy chain) (Fig. 5.22), chromosome 2 (κ light chain), or chromosome 22 (λ light chain). These rearrangements deregulate expression of the Myc protein that is involved in the control of the cell cycle in normal cells. Deregulation of Myc protein expression leads to increased proliferation of B cells, although other mutations elsewhere in the genome are also needed before a B-cell tumor results.

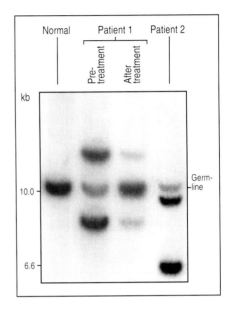

Fig. 5.21 Clonal analysis of B-cell tumors. DNA analysis of white blood cells using Southern blotting techniques can be used to detect lymphoid malignancy. In a sample from a healthy person (left lane), immunoglobulin genes are in the germline configuration in non-B cells, so a digest of their DNA with a suitable restriction endonuclease yields a single germline DNA fragment when probed with an Ig heavy-chain J region probe (J$_H$). Normal B cells present in this sample make many different rearrangements to J$_H$, each so faint that it cannot be seen (see Fig. 3.12). By contrast, in samples from patients with B-cell malignancies (Patient 1 and Patient 2), where a single cell has given rise to all the tumor cells in the sample, two extra predominant bands are seen, which are characteristic of each patient's tumor. These result from the rearrangement of both alleles of the J$_H$ gene in that cell. The intensity of the bands, compared with the germline signal, gives an indication of the abundance of the tumor cells in the sample. When the same patient is analyzed before and after treatment, the intensity of the tumor-specific bands diminish after treatment. Photograph courtesy of T J Vulliamy and L Luzzatto.

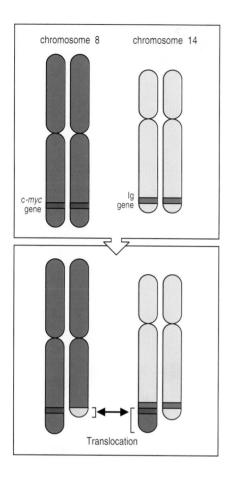

chromosome 8   chromosome 14

c-myc gene

Ig gene

Translocation

Fig. 5.22 Specific chromosomal rearrangements are found in some lymphoid tumors. If a chromosomal rearrangement joins one of the immunoglobulin genes to a cellular proto-oncogene, it can result in the aberrant expression of the proto-oncogene under the control of the immunoglobulin regulatory sequences. Such chromosomal rearrangements are frequently associated with B-cell tumors. In the example shown, from Burkitt's lymphoma, the translocation of the proto-oncogene c-myc from chromosome 8 to the immunoglobulin heavy-chain locus on chromosome 14 results in the deregulated expression of c-myc and the unregulated growth of the B cell. The immunoglobulin gene located on the normal chromosome 14 is usually productively rearranged and the tumors that result from such translocations generally have a mature phenotype and express immunoglobulin.

Other B-cell lymphomas bear a chromosomal translocation of immunoglobulin genes to the proto-oncogene *bcl-2*, increasing production of Bcl-2 protein. The Bcl-2 protein prevents programmed cell death in B-lineage cells, so its abnormal expression allows some B cells to survive and accumulate beyond their normal life span. During this time further genetic changes may occur that lead to malignant transformation. Mice carrying an expressed *bcl-2* transgene tend to develop B-cell lymphomas late in life.

Research into B-cell tumors has therefore provided some fundamental insights into the link between chromosome abnormalities and cancers, and has identified several proto-oncogenes that regulate B-cell growth. Much remains to be learned both about cancer and about normal B-cell development from the careful analysis of B-cell lymphomas and leukemias.

Summary.

B cells are not a single, homogeneous population. Rather, there are two major subpopulations that appear to arise from distinct stem cells and which have distinctive properties. B-1 B cells, many of which bear surface CD5, arise early in ontogeny and, in adults, form a self-renewing population, which is the dominant B-cell population in the pleural and peritoneal cavities. The repertoire of receptors expressed by B-1 B cells is distinctive, and low affinity polyspecific IgM is made by these cells. Conventional B cells, B-2 B cells, appear later in ontogeny and they continue to be generated from the bone marrow throughout the lives of both humans and mice. Conventional B cells can be subdivided into several subpopulations, which represent stages in their maturation, the final stage being the antibody-secreting plasma cell. Mature B-2 B cells migrate through lymphoid tissue in different body sites, and each cell type is found in a distinctive location within the lymphoid tissue, suggesting that important microenvironmental factors act on cells at different stages of development. Our understanding of B-cell development and migratory behavior has been, and will continue to be, aided greatly by studying B-cell tumors. These tumors are readily identified by their unique immunoglobulin gene rearrangements, and their behavior often reflects the normal behavior of the cells from which they arose.

Summary to Chapter 5.

In humans and mice, B cells develop in the bone marrow and are produced throughout life. The development of human B cells is summarized in Fig. 5.23. The stages of B-cell development are marked by a series of

	B cells		Heavy-chain genes	Light-chain genes	Intra-cellular proteins	Surface marker proteins	
ANTIGEN INDEPENDENT	Stem cell		Germline	Germline		CD34 CD45	BONE MARROW
ANTIGEN INDEPENDENT	Early pro-B cell		D–J rearranged	Germline	RAG-1 RAG-2 TdT λ5, VpreB	CD34, CD45 MHC class II CD10, CD19 CD38	BONE MARROW
ANTIGEN INDEPENDENT	Late pro-B cell		V–DJ rearranged	Germline	TdT λ5, VpreB	CD45R MHC class II (Dμ) CD10, CD19 CD38, CD20 CD40	BONE MARROW
ANTIGEN INDEPENDENT	Large Pre-B cell	pre-B receptor	VDJ rearranged	Germline	RAG-1 RAG-2 μ λ5, VpreB	CD45R MHC class II preB-R CD19, CD38 CD20, CD40	BONE MARROW
ANTIGEN INDEPENDENT	Small Pre-B cell	μ	VDJ rearranged	V–J rearrangement	μ	CD45R MHC class II CD19, CD38 CD20, CD40	BONE MARROW
ANTIGEN INDEPENDENT	Immature B cell	IgM	VDJ rearranged. μ heavy chain produced in membrane form	VJ rearranged		CD45R MHC class II IgM CD19, CD20 CD40	BONE MARROW
ANTIGEN DEPENDENT	Mature naive B cell	IgD IgM	VDJ rearranged. μ chain produced in membrane form. Alternative splicing yields μ + δ mRNA	VJ rearranged		CD45R MHC class II IgM, IgD CD19, CD20 CD21, CD40	PERIPHERY
ANTIGEN DEPENDENT	Lympho-blast	IgM	VDJ rearranged. Alternative splicing yields secreted μ chains	VJ rearranged	Ig	CD45R MHC class II CD19, CD20 CD21, CD40	PERIPHERY
ANTIGEN DEPENDENT	Memory B cell	IgG	Isotype switch to Cγ, Cα, or Cε. Somatic hypermutation	VJ rearranged. Somatic hypermutation		CD45R MHC class II IgG, IgA CD19, CD20 CD21, CD40	PERIPHERY
TERMINAL DIFFERENTIATION	Plasma cell	IgG	Isotype switch and alternative splicing yields secreted γ, α, or ε chains	VJ rearranged	Ig	Plasma cell antigen-1 CD38	PERIPHERY

Fig. 5.23 A summary of the development of human conventional B-lineage cells. The stages in B-cell development, their location, the state of the immunoglobulin genes, the expression of some cell-surface molecules, and the expression of some essential intracellular proteins are all shown.

irreversible changes in the immunoglobulin genes, which contribute to the diversity of antibodies, and by changes in immunoglobulin gene expression that depend on the regulation of transcription and RNA splicing (Fig. 5.24). The irreversible genetic rearrangements that assemble complete immunoglobulin genes from the separate V, D, and J gene segments are regulated to ensure the monospecificity of most B cells. Heavy-chain gene segments rearrange first, and as soon as a functional heavy-chain gene is generated its product is expressed at the cell surface with a surrogate light chain, and further heavy-chain gene rearrangement ceases. Light-chain gene rearrangements are similarly halted when either an intact κ or λ chain is produced, and a complete IgM molecule is expressed at the cell surface The generation of diversity in this primary receptor repertoire is independent of encounter with antigen and leads to some cell loss as a result of the joining mechanisms used. Once surface immunoglobulin is expressed, however, it can function as an antigen receptor, and ligand-mediated selection can take place. Immature B cells that bind antigen in the bone marrow may die, change their receptor, or become anergic, thus establishing tolerance to these self antigens. Clonal deletion and anergy may also be induced by antigens contacted by B cells when they first emerge into the periphery. Once in the periphery, B cells appear to need access to the lymphoid follicles to survive, thus anergic B cells and B cells binding soluble self antigens are excluded from the follicles and die. Indeed the majority of the cells that emerge from the bone marrow survive for only a week or less, perhaps because of the competition for follicular access. The repertoire of B cells that survive to form part of the relatively long-lived pool of mature peripheral B cells provides the raw material for clonal selection in the adaptive immune response. These mature naive B cells, which co-express IgM and IgD, circulate through the lymphoid organs, including Peyer's patches in the gut, until they encounter antigen. Upon interacting with antigen and specific helper T cells in the T-cell areas of lymphoid tissue, a B cell is activated to divide, giving rise to both antibody-secreting plasma cells that migrate to local medullary cords and some progeny cells that migrate to a nearby follicle to form a germinal center. Here they proliferate vigorously and undergo changes in their immunoglobulin variable-region genes by somatic hypermutation. Selected B cells then differentiate into plasma cells, which secrete large amounts of antibody, or long-lived memory cells, which contribute to lasting protective immunity.

Fig. 5.24 Changes in immunoglobulin genes that accompany B-cell development and differentiation. Those changes that establish immunological diversity are all irreversible, as they involve changes in B-cell DNA. Switch recombination allows the same variable region to be attached to several functionally distinct heavy-chain constant regions (as explained in Chapter 3) and thereby creates functional diversity in an irreversible manner. Enhancer- and promoter-binding proteins regulate immunoglobulin gene expression and RNA processing; changes arising out of their actions—the expression of IgM versus IgD, and of membrane-bound versus secreted forms of all immunoglobulin types—are therefore reversible.

Event	Process	Nature of change
V-region assembly	Somatic recombination of DNA	Irreversible
Junctional diversity	Imprecise joining, N-sequence insertion in DNA	Irreversible
Transcriptional activation	Activation of promoter by proximity to the enhancer	Irreversible but regulated
Switch recombination	Somatic recombination of DNA	Irreversible
Somatic hypermutation	DNA point mutation	Irreversible
IgM, IgD expression on surface	Differential splicing of RNA	Reversible, regulated
Membrane vs secreted form	Differential splicing of RNA	Reversible, regulated

Many IgG-secreting plasma cells migrate to the bone marrow, while B cells that have differentiated to secrete IgA migrate to the lamina propria of the mucosal surfaces. B-lineage tumors that reflect the properties of their normal counterparts can arise from cells at many of these stages of development and have been useful in studying B-cell development and function. We shall look in more depth at how B cells are clonally selected to function in an adaptive humoral immune response in Chapter 8, but before this can be fully understood, the development and activation of T cells must be described. This will occupy the next two chapters of this book.

General references.

Casali, P., and Silberstein, L.E.S., (eds).: **Immunoglobulin gene expression in development and disease.** *Ann. N.Y. Acad. Sci.* 1995, **764**.

Cumano, A., Kee, B.L., Ramsden, D.A., Marshall, A., Paige, C.J., and Wu, G.E.: **Development of B-lymphocytes from lymphoid committed and uncommitted progenitors.** *Immunol. Rev.* 1994, **137**:5-33.

Goodnow, C.C., Cyster, J.G., Hartley, S.B., Bell, S.E., Cooke, M.P., Healy, J.I., Akkaraju, S., Rathmell, J.C., Pogue, S.L., and Shokat, K.P.: **Self-tolerance checkpoints in B-lymphocyte development.** *Adv. Immunol.* 1995, **59**:279-368.

Hardy, R.R., and Hayakawa, K.: **B-lineage differentiation stages resolved by multiparameter flow-cytometry.** *Ann. N.Y. Acad. Sci.* 1995, **764**:19-24.

Kelsoe, G.: **In-situ studies of the germinal center reaction.** *Adv. Immunol.* 1995, **60**:267-288.

Lemischka, I.R.: **What we have learned from retroviral marking of hematopoietic stem-cells.** *Curr.Top. Microbiol. Immunol.* 1992, **177**:59-71.

Linette, G.P., and Korsmeyer, S.J.: **Differentiation and cell-death—lessons from the immune-system.** *Curr. Opin. Cell Biol.* 1994, **6**:809-815.

Loffert, D., Schaal, S., Ehlich, A., Hardy, R.R., Zou, Y.R., Muller, W., and Rajewsky, K.: **Early B-cell development in the mouse—insights from mutations introduced by gene targeting.** *Immunol. Rev.* 1994, **137**:135-153.

Melchers, F., Haasner, D., Grawunder, U., Kalberer, C., Karasuyama, H., Winkler, T., and Rolink, A.G.: **Roles of Ig H-chain and L-chain and of surrogate H-chain and L-chain in the development of cells of the B-lymphocyte lineage.** *Ann. Rev. Immunol.* 1994, **12**:209-225.

Pfeffer, K., and Mak, T.W.: **Lymphocyte ontogeny and activation in gene targeted mutant mice.** *Ann. Rev. Immunol.* 1994, **12**:367-411.

Rajewsky, K.: **Clonal selection and learning in the antibody system.** *Nature* 1996, **381**:751-758.

Rolink, A., and Melchers, F.: **B-Lymphopoiesis In the Mouse.** *Adv. Immunol.* 1993, **53**:123-156.

Schatz, D.G., Oettinger, M.A., and Schlissel, M.S.: **V(D)J Recombination—molecular biology and regulation.** *Ann. Rev. Immunol.* 1992, **10**:359-383.

Spangrude, G.J.: **Biological and clinical aspects of hematopoietic stem-cells.** *Ann. Rev. Med.* 1994, **45**:93-104.

Section references.

5-1   **B cell development proceeds through several stages.**

Ehrlich, A., and Kuppers, R.: **Analysis of immunoglobulin gene rearrangements in single B cells.** *Curr. Opin. Immunol.* 1995, **7**:281-284.

Kee, B.L., and Paige, C.J.: **Murine B-cell development—commitment and progression from multipotential progenitors to mature B-lymphocytes.** *Intl. Rev. Cytol.—a survey of Cell Biol.* 1995, **157**:129-179.

Ten-Boekel, E., Melchers, F., and Rolink, A.: **The status of Ig loci rearrangements in single cells from different stages of B-cell development.** *Intl. Immunol.* 1995, **7**:1013-1019.

5-2   **The bone marrow provides an essential microenvironment for early B-cell development.**

Funk, P.E., Kincade, P.W., and Witte, P.L.: **Native associations of early hematopoietic stem-cells and stromal cells isolated in bone-marrow cell aggregates.** *Blood* 1994, **83**:361-369.

Jacobsen, K., Kravitz, J., Kincade, P.W., and Osmond, D.G.: **Adhesion receptors on bone-marrow stromal cells—in vivo expression of vascular cell adhesion molecule-1 by reticular cells and sinusoidal endothelium in normal and γ-irradiated mice.** *Blood* 1996, **87**:73-82.

Rosenberg, N., and Kincade, P.W.: **B-lineage differentiation in normal and transformed-cells and the microenvironment that supports it.** *Curr. Opin. Immunol.* 1994, **6**:203-211.

Nagasawa, T., Hirota, S., Tachibana, V., Takakura, N., Nishikawa, S., Kitamura, Y., Yoshida, V., Kikutani, H, Kishimoto, T.: **Defects of B-cell lymphopoiesis and bone-marrow myelopoiesis in mice lacking the CXC chemokine PBSF/SDF-1.** *Nature* 1996, **382**:635-638.

5-3   **The survival of developing B cells depends on the productive, sequential rearrangement of a heavy- and a light-chain gene.**

Prak, E.L., and Weigert, M.: **Light-chain replacement—a new model for antibody gene rearrangement.** *J. Exp. Med.* 1995, **182**:541-548.

Zou, Y.R., Takeda, S., and Rajewsky, K.: **Gene targeting in the Ig-κ locus—efficient generation of λ-chain expressing B-cells, independent of gene rearrangements in Ig-κ.** *EMBO J.* 1993, **12**:811-820.

| 5-4 | The expression of proteins regulating immunoglobulin gene rearrangement and function is developmentally programmed. |

Desiderio, S.: **Lymphopoiesis—transcription factors controlling B-cell development.** *Curr. Biol.* 1995, **5**:605-608.

Khan, W.N., Alt, F.W., Gerstein, R.M., Malynn, B.A., Larsson, I., Rathbun, G., Davidson, L., Muller, S., Kantor, A.B., Herzenberg, L.A., Rosen, F.S., and Sideras, P.: **Defective B-cell development and function in *btk*-deficient mice.** *Immunity* 1995, **3**:283-299.

Mandik, L., Nguyen, K.A.T., and Erikson, J.: **Fas receptor expression on B-lineage cells.** *Eur. J. Immunol.* 1995, **25**:3148-3154.

Neurath, M.F., Stuber, E.R., and Strober, W.: **BSAP—a key regulator of B-cell development and differentiation.** *Immunol. Today* 1995, **16**:564-569.

Opstelten, D.: **B lymphocyte development and transcription regulation *in vivo*.** *Adv. Immunol.* 1996, **63**:197-268.

Russell, S.M., Tayebi, N., Nakajima, H., Riedy, M.C., Roberts, J.L., Aman, M.J., Migone, T.S., Noguchi, M., Markert, M.L., Buckley, R.H., Oshea, J.J., and Leonard, W.J.: **Mutation of Jak3 in a patient with SCID—essential role of Jak3 in lymphoid development.** *Science* 1995, **270**:797-800.

Sideras, P., and Smith, C.I.E.: **Molecular and cellular aspects of X-linked agammaglobulinemia.** *Adv. Immunol.* 1995, **59**:135.

| 5-5 | Immunoglobulin gene rearrangement is closely co-ordinated with gene transcription. |

Sleckman, B.P., Gorman, J.R., and Alt, F.W.: **Accessibility control of antigen receptor variable region gene assembly—role of cis-acting elements.** *Ann. Rev. Immunol.* 1996, **14**:459-481.

Stanhope-Baker, P., Hudson, K.M., Shaffer, A.L., Constantinescu, A., and Schlissel, M.S.: **Cell-type specific chromatin structure determines the targeting of V(D)J recombinase activity *in vitro*.** *Cell* 1996, **85**:887-897.

Xu, Y., Davidson, L., Alt, F.W., and Baltimore, D.: **Deletion of the Ig-κ light-chain intronic enhancer/matrix attachment region impairs but does not abolish Vκ-Jκ rearrangement.** *Immunity* 1996, **4**:377-385.

| 5-6 | Gene rearrangement alters the activity of the immunoglobulin gene promoters. |

Kottmann, A.H., Zevnik, B., Welte, M., Nielsen, P.J., and Kohler, G.: **A 2nd promoter and enhancer element within the immunoglobulin heavy-chain locus.** *Eur. J. Immunol.* 1994, **24**:817-821.

| 5-7 | Cell-surface expression of the products of rearranged immunoglobulin genes act as checkpoints of B-cell development. |

Grawunder, U., Leu, T.M.J., Schatz, D.G., Werner, A., Rolink, A.G., Melchers, F., and Winkler, T.H.: **Down-regulation of *Rag1* and *Rag2* gene expression in pre-B cells after functional immunoglobulin heavy-chain rearrangement.** *Immunity* 1995, **3**:601-608.

Horne, M.C., Roth, P.E., and Defranco, A.L.: **Assembly of the truncated immunoglobulin heavy chain Dμ into antigen receptor-like complexes in pre-B cells but not in B cells.** *Immunity* 1996, **4**:145-158.

| 5-8 | The immunoglobulin gene rearrangement program leads to monospecificity of individual B cells. |

Arakawa, H., Shimizu, T., and Takeda, S.: **Reevaluation of the probabilities for productive rearrangements on the κ-loci and λ-loci.** *Intl. Immunol.* 1996, **8**:91-99.

Gorman, J.R., van der Stoep, N., Monroe, R., Cogne, M., Davidson, L., and Alt, F.W.: **The Igκ 3′ enhancer influences the ratio of Igκ versus Igλ B lymphocytes.** *Immunity* 1996, **5**:241-252.

Loffert, D., Ehlich, A., Muller, W., and Rajewsky, K.: **Surrogate light-chain expression is required to establish immunoglobulin heavy-chain allelic exclusion during early B-cell development.** *Immunity* 1996, **4**:133-144.

Takeda, S., Sonoda, E., and Arakawa, H.: **The κ–λ ratio of immature B cells.** *Immunol. Today* 1996, **17**:200

| 5-9 | Lymphoid follicles are thought to provide a second essential environment for B cells. |

Cyster, J.G., Hartley, S.B., and Goodnow, C.C.: **Competition for follicular niches excludes self-reactive cells from the recirculating B-cell repertoire.** *Nature* 1994, **371**:389-395.

Cyster, J.G., and Goodnow, C.C.: **Protein tyrosine phosphatase-1c negatively regulates antigen receptor signaling in B-lymphocytes and determines thresholds for negative selection.** *Immunity* 1995, **2**:13-24.

| 5-10 | Immature B cells can be eliminated or inactivated by contact with self antigens. |

Cornall, R.J., Goodnow, C.C., and Cyster, J.G.: **The regulation of self-reactive B cells.** *Curr. Opin. Immunol.* 1995, **7**:804-811.

Hartley, S.B., Cooke, M.P., Fulcher, D.A., Harris, A.W., Cory, S., Basten, A., and Goodnow, C.C.: **Elimination of self-reactive B lymphocytes proceeds in two stages—arrested development and cell death.** *Cell* 1993, **72**:325-335.

| 5-11 | Some potentially self-reactive B cells may be rescued by further immunoglobulin gene rearrangement. |

Chen, C., Nagy, Z., Prak, E.L., and Weigert, M.: **Immunoglobulin heavy chain gene replacement—a mechanism of receptor editing.** *Immunity* 1995, **3**:747-755.

Chen, C., Nagy, Z., Radic, M.Z., Hardy, R.R., Huszar, D., Camper, S.A., and Weigert, M.: **The site and stage of anti-DNA B-cell deletion.** *Nature* 1995, **373**:252-255.

Nemazee, D.: **Antigen receptor capacity and the sensitivity of self-tolerance.** *Immunol. Today* 1996, **17**:25-29.

| 5-12 | In some species, most immunoglobulin gene diversification occurs after gene rearrangement. |

Knight, K.L., and Crane, M.A.: **Generating the antibody repertoire in rabbit.** *Adv. Immunol.* 1994, **56**:179-218.

Reynaud, C.A., Bertocci, B., Dahan, A., and Weill, J.C.: **Formation of the chicken B-cell repertoire—ontogeny, regulation of Ig gene rearrangement, and diversification by gene conversion.** *Adv. Immunol.* 1994, **57**:353-378.

Reynaud, C.A., Garcia, C., Hein, W.R., and Weill, J.C.: **Hypermutation generating the sheep immunoglobulin repertoire is an antigen independent process.** *Cell* 1995, **80**:115-125.

Weill, J.C., and Reynaud, C.A.: **Rearrangement/hypermutation/gene conversion—when, where, and why.** *Immunol. Today* 1996, **17**:92-97.

Weinstein, P.D., Anderson, A.O., and Mage, R.G.: **Rabbit *Igh* sequences in appendix germinal centers—V diversification by gene conversion-like and hypermutation mechanisms.** *Immunity* 1994, **1**:647-659.

5-13 **B cells are produced continuously but only some contribute to a relatively stable peripheral pool.**

Deenen, G.J., and Kroese, F.G.M.: **Kinetics of B-cell subpopulations in peripheral lymphoid-tissues—evidence for the presence of phenotypically distinct short-lived and long-lived B-cell subsets.** *Intl. Immunol. 1993,* **5**:735-741.

Fulcher, D.A., and Basten, A.: **Reduced lifespan of anergic self-reactive B cells in a double-transgenic model.** *J. Exp. Med.* 1994, **179**:125-134.

Osmond, D.G.: **The turnover of B-cell populations.** *Immunol. Today* 1993, **14**:34-37.

5-14 **B cells bearing surface CD5 express a distinctive repertoire of receptors.**

Herzenberg, L.A.H., G.A.; Rajewsky, K. (eds).: **CD5 B cells in development and disease.** *Ann. N. Y. Acad. Sci.* 1992, **51**.

Murakami, M., Yoshioka, H., Shirai, T., Tsubata, T., and Honjo, T.: **Prevention of autoimmune symptoms in autoimmune-prone mice by elimination of B-1 cells.** *Intl. Immunol.* 1995, **7**:877-882.

Murakami, M., and Honjo, T.: **Involvement of B-1 cells in mucosal immunity and autoimmunity.** *Immunol. Today* 1995, **16**:534-539.

5-15 **B cells at different developmental stages are found in different anatomical sites.**

Griebel, P.J., and Hein, W.R.: **Expanding the role of Peyer's patches in B-cell ontogeny.** *Immunol. Today* 1996, **17**:30-39.

Jacob, J., Kelsoe, G., Rajewsky, K., and Weiss, U.: **Intraclonal generation of antibody mutants in germinal centers.** *Nature* 1991, **354**:389-392.

Kelsoe, G.: **Life and death in germinal centers (Redux).** *Immunity* 1996, **4**:107-111.

Maclennan, I.C.M.: **Germinal centers.** *Ann. Rev. Immunol.* 1994, **12**:117-139.

5-16 **B-cell tumors often occupy the same site as their normal counterparts.**

Cotran, R.S., Kumar, V., Robbins, S.L.: *Diseases of white cells, lymph nodes, and spleen. Pathologic basis of disease,* 5th edn. W.B. Saunders, 1994, 629-672.

5-17 **Malignant B cells frequently carry chromosomal translocations that join immunoglobulin loci to genes regulating cell growth.**

Corral, J., Lavenir, I., Impey, H., Warren, A.J., Forster, A., Larson, T.A., Bell, S., McKenzie, A.N.J., King, G., and Rabbitts, T.H.: **An Mll-AF9 fusion gene made by homologous recombination causes acute leukemia in chimeric mice—a method to create fusion oncogenes.** *Cell* 1996, **85**:853-861.

Cory, S.: **Regulation of lymphocyte survival by the *Bcl-2* gene family.** *Ann. Rev. Immunol.* 1995, **13**:513-543.

Rabbitts, T.H.: **Chromosomal translocations in human cancer.** *Nature* 1994, **372**:143-149.

Yang, E., and Korsmeyer, S.J.: **Molecular thanatopsis—a discourse on the *Bcl-2* family and cell death.** *Blood* 1996, **88**:386-401.

The Thymus and the Development of T Lymphocytes

6

T-cell development has much in common with B-cell development. Like B cells, T cells derive from bone marrow stem cells and undergo gene rearrangements in a specialized microenvironment to produce a unique antigen receptor on each cell. However, unlike B cells, T cells do not differentiate in the bone marrow but rather migrate at a very early stage to the **thymus**, a central lymphoid organ that provides the specialized microenvironment where receptor gene rearrangement and the maturation of T cells occur. There is a further crucial difference in T- and B-cell development that reflects the distinct ways in which T cells and B cells recognize antigen. As we learned in Chapter 4, T cells recognize antigen in the form of peptide fragments bound to molecules encoded by the MHC. Since T cells are MHC restricted, only those T cells able to recognize the body's own MHC molecules will be capable of contributing to adaptive immune responses. It is thus essential that each individual's T cells be able to react against foreign antigenic peptides when they are bound to his or her own MHC molecules; that is, that they should be self MHC restricted. It is equally important, however, that T cells should be unable to respond to self peptides bound to self MHC molecules; that is, they must also be self tolerant.

T cells are selected to fulfill these dual requirements for self MHC restriction and self tolerance during their maturation in the thymus. Here, once the immature T cells have rearranged their antigen-receptor genes and the receptor is expressed on the cell surface, they are screened by the two selective processes known as **positive selection**, in which they are selected for self MHC restriction, and **negative selection**, which eliminates those cells that are specific for self peptides bound to self MHC molecules.

How T cells are selected for self restriction but not self reactivity during T-cell maturation is one of the most intriguing problems in immunobiology and, in consequence, one of the most active areas of research. In this chapter we shall describe what is known about the development of T cells and what mechanisms might explain positive and negative selection. As developmental studies depend largely on experimental manipulation, virtually all the information that we have about T-cell development in the thymus has been gained from experiments with mice. We shall comment on the development of human T cells where information exists.

The development of T cells in the thymus.

T cells develop from bone marrow stem cells but their progenitors migrate to the thymus where they mature (Fig. 6.1): for that reason they are called **thymus-dependent (T) lymphocytes** or **T cells**. In the thymus, the immature T cells, or **thymocytes**, proliferate and differentiate, passing through a series of discrete phenotypic stages that can be identified by distinctive patterns of expression of various cell-surface proteins. It is during their development as thymocytes that the cells undergo the gene rearrangements that produce the T-cell receptor, and the positive and negative selection that shapes the mature receptor repertoire. These processes depend upon interactions of the developing cells with the cells of the thymic microenvironment. We shall therefore begin with a general overview of the stages of thymocyte development and its relationship to thymic architecture, before going on in the later sections of this chapter to consider the rearrangement of the T-cell receptor genes and the selection of the receptor repertoire.

Fig. 6.1 T-cell precursors migrate to the thymus to mature. T cells derive from bone marrow stem cells, whose progeny migrate from the bone marrow to the thymus (left panel), where the development of T cells occurs. Mature T cells leave the thymus and recirculate from the bloodstream through secondary lymphoid tissues (right panel) such as lymph nodes, spleen or Peyer's patches, where they may encounter antigen. It is the developmental process within the thymus that is the subject of this chapter.

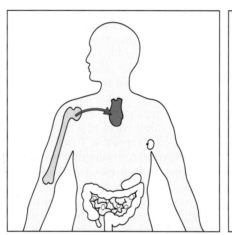 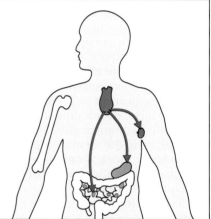

| 6-1 | **T cells develop in the thymus.** |

T lymphocytes develop in the thymus, a lymphoid organ in the upper anterior thorax, just above the heart. In young individuals, the thymus contains many developing T-cell precursors embedded in an epithelial network known as the **thymic stroma**, which provides a unique microenvironment for T-cell development. The thymus consists of numerous lobules, each clearly differentiated into an outer cortical region—the **thymic cortex**—and an inner **medulla**. The thymic stroma arises early in embryonic development from the endodermal and ectodermal layers of the embryonic structures known as the third pharyngeal pouch and third branchial cleft. From studies in embryonic mice it appears that the ectodermal layers give rise to epithelial cells in the thymic cortex, while the endodermal layers give rise to the epithelial component of the medulla. Together these epithelial tissues form a rudimentary thymus, or **thymic anlage** (Fig. 6.2). The thymic anlage then attracts cells of hematopoietic origin, which colonize it; these give rise to both thymocytes committed to the T-cell lineage and intrathymic dendritic cells; the thymus is also independently colonized by numerous macrophages of hematopoietic origin.

The human thymus is fully developed before birth. Like the mouse thymus, it consists of a thymic stroma of medullary epithelia and connective tissue, which is populated by very large numbers of bone marrow derived cells. The bone marrow derived cells are differentially distributed between the thymic cortex and medulla; the cortex contains only immature thymocytes and scattered macrophages, whereas more mature thymocytes, along with the dendritic cells and most of the macrophages, are found in the medulla (Fig. 6.3). We shall see that this reflects the different developmental events that occur in these two compartments.

The rate of T-cell production by the thymus is greatest before puberty. After puberty, the thymus begins to shrink and the production of new T cells in adults is lower. However, in both mice and humans, removal of the thymus is not accompanied by any notable loss of T-cell function although adult thymectomy in mice is accompanied by some loss of T cells. Thus, it seems that once the T-cell repertoire is established, immunity can be sustained without the production of large numbers of new T cells.

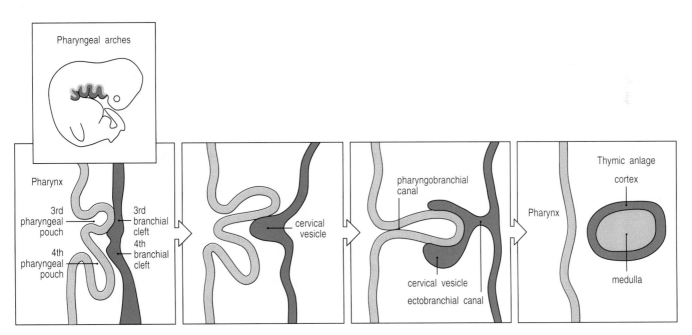

Fig. 6.2   The thymus forms from a fold of tissue in the pharyngeal region of the embryo, here illustrated for the mouse. Two discrete layers of embryonic tissues are involved, the ectoderm (blue) of the third branchial cleft and the endoderm (orange) of the third pharyngeal pouch (first panel). Starting at about 9 days (second panel), the endoderm of the third pharyngeal pouch and the ectoderm of the branchial cleft grow inwards, forming a structure known as the cervical vesicle. With the continued invagination of these structures the two layers come together and the ectodermal layer begins to surround the endodermal layer (third panel). At this stage, by about 11 days, the invaginations close, eventually isolating the thymic rudiment (last panel). Comparisons of thymus development in normal mice and in mutant (*nude*) mice which lack a normal thymus, suggest that the ectodermal layer forms the cortical epithelial tissues of the thymus, while the endodermal layer forms the medullary tissues.

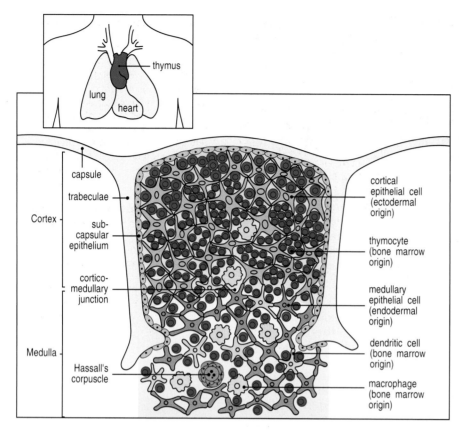

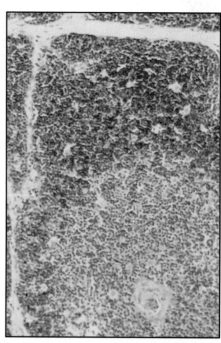

Fig. 6.3 The cellular organization of the thymus. The thymus, which lies in the midline of the body, above the heart, is made up from several lobules, each of which contains discrete cortical (outer) and medullary (central) regions. The cortex consists of immature thymocytes (dark blue), branched cortical epithelial cells (pale blue), with which the immature cortical thymocytes are closely associated, and scattered macrophages (yellow) involved in clearing apoptotic thymocytes. The medulla consists of mature thymocytes (dark blue), and medullary epithelial cells (orange), along with macrophages (yellow) and dendritic cells (yellow) of bone marrow origin. Hassall's corpuscles found in the human thymus are probably also sites of cell destruction. The thymocytes in the outer cortical cell layer are proliferating immature cells, while the deeper cortical thymocytes are mainly cells undergoing thymic selection. The photograph shows the equivalent section of a human thymus, stained with hematoxylin and eosin. Photograph courtesy of C J Howe.

6-2   The thymus is required for T-cell maturation.

The importance of the thymus in T-cell development was first discovered through observations of immunodeficient children, and much evidence has accumulated since to confirm and extend these observations. Thus, for example, in the **DiGeorge syndrome** in humans, and in mice with the *nude* mutation (which also causes hairlessness), the thymus fails to form and the affected individual produces B lymphocytes but few T lymphocytes. Surgical removal of the thymus (thymectomy) of mice at birth, when few T cells have left the thymus, likewise results in a mouse with B cells but few T cells.

The crucial role of the thymic stroma in inducing the differentiation of bone marrow-derived precursor cells can be demonstrated using two mutant mice, each lacking mature T cells for a different reason. In *nude* mice, the thymic epithelium fails to differentiate; while in *scid* mice, which we encountered in Section 3-17, the thymic stroma is normal but both B and T lymphocytes fail to develop because of a defect in receptor gene recombination. Reciprocal grafts of thymus and bone marrow between these immunodeficient strains show that *nude* bone marrow precursors develop normally in a *scid* thymus (Fig. 6.4). We shall see

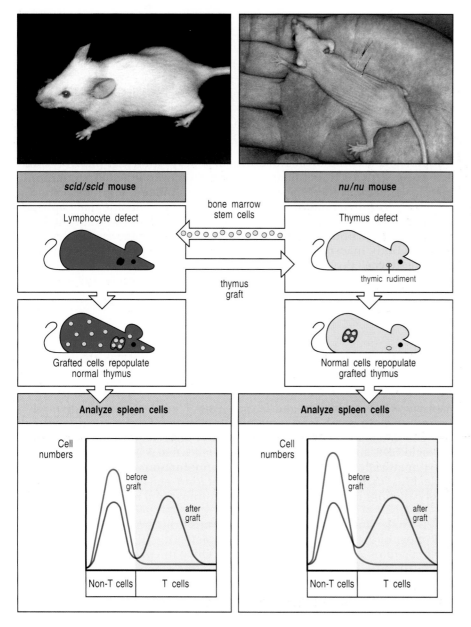

Fig. 6.4 The thymus is critical for the maturation of bone marrow derived cells into T cells. Mice with the *scid* mutation (upper left) have a defect that prevents lymphocyte maturation, while mice with the *nude* mutation (upper right) have a defect that affects the development of the cortical epithelium of the thymus. T cells do not develop in either strain of mouse: this can be demonstrated by staining spleen cells with antibodies specific for mature T cells and analyzing them in a flow cytometer (see Fig. 2.28), as represented by the graphs in the bottom panels. Bone marrow cells from *nude* mice can restore T cells to *scid* mice, showing that, in the right environment, the *nude* bone marrow cells are intrinsically normal, and capable of producing T cells. Thymic epithelial cells from *scid* mice can induce the maturation of T cells in *nude* mice, demonstrating that the thymus is the essential environment for T-cell development.

later that thymic grafts between different strains of mice have been instrumental in defining the role of the thymus in selecting the mature T-cell repertoire.

6-3   Developing T cells proliferate in the thymus but most die there.

T-cell precursors arriving in the thymus from the bone marrow spend up to a week differentiating there before they enter a phase of intense proliferation. In a young adult mouse, where the thymus contains around $1–2 \times 10^8$ thymocytes, about 5×10^7 cells are newly generated each day. However, only about 10^6 (roughly 2%) of these will leave the thymus in the same period as mature T cells. Despite the disparity between the numbers of T cells generated daily in the thymus and the number leaving, the thymus does not continue to grow in size or in cell number. This is because approximately 98% of the thymocytes generated each day die within the thymus. No widespread damage is seen, indicating that death is occurring by apoptosis rather than necrosis.

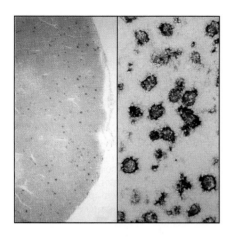

Fig. 6.5 Developing T cells that undergo apoptosis are ingested by macrophages in the thymic cortex. The photographs show thymic sections in which cells are stained for apoptosis with a red dye, and in blue either for a macrophage marker (left panel) or for a cortical epithelial cell marker (right panel). The figure shows many cells undergoing apoptosis in the cortex of a thymus. Apoptosis changes the surface properties of cells so that they are readily ingested by macrophages. Photographs courtesy of J Sprent and C Suhr.

Apoptosis is a common feature of many developmental pathways and one of its features is that changes in the membrane of cells undergoing apoptosis leads to their rapid phagocytosis. Indeed, apoptotic bodies, which are residual condensed chromatin, are seen inside macrophages throughout the thymic cortex (Fig. 6.5); as a result of the ready staining of the apoptotic bodies these macrophages are sometimes referred to as 'tingible body macrophages'. The apparently profligate wastefulness of this massive cell death is a crucial part of T-cell development, as it reflects the intensive screening that each new T cell undergoes for self MHC restriction and self tolerance.

6-4   **Successive stages in the development of thymocytes are marked by changes in cell-surface molecules.**

As thymocytes proliferate and mature into T cells, they pass through a series of distinct phases marked by changes in the status of T-cell receptor genes and in the expression of the T-cell receptor, the co-receptors CD4 and CD8, and other cell-surface molecules that reflect the state of functional maturation of the cell. Specific combinations of these cell-surface molecules, can thus be used as markers for T cells at different stages of differentiation: the principal stages are summarized in Fig. 6.6.

When progenitor cells first enter the thymus from the bone marrow, they lack most of the surface molecules characteristic of mature T cells and their receptor genes are unrearranged. Once the progenitor cell arrives in the thymus, interactions with the thymic stroma trigger differentiation, proliferation and the expression of the first T-cell specific surface molecules, CD2, and (in mice) Thy-1. At the end of this phase, which can last about 1 week, the immature thymocytes bear distinctive markers of the T-cell developmental lineage but they do not express any of the three cell-surface markers that define mature T cells, namely the CD3:T-cell receptor complex, CD4, and CD8. Owing to the absence of CD4 and CD8, such cells are called **'double-negative'** thymocytes.

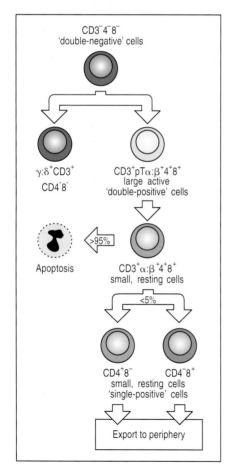

CD3⁻4⁻8⁻ 'double-negative' cells

γ:δ⁺CD3⁺ CD4⁻8⁻

CD3⁺pTα:β⁺4⁺8⁺ large active 'double-positive' cells

>95%

Apoptosis

CD3⁺α:β⁺4⁺8⁺ small, resting cells

<5%

CD4⁺8⁻   CD4⁻8⁺ small, resting cells 'single-positive' cells

Export to periphery

Fig. 6.6 Changes in cell-surface molecules allow thymocyte populations at different stages of maturation to be distinguished. The most important cell-surface molecules for identifying thymocyte subpopulations have been the CD4, CD8, and T-cell receptor molecules. The earliest cell population in the thymus does not express any of these. Since these cells do not express CD4 or CD8, they are called 'double-negative' cells. (In the thymus, γ:δ T cells do not express CD4 or CD8 but these are a minor population.) Maturation of α:β T cells occurs through a stage where both CD4 and CD8, as well as low levels of the T-cell receptor, are expressed by the same cell. These cells are known as 'double-positive' thymocytes. Most (>95%) of these cells become small double-positive cells and die within the thymus. Those whose receptors bind self MHC molecules lose expression of either CD4 or CD8 and increase the level of expression of the T-cell receptor. The outcome of this process is the mature, 'single-positive' T cell that is exported from the thymus.

In the fully developed thymus, these immature double-negative cells form part of a small, highly heterogeneous pool of cells (about 5% of thymocytes) that includes two populations of cells belonging to minority lineages. One of these, representing about 20% of all the double-negative cells in the thymus, comprises cells that have rearranged and are expressing the genes encoding the rare γ:δ receptor; we shall return to these cells in Section 6-7. The second, also representing about 20% of all double negatives, includes cells bearing α:β T-cell receptors of a very limited diversity, which are activated as part of the early response to many infections. We shall use the term 'double-negative thymocyte' to describe the remaining 60% of early thymocytes that are committed to the major α:β T-cell lineage but have not yet rearranged their α or β T-cell receptor genes.

These cells can be further subdivided on the basis of expression of the adhesion molecule CD44 and the α chain of the IL-2 receptor, CD25. In the first step, thymocytes express CD44 but not CD25; in these cells, the genes encoding the β chain of the T-cell receptor are in the germline configuration. As the thymocytes mature further, they begin to express CD25 on their surface, and still later, expression of CD44 is reduced. In these latter cells, which are known as CD44^{low}CD25$^+$ cells, rearrangement of the T-cell receptor β-chain gene occurs. Cells that fail to make a successful rearrangement of the β-chain gene remain in the CD44^{low}CD25$^+$ stage, while cells that make productive β-chain gene rearrangements lose expression of CD25 once again (Fig. 6.7). The functional significance of the transient expression of CD25 is unclear: T cells develop normally in mice in which the IL-2 gene has been deleted by gene knock-out (see Section 2-37).

The β chain expressed by such CD44^{low}CD25$^+$ thymocytes reaches the cell surface by pairing with a surrogate α chain called pTα (pre-T-cell α), together with the CD3 molecules. Expression of this complex leads to cell proliferation and the arrest of further β-chain gene rearrangements, and eventually results in the expression of both CD8 and CD4 (see Fig. 6.7). Cells at this stage are therefore called 'double-positive' thymocytes. While the cells are proliferating, the enzymes responsible for gene rearrangements are suppressed, so there is no gene rearrangement in these cycling cells. Once the cells cease to proliferate and become small double-positive cells, these enzymes are reactivated. This then allows the α-chain genes to rearrange, ultimately producing a complete α:β T-cell receptor.

Small double-positive thymocytes express only low levels of the T-cell receptor, and most (more than 95%) are destined to die. These are the cells that express receptors that cannot recognize self MHC and thus fail positive selection. Those double-positive cells that recognize self MHC, however, mature to express high levels of T-cell receptor and subsequently cease to express one or other of the two co-receptor molecules, becoming either CD4 or CD8 'single-positive' thymocytes (see Fig. 6.7). Thymocytes also undergo negative selection during and after the double-positive stage in development. Those that survive this dual screening mature to single-positive T cells that are rapidly exported from the thymus to join the peripheral T-cell repertoire.

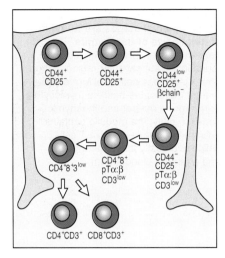

Fig. 6.7 The pathway of α:β T-cell development. During the 3 weeks that α:β thymocytes are maturing in the thymus, they undergo a series of phenotypic and proliferative changes. The earliest thymic emigrants spend up to a week slowly dividing in the subcapsular region, before showing signs of maturation. At this stage, these cells can give rise to intrathymic dendritic cells as well as the α:β and γ:δ thymocytes. Later, they begin to express markers associated with T cells, such as CD2 or Thy-1 (mouse). Then they express CD44 and, at a later stage, the α chain of the IL-2 receptor, CD25. After this, the CD44$^+$ CD25$^+$ cells begin to rearrange their β chain genes, becoming CD44^{low} as this occurs. The cells are then arrested in the CD44^{low} CD25$^+$ stage until they productively rearrange their β-chain genes, allowing the in-frame β chain to pair with pTα which triggers their entry into the cell cycle. Expression of pTα:β on the cell surface is associated with small amounts of CD3, and causes the loss of CD25, cessation of β-chain gene rearrangement, cell proliferation, expression of CD4 and CD8, and ultimately the rearrangement of the α-chain genes. The cells then express low levels of an α:β T-cell receptor and the associated CD3 complex and are ready for selection. Most cells die by failing to be positively selected but some are selected to mature into CD4 or CD8 single-positive cells and leave the thymus.

| 6-5 | **Thymocytes at different developmental stages are found in distinct parts of the thymus.** |

We have seen that the thymus is divided into two main regions, a peripheral cortex and a central medulla (see Fig. 6.3). Most T-cell development takes place in the cortex; only mature single-positive thymocytes are seen in the medulla. At the outer edge of the cortex, in the subcapsular

Fig. 6.8 Thymocytes of different developmental stages are found in distinct parts of the thymus. The earliest cells to enter the thymus are found in the subcapsular region of the cortex. As these cells proliferate and mature into double-positive thymocytes, they migrate deeper into the thymic cortex. Finally, the medulla contains only mature single-positive T cells, which eventually leave the thymus and enter the bloodstream.

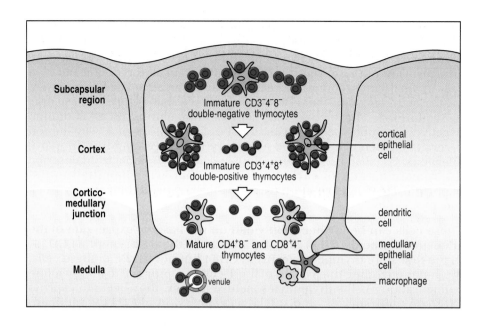

region of the thymus, large immature double-negative thymocytes proliferate vigorously (Fig. 6.8); these cells are thought to represent the thymic progenitors and their immediate progeny. These cells will give rise to all subsequent thymocyte populations. Deeper in the cortex, most of the thymocytes are small double-positive cells. The stroma of the cortex is composed of epithelial cells with long branching processes that express MHC class II as well as MHC class I molecules on their surface. The thymic cortex is densely packed with thymocytes, and the branching processes of the thymic cortical epithelial cells make contact with most cortical thymocytes. Contact between the MHC molecules on thymic cortical epithelial cells and the receptors of developing T cells plays a crucial part in positive selection, as we shall see later in this chapter.

The medulla of the thymus is less well characterized. It contains relatively few thymocytes, and those that are present are single-positive cells resembling mature T cells. These cells may be newly mature T cells that are leaving the thymus through the medulla, or they may represent some other population of mature T cells that remain within the medulla or return to it from the periphery to perform some specialized function, such as elimination of infectious agents within the thymus. At some point during their development in the thymic cortex and before their appearance in the medulla, therefore, the developing thymocytes must undergo negative selection. We shall see that this selective process is mainly carried out by the dendritic cells, which are particularly numerous at the cortico-medullary junction, and by the macrophages which are scattered in the cortex but are also abundant in the thymic medulla. Before discussing in more detail the succession of interactions whereby double-negative thymocytes mature into a population of self MHC-restricted and self-tolerant T cells, we must turn to the gene rearrangements that generate the random receptor repertoire on which positive and negative selection act.

Summary.

The thymus provides a sequestered and architecturally organized microenvironment for the development of mature T cells. Precursors of T cells migrate from the bone marrow and mature in the thymus, passing through a series of stages that can be distinguished by the differential expression of CD44 and CD25, the CD3:T-cell receptor complex proteins, and the co-receptor proteins, CD4 and CD8. T-cell development is accompanied by extensive cell death, reflecting the intense selection of T cells and the elimination of those with inappropriate receptor specificities. Most steps in T-cell differentiation occur in the cortex of the thymus. The thymic medulla contains only mature cells.

T-cell receptor gene rearrangements and receptor expression.

In the early stages of thymocyte maturation, the receptor genes of T cells go through a programmed series of rearrangements that produce large numbers of immature T cells each expressing receptors of a single specificity. This process is similar in many ways to that which occurs in B cells, with two important differences. First, rearrangement of two different sets of receptor genes distinguishes two T-cell lineages, one expressing $\alpha:\beta$ and the other $\gamma:\delta$ receptors. Second, there is much greater scope for repeated rearrangements of T-cell receptor genes, particularly at the α locus, allowing rescue of many cells in which the initial rearrangements have been non-productive. The end result of this process in the $\alpha:\beta$ T-cell lineage is a double-positive thymocyte expressing T-cell receptors on which positive and negative selection can then act.

6-6   T cells with $\alpha:\beta$ or $\gamma:\delta$ receptors arise from a common progenitor.

T cells bearing $\gamma:\delta$ receptors differ from $\alpha:\beta$ T cells in their specificity, the pattern of expression of the CD4 and CD8 co-receptors, and in their anatomical distribution. The two types of T cells also differ in function, although relatively little is known about the function of $\gamma:\delta$ T cells. Nonetheless, studies of the gene rearrangements found in thymocytes and mature $\gamma:\delta$ and $\alpha:\beta$ T cells show that they diverge from a common precursor at a relatively late stage of their development, when gene rearrangements have already occurred. Mature $\gamma:\delta$ T cells can be found to have productively rearranged β-chain genes, while mature $\alpha:\beta$ T cells often contain rearranged, but mostly out-of-frame, γ- and δ-chain genes.

At present, the commitment of a common T-cell precursor to one or the other of these lineages is thought to depend simply upon whether productive rearrangements of a γ and a δ chain gene have occurred in the same cell. The β, γ, and δ genes undergo rearrangement almost simultaneously in developing thymocytes and it appears that successful rearrangement of the γ and δ genes leads to the expression of a functional $\gamma:\delta$ T-cell receptor that signals the cell to differentiate along the $\gamma:\delta$ lineage. In the majority of precursors, however, there is a successful rearrangement of a β-chain gene before successful rearrangement of both γ and δ genes can occur. A functional β-chain protein pairs with pTα, arresting further rearrangements and signaling the cell to proliferate, to express their co-receptor genes, and to start transcribing the α-chain genes.

These cells have taken a further maturational step towards becoming $\alpha:\beta$ cells but they are not yet committed to this lineage. Once the proliferative burst is over, the enzymes responsible for gene rearrangements are reactivated and, in some cells, successful completion of $\gamma:\delta$ rearrangement will lead to the emergence of more $\gamma:\delta$ T cells. In most cases, however, rearrangements at the α locus will delete the intervening δ gene as an extrachromosomal circle and a functional α chain will be expressed. The further maturation of α:β T cells depends on positive selection for the ability to recognize self MHC molecules. The signals that drive a γ:δ T cell to mature are unknown. Certainly, γ:δ T cells seem able to develop in the absence of a functioning thymus and are present in, for example, *nude* mice.

6-7 | **Cells expressing particular γ:δ genes arise first in embryonic development.**

The first T cells to appear during embryonic development carry γ:δ T-cell receptors (Fig. 6.9). In the mouse, where the development of the immune system can be studied in detail, γ:δ T cells first appear in discrete waves or bursts, with the T cells in each wave homing to distinct sites in the adult animal.

The first wave of γ:δ T cells homes specifically to the epidermis, where they are called **dendritic epidermal T cells (dETC)**, whereas the second

Fig. 6.9 The rearrangement of T-cell receptor γ and δ genes in the mouse proceeds in waves of cells expressing different V gene segments. At about 2 weeks of gestation, the $C_\gamma 1$ locus is expressed with its closest V gene ($V_\gamma 5$; also known as $V_\gamma 3$ *). After a few days $V_\gamma 5$-bearing cells decline (upper panel) and are replaced by cells expressing the next most proximal gene, $V_\gamma 6$. Both these rearranged γ chains are expressed with the same rearranged δ-chain gene, as shown in the lower panels, and there is no junctional diversity. As a consequence, all of the γ:δ T cells produced in each of these early waves have the same specificity, although the nature of the antigen recognized by the early γ:δ T cells is not yet known. The $V_\gamma 5$-bearing cells migrate selectively to the epidermis while the $V_\gamma 6$-bearing cells migrate to the epithelium of the reproductive tract. After birth, the α:β T-cell lineage becomes dominant and while γ:δ T cells are still produced, they are a much more heterogeneous population, with a high level of junctional diversity.
*The nomenclature of V_γ gene segments is a source of confusion, as there are two different nomenclatures. One system specifies $V_\gamma 1.1$, $V_\gamma 1.2$, and $V_\gamma 1.3$, while the other refers to these as $V_\gamma 1$, $V_\gamma 2$, and $V_\gamma 3$. Thus, $V_\gamma 2$, $V_\gamma 3$, $V_\gamma 4$, and $V_\gamma 5$ in the first system become $V_\gamma 4$, $V_\gamma 5$, $V_\gamma 6$, and $V_\gamma 7$ in the second. In this book, we use the latter nomenclature.

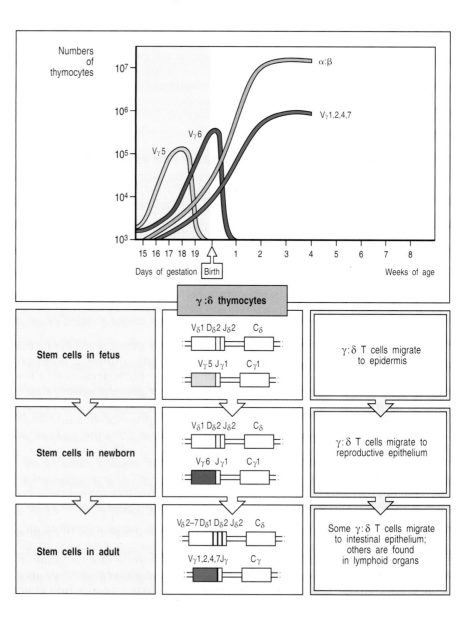

wave homes to the epithelial layers of the reproductive tract. The receptors expressed by these early waves of γ:δ T cells are essentially homogeneous: all the cells in each wave express the same rearranged V_γ and V_δ sequences and the same J regions. There are no N-nucleotides to contribute additional diversity at the junctions between V, D, and J gene segments, reflecting the absence of the enzyme terminal deoxynucleotidyl transferase (TdT) in these early T cells.

Later in development, T cells are produced continuously rather than in waves, and α:β T cells predominate, making up more than 95% of thymocytes. The γ:δ T cells produced at this stage are different from those of the early waves, with considerably more diverse receptors containing several different V gene segments and abundant N-region additions. Most of these γ:δ T cells, like α:β T cells, are found in peripheral lymphoid tissues rather than in the specific epithelial sites to which the early γ:δ T cells preferentially home.

The developmental changes in V gene segment usage and N-nucleotide additions in γ:δ T cells parallel changes in B-cell populations during fetal development (see Section 5-13). The functional significance of the early γ:δ T cells, like the functional significance of the γ:δ T cells themselves, is unclear.

It should be emphasized that most of what we know about γ:δ T-cell development comes from studies in mice and we do not know whether similar changes in the pattern of receptors expressed by γ:δ T cells occur in humans. Certainly, the γ:δ T cells that home to the skin of mice, namely the dendritic epidermal T cells, do not seem to have exact human counterparts, although there are γ:δ T cells in the human reproductive and gastrointestinal tracts.

6-8 Productive β-chain gene rearrangement triggers rapid proliferation and the cessation of β-chain gene rearrangement.

T cells expressing α:β receptors first appear a few days after the earliest γ:δ T cells and rapidly become the most abundant type of thymocyte (see Fig. 6.9). The rearrangement of β- and α-chain genes during T-cell development is summarized in Fig. 6.10 and closely parallels the rearrangement of immunoglobulin heavy- and light-chain genes during B-cell development (see Section 5-2). The β-chain genes rearrange first. D_β gene segments rearrange to J_β gene segments, and this is followed by V_β to DJ_β rearrangement. If no functional β chain can be synthesized from these rearrangements, the cell will not be able to produce a pre-T-cell receptor and will die unless it successfully rearranges both γ and δ genes. However, unlike B cells with non-productive immunoglobulin heavy-chain gene rearrangements, thymocytes with non-productive β-chain VDJ rearrangements can be rescued by subsequent β-chain gene rearrangements, because of the organization of the D_β and J_β gene segments into two clusters upstream of two C_β constant-region genes. This increases the likelihood of a productive VDJ join from 55% for immunoglobulin heavy chains to more than 80% for T-cell receptor β-chain genes (Fig. 6.11).

Once a productive β-chain gene rearrangement has occurred, the β-chain protein is expressed on the cell surface together with the invariant partner chain pTα (see Fig. 6.10). Like the pre-B-cell receptor complex in B-cell development, this β:pTα heterodimer is a functional pre-T-cell receptor that must reach the cell surface for further development to occur. Expression of the pre-T-cell receptor triggers rapid proliferation of the cells; it also halts β-chain gene rearrangement and eventually induces the expression of the co-receptor proteins CD4 and CD8. All these

Fig. 6.10 The stages of gene rearrangement in α:β T cells. The sequence of gene rearrangements is shown, together with an indication of the stage at which the events take place and the nature of the cell-surface receptor molecules expressed at each stage. The T-cell receptor (TCR) β-chain genes rearrange first, in CD4⁻ CD8⁻ double-negative thymocytes expressing CD25 and low levels of CD44. As with immunoglobulin heavy-chain genes, D to J gene segments rearrange before V gene segments rearrange to DJ (second and third panels). Since there are four D gene segments and two sets of J gene segments, it is possible to make up to four attempts to generate a productive rearrangement of the β-chain genes. The productively rearranged gene is expressed initially within the cell and then at low levels on the cell surface in a complex with the CD3 chains as a pTα:β heterodimer (fourth panel), where pTα is a 33 kDa surrogate α chain equivalent to λ5 in B-cell development. The expression of the pre-T-cell receptor signals the developing thymocytes via the tyrosine kinase Lck to halt β-chain gene rearrangement, and to undergo multiple cycles of division. These events may be triggered as a consequence of the pre-T-cell receptor engaging the CD81 molecule, which is expressed on thymic stromal cells, as they are blocked by antibody to CD81. At the end of this proliferative burst, the CD4 and CD8 molecules are expressed, the cell ceases cycling, and the α chain is now able to undergo rearrangement. The first α-chain gene rearrangement deletes all δ chain D, J, and C gene segments on that chromosome, although these are retained as a circular DNA, proving that these are non-dividing cells (bottom panel). This inactivates the δ-chain genes. α-chain gene rearrangement can proceed through many cycles, because of the large number of V_α and J_α gene segments, until a functional α chain is produced that pairs efficiently with the β chain. Finally, with the expression of a functional α:β receptor capable of recognizing peptides in association with self MHC molecules, the CD3^low CD4⁺CD8⁺ thymocyte is ready to undergo selection.

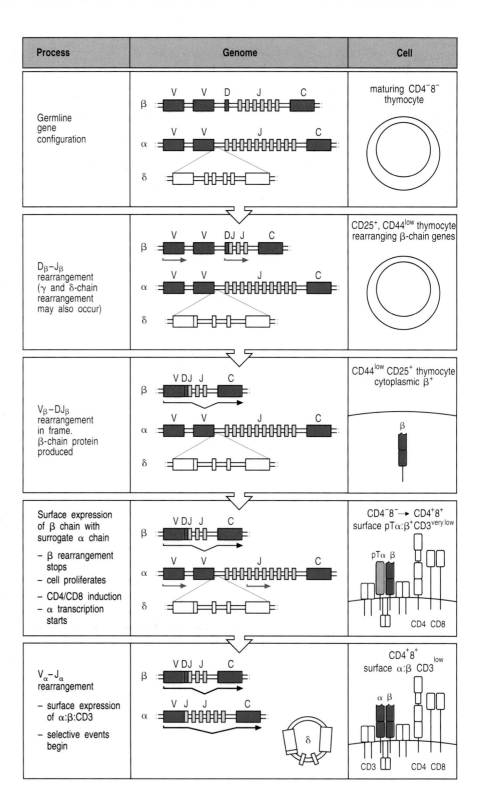

events can be blocked by an antibody to CD81, a transmembrane molecule that is expressed on thymic stromal cells. It is possible that CD81, which we have previously encountered as the TAPA-1 element of the B-cell co-receptor complex (see Section 3-26) delivers the signal for these events by interacting directly with the β:pTα receptor, but this is not yet known.

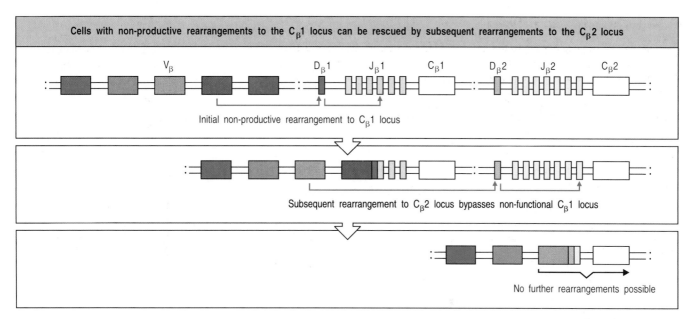

Fig. 6.11 Rescue of non-productive β-chain gene rearrangements. Successive rearrangements can rescue an initial non-productive β-chain gene rearrangement only if that rearrangement involved the $C_\beta1$ locus. A second rearrangement is then possible in which a second V_β gene segment rearranges to a DJ segment in the $C_\beta2$ locus, deleting the $C_\beta1$ locus and the non-productively rearranged gene.

The induction of proliferation, the arrest of β-chain gene rearrangement, and the eventual induction of CD4 and CD8 expression all require the protein tyrosine kinase Lck, which later associates with the co-receptor proteins. In $p56^{lck}$-deficient mice, T-cell development is arrested before the double-positive stage. The role of the expressed β chain in suppressing further β-chain gene rearrangement can be demonstrated in transgenic mice containing a rearranged β-chain transgene: these mice express the transgenic β chain on most or all their T cells and rearrangement of the endogenous β-chain genes is strongly suppressed.

During the proliferative phase triggered by the expression of the pre-T cell receptor, the *RAG-1* and *RAG-2* genes that mediate receptor gene segment recombination are repressed and RAG-2 protein is not active because it is phosphorylated and degraded in the rapidly cycling cells. Hence, no rearrangement of α-chain genes occurs until the proliferative phase ends, allowing *RAG-1* and *RAG-2* mRNA and RAG-2 protein to accumulate again. This ensures that each successful rearrangement of a β-chain gene gives rise to many CD4, CD8 double-positive thymocytes, each of which can independently rearrange its α-chain genes once the cells stop dividing, so that a single β chain is associated with many different α chains in the resulting progeny. During the period of α-chain gene rearrangement, α:β heterodimeric T-cell receptors are first expressed, and selection by peptide:MHC complexes in the thymus can begin. The events leading to this point are summarized in Figure 6.10.

6-9   T-cell receptor α-chain genes can undergo several successive rearrangements.

The T-cell receptor α-chain genes are comparable with the immuno-globulin κ light-chain genes, in that they do not have D gene segments and are the second of the two receptor-chain genes to undergo rearrangement

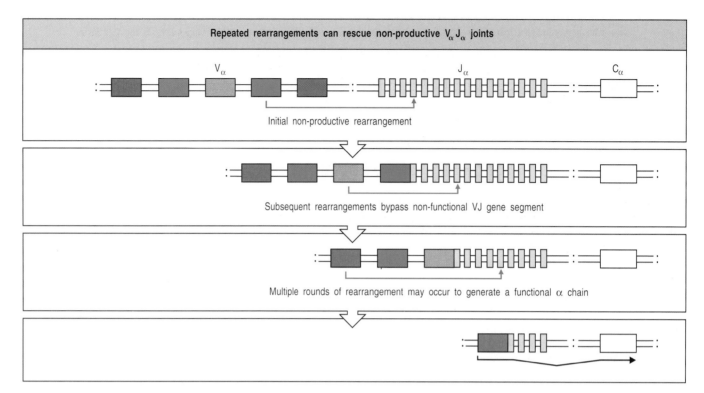

Fig. 6.12 Several successive gene rearrangement events can allow the replacement of one T-cell receptor α chain by another. For the T-cell receptor α chains, the multiplicity of V and J gene segments allows successive rearrangement events to 'leapfrog' over non-productively rearranged VJ segments, deleting any intervening gene segments. This process can continue until either a productive rearrangement occurs or there are no more V or J gene segments available for rearrangement, or the cell dies. The α-chain rescue pathway resembles that of immunoglobulin κ light-chain genes (see Section 5-3).

during normal T-cell development. However, the presence of multiple V_α gene segments and at least 50 J_α gene segments spread over some 80 kilobases of DNA allows many successive VJ_α gene rearrangements, conferring a far greater capacity to rescue cells with non-productive rearrangements than is the case for κ-chain genes (Fig. 6.12).

The potential for successive α-chain gene rearrangements on both chromosomes virtually guarantees that α-chain proteins will be produced in every developing T cell. Indeed, many T cells have in-frame rearrangements on both chromosomes and produce two α-chain proteins. This is possible because the rearrangement of α-chain genes can continue even after production of a cell-surface receptor. This phase of gene rearrangement lasts 3–4 days in the mouse and it only ceases when positive selection has occurred or the cell dies. Thus, in the strict sense, T-cell receptor α chains are not subject to allelic exclusion (see Section 5-8). However, as we shall see in the next part of this chapter, even T cells with two cell-surface α:β T-cell receptors have only a single receptor that can recognize peptide:self MHC complexes, and the cell therefore effectively expresses only a single receptor specificity.

Summary.

In differentiating T cells, receptor genes rearrange according to a defined program, which is similar to that in B cells, with the added complication that individual precursor cells can follow one of two distinct lines of development leading to cells bearing either γ:δ receptors or α:β receptors.

Early in ontogeny, γ:δ T cells predominate, but from birth onwards more than 90% of thymocytes express α:β receptors. The two T-cell lineages home to different tissues and perform different functions, although the function of γ:δ T cells is not yet fully established. In precursors destined to become γ:δ T cells, the γ and δ genes seem to rearrange virtually simultaneously and, when they produce a functional receptor protein, this appears to determine lineage commitment. When this fails, cells enter the α:β lineage. In cells destined to become α:β T cells, β-chain genes rearrange first. The expression of a functional β chain at the cell surface in the form of a pre-T-cell receptor signals the cell to proliferate, to arrest β-chain gene rearrangement, to express CD4 and CD8, and eventually to rearrange the α-chain gene in CD4, CD8 double-positive thymocytes. In α:β T cells, α-chain gene rearrangement continues until positive selection occurs. This means that mature T cells often express two α chains, although because of positive selection there is nonetheless only one receptor restricted to self MHC in any one cell.

Positive and negative selection of T cells.

We saw in the first section of this chapter that T cells first enter the thymus as double-negative cells, expressing neither the T-cell receptor nor either of the two co-receptor molecules, CD4 and CD8. During a phase of vigorous proliferation in the subcapsular zone, these immature thymocytes differentiate into double-positive cells, expressing low levels of the T-cell receptor and both co-receptor molecules, and move on to the deeper layers of the thymic cortex. Here they undergo positive selection for self MHC-restriction and start to lose one of their two co-receptor molecules. The double-positive cells must also undergo negative selection in which potentially self-reactive cells are eliminated. By the time single-positive thymocytes are ready to emigrate, autoreactive T cells have been deleted. This sequence of events is summarized in Fig. 6.13.

Most of the evidence on the role of the thymus in the selection of the T-cell receptor repertoire has come from studies on chimeric or transgenic mice (see Sections 2-32 and 2-36). In this section, we shall see how these studies have defined the crucial interactions between developing thymocytes and the different thymic components that contribute to the selection of the mature T-cell repertoire, and will discuss the mechanisms by which these distinctive selective processes generate a self MHC-restricted and self-tolerant repertoire of T cells.

| 6-10 | **Only T cells specific for peptides bound to self MHC molecules mature in the thymus.** |

Positive selection was first shown clearly by transferring bone marrow cells from a mouse of one MHC genotype into an irradiated mouse of a different MHC genotype. Irradiation destroys all the lymphocytes and bone marrow progenitor cells in the host animal, so that all the cells derived from bone marrow are of the donor genotype. This includes all lymphocytes and antigen-presenting cells. Mice whose bone marrow derived cells have been replaced by those of a donor mouse are

Fig. 6.13 The development of T cells can be considered as a series of discrete phases. Thymocyte progenitors enter the thymus in the subcapsular region. At this stage, they express neither the antigen receptor nor either of the two co-receptors CD4 and CD8, and are known as double-negative cells. As double-negative cells, the thymocytes proliferate and begin the process of gene rearrangement that culminates in the expression of the pre-T-cell receptor along with the co-receptors CD4 and CD8 on the cell surface, to produce double-positive cells. As the cells mature, they move deeper into the thymus. These cells then rearrange α-chain genes and become sensitive to peptide:MHC complexes. These double-positive cells are found in the thymic cortex where they undergo positive selection and negative selection. Negative selection is thought to be most stringent at the corticomedullary junction, where nearly mature thymocytes encounter plentiful dendritic cells derived from the same intrathymic precursors that gave rise to the thymocytes. Finally, surviving thymocytes mature and exit to the peripheral circulation from the medulla.

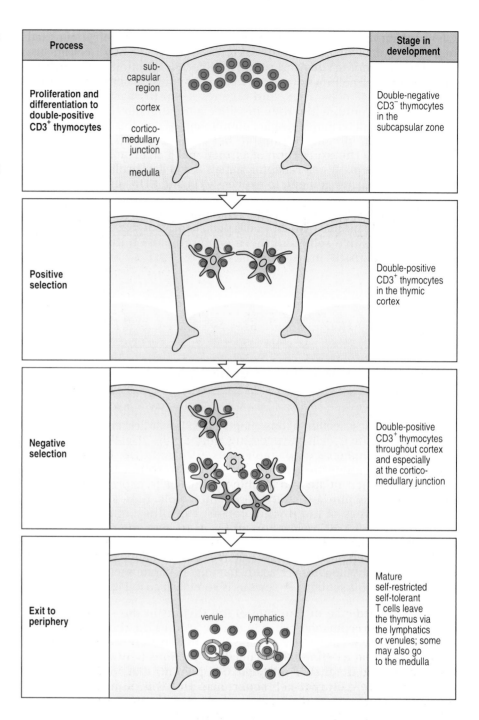

Process		Stage in development
Proliferation and differentiation to double-positive CD3+ thymocytes	sub-capsular region / cortex / cortico-medullary junction / medulla	Double-negative CD3⁻ thymocytes in the subcapsular zone
Positive selection		Double-positive CD3+ thymocytes in the thymic cortex
Negative selection		Double-positive CD3+ thymocytes throughout cortex and especially at the cortico-medullary junction
Exit to periphery	venule lymphatics	Mature self-restricted self-tolerant T cells leave the thymus via the lymphatics or venules; some may also go to the medulla

known as **bone marrow chimeras** (see Section 2-32). The donor mice used in the experiments on positive selection were F1 hybrids derived from MHC^a and MHC^b parents, and thus were of the MHC^{axb} genotype, while the irradiated recipients were one of the parental strains, either MHC^a or MHC^b (Fig. 6.14).

Individual T cells in MHC^{axb} F1 hybrid mice will recognize antigen presented by either MHC^a or MHC^b, but not both, because their receptors are MHC restricted in antigen recognition. When T cells of MHC^{axb} genotype develop in a parental MHC^a thymus and are then immunized, they will be presented with antigen bound to both MHC^a and MHC^b, as the antigen-presenting cells in the chimera are of bone marrow origin and

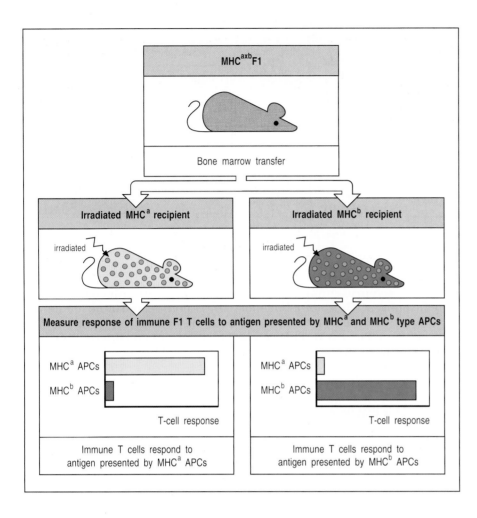

MHC^{axb}F1

Bone marrow transfer

Irradiated MHC^a recipient

irradiated

Irradiated MHC^b recipient

irradiated

Measure response of immune F1 T cells to antigen presented by MHC^a and MHC^b type APCs

MHC^a APCs

MHC^b APCs

T-cell response

MHC^a APCs

MHC^b APCs

T-cell response

Immune T cells respond to antigen presented by MHC^a APCs

Immune T cells respond to antigen presented by MHC^b APCs

Fig. 6.14 Positive selection is revealed by bone marrow chimeric mice.
T cells in MHC^{axb}F1 mice can be primed to respond to antigen presented by antigen-presenting cells (APCs) from both MHC^a and MHC^b mice. If bone marrow from such an F1 hybrid mouse is transferred to a lethally irradiated recipient mouse of either parental MHC type (MHC^a or MHC^b), the T cells that mature are positively selected in that recipient's thymus, as shown by their response to antigen. When these animals are immunized with antigen, the antigen can be presented by the bone marrow derived antigen-presenting cells in association with both MHC^a and MHC^b molecules. However when tested *in vitro* with APCs of MHC^a or MHC^b, T cells from such chimeric animals only respond to antigen presented by the MHC molecules of the recipient MHC type, as shown in the bottom panel.

thus MHC^{axb}. However, these T cells recognize antigen only when it is presented by MHC^a molecules (see Fig. 6.14). This experiment thus shows clearly that the environment in which the T cells mature determines the MHC molecules to which they become restricted.

A further experiment demonstrates that the host component responsible for the positive selection of developing T cells is the thymic stroma. For this experiment, the recipient animals were athymic *nude* or thymectomized mice of the MHC^{axb} genotype with thymic stromal grafts of the MHC^a genotype, so that all of their cells carried both MHC^a and MHC^b except those of the thymic stroma. The MHC^{axb} bone marrow cells of these mice also mature into T cells that recognize antigens presented by MHC^a but not antigens presented by MHC^b. Thus, what mature T cells consider to be self MHC is determined by the MHC molecules expressed by the thymic stromal cells they encounter during intrathymic development. We shall see later that the thymic cortical epithelial cell is the critical cell that governs the specificity of positive selection.

The chimeric mice used to demonstrate positive selection produce normal T-cell responses to foreign antigens. By contrast, chimeras made by injecting MHC^a bone marrow cells into MHC^b animals cannot make normal T-cell responses. This is because the T cells in these animals have been selected to recognize peptides only when they are presented by MHC^b, while the antigen-presenting cells that they encounter as mature T cells in the periphery are bone marrow derived MHC^a cells. The T cells will therefore fail to recognize antigen presented by antigen-presenting cells of their own MHC type, and T cells can be activated in these animals

Fig. 6.15 Summary of T-cell responses to immunization in bone marrow chimeric mice. T cells can make immune responses only if the antigen-presenting cells (APCs) present in the host at the time of priming share at least one MHC molecule with the thymus in which the T cells developed.

Bone marrow donor	*In vivo* immunized recipient	Mice contain APC of type:	Secondary T-cell responses to antigen presented *in vitro* by APC of type:	
			MHC^a APC	MHC^b APC
MHC^{axb}	MHC^a	MHC^{axb}	Yes	No
MHC^{axb}	MHC^b	MHC^{axb}	No	Yes
MHC^a	MHC^b	MHC^a	No	No
MHC^a	MHC^b + MHC^b APC	MHC^a + MHC^b	No	Yes

only if antigen-presenting cells of the MHC^b type are injected together with the antigen. Thus, for a bone marrow graft to reconstitute immunity, there must be at least one MHC molecule in common between donor and recipient (Fig. 6.15). This can be an important consideration when bone marrow grafts are used in the treatment of human diseases such as leukemias.

6-11   Cells that fail positive selection die in the thymus.

Bone marrow chimeras and thymic grafting provided the first crucial evidence for the central importance of the thymus in positive selection but more detailed investigation of the process has generally required the use of mice transgenic for T-cell receptor genes. When rearranged T-cell receptor genes of known specificity are introduced into the genome of a mouse, rearrangement of the endogenous genes are inhibited, so that most developing T cells express the receptor encoded by the α- and β-chain transgenes. By introducing the transgenes into mice of known MHC genotype, it is possible to establish the effect of MHC molecules on the maturation of thymocytes with known recognition properties. Such a T-cell receptor transgenic mouse was used to establish the fate of T cells that fail positive selection. In this case, rearranged receptor genes from a mature T cell restricted to a particular MHC molecule were introduced into a recipient mouse lacking that molecule, and the fate of the thymocytes was investigated directly by staining with clonotypic antibodies specific for the transgenic receptor. Antibodies to other molecules such as CD4 and CD8 were used at the same time to mark the stages of T-cell development. In this way it was shown that cells that do not encounter their restricting MHC molecule on the thymic epithelium never progress further than the double-positive stage and die in the thymus within 3 or 4 days of their last division.

The total potential receptor repertoire must be capable of recognizing all of the hundreds of different allelic variants of MHC molecules present in the population, since the genes for the T-cell receptor α and β chains segregate in the population independently from those of the MHC. In any individual the thymus will express only a few of these many distinct MHC molecules, so only a relatively small proportion of the thymocytes will be capable of recognizing an MHC molecule. Most of the 50×10^6 thymocytes that die each day in the thymus presumably do so because they fail positive selection. It has been estimated that 95% of thymocytes die because they are not rescued by a signal received from their T-cell receptor.

6-12   Positive selection also regulates α-chain gene rearrangement.

We have seen that in B cells, the expression of a receptor on the cell surface shuts off further rearrangement of the receptor genes; this is accompanied by the disappearance of the expression of *RAG-1* and *RAG-2* genes. In the case of T cells, however, receptor expression is not sufficient to shut off gene rearrangement. Instead, the rearrangement machinery, including *RAG-1*, *RAG-2*, and TdT, remains active, and rearrangement of the α-chain genes continues until the cells are positively selected or die. In this way, several different α chains can be tested for self MHC recognition in partnership with the single β chain of each developing T cell. If positive selection does not occur within 3–4 days of the initial expression of an α:β receptor, the cell dies.

Thus, positive selection not only selects cells for further maturation, but it also regulates the rearrangement of T-cell receptor α-chain genes. The ability of a single developing thymocyte to express several different rearranged α-chain genes during the time it is susceptible to positive selection must increase the yield of useful T cells significantly. Without this mechanism even more thymocytes would die because they fail positive selection.

Since α-chain gene rearrangement can occur simultaneously on both chromosomes and because positive selection is such a rare event, it seemed likely that a significant percentage of mature T cells would express two T-cell receptors, sharing a β chain but differing in α-chain expression. Indeed, one can predict that if positive selection is sufficiently rare, roughly one cell in three would have two α chains at the cell surface. This was confirmed recently for human and mouse T cells. However, while both of these α chains were functional in response to antibodies specific for α chains, only one of the two T-cell receptors could recognize peptide presented by self MHC.

6-13   The expression of CD4 and CD8 on mature T cells and the associated T-cell functions are determined by positive selection.

At the time of positive selection, the thymocyte expresses both the CD4 and the CD8 co-receptor molecules. At the end of the selection process, mature thymocytes ready for export to the periphery express only one of these two co-receptors. Moreover, almost all mature T cells that express CD4 have receptors that recognize peptides bound to self MHC class II molecules and are programmed to become cytokine-secreting cells, whereas most of those that express CD8 have receptors that recognize peptides bound to self MHC class I molecules and are programmed to become cytotoxic effector cells. Thus, positive selection also determines the cell-surface phenotype and functional potential of the mature T cell, selecting the co-receptor that it requires for efficient antigen recognition and programming it for appropriate functional differentiation upon activation in an immune response. Again, experiments with mice made transgenic for rearranged T-cell receptor genes show clearly that it is the specificity of the T-cell receptor for self MHC molecules that determines which co-receptor a mature T cell will express. If the T-cell receptor transgenes encode a receptor specific for antigen presented by self MHC class I molecules, mature T cells that express the transgenic receptor are also CD8 T cells. Similarly, in mice made transgenic for a receptor that recognizes antigen with self MHC class II molecules, mature T cells that express the transgenic receptor also express CD4 (Fig. 6.16).

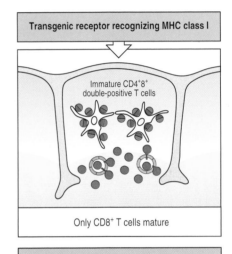

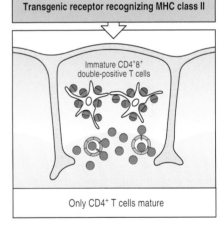

Fig. 6.16 Positive selection determines co-receptor specificity. In mice transgenic for T-cell receptors restricted by an MHC class I molecule (top panel), the only mature T cells to develop have the CD8 (red) phenotype. In mice transgenic for receptors restricted by an MHC class II molecule (bottom panel), all the mature T cells have the CD4 (blue) phenotype. In both cases, normal numbers of immature, double-positive thymocytes are found. The specificity of the T-cell receptor determines the outcome of the developmental pathway, ensuring that the only T cells that mature are those equipped with a co-receptor that is able to bind the same self MHC molecule as the T-cell receptor.

The importance of MHC molecules in such selective events can also be seen in the class of human immunodeficiency diseases known as **bare lymphocyte syndromes**, which are caused by mutations that lead to absence of MHC molecules on lymphocytes and thymic epithelial cells. People who selectively lack MHC class II molecules have CD8 T cells but only a few highly abnormal CD4 T cells; a similar result has been obtained in mice in which MHC class II expression has been eliminated by targeted gene disruption (see Section 2-37). Likewise, mice and humans that lack MHC class I molecules lack CD8 T cells. Thus, MHC class II molecules are required for CD4 T-cell development, while MHC class I molecules are required for CD8 T-cell development.

| 6-14 | Thymic cortical epithelial cells mediate positive selection. |

The ability of thymic stromal cells to determine co-receptor specificity has been used as the basis for experiments aimed at identifying the stromal cell type that is critical in positive selection of thymocytes. An obvious candidate, on the basis of much circumstantial evidence, is the thymic cortical epithelial cell. Thymic cortical epithelial cells form a web of processes that make close contacts with the double-positive T cells undergoing positive selection and at these sites of contact, T-cell receptors can be seen clustering with MHC molecules. Direct evidence that thymic cortical epithelial cells mediate positive selection comes from an ingenious manipulation of mice whose MHC class II genes have been eliminated by targeted gene disruption.

As we have already seen, mutant mice that lack MHC class II molecules do not produce CD4 T cells. To test the role of the thymic epithelium in positive selection therefore, an MHC class II transgene was introduced into such mutant mice. The MHC class II coding region of the transgene was placed under the control of a promoter that restricted its expression to thymic cortical epithelial cells. In these mice, CD4 T cells develop normally. A further variant on this experiment shows that, in order to promote the normal development of CD4 T cells, the MHC class II molecule on the thymic epithelial cells must bind CD4. Thus, when the MHC class II transgene expressed in the thymus contains a mutation that prevents it from binding to CD4, very few CD4 T cells develop (Fig. 6.17).

The experiments with T-cell receptor transgenic animals show that the specificity of the T cell-receptor for class I or class II MHC molecules determines which co-receptor will be selected, whereas experiments with mutant MHC class II molecules, and equivalent studies of CD8 interaction with MHC class I molecules show that co-receptor binding is necessary for normal positive selection to occur. However, the mechanism whereby antigen receptor and co-receptor selection are coordinated remains to be established.

There are two broad theories for how this might be accomplished: the **instructive model**; and the **stochastic/selection model**. According to the instructive model, the two co-receptors deliver distinct intracellular signals: the signal for CD4 shuts off the expression of the CD8 gene, while the signal from CD8 silences the CD4 gene. In the stochastic/selection model, by contrast, cells randomly inactivate either the CD4 or CD8 gene, and the thymocytes are then tested for the correct match of co-receptor with the specificity of the T-cell receptor. Cells in which the specificity of the co-receptor is mismatched with that of the antigen receptor die, while those with correct matching of CD4 and MHC class II recognition, or of CD8 and MHC class I recognition, survive, mature, and leave the thymus. At the present time there is experimental evidence supporting both models and each may prove correct some of the time.

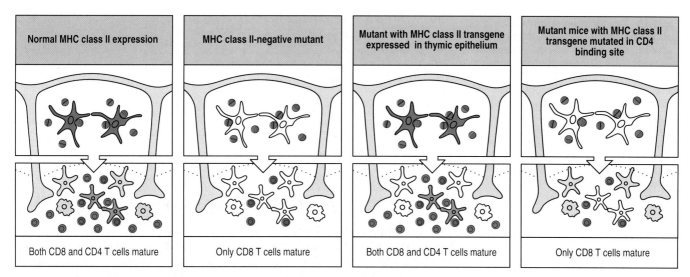

Normal MHC class II expression	MHC class II-negative mutant	Mutant with MHC class II transgene expressed in thymic epithelium	Mutant mice with MHC class II transgene mutated in CD4 binding site
Both CD8 and CD4 T cells mature	Only CD8 T cells mature	Both CD8 and CD4 T cells mature	Only CD8 T cells mature

Fig. 6.17 Mice lacking MHC class II molecules fail to develop CD4 T cells. The expression of MHC class II molecules in the thymus of normal and mutant strains of mice is shown by coloring the stromal cells only if they are expressing MHC class II molecules. In the thymus of normal mice (first panels), which express MHC class II molecules on epithelial cells in the thymic cortex (blue) as well as on medullary epithelial cells (orange) and bone marrow derived cells (yellow), both CD4 (blue) and CD8 (red) T cells mature. Double-positive thymocytes are shown as half red/half blue. The second panels represent mutant mice in which MHC class II expression has been eliminated by targeted gene disruption; in these mice, few CD4 T cells develop, although CD8 T cells develop normally. In MHC class II-negative mice containing an MHC class II transgene engineered so that it is expressed only on the epithelial cells of the thymic cortex (third panels), normal numbers of CD4 T cells mature. In MHC class II-negative mice bearing a mutant MHC class II transgene defective in its CD4 binding site (fourth panels), no CD4 T cells develop. Thus, the cortical epithelial cells are the critical cell type mediating positive selection.

6-15   T cells specific for ubiquitous self antigens are deleted in the thymus.

When a mature T cell in the periphery encounters its corresponding antigen on a professional antigen-presenting cell, it is activated to proliferate and produce effector T cells. In contrast, when a developing thymocyte encounters its corresponding antigen on thymic stromal or bone marrow derived cells, it dies by apoptosis. This response to antigen is the basis of negative selection and has been demonstrated in mice expressing a transgenic T-cell receptor specific for a peptide of ovalbumin bound to the MHC class II molecule I-A^d. When such a mouse is injected with the appropriate ovalbumin peptide, its peripheral CD4 T cells become activated, but all the intrathymic cells die (Fig. 6.18). Similar results are obtained in thymic organ culture with T cells from normal or transgenic mice, showing that secondary effects of the induction of cytokines or corticosteroids cannot account for these results.

In unmanipulated mice, T cells developing in the thymus will encounter a large selection of self peptides bound to self MHC molecules on thymic cells of various types, and cells that would be reactive to such peptides are eliminated by these encounters. The profound effect on the T-cell receptor repertoire of peptides bound to MHC class II molecules has been demonstrated in experiments in which H-2M, the mouse homolog of human HLA-DM, is disrupted. In mice lacking a functional H-2Mα molecule, the CLIP fragment of the invariant chain (see Fig. 4.16) is not released from the newly synthesized MHC class II molecules. These CLIP-associated MHC class II molecules are unable to bind the usual array of self peptides that are normally acquired in the peptide loading compartment of the cells and thus the only peptide expressed by MHC class II molecules on the surface of the thymic epithelium is the invariant CLIP peptide. In these mice, the total number of CD4 T cells is

Fig. 6.18 T cells specific for self antigens are deleted in the thymus. In mice transgenic for a T-cell receptor that recognizes a known peptide antigen with self MHC, all of the T cells have the same specificity; in the absence of the peptide, their thymocytes mature (bottom left panel) and migrate to the periphery. When the mice are injected with the specific peptide antigen, immature T cells in the same animal (bottom right panel) undergo apoptosis and die. Photographs courtesy of K Murphy.

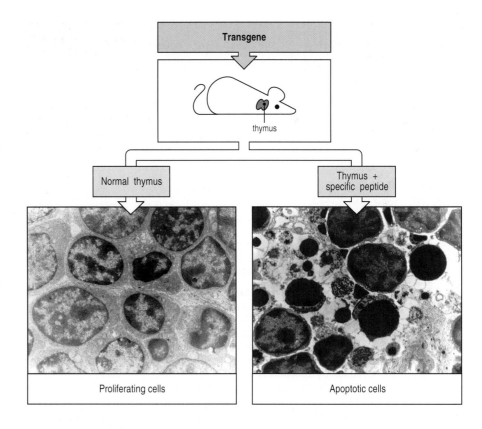

reduced two- to three-fold, and there is a striking increase in the number of cells reactive against stimulator cells from wild-type mice of the same MHC genotype (Fig. 6.19). The reduced number of CD4 T cells is probably due to the positive selection of a narrower range of T-cell receptors in the absence of the normal diverse array of peptide:MHC class II complexes in the thymuses of these mice. The high frequency of cells reactive to non-mutant cells of the same MHC genotype, which bind a wide variety of self peptides, probably reflects the combined effects of positive selection for self MHC recognition and the absence of effective negative selection for self MHC class II binding self peptides.

These experiments also illustrate the principle that self peptide:self MHC complexes encountered in the thymus purge the T-cell repertoire of cells bearing self-responsive receptors during development. However, not all proteins are expressed in the thymus, and those that appear in the periphery, or are expressed at different stages in development, such as after puberty, must encounter mature T cells that have the potential to respond to them. That they do not respond to such proteins in most cases suggests that some other mechanism or mechanisms must prevent T-cell responses to such antigens. The induction of self tolerance in the periphery will be discussed in the next chapter (see Section 7-10).

6-16   Negative selection is driven most efficiently by antigen-presenting cells.

Whereas thymic cortical epithelial cells mediate positive selection, negative selection in the thymus can be mediated by several different cell types. The most important of these are the bone marrow derived dendritic cells, and macrophages. These are the professional antigen-presenting cells that also activate mature T cells in peripheral lymphoid tissues. The self antigens presented by these cells are, therefore, the most important

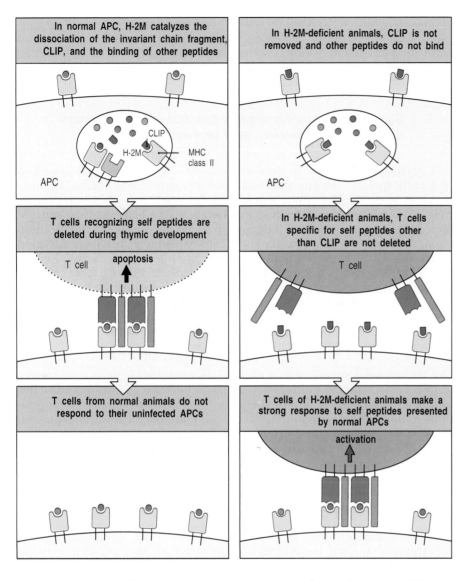

Fig. 6.19 The effect of peptides bound to MHC class II molecules in setting the T-cell receptor repertoire.
Mice with their H-2Mα gene disrupted by targeted mutagenesis express MHC class II molecules dominated by the CLIP peptide of the invariant chain (top panel). Their APCs have the same defect and thus present only the CLIP peptide to T cells maturing in the thymus. This means that T cells not specific for the CLIP peptide will not be deleted (middle right panel). Mature T cells from such mice respond strongly to MHC-identical APCs, which express the normal array of self peptides (bottom right panel), showing that, despite the dominance of a single MHC:peptide complex, CD4 T cells with a diverse repertoire of specificities have been selected. The total number of CD4 T cells is however reduced two- to three-fold.

source of potential autoimmune responses, and T cells responding to such self peptides must be eliminated in the thymus.

Bone marrow chimera experiments have shown clearly the role of thymic macrophages and dendritic cells in negative selection. Thus, if MHC^{axb} F1 bone marrow is grafted into the parental strains (MHC^a or MHC^b), T cells developing in the grafted animals will tolerate skin grafts from animals of both MHC^a and MHC^b strains (Fig. 6.20). This means they must have become tolerant not only to host MHC^a antigens but also to the donor-specific MHC^b antigens carried on cells derived from the grafted marrow. As the only cells that could present donor antigens are the bone marrow derived cells, these cell types are assumed to have a crucial role in negative selection.

It is interesting to note that in some mouse strain combinations, such skin grafts are rejected. This occurs because some proteins expressed in skin are not expressed by bone marrow derived cells and hence the mouse is not tolerant to peptides derived from them. We shall see in Chapter 12 that responses to such **minor histocompatibility antigens** are important in human tissue transplantation. Although bone marrow derived cells are the principal mediators of negative selection, both thymocytes themselves and thymic epithelial cells also have the ability to cause the deletion of self-reactive cells. Such reactions may normally be

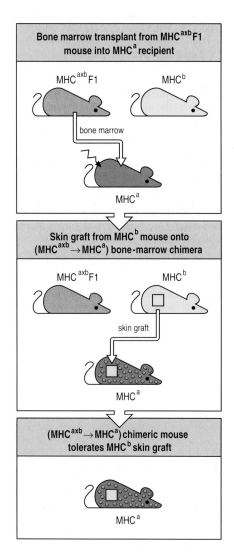

Fig. 6.20 Bone marrow derived cells mediate negative selection in the thymus. When MHC^{axb}F1 bone marrow is injected into an irradiated strain A mouse, the T cells mature on thymic epithelium expressing only type a MHC molecules (MHC^a). Nonetheless, the chimeric mice are tolerant to skin grafts expressing MHC^b molecules. This implies that the T cells whose receptors recognize self antigens presented by MHC^b have been eliminated in the thymus. Since the transplanted MHC^{axb}F1 bone marrow cells are the only source of MHC^b molecules in the thymus, bone marrow derived cells must be able to induce negative selection.

The boxes in the figure read:

Bone marrow transplant from MHC^{axb}F1 mouse into MHC^a recipient

MHC^{axb}F1   MHC^b

bone marrow

MHC^a

Skin graft from MHC^b mouse onto (MHC^{axb}→MHC^a) bone-marrow chimera

MHC^{axb}F1   MHC^b

skin graft

MHC^a

(MHC^{axb}→MHC^a) chimeric mouse tolerates MHC^b skin graft

MHC^a

of little significance. In patients undergoing bone marrow transplantation from an unrelated donor, however, where all the thymic macrophages and dendritic cells are of donor type, negative selection mediated by thymic epithelial cells may assume a special importance in maintaining tolerance to the recipient's own self tissue antigens.

6-17   Superantigens mediate negative selection of T-cell receptors derived from particular Vβ gene segments.

It is virtually impossible to demonstrate directly the negative selection of T cells specific for any particular self antigen in the normal thymus because such T cells will be too few to detect. There is, however, one case in which negative selection can be seen on a large scale in normal mice and the point at which it occurs in T-cell development can be identified. In the most striking examples, T cells expressing receptors encoded by particular Vβ gene segments are virtually eliminated in the affected mouse strains. This occurs as the consequence of the interaction of immature thymocytes with endogenous superantigens present in those strains. We learned in Chapter 4 that superantigens are viral or bacterial proteins that bind tightly to both MHC class II molecules and particular Vβ domains, irrespective of the antigen specificity of the receptor and the peptide bound by the MHC molecule (see Fig. 4.32).

The endogenous superantigens of mice are encoded by mouse mammary tumor virus (MMTV) genomes that have become integrated into the mouse chromosomes, where they are inherited by successive generations of mice along with mouse genes. Like the bacterial superantigens, these viral antigens induce strong T-cell responses; indeed, they were originally designated **minor lymphocyte stimulating (Mls)** antigens because, although they are not major histocompatibility complex proteins (hence minor), they stimulate exceptionally strong primary T-cell responses when T cells from a strain lacking the superantigen gene are stimulated by B cells from MHC-identical mice that express it.

T-cell receptors containing Vβ regions to which the Mls proteins bind are signaled during intrathymic maturation in Mls$^+$ strains, causing apoptosis and thus elimination of such T cells. For example, one variant of the Mls antigen (Mls-1^a) deletes all thymocytes expressing the Vβ6 variable region (and also those expressing Vβ8.1 and Vβ9), whereas such cells are not deleted in mice that lack Mls-1^a. Thus, the expression of endogenous superantigens in mice has a profound impact on the repertoire of T-cell receptors. This sort of deletion has not yet been seen in any other species, including humans, despite the presence of retroviral sequences in the genomes of many mammals.

In mice that express the superantigen and are thus tolerant to it, cells expressing T-cell receptors responsive to superantigens are found among double-positive thymocytes, and are abundant in thymic cortex but absent from the thymic medulla and the periphery. This suggests that superantigens may delete relatively mature cells as they migrate out of the cortex into the medulla, where a particularly dense network of dendritic cells marks the corticomedullary junction (Fig. 6.21).

Although clonal deletion by superantigens is a powerful tool for examining negative selection in normal mice, it must be remembered that superantigen-driven clonal deletion may not be representative of clonal deletion by self peptide:self MHC complexes. What is clear is that clonal deletion by either superantigens or self peptide:self MHC complexes generates a repertoire of T cells that does not respond to the self-antigens expressed by its own professional antigen-presenting cells.

Fig. 6.21 Clonal deletion by Mls-1^a occurs late in the development of thymocytes. T cells with Mls-1^a responsive receptors encoded by V$_\beta$6 are seen in both the cortex and medulla of Mls-1^b mice (top panel, cells stained with anti-V$_\beta$6 antibody). Note that the mature cells in the medulla express higher levels of the receptor and thus stain more darkly than the immature cells in the cortex. In Mls-1^a mice, the mature cells are not found; instead only the immature, cortical cells express the V$_\beta$6 receptor (lower panel). Photographs courtesy of H Hengartner.

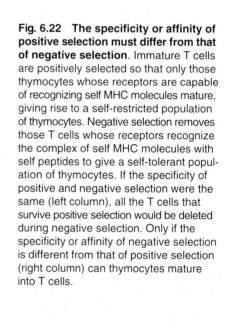

6-18 The signals for negative and positive selection must differ.

In the preceding sections we have described some of the experiments that have contributed to the large body of evidence that T cells are selected both for self MHC restriction and for self tolerance by MHC molecules expressed on cells in the thymus. We now turn to the central question posed by positive and negative selection: how can interactions with the same thymic MHC:peptide complexes lead both to further maturation during positive selection, and to cell death during negative selection?

There are two issues to be resolved. First, the interactions of the T-cell receptor with self peptide:MHC complexes that lead to positive selection must embrace a wider range of receptor specificities than those that lead to negative selection. Were this not so, all the cells that are positively selected in the thymic cortex would subsequently be eliminated by negative selection and no T cells would ever leave the thymus (Fig. 6.22). Second, the consequences of the interaction must differ,

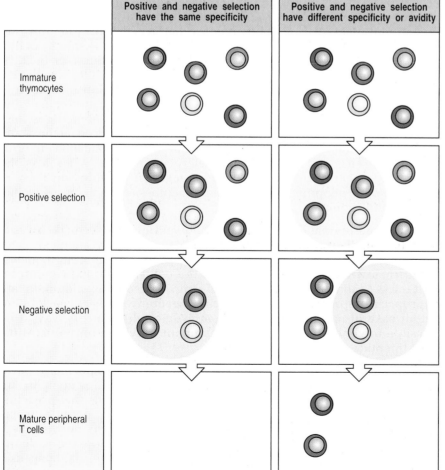

Fig. 6.22 The specificity or affinity of positive selection must differ from that of negative selection. Immature T cells are positively selected so that only those thymocytes whose receptors are capable of recognizing self MHC molecules mature, giving rise to a self-restricted population of thymocytes. Negative selection removes those T cells whose receptors recognize the complex of self MHC molecules with self peptides to give a self-tolerant population of thymocytes. If the specificity of positive and negative selection were the same (left column), all the T cells that survive positive selection would be deleted during negative selection. Only if the specificity or affinity of negative selection is different from that of positive selection (right column) can thymocytes mature into T cells.

so that the cells which recognize self MHC on cortical epithelial cells mature, whereas those whose receptors might confer autoreactivity are negatively selected and die.

Two main hypotheses have been proposed to account for these differences between positive and negative selection. The first is the **avidity hypothesis**, which states that the outcome of MHC:peptide binding by T-cell receptors of thymocytes depends upon the strength of the signal delivered by the receptor on binding, and that this will, in turn, depend upon both the affinity of the T-cell receptor for the MHC:peptide complex and the density of the complex on the antigen-presenting cell (usually a thymic cortical epithelial cell). Thymocytes that are signaled weakly are rescued from programmed cell death and therefore positively selected, whereas thymocytes that are signaled strongly are driven to programmed cell death and therefore negatively selected.

Alternatively, self peptides that deliver incomplete activating signals could account for positive selection: we shall call this the **differential signaling hypothesis**. Under this hypothesis, it is the nature of the signal delivered by the receptor, rather than the number of receptors engaged, that distinguishes positive from negative selection. Thus, the avidity hypothesis would predict that the same MHC:peptide complex could drive positive or negative selection of the same T-cell receptor depending on its density on the cell surface, whereas the differential signaling hypothesis would predict that this could not occur, because it proposes that the interactions leading to positive and negative selection are qualitatively different.

A new approach to testing these hypotheses has opened up with the recent description of antagonist peptides. Antagonist peptides, which we discussed in Chapter 4 (see Section 4-30), are variants of the peptide component of an MHC:peptide complex that, when substituted for the original peptide, bind the T-cell receptor and block the response of the T cell to the original MHC:peptide complex. Some peptide variants that act as antagonists may deliver a partial signal to the T cell that produces a subset of the full response (for example, proliferation or cytokine secretion but not both). Since positive selection is thought to entail the delivery of a weak signal to developing thymocytes, it seemed possible that antagonist peptides that deliver partial signals might reflect the same mechanism that operates in positive selection. Using thymic lobe cultures from mice transgenic for a known T-cell receptor, it has been possible to test the effect of both agonist and antagonist peptides on thymic selection of developing T cells bearing receptors recognizing a specific MHC:peptide complex.

The cultured thymic lobes used for the experiments were taken from so-called knock-out mice (see Section 2-37), genetically engineered to lack either β_2-microglobulin or the TAP transporter, and therefore unable to express MHC class I molecules on the cell surface. Expression of MHC class I can be restored to such thymic tissue by the addition of an appropriate peptide alone, or of peptide together with β_2-microglobulin in the case of mice deficient in β_2-microglobulin. In this way, it is possible to generate a thymic environment in which only one MHC class I:peptide complex is displayed.

Using this system, developing thymocytes of known specificity have been tested for their response to four types of MHC:peptide complex. In each case the MHC molecule was the self MHC molecule that presents peptide to the T-cell receptor being tested. If the added peptides were unrelated to the peptide recognized by the cells, the thymocytes died because they failed positive selection. If the added peptides were identical to the peptide recognized by the cells, the thymocytes died because they were negatively selected. If, however, they were antagonist or partial

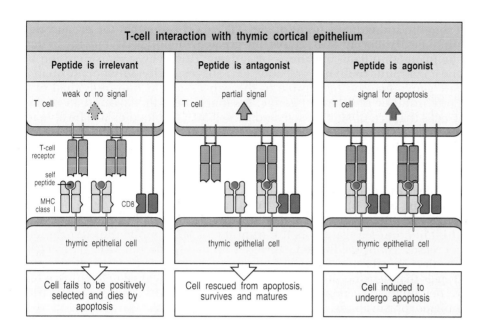

T-cell interaction with thymic cortical epithelium

Peptide is irrelevant	Peptide is antagonist	Peptide is agonist
weak or no signal	partial signal	signal for apoptosis
thymic epithelial cell	thymic epithelial cell	thymic epithelial cell
Cell fails to be positively selected and dies by apoptosis	Cell rescued from apoptosis, survives and matures	Cell induced to undergo apoptosis

Fig. 6.23 Effects of peptides acting as agonists, antagonists or neither on thymic selection. Thymocytes encounter self-MHC: self peptide complexes that have different effects depending upon the specificity of the T-cell receptor. For some receptors, no self peptide bound to self-MHC molecules will signal at all (left panel), and cells with these receptors undergo programmed cell death by apoptosis (death by neglect). For other receptors, a self peptide bound by self-MHC acts as an agonist, triggering apoptosis (right panel) (death as a result of activation). Some cells, however, bear receptors that are partially signaled by self peptides bound to self-MHC molecules. These peptides are equivalent to antagonist peptides and, by positive selection, rescue the cells from programmed cell death.

agonist variants of the peptide for which the cells were specific, the thymocytes were positively selected and survived (Fig. 6.23).

In some experiments, attempts have been made directly to test the avidity hypothesis by varying the dose of agonist or partial agonist peptides and showing that, at high doses of peptide, the cells died, whereas at lower doses they could survive. However, it is not clear whether or not the surviving cells in these experiments are functional: in some experiments aimed at addressing this question it has been shown that although the cells may appear to mature, they express a low level of CD8 and cannot respond to complexes containing the peptide with which they were cultured.

Antagonist or partial agonist peptides, as we saw in Chapter 4, seem to be unable to deliver a full activating signal to T cells. These experiments therefore imply that in a normal animal, thymocytes may be positively selected by an MHC:peptide complex that delivers only a partial or weak activating signal but negatively selected by one that delivers a full or strong activating signal. Whether the strength of the signal is determined by the avidity of binding, as predicted by the avidity hypothesis, or by some special characteristic of the peptide, as predicted by the differential signaling hypothesis, remains to be determined.

6-19 The requirements of T-cell activation and of thymic selection may explain why the MHC is highly polymorphic and not highly polygenic.

As we saw in Chapter 4, the MHC genes are highly polymorphic, with loci having over a hundred different allelic variants within the human population. There are several different genes for each class of MHC molecule (each of which is highly polymorphic), and so the MHC is also somewhat polygenic. All these allelic and non-allelic MHC variants preferentially bind different antigenic peptides. The polymorphism and polygeny of the MHC is believed to reflect both the selective advantage to the species of individuals able to bind different sets of peptides, and the selective advantage to each individual of expressing several variants able to bind peptides from a broad range of pathogens.

From the individual's point of view, it would seem that the greater the number of different MHC genes, the greater the polygeny, and the better the protection from infectious organisms. However, a consideration of the constraints of thymic selection also suggests why polymorphism in a few genes may be preferable to the expression in one individual of a large number of different genes. It seems likely that around 5% of the T cells that are positively selected by self MHC molecules will be able to recognize self peptides presented by these self MHC molecule and must therefore be deleted in the thymus to avoid reactivity to self. This estimate is based on the frequency of T cells that respond to a given non-self MHC molecule (see Section 4-19). Thus, each new MHC molecule expressed will cost the animal 5% of its T-cell receptor repertoire. The counterbalancing effect of gaining new MHC molecules that can drive positive selection offers a net advantage up to a point but this diminishes and then becomes negative as the number of MHC molecules expressed increases. A normal human expresses up to 15 different MHC molecules, and thus may delete a substantial portion (up to 75%) of the positively selected T cells that develop. It seems unlikely that the individual will improve his or her ability to respond to pathogens by adding MHC genes. Instead, MHC polymorphism appears to be the dominant effect.

6-20 | **A range of tumors of immune system cells throws light on different stages of T-cell development.**

We saw in Chapter 5 that tumors of lymphoid cells corresponding in phenotype to intermediate stages in the development of the B cell can provide an invaluable tool in the analysis of B-cell differentiation. Tumors of T cells and other cells involved in T-cell development have been identified but, unlike the malignancies of B cells, few that correspond to intermediate stages in T-cell development have been identified in humans. Instead, the tumors resemble either mature T cells or, in the case of common **acute lymphoblastic leukemia**, the earliest type of lymphoid progenitor (Fig. 6.24). One possible reason for the rarity of tumors corresponding to intermediate stages is that immature T cells are programmed to die unless rescued within a very narrow time window by positive selection (see Section 6-11). It may therefore be that thymocytes simply do not linger long enough at the intermediate stages of their development to provide an opportunity for malignant transformation. Thus, only cells that are already transformed at earlier stages, or that do not become transformed until the T cell has matured, are ever seen as tumors.

An understanding of the normal development of the immature T cell may help in understanding the pathology of the tumors that arise from such cells. For example, **cutaneous T-cell lymphomas**, which home to the skin and proliferate slowly, are clonal outgrowths of a CD4 T cell that, when activated, homes to the skin. The most complex lymphoid tumor is known as **Hodgkin's disease**, and appears in several forms. The malignantly transformed cell seems to be an antigen-presenting cell, and in some patients the disease is dominated by T cells that are stimulated by the tumor cells. This form of the disease is called Hodgkin's lymphoma. Other patients have no lymphocytic abnormalities and show a proliferation of a reticular cell, a condition known as nodular sclerosis. The differences between these two manifestations of Hodgkin's disease may reflect a real heterogeneity in the transformed cell or, more probably, differences in the T-cell responses of individual patients to the transformed cells. The prognosis for Hodgkin's lymphoma is far better than that for nodular sclerosis, suggesting that the responding cells may be controlling tumor growth. Control of tumors by the immune response will be considered in Chapter 13.

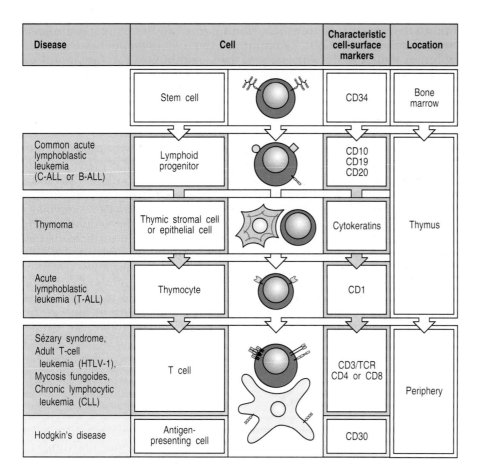

Disease	Cell		Characteristic cell-surface markers	Location
	Stem cell		CD34	Bone marrow
Common acute lymphoblastic leukemia (C-ALL or B-ALL)	Lymphoid progenitor		CD10 CD19 CD20	
Thymoma	Thymic stromal cell or epithelial cell		Cytokeratins	Thymus
Acute lymphoblastic leukemia (T-ALL)	Thymocyte		CD1	
Sézary syndrome, Adult T-cell leukemia (HTLV-1), Mycosis fungoides, Chronic lymphocytic leukemia (CLL)	T cell		CD3/TCR CD4 or CD8	Periphery
Hodgkin's disease	Antigen-presenting cell		CD30	

Fig. 6.24 T-cell tumors represent monoclonal outgrowths of normal cell populations. Each distinct T-cell tumor has a normal equivalent, as also seen with B-cell tumors, and retains many of the properties of the cell from which it develops. Some of these tumors represent massive outgrowth of a rare cell type with, for example, common acute lymphoblastic leukemia being derived from the lymphoid progenitor cell. Thus, T-cell tumors provide valuable information about the phenotype, homing properties and receptor gene rearrangements of normal cell types. Two T-cell related tumors are also included. Thymomas derive from thymic stromal or epithelial cells, while the malignantly transformed cell in Hodgkin's disease is thought to be an antigen-presenting cell. Some characteristic cell-surface markers for each stage are also shown. For example, CD10 (common acute lymphoblastic leukemia antigen or CALLA) is a widely-used marker for acute lymphoblastic leukemia. Note that T-cell chronic lymphocytic leukemia (CLL) cells express CD8, while the other T-cell tumors mentioned express CD4.

As with B-cell tumors, T-cell lymphomas can be shown to be monoclonal outgrowths of a single transformed cell by examination of the rearrangements of their receptor genes (Fig. 6.25). When tissues or cells from patients are examined, the proportion of cells showing the same rearrangements is a measure of the proportion of transformed cells in the sample. The sensitivity of this approach can be increased by using the polymerase chain reaction (see Section 2-27) to identify the tumor-specific rearrangement, allowing the identification of very small numbers of tumor cells remaining in a tissue. This can be of particular importance in cases where a patient's own bone marrow has been taken for re-injection after radiotherapy. If the marrow contains any transformed cells, then returning

Fig. 6.25 The unique rearrangement events in each T cell can be used to identify tumors of T cells. Tumors are the outgrowth of a single transformed cell. Thus, each cell in a tumor will have an identical pattern of rearranged T-cell receptor genes. These panels show the migration in gel electrophoresis of DNA fragments containing the T-cell receptor β-chain constant regions; the DNA is either obtained from the placenta (lane P), a tissue in which the T-cell receptor genes are not rearranged, or from peripheral blood lymphocytes from two patients suffering from T-cell tumors (lanes T_1 and T_2). Bands corresponding to the unrearranged $C_\beta 1$ and $C_\beta 2$ genes can be seen in all lanes. Additional bands corresponding to specific rearrangements (arrowed) can be seen in each of the tumor samples, indicating that a large proportion of the cells in the sample carry an identical rearrangement. Note that these are the only discrete additional bands that can be seen in these samples; no bands deriving from rearranged genes in the normal lymphocytes also present in the patients' samples can be seen, as no one rearranged band is present at sufficient concentration to be detected in this assay. Photograph courtesy of T Diss.

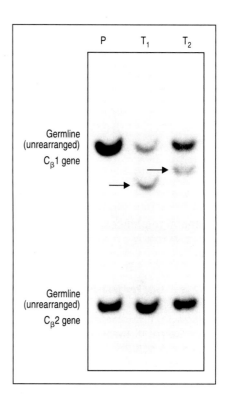

P T_1 T_2

Germline (unrearranged) $C_\beta 1$ gene

Germline (unrearranged) $C_\beta 2$ gene

the marrow would re-transplant the tumor into the patient and defeat the object of the therapy. Techniques exist to deplete the bone marrow of tumor cells and the efficiency of these techniques can be monitored by determining the persistence of the tumor-specific gene rearrangement.

Summary.

T-cell development involves two types of selection: positive selection for recognition of self MHC:self peptide complexes that provide a still ill-defined positive survival signal; and negative selection for cells bearing receptors for recognition of self peptide:self MHC complexes that would trigger the T cell in the periphery. The first process is normally mediated exclusively by thymic epithelial cells and the second largely by dendritic cells and macrophages. Positive selection ensures that all mature T cells are able to respond to foreign peptides presented by self MHC molecules on antigen-presenting cells, and negative selection eliminates self-reactive cells. The paradox that recognition of the same set of ligands by the same basic receptor can lead to two conflicting effects, namely positive and negative selection, is one of the central mysteries of immunology. Its solution will rest in understanding the ligands, the receptors, the signal transduction mechanisms, and the physiology of each step of the process.

Summary to Chapter 6.

T-cell development occurs in the special inductive microenvironment of the thymic cortex. In this location, T-cell receptor genes rearrange to generate the two lineages of T cells, the $\gamma{:}\delta$ T cells, whose function remains mysterious, and the $\alpha{:}\beta$ T cells that are the primary mediators of the adaptive immune response. The specialized environment of the thymus selects for the maturation of those $\alpha{:}\beta$ T cells having useful receptors, by contact of the receptor and its co-receptor with self MHC molecules on thymic cortical epithelial cells. Also within the thymus, professional antigen-presenting cells of bone marrow origin delete all T cells whose receptors recognize self antigens normally expressed by these cells, thus assuring self tolerance. In this way, a useful and non-damaging repertoire of T-cell receptors is generated.

General references.

Moller, G (ed).: **Positive T-cell selection in the thymus.** *Immunol. Rev.* 1993, **135**:5-242.

Nossal, G.J.V.: **Negative Selection of Lymphocytes.** *Cell 1994*, **76**:229-239.

von Boehmer, H.: **The developmental biology of T lymphocytes.** *Ann. Rev. Immunol.* 1993, **6**:309-326.

von Boehmer, H.: **Positive Selection of Lymphocytes.** *Cell* 1994, **76**:219-228.

Section references.

6-1   T cells develop in the thymus.

Cordier, A.C., and Haumont, S.M.: **Development of thymus, parathyroids, and ultimobranchial bodies in NMRI and nude mice.** *Am. J. Ana.* 1980, **157**:227.

Nehls, M., Kyewski, B., Messerle, M., Waldschütz, R., Schüddekopf, K., Smith, A.J.H., Boehm, T.: **Two Genetically Separable Steps in the Differentiation of Thymic Epithelium.** *Science* 1996, **272**:886-889.

van Ewijk, W.: **T-cell differentiation is influenced by thymic microenvironments.** *Ann. Rev. Immunol.* 1991, **9**:591-615.

6-2 The thymus is required for T-cell maturation.

Anderson, G., Moore, N.C., Owen, J.J.T., Jenkinson, E.J.: **Cellular Interactions in Thymocyte Development.** *Ann. Rev. Immunol.* 1996, **14**:73-99.

Zúñiga-Pflücker, J.C., Lenardo, M.J.: **Regulation of thymocyte development from immature progenitors.** *Curr. Opin. Immunol.* 1996, **8**:215-224.

6-3 Developing T cells proliferate in the thymus but most die there.

Shortman, K., Egerton, M., Spangrude, G.J., and Scollay, R.: **The generation and fate of thymocytes.** *Semin. Immunol.* 1990, **2**:3-12.

Strasser, A.: **Life and death during lymphocyte development and function: evidence for two distinct killing mechanisms.** *Curr. Opin. Immunol.* 1995, **7**:228-234.

6-4 Successive stages in the development of thymocytes are marked by changes in cell-surface molecules.

Petrie, H.T., Hugo, P., Scollay, R., and Shortman, K.: **Lineage relationships and developmental kinetics of immature thymocytes: CD3, CD4, and CD8 acquisition** *in vivo* **and** *in vitro*. *J. Exp. Med.* 1990, **172**:1583-1588.

Shortman, K., Wu, L.: **Early T Lymphocyte Progenitors.**: *Ann. Rev. Immunol.* 1996, **14**:29-47.

6-5 Thymocyes at different developmental stages are found in distinct parts of the thymus.

Picker, L.J., and Siegelman, M.H.: **Lymphoid Tissues and Organs.** In: *Fundamental Immunology,* 1993, 3rd edn. Raven Press Ltd., New York, (Paul, W.E., Ed.), pp 152-161.

6-6 T cells with α:β or γ:δ receptors arise from a common progenitor.

Lauzurica, P., and Krangel, M.S.: **Temporal and lineage-specific control of T- cell receptor** α/δ **gene rearrangement by T-cell receptor** α **and** δ **enhancers.** *J. Exp. Med.* 1994, **179**:193-1921.

Livak, F., Petrie, H.T., Crispe, I.N., and Schatz, D.G.: **In-frame TCR** δ **gene rearrangements play a critical role in the** αβ/γδ **T cell lineage decision.** *Immunity* 1995, **2**:617-627.

6-7 Cells expressing particular γ:β genes arise first in embryonic development.

Havran, W.L., Boismenu, R.: **Activation and function of** γδ **T cells**. *Curr. Opin. Immunol.* 1994, **6**:442-446.

Itohara, S., Nakanishi, N., Kanagawa, O., Kubo, R., and Tonegawa, S.: **Monoclonal antibodies specific to native murine T cell receptor** γδ **analysis of** γδ **T cells in thymic ontogeny and peripheral lymphoid organs**. *Proc. Natl. Acad. Sci. 1989*, **86**:5094-5098.

6-8 Productive β-chain gene rearrangement triggers rapid proliferation and the cessation of β-chain gene rearrangement.

Boismenu, R., Rhein, M., Fischer, W.H., Havran, W.L.: **A role for CD81 in Early T Cell Development**. *Science* 1996, **271**:198-200.

Borst, J., Jacobs, H., Brouns, G.: **Composition and function of T-cell receptor and B-cell receptor complexes on precursor lymphocytes.** *Curr. Opin. Immunol.* 1996, **8**:181-190.

Dudley, E.C., Petrie, H.T., Shah, L.M., Owen, M.J., and Hayday, A.C.: **T-cell receptor** β **chain gene rearrangement and selection during thymocyte development in adult mice.** *Immunity* 1994, **1**:83-93.

Philpott, K.I., Viney, J.L., Kay, G., Rastan, S., Gardiner, E.M., Chae, S., Hayday, A.C., and Owen, M.J.: **Lymphoid development in mice congenitally lacking T cell receptor** α β**-expressing cells.** *Science* 1992, **256**:1448-1453.

Saint-Ruf, C., Ungewiss, K., Groetrrup, M., Bruno, L., Fehling, H.J., and von Boehmer, H.: **Analysis and expression of a cloned pre-T-cell receptor gene.** *Science* 1994, **266**:1208.

6-9 T-cell recepor α-chain genes can undergo several successive rearrangements.

Hardardottir, F., Baron, J.L., and Janeway, C.A. Jr.: **T cells with two functional antigen-specific receptors.** *Proc. Natl. Acad. Sci.* 1995, **92**:354-358.

Padovan, E., Casorati, G., Dellabona, P., Meyer, S., Brockhaus, M., and Lanzavecchia, A.: **Expression of two T-cell receptor** α **chains: Dual receptor T cells.** *Science* 1993 **262**:422-424.

Petrie, H.T., Livak, F., Schatz, D.G., Strasser, A., Crispe, I.N., and Shortman, K.: **Multiple rearrangements in T-cell receptor** α**-chain genes maximize the production of useful thymocytes.** *J. Exp. Med.* 1993, **178**:615-622.

6-10 Only T cells specific for peptides bound to self MHC molecules mature in the thymus.

Fink, P.J., and Bevan, M.J.: **H-2 antigens of the thymus determine lymphocyte specificity.** *J. Exp. Med.* 1978, **148**:766-775.

Zinkernagel, R.M., Callahan, G.N., Klein, J., and Dennert, G.: **Cytotoxic T cells learn specificity for self H-2 during differentiation in the thymus.** *Nature* 1978, **271**:251-253.

6-11 Cells that fail positive selection die in the thymus.

Huessman, M., Scott, B., Kisielow, P., and von Boehmer, H.: **Kinetics and efficacy of positive selection in the thymus of normal and T-cell receptor transgenic mice.** *Cell* 1991, **66**:533-562.

Surh, C.D. and Sprent, J.: **T-cell apoptosis detected** *in situ* **during positive and negative selection in the thymus.** *Nature* 1994, **372**:100-103.

6-12 Positive selection also regulates α-chain gene rearrangement.

Borgulya, P., Kishi, H., Uematsu, Y., and von Boehmer, H.: **Exclusion and inclusion of** α **and** β **T-cell receptor alleles.** *Cell* 1992, **65**:529-537.

Malissen, M., Trucy, J., Jouvin-Marche, E., Cazenave, P.A., Scollay, R., and Malissen, B.: **Regulation of TCR** α **and** β **chain gene allelic exclusion during T-cell development.** *Immunol. Today* 1992, **13**:315-322.

Petrie, H.T., Livak, F., Burtrum. D., and Mazel, S.: **T cell receptor gene recombination patterns and mechanisms—cell death, rescue and T cell production.** *J. Exp. Med.* 1995, **182**:121-127.

6-13 The expression of CD4 and CD8 on mature T cells and the associated T-cell functions are determined by positive selection.

Kaye, J., Hsu, M.L., Sauvon, M.E., Jameson, S.C., Gascoigne, N.R.J., and Hedrick, S.M.: **Selective development of CD4[+] T cells in transgenic mice expressing a class II MHC-restricted antigen receptor.** *Nature* 1989, **341**:746-748.

Lundberg, K., Heath, W., Kontgen, F., Carbone, F.R., and Shortman, K.: **Intermediate steps in positive selection: Differentiation of CD4⁺8ⁱⁿᵗTCRⁱⁿᵗ thymocytes into CD4⁻8⁻TCRʰⁱ thymocytes.** *J. Exp. Med.* 1995, **181**:1643-1651.

von Boehmer, H., Kisielow, P., Lishi, H., Scott, B., Borgulya, P., and Teh, H.S.: **The expression of CD4 and CD8 accessory molecules on mature T cells is not random but correlates with the specificity of the αβ receptor for antigen.** *Immunol. Rev.* 1989, **109**:143-151.

6-14   Thymic cortical epithelial cells mediate positive selection.

Cosgrove, D., Chan, S.H., Waltzinger, C., Benoist, C., and Mathis, D.: **The thymic compartment responsible for positive selection of CD4⁺ T cells.** *Intl. Immunol.* 1992, **4**:707-710.

Fowlkes, B.J., Schweighoffer, E.: **Positive selection of T cells.** *Curr. Opin. Immunol.* 1995, **7**:188-195.

6-15   T cells specific for ubiquitous self antigens are deleted in the thymus.

Kruisbeek, A.M., Amsen, D.: **Mechanisms underlying T-cell tolerance.** *Curr. Opin. Immunol.* 1996, **8**:233-244.

Zal, T., Volkmann, A., and Stockinger, B.: **Mechanisms of tolerance induction in major histocompatibility complex class II-restricted T cell specific for a blood-borne self antigen.** *J. Exp. Med.* 1994, **180**:2089-2099.

6-16   Negative selection is driven most efficiently by antigen-presenting cells.

Matzinger, P., and Guerder, S.:**Does T cell tolerance require a dedicated antigen-presenting cell?** *Nature* 1989. **338**:74-76.

Sprent, J., and Webb, S.R.: **Intrathymic and extrathymic clonal deletion of T cells.** *Curr. Opin. Immunol.* 1995, **7**:196-205.

6-17   Superantigens mediate negative selection of T-cell receptors derived from particular Vᵦ gene segments.

Kappler, J.W., Roehm, N., and Marrack, P.: **T-cell tolerance by clonal elimination in the thymus.** *Cell* 1987, **49**:273-280.

MacDonald, H.R., Schneider, R., Lees, R.K., Howe, R.C., Acha-Orbea, H., Festenstein, H., Zinkernagel, R.M., and Hengartner, H.: **T-cell receptor Vᵦ use predicts reactivity and tolerance to Mlsª-encoded antigens.** *Nature* 1988, **332**:40-45.

6-18   The signals for negative and positive selection must differ.

Ashton-Rickardt, P.G., Bandeira, A., Delaney, J.R., Van Kaer, L., Pircher, H.P., Zinkernagel, R.M., and Tonegawa, S.: **Evidence for a differential avidity model of T-cell selection in the thymus.** *Cell* 1994, **74**:577.

Hogquist, K.A., Jameson, S.C., Heath, W.R., Howard, J.L., Bevan, M.J., and Carbane, F.R.: **T-cell receptor antagonist peptides induce positive selection.** *Cell* 1994, **76**:17-27.

Jameson, S.C., Hogquist, K.A., and Bevan, M.J:**Specificity and flexibility in thymic selection.** *Ann. Rev. Immunol.* 1994, **369**:750-753.

6-19   The requirements of T-cell activation and of thymic selection may explain why the MHC is highly polymorphic and not highly polygenic.

Alberola-lla, J., Forbush, K.A., Seger, R., Krebs, E.G., Perlmutter, R.M.: **Selective requirement for MAP kinase activation in thymocyte differentiation.** *Nature* 1995, **373**:620-623

Demotz, S., Grey, H.M., and Sette, A.: **The minimal number of class II MHC-antigen complexes needed for T cell activation.** *Science* 1990, **249**:1028-1030.

Harding, C.V., and Unanue, E.R.: **Quantitation of antigen-presenting cell MHC class II/peptide complexes necessary for T cell stimulation.** *Nature* 1990, **346**:574-576.

Liao, X.C., and Littman, D.R.: **Altered T cell receptor signaling and disrupted T cell development in mice lacking Itk.** *Immunity* 1995, **3**:757-769.

Valitutti, S., Muller, S., Cella, M., Padovan, E., and Lanzavecchia, A.: **Serial triggering of many T-cell receptors by a few peptide-MHC complexes.** *Nature.* 1995, **375**:148-151.

Wang, C-R., Hashimoto, K., Kubo, S., Yokochi, T., Kubo, M., Suzuki, M., Suzuki, K., Tada, T., Nakayama, T.: **T cell receptor-mediated signaling events in CD4⁺CD8⁺ thymocytes undergoing thymic selection: requirement of calcineurin activated for thymic positive selection but not negative selection.** *J. Exp. Med.* 1995, **181**:927-941.

6-20   A range of tumors of immune system cells throws light on different stages of T-cell development.

Hwang, L-Y., Baer, R.J.: **The role of chromosome translocations in T cell acute leukemia.** *Curr. Opin. Immunol.* 1995, **7**:659-664.

Rabbitts, T.H.: **Chromosomal translocations in human cancer.** *Nature* 1994, **372**:143-149.

PART IV

THE ADAPTIVE IMMUNE RESPONSE

T-Cell Mediated Immunity

Once they have completed their development in the thymus, T cells enter the bloodstream, from which they migrate through the peripheral lymphoid organs, returning to the bloodstream to recirculate until they encounter antigen. To participate in an adaptive immune response, these **naive T cells** must be induced to proliferate and differentiate into cells capable of contributing to the removal of pathogens; we shall term these **armed effector T cells** because they can act immediately or very rapidly after encountering specific antigen on other cells. The cells on which armed effector T cells act will be referred to as **target cells**.

In this chapter, we shall see how naive T cells are activated to proliferate and differentiate into armed effector cells the first time they encounter their specific antigen on the surface of a **professional antigen-presenting cell** (APC). These specialized antigen-presenting cells are distinguished by surface molecules that synergize with specific antigen in the activation of naive T cells. Professional antigen-presenting cells are concentrated in the peripheral lymphoid organs, to which they migrate after trapping antigen in the periphery. They present peptide fragments of protein antigens to recirculating naive T cells. The most important professional antigen-presenting cells are the highly specialized **dendritic cells**, whose only known function is to present antigen, and **macrophages**, which are also important as phagocytic cells in providing a first line of defense against infection and as targets for activation by armed effector T cells. B cells can also serve as professional antigen-presenting cells in some circumstances.

Effector T cells, as we learned in Chapter 4, fall into three functional classes that detect peptide antigens derived from different types of pathogens. Peptides derived from pathogens that multiply within the cytoplasm of the cell are carried to the cell surface by MHC class I molecules and presented to CD8 T cells, which differentiate into **cytotoxic T cells** that kill infected target cells. Peptide antigens derived from pathogens multiplying in intracellular vesicles, and those derived from ingested extracellular bacteria and toxins, are carried to the cell surface by MHC class II molecules and presented to CD4 T cells that can differentiate into two types of effector T cell. Pathogens that accumulate in large numbers inside macrophage vesicles tend to stimulate differentiation of T_H1 cells, whereas extracellular antigens tend to stimulate the production of T_H2 cells. T_H1 cells activate the microbicidal properties of macrophages and induce B cells to make IgG antibodies that are very effective at opsonizing extracellular pathogens for uptake by phagocytic cells. T_H2 cells initiate the humoral immune response by activating naive antigen-specific B cells to produce IgM antibodies, and may subsequently stimulate the production of different isotypes, including IgA and IgE, as well as neutralizing and/or weakly opsonizing subtypes of IgG (Fig. 7.1).

Fig. 7.1   The role of effector T cells in cell-mediated and humoral immunity to representative pathogens.
Cell-mediated immunity involves the destruction of infected cells by cytotoxic T cells, or the destruction of intracellular pathogens by macrophages activated by T_H1 cells, and is directed principally at intracellular parasites. However, T_H1 cells can also contribute to humoral immunity by inducing the production of strongly opsonizing antibodies, while T_H2 cells activate naive B cells to secrete IgM and induce the production of other antibody isotypes including weakly opsonizing antibodies like IgG1 and IgG3 (mouse), and IgG2 and IgG4 (human), as well as IgA and IgE (mouse and human). All types of antibody contribute to humoral immunity, which is directed principally at extracellular pathogens. Note, however, that both cell-mediated and humoral immunity play a role in many infections, such as the response to *Pneumocystis carinii*, which requires antibody for ingestion by phagocytes and macrophage activation for effective destruction of the ingested pathogen.

	Cell-mediated immunity		Humoral immunity
Typical pathogens	Vaccinia virus Influenza virus Rabies virus *Listeria*	*Mycobacterium tuberculosis Mycobacterium leprae Leishmania donovani Pneumocystis carinii*	*Clostridium tetani Staphylococcus aureus Streptococcus pneumoniae* Polio virus *Pneumocystis carinii*
Location	Cytosol	Macrophage vesicles	Extracellular fluid
Effector T cell	Cytotoxic CD8 T cell	T_H1 cell	T_H1/T_H2 cell
Antigen recognition	Peptide:MHC class I on infected cell	Peptide:MHC class II on infected macrophage	Peptide:MHC class II on specific B cell
Effector action	Killing of infected cell	Activation of infected macrophages	Activation of specific B cell to make antibody

The first encounter of naive T cells with antigen on a professional antigen-presenting cell results in a **primary immune response**, and at the same time generates immunological memory, which provides protection from subsequent challenge by the same pathogen. The generation of memory T cells—long-lived cells that respond to antigen with an accelerated reponse—is much less well understood than the generation of effector T cells, and will be dealt with in Chapter 9. Memory T cells differ in several ways from naive T cells but like naive T cells they are quiescent, and require activation by professional antigen-presenting cells to regenerate effector T cells.

Armed effector T cells differ in many ways from their naive precursors, and these changes equip them to respond quickly and efficiently when they encounter antigen on their target cells. In the final sections of the chapter, we shall describe the specialized mechanisms of T-cell mediated cytotoxicity and of macrophage activation by armed effector T cells, the major components of **cell-mediated immunity**. We shall leave the activation of B cells by helper T cells until Chapter 8, where the humoral or antibody-mediated immune response is discussed.

The production of armed effector T cells.

Activation of naive T cells requires recognition of a foreign peptide fragment bound to a self MHC molecule, but this is not on its own sufficient for activation—it also requires the simultaneous delivery of a **co-stimulatory signal** by a specialized antigen-presenting cell. Only professional antigen-presenting cells are able to express both classes of MHC molecules as well as the co-stimulatory surface molecules that drive the clonal expansion of naive T cells and their differentiation into armed effector T cells. The activation of naive T cells on initial encounter with antigen on the surface of a professional antigen-presenting cell is often called **priming**, to distinguish it from the responses of armed effector T cells to antigen on their target cells, and the responses of primed memory T cells.

7-1 The initial interaction of naive T cells with antigen occurs in peripheral lymphoid organs.

Adaptive immune responses are not initiated at the site where a pathogen first establishes a focus of infection. They occur in the organized peripheral lymphoid tissues, such as the lymph nodes, to which the pathogen or its products are transported in the lymph, which is produced continuously by filtration of extracellular fluid from the blood. Pathogens infecting peripheral sites will be trapped in the lymph nodes directly downstream of the site of infection; those that enter the blood will be trapped in the spleen; and pathogens infecting mucosal surfaces will accumulate in Peyer's patches or tonsils (see Chapter 1). All these lymphoid organs contain antigen-presenting cells specialized for capturing antigen and activating T cells. Some of these cells have captured antigen at the site of infection and then migrated to the downstream lymph node. Naive T lymphocytes circulate continuously from the bloodstream to the lymphoid organs, and back to the blood, making contact with many antigen-presenting cells every day. This ensures that each naive T cell has a high probability of encountering antigens derived from pathogens at any site of infection.

Naive T cells leave the blood by crossing the walls of specialized venules known as **high endothelial venules** (**HEV**), which deliver them to the cortical region of a lymph node. The continual passage of naive T cells past antigen-presenting cells in the lymph node is crucial for adaptive immunity. As only one naive T cell in 10^4–10^6 is likely to be specific for a particular antigen, most of the passing T cells will not recognize the antigen. These T cells eventually reach the medulla of the lymph node and are carried by the efferent lymphatics back to the blood to continue recirculating through other lymphoid organs. Naive T cells that recognize their specific antigen on the surface of a professional antigen-presenting cell cease to migrate, and embark on the steps that will lead to the generation of armed effector cells (Fig. 7.2).

The three main types of specialized antigen-presenting cells present in the peripheral lymphoid organs are dendritic cells, macrophages, and B cells. Each of these cell types is specialized to process and present antigens from different sources to T cells. Dendritic cells appear to function exclusively as antigen-presenting cells, whereas macrophages and B cells are also the targets of subsequent actions of armed effector T cells. Only these three cell types express the specialized co-stimulatory molecules required to activate naive T cells; furthermore, macrophages and B cells express these molecules only when suitably activated by infection.

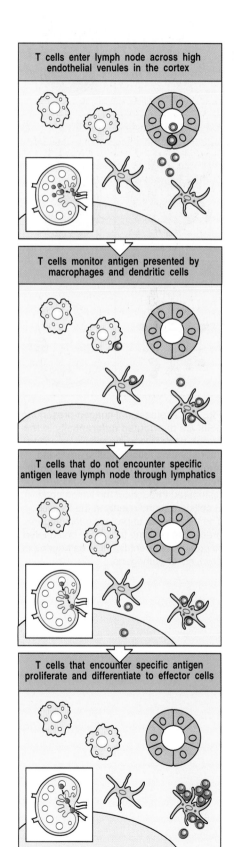

Fig. 7.2 Naive T cells encounter antigen during their recirculation through peripheral lymphoid organs. Naive T cells recirculate through peripheral lymphoid organs, such as the lymph node shown here, entering through specialized regions of vascular endothelium called high endothelial venules. On leaving the blood vessel, the T cells enter the cortex of the lymph node, where they encounter many antigen-presenting cells (mainly dendritic cells and macrophages). T cells that do not encounter their specific antigen (green) leave the lymph node through the lymphatics and eventually return to the circulation. T cells that encounter antigen (blue) on the antigen-presenting cells are activated to proliferate and to differentiate into effector cells. Once this process is completed, these armed effector T cells also leave the lymph node via the efferent lymphatics and enter the circulation.

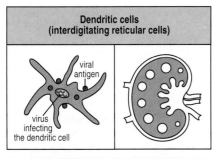

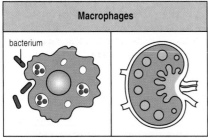

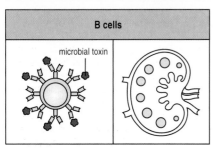

Fig. 7.3 Professional antigen-presenting cells are distributed differentially in the lymph node. Dendritic cells, also called interdigitating reticular cells, are found throughout the cortex of the lymph node in the T-cell areas. Macrophages are distributed throughout the lymph node. B cells are found mainly in the follicles. The three types of professional antigen-presenting cells are thought to be adapted to present different types of pathogens or products of pathogens.

The three types of antigen-presenting cell are distributed differently in the lymphoid organs (Fig. 7.3). Macrophages are found in all areas of the lymph node and actively ingest microbes and particulate antigens. As most pathogens are particulate, macrophages stimulate immune responses to many sources of infection. Dendritic cells, which in lymphoid tissues are also known as **interdigitating reticular cells**, are present only in the T-cell areas of the lymph node. These cells, which were mentioned in Chapter 6 because of their role in negative selection of thymocytes, are the most potent antigen-presenting cells for naive T cells, and are thought to be especially important in presenting viral antigens. Finally, the B cells in the lymphoid follicles are particularly efficient at taking up soluble antigens, such as bacterial toxins, by the specific binding of the antigens to the B-cell surface immunoglobulin molecules. Degraded fragments of these antigens can return to the B-cell surface complexed with MHC class II molecules, thus enabling B cells to play a part in the activation of naive CD4 T cells.

The generation of effector cells from a naive T cell takes several days. At the end of this period, the armed effector T cells leave the lymphoid organ and re-enter the bloodstream so that they can migrate to sites of infection.

7-2   **Lymphocyte migration, activation, and effector function depend on cell-adhesion molecules.**

The migration of naive T cells through the lymph nodes, and their initial interactions with antigen-presenting cells, involves antigen non-specific binding to other cells. Similar interactions eventually guide the effector T cells into the peripheral tissues, and play an important part in their interactions with target cells. Binding of T cells to other cells is controlled by an array of adhesion molecules on the surface of the T lymphocyte. These cell-surface proteins recognize a complementary array of adhesion molecules on the surfaces of the cells with which the T cell interacts. The main classes of adhesion molecules involved in lymphocyte interactions are the selectins, the integrins, the immunoglobulin superfamily, and some mucin-like molecules. Some of these molecules are concerned mainly with lymphocyte homing and migration, which we shall describe in more detail in Chapter 9, where we present an integrated view of the immune response; others have broader roles in the generation of immune responses and the interactions of armed effector T cells with their target cells, which will be discussed here.

The nomenclature of the adhesion molecules is confusing, because most were first defined either as cell-surface molecules recognized by monoclonal antibodies or in functional assays of cell–cell interactions, and were only subsequently characterized biochemically. For this reason, the names of many of the adhesion molecules bear no relationship to the structural families to which they belong. A brief explanation of the terminology can be found in the legend to Fig. 7.4, where the main classes of leukocyte adhesion molecules are summarized. We begin our discussion, however, with the **selectins**, which all belong to the same small protein family.

The selectins (CD62) are particularly important for leukocyte homing to specific tissues, and can be expressed either on leukocytes (**L-selectin, CD62L**) or on vascular endothelium (**P-selectin, CD62P,** and **E-selectin, CD62E,** which are discussed in Chapter 9). Selectins are cell-surface molecules with a common core structure, distinguished from each other by the presence of different lectin-like domains in their extracellular

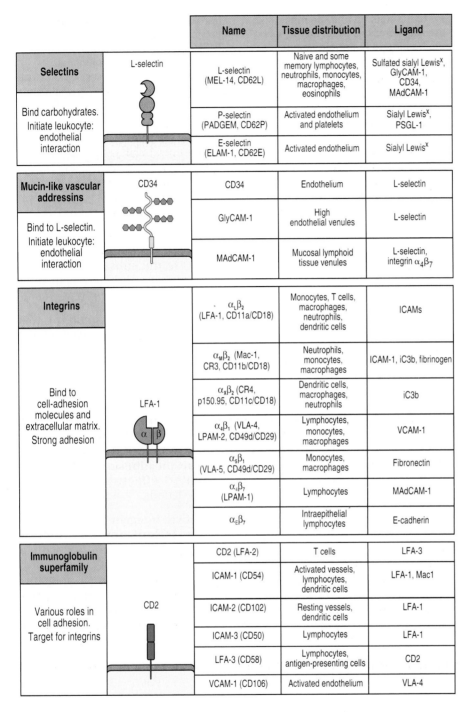

	Name	Tissue distribution	Ligand
Selectins Bind carbohydrates. Initiate leukocyte: endothelial interaction	L-selectin (MEL-14, CD62L)	Naive and some memory lymphocytes, neutrophils, monocytes, macrophages, eosinophils	Sulfated sialyl Lewis^x, GlyCAM-1, CD34, MAdCAM-1
	P-selectin (PADGEM, CD62P)	Activated endothelium and platelets	Sialyl Lewis^x, PSGL-1
	E-selectin (ELAM-1, CD62E)	Activated endothelium	Sialyl Lewis^x
Mucin-like vascular addressins Bind to L-selectin. Initiate leukocyte: endothelial interaction	CD34	Endothelium	L-selectin
	GlyCAM-1	High endothelial venules	L-selectin
	MAdCAM-1	Mucosal lymphoid tissue venules	L-selectin, integrin $\alpha_4\beta_7$
Integrins Bind to cell-adhesion molecules and extracellular matrix. Strong adhesion	$\alpha_L\beta_2$ (LFA-1, CD11a/CD18)	Monocytes, T cells, macrophages, neutrophils, dendritic cells	ICAMs
	$\alpha_M\beta_2$ (Mac-1, CR3, CD11b/CD18)	Neutrophils, monocytes, macrophages	ICAM-1, iC3b, fibrinogen
	$\alpha_X\beta_2$ (CR4, p150.95, CD11c/CD18)	Dendritic cells, macrophages, neutrophils	iC3b
	$\alpha_4\beta_1$ (VLA-4, LPAM-2, CD49d/CD29)	Lymphocytes, monocytes, macrophages	VCAM-1
	$\alpha_5\beta_1$ (VLA-5, CD49d/CD29)	Monocytes, macrophages	Fibronectin
	$\alpha_4\beta_7$ (LPAM-1)	Lymphocytes	MAdCAM-1
	$\alpha_E\beta_7$	Intraepithelial lymphocytes	E-cadherin
Immunoglobulin superfamily Various roles in cell adhesion. Target for integrins	CD2 (LFA-2)	T cells	LFA-3
	ICAM-1 (CD54)	Activated vessels, lymphocytes, dendritic cells	LFA-1, Mac1
	ICAM-2 (CD102)	Resting vessels, dendritic cells	LFA-1
	ICAM-3 (CD50)	Lymphocytes	LFA-1
	LFA-3 (CD58)	Lymphocytes, antigen-presenting cells	CD2
	VCAM-1 (CD106)	Activated endothelium	VLA-4

Fig. 7.4 Adhesion molecules in leukocyte interactions. Several structural families of adhesion molecules play a part in leukocyte migration, homing and cell–cell interactions: the selectins; mucin-like vascular addressins; the integrins; and proteins of the immunoglobulin superfamily. The figure shows schematic representations of an example from each family, a list of other family members that participate in leukocyte interactions, their cellular distribution, and their partners (ligands) in adhesive interactions. The family members shown here are limited to those we consider in this text but include some that will not be encountered until Chapter 9. The nomenclature of the different molecules in these families is confusing because it often reflects the way in which the molecules were first identified rather than their related structural characteristics. Thus while all the ICAMs are immunoglobulin-related, and all the VLA molecules are β_1 integrins, the CD nomenclature reflects the characterization of leukocyte cell-surface molecules by raising monoclonal antibodies against them (Appendix I contains details of all the CD molecules mentioned in this book). Thus CD molecules comprise a large and diverse collection of cell-surface molecules, which includes adhesion molecules in all the structural families. The LFA molecules were defined through experiments in which cytotoxic T-cell killing could be blocked by monoclonal antibodies against cell-surface molecules on the interacting cells, and there are LFA molecules in both the integrin and the immunoglobulin families. Alternative names for each of the adhesion molecules are given in parentheses. Sialyl Lewis^x, which is recognized by P- and E-selectin, is an oligosaccharide present on cell-surface glycoproteins of circulating leukocytes. Adhesion molecules expressed on monocytes are also expressed on their mature form, tissue macrophages.

portion (Fig. 7.5). Lectins bind to specific sugar groups, and each selectin binds to a cell-surface carbohydrate. L-selectin is expressed on naive T cells. It binds to the carbohydrate moiety, sulfated sialyl Lewis^x, of mucin-like molecules called **vascular addressins**, which are expressed on vascular endothelium. Two of these addressins, **CD34** and **GlyCAM-1**, are expressed as sulfated sialyl Lewis^x molecules on high endothelial venules in lymph nodes. A third, **MAdCAM-1**, is expressed on endothelium in mucosa, and guides lymphocyte entry into mucosal lymphoid tissue such as that of the gut (see Fig. 7.5).

The interaction between L-selectin and the vascular addressins is responsible for the specific homing of naive T cells to lymphoid organs but does not, on its own, enable the cell to cross the endothelial barrier

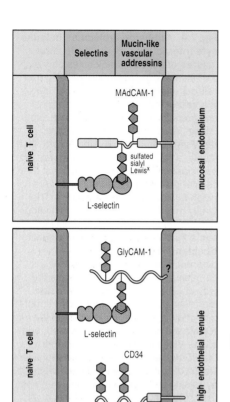

Fig. 7.5 L-selectin and the mucin-like vascular addressins direct naive lymphocyte homing to lymphoid tissues. L-selectin is expressed on naive T cells, which bind to sulfated sialyl Lewis^x moieties on the vascular addressins CD34 and GlyCAM-1 on high endothelial venules in order to enter lymph nodes. The relative importance of CD34 and GlyCAM-1 in this interaction is unclear. GlyCAM-1 is expressed exclusively on high endothelial venules but has no transmembrane region and it is unclear how it is attached to the membrane; CD34 has a transmembrane anchor and is expressed in its appropriately glycosylated form only on high endothelial venule cells, although it is found in other forms on other endothelial cells. The addressin MAdCAM-1 is expressed on mucosal endothelium and guides entry into mucosal lymphoid tissue. L-selectin recognizes the carbohydrate moieties on the vascular addressins.

into the lymphoid tissue; for this, molecules of two other families, the integrins and the immunoglobulin superfamily, are required. Proteins of these two families also play a critical part in the subsequent interactions of lymphocytes with antigen-presenting cells and later with their target cells.

The **integrins** comprise a large family of cell-surface proteins that mediate adhesion between cells, and between cells and the extracellular matrix, in immune and inflammatory responses. They are also important in many aspects of tissue organization and cell migration during development. An integrin molecule consists of a large α chain that pairs non-covalently with a smaller β chain. There are several subfamilies of integrins, broadly defined by their common β chains. We shall be concerned chiefly with the **leukocyte integrins**, which have a common β2 chain with distinct α chains (Fig. 7.6). All T cells express a leukocyte integrin known as **lymphocyte function-associated antigen-1 (LFA-1)**. This is thought to be the most important adhesion molecule for lymphocyte activation as antibodies to LFA-1 effectively inhibit the activation of both naive and armed effector T cells.

LFA-1 and two other members of the leukocyte integrin family are also expressed on neutrophils and macrophages. In **leukocyte adhesion deficiency**, an inherited immunodeficiency disease resulting from a defect in the synthesis of the common β2 chain, immunity to infection with extracellular bacteria is severely impaired because of defective neutrophil and macrophage function. Surprisingly, T-cell responses can be normal in such patients. This is probably because T cells also express other adhesion molecules, including CD2 and members of the β1 integrin family, which may be able to compensate for the absence of LFA-1. Expression of the β1 integrins increases significantly at a late stage in T-cell activation, and they are thus often called **VLA**s for

Fig. 7.6 Integrins are important in leukocyte adhesion. Integrins are heterodimeric proteins containing a β chain, which defines the class of integrin, and an α chain, which defines the different integrins within a class. The α chain is larger than the β chain and contains binding sites for divalent cations that may be important in signaling. Most integrins expressed on leukocytes have a common β chain, β2, but different α chains. LFA-1, and VLA-4 (which is a β1 integrin), are upregulated on armed effector T cells and are important in the migration and activation of these cells. Macrophages and neutrophils express all three members of the β2 integrin family. Like LFA-1, Mac-1 binds the immunoglobulin superfamily ICAM molecule, but in addition Mac-1 is a complement receptor whose function will be discussed in Chapter 8; other functions of p150.95, which also binds complement, are unknown.

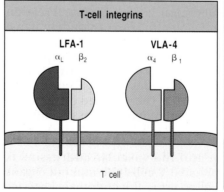

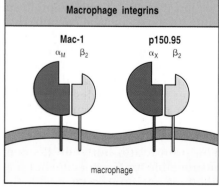

very late activation antigens; we shall see in Chapter 9 that they play an important part in directing armed effector T cells to their target tissues.

Many cell-surface adhesion molecules are members of the immunoglobulin superfamily, which also includes the antigen receptors of T and B cells, the co-receptors CD4, CD8, and CD19, and the invariant domains of MHC molecules. At least six adhesion molecules of the immunoglobulin superfamily are especially important in T-cell activation (Fig. 7.7). Three very similar **intercellular adhesion molecules (ICAMs)**—**ICAM-1**, **ICAM-2**, and **ICAM-3**—all bind to the T-cell integrin LFA-1. ICAM-1 and ICAM-2 are expressed on endothelium as well as on antigen-presenting cells; binding to these molecules enables lymphocytes to migrate through blood vessel walls. ICAM-3 is expressed only on leukocytes and is thought to play an important part in adhesion between T cells and antigen-presenting cells. The interaction of LFA-1 with ICAM-1 and ICAM-2 synergizes with a second adhesive interaction involving the immunoglobulin superfamily members **CD2** and **LFA-3**; CD2 is expressed on the T-cell surface, and LFA-3 is expressed on the antigen-presenting cell (see Fig. 7.7).

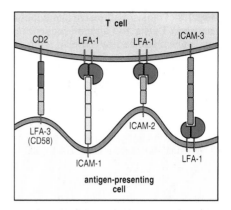

Fig. 7.7 Cell-surface molecules of the immunoglobulin superfamily are important in the interactions of lymphocytes with antigen-presenting cells. In the initial encounter of T cells with antigen-presenting cells, CD2 binding to LFA-3 on the antigen-presenting cell synergizes with LFA-1 binding to ICAM-1 and ICAM-2 on the antigen-presenting cell. ICAM-3 expressed on the T cell binds to LFA-1 on the antigen-presenting cell. Similar adhesive interactions occur between effector T cells and their targets (not shown).

7-3 **The initial interaction of T cells with antigen-presenting cells is also mediated by cell-adhesion molecules.**

As they migrate through the cortical region of the lymph node, naive T cells bind transiently to each antigen-presenting cell they encounter. Professional antigen-presenting cells, and dendritic cells in particular, bind naive T cells very efficiently through interactions between LFA-1, CD2, and ICAM-3 on the T cell, and ICAM-1, ICAM-2, LFA-1, and LFA-3 on the antigen-presenting cell. These molecules synergize in the binding of lymphocytes to antigen-presenting cells and the exact role of each has been difficult to distinguish. People lacking LFA-1 can have normal T-cell responses, and this also seems to be the case for genetically engineered mice lacking CD2. It would not be surprising if there was sufficient redundancy in the molecules mediating T-cell adhesive interactions to enable immune responses to occur in the absence of any one of them; such molecular redundancy has been observed in other complex biological processes.

The transient binding of naive T cells to professional antigen-presenting cells is crucial in providing time for T cells to sample large numbers of MHC molecules on the surface of each antigen-presenting cell for the presence of specific peptide. In those rare cases in which a naive T cell recognizes its specific peptide:MHC ligand, signaling through the T-cell receptor induces a conformational change in LFA-1, which greatly increases its affinity for ICAM-1 and ICAM-2. The mechanism of this conformational change in LFA-1 is not known. These changes stabilize the association between the antigen-specific T cell and the antigen-presenting cell (Fig. 7.8). The association can persist for several days during which the naive T cell proliferates and its progeny, which also adhere to the antigen-presenting cell, differentiate into armed effector T cells.

Most T-cell encounters with antigen-presenting cells, however, do not result in recognition of specific antigen. In these encounters, the T cells must be able to separate efficiently from the antigen-presenting cells so that they can continue to migrate through the lymph node, eventually leaving via the efferent lymphatic vessels to re-enter the blood and continue recirculating. Dissociation, like stable binding, may also involve signaling between the T cell and the antigen-presenting cells but little is known of its mechanism.

Fig. 7.8 Transient adhesive interactions between T cells and antigen-presenting cells are stabilized by specific antigen recognition. When a T cell binds to its specific ligand on an antigen-presenting cell (APC), intracellular signaling through the T-cell receptor (TCR) induces a conformational change in LFA-1 that causes it to bind with higher affinity to ICAMs on the antigen-presenting cell. The T cell shown here is a CD4 T cell.

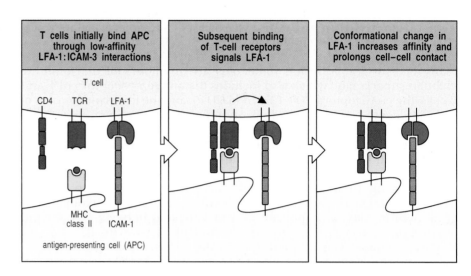

| T cells initially bind APC through low-affinity LFA-1:ICAM-3 interactions | Subsequent binding of T-cell receptors signals LFA-1 | Conformational change in LFA-1 increases affinity and prolongs cell–cell contact |

7-4   Both specific ligand and co-stimulatory signals provided by a professional antigen-presenting cell are required for the clonal expansion of naive T cells.

We saw in Chapter 4 that effector T cells are triggered when their antigen-specific receptors and either the CD4 or the CD8 co-receptors bind to peptide:MHC complexes. Nevertheless ligation of the T-cell receptor and co-receptor does not, on its own, stimulate naive T cells to proliferate and differentiate into armed effector T cells. The antigen-specific clonal expansion of naive T cells requires a second, co-stimulatory, signal (Fig. 7.9), which must be delivered by the same antigen-presenting cell on which the T cell recognizes its specific antigen. CD8 T cells appear to require a stronger co-stimulatory signal than CD4 cells and, as we shall see later, their clonal expansion may be aided by CD4 cells interacting with the same antigen-presenting cell.

The best characterized co-stimulatory molecules on antigen-presenting cells are the structurally related glycoproteins **B7.1 (CD80)** and **B7.2 (CD86)**, which we shall call **B7 molecules** in the subsequent text, as functional differences between them have yet to be defined. The B7 molecules are homodimeric members of the immunoglobulin super-family found exclusively on the surface of cells capable of stimulating T-cell growth. Their role in co-stimulation has been demonstrated by transfecting fibroblasts that express a T-cell ligand with genes encoding B7 molecules and showing that the fibroblasts could then stimulate growth of naive T cells. The receptor for B7 molecules on the T cell is **CD28**, yet another member of the immunoglobulin superfamily (Fig. 7.10). Ligation of CD28 by B7 molecules or by anti-CD28 antibodies will co-stimulate the growth of naive T cells, while antibodies to the B7 molecules, which inhibit their binding to CD28, inhibit T-cell responses.

On naive T cells, CD28 is the only receptor for B7 molecules. Once T cells are activated, however, they express an additional receptor called **CTLA-4**. CTLA-4 closely resembles CD28 in sequence, and the two molecules are encoded by closely linked genes. CTLA-4 binds B7 molecules about 20 times more avidly than CD28 and appears to deliver a negative signal to the activated T cell (Fig. 7.11). This makes the activated progeny of a naive T cell less sensitive to stimulation by the antigen-presenting cell and limits the amount of the T-cell growth factor **interleukin-2 (IL-2)** produced. Thus, binding of CTLA-4 to B7 molecules plays an essential role in limiting the proliferative response of activated T cells to antigen and B7 on the surface of antigen-presenting cells. This

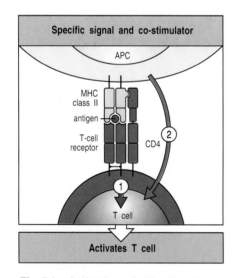

Fig. 7.9 Activation of naive T cells requires two independent signals. Binding of the peptide:MHC complex by the T-cell receptor and, in this example, the CD4 co-receptor, transmits a signal (arrow 1) to the T cell that antigen has been recognized. Activation of naive T cells requires a second signal (arrow 2), the co-stimulatory signal, to be delivered by the same antigen-presenting cell (APC).

Fig. 7.10 The principal co-stimulatory signals expressed on professional antigen-presenting cells (APCs) are B7 molecules, which bind the T-cell protein CD28. Binding of the T-cell receptor (TCR) and its co-receptor CD4 to the peptide:MHC class II complex delivers a signal (arrow 1) that can only induce clonal expansion of T cells when the co-stimulatory signal (arrow 2) is given by binding of CD28 to B7 molecules. Both CD28 and B7 molecules are members of the immunoglobulin superfamily. B7.1 and B7.2 are homodimers, each of whose chains have one V-like domain and one C-like domain. CD28 is a disulfide-linked homodimer in which each chain has one domain resembling an immunoglobulin V-domain.

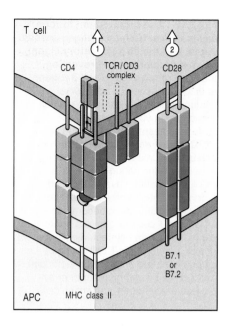

was confirmed by producing mice with a disrupted CTLA-4 gene; such mice develop a fatal disorder characterized by massive lymphocyte proliferation. Although other molecules have been reported to co-stimulate naive T cells, to date only B7.1 and B7.2 binding to CD28 has been shown definitively to provide co-stimulatory signals in normal immune responses.

The requirement for simultaneous delivery of antigen-specific and co-stimulatory signals by one cell in the activation of naive T cells means that only professional antigen-presenting cells can initiate T-cell responses. This is important because not all potentially self-reactive T cells are deleted in the thymus; peptides derived from proteins made only in specialized cells in the peripheral tissues may not be encountered during the negative selection of thymocytes. Self tolerance could be broken if naive autoreactive T cells could recognize self antigens on tissue cells and then be co-stimulated by a professional antigen-presenting cell, either locally or at a distant site. Thus, the requirement that the same cell presents both the specific antigen and the co-stimulatory signal is important in preventing destructive immune responses to self tissues. Indeed, antigen binding to the T-cell receptor in the absence of co-stimulation not only fails to activate the cell but also leads to a state called **anergy**, in which the T cell becomes refractory to activation (Fig. 7.12).

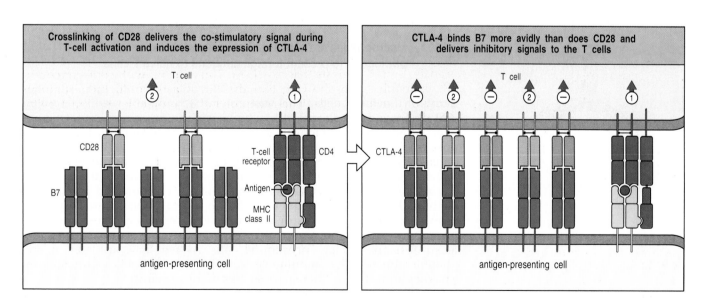

Fig. 7.11 T-cell activation through the T-cell receptor and CD28 leads to increased expression of CTLA-4, an inhibitory receptor for B7 molecules. CTLA-4 has a higher affinity for B7 molecules than does CD28 and thus binds most or all the B7 molecules, effectively shutting down the response. Signaling through CTLA-4 inhibits T-cell activation.

Fig. 7.12   The requirement for one cell to deliver both the antigen-specific signal and the co-stimulatory signal plays a crucial role in preventing immune responses to self antigens. In this example of the initiation of an immune response to a virus, a T cell recognizes a viral peptide on a professional antigen-presenting cell (APC) and is activated to proliferate and differentiate into an effector cell capable of eliminating any virus-infected cell (upper panels). Naive T cells that recognize antigen on cells that cannot provide co-stimulation become anergic, as when a T cell recognizes a self antigen expressed by an uninfected epithelial cell (lower panels). This T cell does not differentiate into an armed effector cell, and cannot be stimulated further by professional antigen-presenting cells.

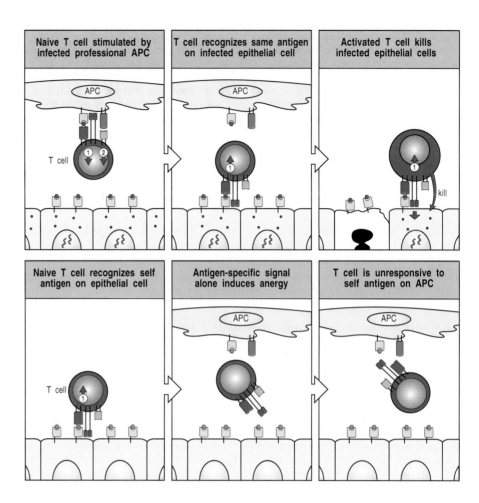

As well as B7.1 and B7.2, professional antigen-presenting cells must express adhesion molecules like ICAM-1, ICAM-2, and LFA-3, and they must be able to process antigen for presentation on both classes of MHC molecules. The three types of antigen-presenting cells differ both in their co-stimulatory and in their antigen-processing properties, and thus have distinctive functions in initiating immune responses.

7-5   Macrophages are scavenger cells that can be induced by pathogens to present foreign antigens to naive T cells.

Many of the microorganisms that enter the body are readily engulfed and destroyed by phagocytes, which provide an innate, antigen non-specific first line of defense against infection. Microorganisms that are destroyed by phagocytes without additional help from T cells do not cause disease and do not require an adaptive immune response. Pathogens, by definition, have developed mechanisms to avoid elimination by innate immune mechanisms, and the recognition and removal of such pathogens is the function of the adaptive immune response. Mononuclear phagocytes or macrophages, in which ingested microorganisms persist, contribute to the adaptive immune response by acting as professional antigen-presenting cells. As we shall see later in this chapter, the adaptive immune response is in turn able to stimulate the phagocytic and microbicidal capacities of these cells.

Professional antigen-presenting cells must be able to present peptide fragments of the antigen on both classes of MHC molecule, and to deliver a co-stimulatory signal, probably through B7 molecules. Resting macrophages, however, have few or no MHC class II molecules on their surface, and do not express B7. Expression of both MHC class II and B7 molecules is induced in these cells by the ingestion of microorganisms.

Macrophages have a variety of receptors for microbial constituents, including the macrophage mannose receptor and the scavenger receptor (see Chapter 9). Once bound, the microorganisms are engulfed and degraded in the endosomes and lysosomes, generating peptides that can be presented by MHC class II molecules on the cell surface. At the same time, MHC class II and B7 molecules are induced on the surface of the macrophage. The receptors that recognize microbial constituents probably also mediate the induction of co-stimulatory activity, since exposure to a single microbial constituent can induce B7 molecules on most macrophages. It seems likely that these receptors evolved originally to allow the phagocytic cells in primitive eukaryotic organisms to recognize microorganisms by binding to structures such as bacterial carbohydrates or lipopolysaccharide that are not found in eukaryotes. Macrophage receptors still serve this function in innate immunity as well as playing an important part in the initiation of adaptive immune responses.

The induction of co-stimulator activity by common microbial constituents is believed to allow the immune system to distinguish antigens borne by infectious agents from antigens associated with innocuous proteins, including self proteins. Indeed, many foreign proteins do not induce an immune response when injected on their own, presumably because they fail to induce co-stimulatory activity in antigen-presenting cells. When such protein antigens are mixed with bacteria, however, they become immunogenic, because the bacteria induce the essential co-stimulatory activity in cells that ingest the protein (Fig. 7.13). Bacteria used in this way are known as adjuvants (see Section 2-4). We shall see in Chapter 12 how self tissue proteins mixed with bacterial adjuvants can induce autoimmune diseases, illustrating the crucial importance of the regulation of co-stimulatory activity in self:non-self discrimination.

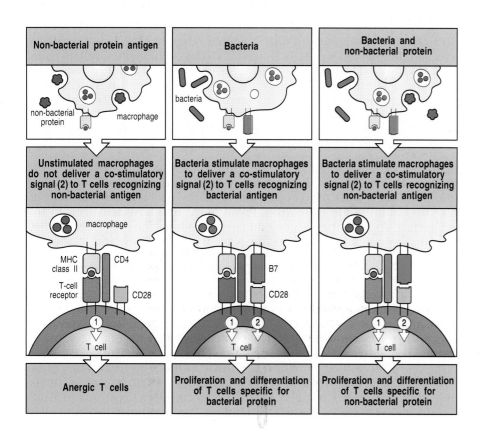

Fig. 7.13 Microbial substances can induce co-stimulatory activity in macrophages. If protein antigens are taken up and presented by macrophages in the absence of bacterial components that induce co-stimulatory activity in the macrophage, T cells specific for the antigen will become anergic (refractory to activation). Many bacteria induce expression of co-stimulators by antigen-presenting cells, and macrophages can present peptide antigens derived by degradation of such bacteria. When bacteria are mixed with protein antigens, the protein antigens are rendered immunogenic because the bacteria induce co-stimulatory activity (for example, the expression of B7 molecules) in the antigen-presenting cells. Such added bacteria act as adjuvants.

As macrophages continuously scavenge dead or senescent cells, it is particularly important that they should not normally be capable of activating T cells in the absence of microbial infection. The Küpffer cells of the liver sinusoids and the macrophages of the splenic red pulp, in particular, remove large numbers of dying cells from the blood daily. Küpffer cells express little MHC class II and its expression is not increased by ingestion of dead cells in the absence of infection or inflammation. Moreover, Küpffer cells are not located at sites through which large numbers of naive T cells pass. Thus, although they generate large amounts of self peptides in their endosomes and lysosomes, these macrophages are not likely to elicit an autoimmune response.

7-6 Dendritic cells are highly efficient inducers of T-cell activation.

It is of crucial importance that all infections be detected by T cells but many dangerous pathogens do not directly induce co-stimulatory molecules and MHC class II on macrophages. Viruses use the biosynthetic machinery of the host to synthesize their proteins, nucleic acids, carbohydrates, and membranes, and are therefore more difficult to distinguish from self than are bacteria. It seems likely that dendritic cells, which are found in the T-cell areas of lymphoid tissues, evolved to cope with this potential chink in the armor of the body. These cells arise from a lymphoid-specific progenitor upon culture with the cytokines IL-4 and GM-CSF (see Section 7-17). This suggests that dendritic cells may have appeared after T and B lymphocytes in evolution and is consistent with their apparently exclusive function of presenting antigen to T cells. Several specializations equip them for this function.

The dendritic cells that are concentrated in the lymphoid tissues express high levels of MHC class I and MHC class II molecules as well as the co-stimulatory B7 molecules, and the adhesion molecules ICAM-1, ICAM-2, LFA-1, and LFA-3 (Fig. 7.14). Not surprisingly, they are very potent activators of naive T cells.

Most cells are susceptible to only a limited range of viruses but dendritic cells can be infected by many different viruses. They efficiently present peptides derived from the viral proteins on their abundant surface MHC molecules. These peptides may be presented either on MHC class I molecules, where they are recognized by naive CD8 T cells (which will differentiate into cytotoxic effector cells), or on MHC class II molecules, where they are recognized by CD4 T cells, which differentiate into either T$_H$1 or T$_H$2 cells or most often, into both.

Most viral proteins are produced in the cytosol; peptides derived from them are transported to the surface by MHC class I molecules for recognition by CD8 T cells. However, viral envelope proteins are translocated into the endoplasmic reticulum. From there they are delivered to the cell surface and can then enter endosomes, where they encounter MHC class II molecules. Peptides of these proteins are delivered to the cell surface by MHC class II molecules and stimulate CD4 T cells. Thus, in many viral infections, dendritic cells are able to prime both CD8 and CD4 T cells.

Cells that resemble dendritic cells are found in many sites in the body, especially in surface epithelia, including the skin, gut and respiratory tract linings. The interdigitating reticular dendritic cells of the lymphoid tissues are mature forms of these tissue dendritic cells. The best studied tissue dendritic cells are the **Langerhans' cells** of the skin. They differ from dendritic cells found in lymphoid tissues in two crucial respects. First, they can ingest antigen both by macropinocytosis and through various cell-surface receptors, including the mannose receptor first

---

Dendritic cell

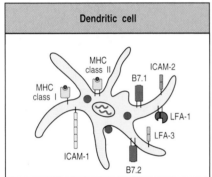
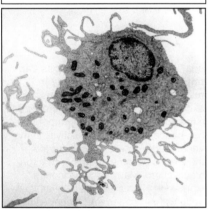

Fig. 7.14 Dendritic cells in lymphoid tissue have high levels of co-stimulatory activity. To activate naive T cells, antigen-presenting cells must be capable of processing antigen from extracellular and intracellular pathogens and presenting it on MHC class I and MHC class II molecules, and they must also express co-stimulatory molecules, probably in the form of B7.1 and B7.2. Dendritic cells in lymphoid tissue express all these surface molecules as well as high levels of the adhesion molecules ICAM-1, ICAM-2, LFA-1, and LFA-3. However, at this mature stage in their development, their ability to take up antigen is limited. Photograph courtesy of J Barker.

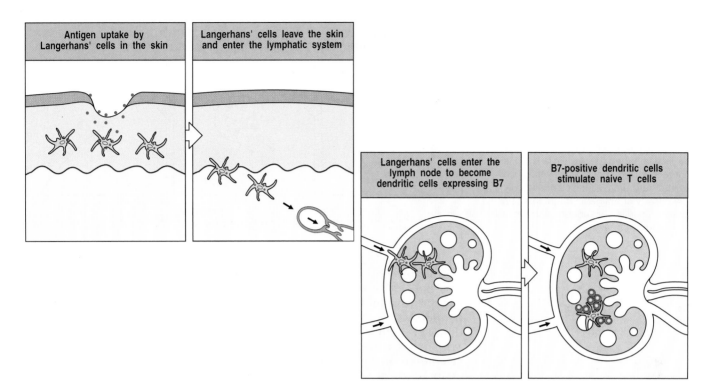

Fig. 7.15   Langerhans' cells can take up antigen in the skin and migrate to lymphoid organs where they present it to T cells. Langerhans' cells can ingest antigen by several means, but have no co-stimulatory activity. In the presence of infection, they take up antigen locally in the skin and then migrate to the lymph nodes. There they differentiate into dendritic cells that can no longer ingest antigen but now have co-stimulatory activity.

identified on macrophages; second, they lack co-stimulatory activity. These cells can be triggered by infection to migrate through the lymph to the lymphoid organs, where they lose the ability to ingest antigen as they differentiate into mature dendritic cells with potent co-stimulatory activity (Fig. 7.15). The role of tissue dendritic cells in physiological immune responses is likely to be in the transport of antigen from sites of infection to the lymphoid tissues, where they can activate naive T lymphocytes.

Once in the lymphoid tissue, it is important that dendritic cells do not readily take up extracellular antigens or scavenge self cells or protein, since their constitutively expressed co-stimulatory activity enables them to present to T cells any antigen they can internalize or synthesize. Dendritic cells do, of course, efficiently present peptides derived from their own proteins. However, these do not elicit autoimmune responses because, as we saw in Section 6-16, dendritic cells in the thymus efficiently delete developing T cells specific for these peptides.

Much of the evidence for the importance of tissue dendritic cells comes from their role in inducing the rejection of tissue grafts, as we shall see in Chapter 12. In experimental animals, grafts depleted of dendritic cells are well tolerated by recipients, at least until repopulated by host antigen-presenting cells.

7-7   B cells are highly efficient at presenting antigens that bind to their surface immunoglobulin.

Macrophages cannot take up soluble antigens efficiently, but dendritic cells can take up large amounts of antigen, although mainly by non-specific means. B cells, by contrast, are uniquely adapted to bind specific

Fig. 7.16 B cells can use their immunoglobulin receptor to present specific antigen very efficiently to T cells. Surface immunoglobulin allows B cells to bind and internalize specific antigen very efficiently. The internalized antigen is processed in cellular vesicles where it binds to MHC class II molecules, which transport the antigenic fragments to the cell surface where they can be recognized by T cells. When the protein antigen is not recognized specifically by the B cell, its internalization is inefficient and only a low density of antigenic fragments of any given protein is subsequently presented at the B-cell surface.

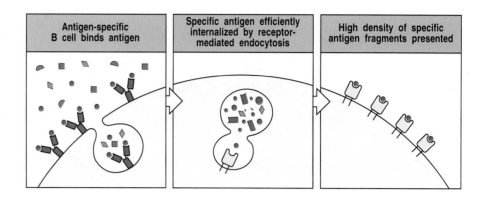

| Antigen-specific B cell binds antigen | Specific antigen efficiently internalized by receptor-mediated endocytosis | High density of specific antigen fragments presented |

soluble molecules through their cell-surface immunoglobulin. B cells internalize the soluble antigens bound by their surface immunoglobulin receptors and then display peptide fragments of these antigens as peptide:MHC complexes (see Chapter 8). Since this mechanism of antigen uptake is highly efficient and B cells constitutively express high levels of MHC class II molecules, high levels of specific peptide:MHC class II complexes are generated at the B-cell surface (Fig. 7.16). This pathway of antigen presentation allows B cells to be targeted by antigen-specific CD4 T cells, which drive their differentiation, as we shall see in Chapter 8. In circumstances in which the presenting B cell is induced to express co-stimulatory activity, it also allows B cells to activate naive T cells.

B cells do not constitutively express co-stimulatory activity but they can be induced by various microbial constituents to express B7.1 and especially B7.2. Indeed, B7.1 was first identified as a molecule expressed on B cells activated by microbial lipopolysaccharide. These observations help explain why it is essential to co-inject bacterial adjuvants in order to produce an immune response to soluble proteins, which seem to require B cells as antigen-presenting cells such as ovalbumin, hen egg-white lysozyme, and cytochrome *c*.

The requirement for induced co-stimulatory activity also helps to explain why, although B cells efficiently present soluble proteins, they are unlikely to initiate responses to soluble self proteins in the absence of infection; in the absence of co-stimulatory activity, antigen not only fails to activate naive T cells but causes them to become anergic, or non-responsive (see Fig. 7.12). This provides an additional safeguard to the mechanisms discussed in Chapters 5 and 6 whereby potentially self-reactive T and B cells are eliminated or inactivated as they develop in the thymus and bone marrow.

Although much of what we know about the immune system in general, and about T-cell responses in particular, has been learned from the study of immune responses to soluble protein immunogens presented by B cells, it is not clear how important a role B cells play in priming naive T cells in natural immune responses. Soluble protein antigens are not abundant during natural infections; most natural antigens, such as bacteria and viruses, are particulate, while soluble bacterial toxins act by binding to cell surfaces and are thus present only at low concentrations in solution. However, there are some natural immunogens that enter the body as soluble molecules; examples are insect toxins, anticoagulants injected by blood-sucking insects, snake venoms, and many allergens.

Thus T-cell responses are primed by three distinct classes of professional antigen-presenting cell. Each is optimally equipped to present a particular

	Macrophages	Dendritic cells	B cells
	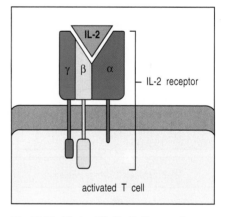		
Antigen uptake	Phagocytosis +++	+++ Phagocytosis by tissue dendritic cells. ++++ Viral infection	Antigen-specific receptor (Ig) ++++
MHC expression	Inducible by bacteria and cytokines – to +++	Constitutive ++++	Constitutive. Increases on activation +++ to ++++
Co-stimulator delivery	Inducible – to +++	Constitutive; by mature non-phagocytic lymphoid dendritic cells ++++	Inducible – to +++
Antigen presented	Particulate antigens. Intracellular and extracellular pathogens	Peptides Viral antigens (allergens?)	Soluble antigens. Toxins. Viruses
Location	Lymphoid tissue. Connective tissue. Body cavities	Lymphoid tissue. Connective tissue. Epithelia	Lymphoid tissue. Peripheral blood

Fig. 7.17 The properties of professional antigen-presenting cells. Macrophages, dendritic cells, and B cells are the main cell types involved in the initial presentation of exogenous antigens to naive T cells. These cells vary in their means of antigen uptake, MHC class II expression, co-stimulator expression, the antigens that appear to be crucial for presenting, and their locations in the body.

class of antigen to naive T cells: those that can present ingested antigens express co-stimulatory activity only when this is induced by microbial particles; only mature dendritic cells constitutively express co-stimulatory activity. These properties allow professional antigen-presenting cells to present peptides of pathogens while avoiding immunization against self (Fig. 7.17).

7-8   Activated T cells synthesize the T-cell growth factor interleukin-2 and its receptor.

Naive T cells can live for many years without dividing. These small resting cells have condensed chromatin and a scanty cytoplasm and synthesize little RNA or protein. On activation, they must re-enter the cell cycle and divide rapidly to produce large numbers of progeny that will differentiate into armed effector T cells. Their proliferation and differentiation is driven by a protein growth factor or cytokine called **interleukin-2 (IL-2)**, which is produced by the activated T cell itself.

The initial encounter with specific antigen in the presence of the required co-stimulatory signal triggers the entry of the T cell into the G1 phase of the cell cycle and, at the same time, induces the synthesis of IL-2 along with the α chain of the IL-2 receptor. The IL-2 receptor has three chains: α, β, and γ (Fig. 7.18). Resting T cells express a form of this receptor composed of β and γ chains that binds IL-2 with low affinity. Association of the α chain with the β and γ chains creates a receptor with a much higher affinity for IL-2. Binding of IL-2 to the high-affinity receptor then triggers progression through the rest of the cell cycle. T cells activated in this way can divide two to three times a day for several days, allowing

Fig. 7.18 High-affinity IL-2 receptors are three-chain structures composed of a γ, a β, and an α chain, which is expressed only on activated T cells. On resting T cells, only the β and γ chains are expressed. They bind IL-2 with moderate affinity, allowing resting T cells to respond to very high concentrations of IL-2. Activation of T cells induces the synthesis of the α chain and the formation of the heterotrimeric receptor, which has a high affinity for IL-2 and allows the T cell to respond to very low concentrations of IL-2. The β and γ chains show amino acid similarities to cell-surface receptors for growth hormone and prolactin, all of which regulate cell growth and differentiation.

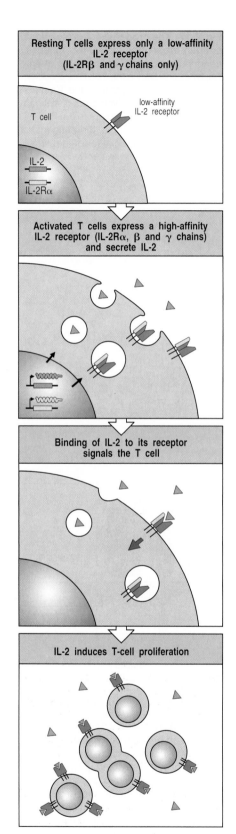

Resting T cells express only a low-affinity IL-2 receptor (IL-2Rβ and γ chains only)

T cell

low-affinity IL-2 receptor

IL-2

IL-2Rα

Activated T cells express a high-affinity IL-2 receptor (IL-2Rα, β and γ chains) and secrete IL-2

Binding of IL-2 to its receptor signals the T cell

IL-2 induces T-cell proliferation

Fig. 7.19 Activated T cells secrete and respond to interleukin-2 (IL-2). Activation of naive T cells by the recognition of a peptide:MHC complex accompanied by co-stimulation induces expression and secretion of IL-2 and the expression of high-affinity IL-2 receptors. IL-2 binds to the IL-2 receptors to promote T-cell growth in an autocrine fashion.

one cell to give rise to thousands of progeny, all bearing an identical receptor for antigen. IL-2 also promotes the differentiation of these cells into armed effector T cells (Fig. 7.19).

Activation also causes the expression on the T-cell surface of the molecule that is called **CD40 ligand**, because it binds to the B-cell surface molecule **CD40**. The binding of CD40 ligand to CD40 activates CD40-positive cells and induces surface expression of B7.1 and B7.2 on the B cell, further driving the T-cell response.

7-9   The co-stimulatory signal is necessary for the synthesis and secretion of IL-2.

The production of IL-2 determines whether a T cell will proliferate and become an armed effector cell, and the most important function of the co-stimulatory signal is to promote the synthesis of IL-2. Antigen recognition by the T-cell receptor ultimately induces several transcription factors (see Chapter 4). One of these factors, **NF-AT (nuclear factor of activation in T cells)**, binds to the promoter region of the IL-2 gene and is necessary to activate its transcription. IL-2 gene transcription on its own, however, does not lead to the production of IL-2, which additionally requires CD28 ligation by B7. One effect of signaling through CD28 is thought to be the stabilization of IL-2 mRNA. Cytokine mRNAs are very unstable because of an 'instability' sequence in their 3' untranslated region, as we shall see later in this chapter. This instability prevents sustained cytokine production and release, and enables cytokine activity to be tightly regulated. The stabilization of IL-2 mRNA increases IL-2 synthesis by 20- to 30-fold. A second effect of CD28 ligation is to activate transcription factors (AP-1 and NF-κB) which increase transcription of IL-2 mRNA by about 3-fold. These two effects together increase IL-2 production by 100-fold. When a T cell recognizes specific antigen in the absence of co-stimulation through its CD28 molecule, little IL-2 is produced and the T cell does not induce its own proliferation.

The requirements for expression of the IL-2 receptor are less stringent than those for IL-2 synthesis. For example, T-cell receptor ligation alone is frequently sufficient to induce expression of high-affinity IL-2 receptors on T cells. This can allow IL-2 made by one cell to act on IL-2 receptors expressed on neighboring antigen-specific cells. Later in this chapter we shall see how this may be important in the priming of CD8 T cells.

The central importance of IL-2 in initiating adaptive immune responses is well illustrated by the drugs that are most commonly used to suppress undesirable immune responses such as the rejection of tissue grafts. The immunosuppressive drugs cyclosporin A and FK506 or tacrolimus inhibit IL-2 production by disrupting signaling through the T-cell receptor, while rapamycin inhibits signaling through the IL-2 receptor. Cyclosporin A and rapamycin act synergistically to inhibit immune responses by preventing the IL-2 driven clonal expansion of T cells. The mode of action of these drugs will be considered in detail in Chapter 13.

| 7-10 | **Antigen recognition in the absence of co-stimulation leads to T-cell tolerance.** |

Antigen recognition in the absence of co-stimulation inactivates naive T cells, inducing a state known as anergy (Fig. 7.20). The most important change in anergic T cells is their inability to produce IL-2. This prevents them from proliferating and differentiating into effector cells when they encounter antigen, even if the antigen is subsequently presented by professional antigen-presenting cells. This helps ensure tolerance of T cells to self-tissue antigens.

As we saw in Section 6-16, any protein synthesized by all cells will be presented by professional antigen-presenting cells in the thymus and will cause clonal deletion of T cells reactive to these ubiquitous self proteins. However, many proteins have specialized functions and are made only by the cells of certain tissues. Since MHC class I molecules present only those peptides derived from proteins synthesized within the cell, such tissue-specific peptides will not be displayed on the MHC molecules of thymic cells and cells recognizing them are unlikely to be deleted in the thymus. An important factor in avoiding autoimmune responses to such tissue-specific proteins is the absence of co-stimulator activity on tissue cells. Naive T cells recognizing self peptides on tissue cells are not activated; instead they may be induced to enter a state of anergy.

While deletion of potentially autoreactive T cells is readily understood as a simple way to maintain self tolerance, the retention of anergic T cells specific for tissue antigens is less easy to understand. It would seem more economical and efficient to eliminate such cells; indeed, binding of the T-cell receptor on peripheral T cells in the absence of co-stimulators can lead to programmed cell death as well as to anergy. Nevertheless, some T cells persist in an anergic state *in vivo*. One possible explanation for this is that such anergic T cells have a role in preventing responses by naive, non-anergic T cells to foreign antigens that mimic self -peptide:self-MHC complexes. The persisting anergic T cells could recognize and bind to such peptide:MHC complexes on professional antigen-presenting cells without responding, and thus could compete with naive, potentially autoreactive cells of the same specificity. In this way, anergic T cells could serve to prevent the accidental activation of autoreactive T cells by infectious agents, thus actively contributing to tolerance.

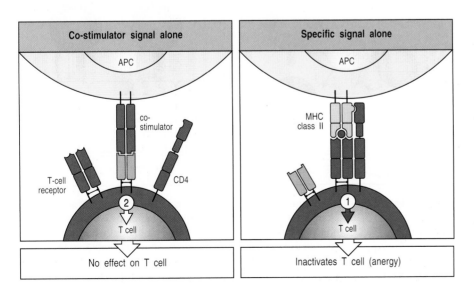

Fig. 7.20 T-cell tolerance to antigens expressed on tissue cells results from antigen recognition in the absence of co-stimulation. Antigen-presenting cells (APC) neither activate nor inactivate T cells if specific antigen is not present on their surface, even if they express a co-stimulatory molecule and can deliver signal 2. However, when T cells recognize antigen in the absence of co-stimulatory molecules, they receive signal 1 alone and are inactivated. This allows self antigens expressed on tissue cells to induce tolerance in T cells.

7-11   Proliferating T cells differentiate into armed effector T cells that do not require co-stimulation to act.

The combination of antigen and co-stimulator induces naive T cells to express IL-2 and its receptor; IL-2 then induces clonal expansion of the naive T cell and the differentiation of its progeny into armed effector T cells. Late in the proliferative phase of the response, after 4–5 days of rapid growth, these T cells differentiate into armed effector T cells that are able to synthesize all the proteins required for their specialized functions as helper or cytotoxic T cells. As well as acquiring the capacity to synthesize the appropriate arsenal of specialized effector molecules when they encounter antigen on target cells, all classes of armed effector T cells undergo several changes that distinguish them from naive T cells. One of the most critical is in their activation requirements; once a T cell has differentiated into an armed effector cell, further encounter with its specific antigen results in immune attack without the need for co-stimulation (Fig. 7.21).

This change applies to all classes of armed effector T cells. Its importance is particularly easy to understand in the case of cytotoxic CD8 T cells, which must be able to act on any cell infected with a virus, whether or not the infected cell can express co-stimulatory molecules. However, B cells and macrophages that have taken up antigen often have too little co-stimulatory activity to activate a naive CD4 T cell. Effector CD4 T cells must be able to activate these B cells and macrophages efficiently, and the change from co-stimulator dependence to independence ensures that any cell displaying antigen can trigger an appropriate T-cell response. Armed effector T cells also express higher levels of the cell-adhesion molecules LFA-1 and CD2.

Finally, most armed effector T cells lose their cell-surface L-selectin and thus cease to recirculate through lymph nodes. Instead, they express the integrin VLA-4, which allows them to bind to vascular endothelium at sites of inflammation. The T cells are now able to migrate to sites of infection in the peripheral tissues where their armory of effector proteins can be put to use. These changes in the T-cell surface are summarized in Fig. 7.22.

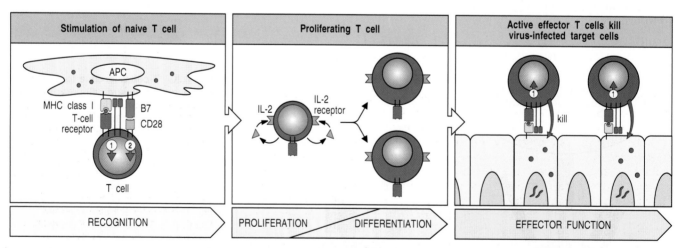

Fig. 7.21   Clonal expansion precedes differentiation to effector function. A naive T cell that recognizes antigen on the surface of a professional antigen-presenting cell (APC) and receives the required two signals (arrows 1 and 2, left panel) becomes activated, and both secretes and responds to IL-2. IL-2 driven clonal expansion (middle panel) is followed by the differentiation of the T cells to armed effector cell status. Once the cells have differentiated into effector T cells, any encounter with specific antigen triggers their effector actions without the need for co-stimulation. Thus, as illustrated here, a cytotoxic T cell can kill targets that express only the peptide:MHC ligand and not co-stimulatory signals (right panel).

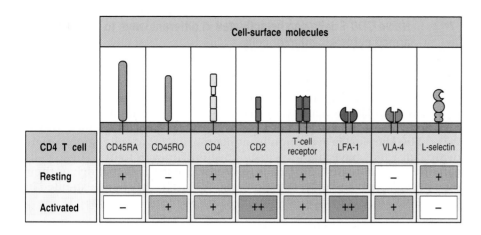

Fig. 7.22 Activation of T cells changes the expression of several cell-surface molecules. Resting naive T cells express L-selectin, through which they home to lymph nodes, with relatively low expression levels of other adhesion molecules such as CD2 and LFA-1. Upon activation of the T cell, the expression of these molecules changes. Activated T cells express higher densities of the adhesion molecules CD2 and LFA-1, increasing the avidity of the interaction of the activated T cell with potential target cells. Expression of the L-selectin homing receptor is lost and instead, increased amounts of the integrin VLA-4 are expressed. VLA-4 acts as a homing receptor for vascular endothelium in sites of inflammation and ensures that activated T cells recirculate through peripheral tissues where they may encounter sites of infection. Finally, the isoform of the CD45 molecule expressed by activated cells changes, by alternative splicing of the RNA transcript of the CD45 gene, so that activated T cells now express the CD45RO isoform that associates with the T-cell receptor and CD4, the co-receptor in this example. The consequences of this change in CD45 make the T cell more sensitive to stimulation by low concentrations of peptide:MHC complexes.

7-12   The differentiation of CD4 T cells into T$_H$1 or T$_H$2 cells determines whether humoral or cell-mediated immunity will predominate.

Naive CD8 T cells emerging from the thymus are already predestined to become cytotoxic cells, even though they are not yet expressing any of the differentiated functions of armed effector cells. The case of CD4 T cells, however, is more complex. Naive CD4 T cells can differentiate upon activation into either T$_H$1 or T$_H$2 cells, which differ in the cytokines they produce upon their stimulation and thus in their function. The decision on which fate a naive CD4 T cell will follow is made during its first encounter with antigen (Fig. 7.23).

The factors that determine whether a proliferating CD4 T cell will differentiate into a T$_H$1 or a T$_H$2 cell are not fully understood. The cytokines elicited by infectious agents (principally the interleukins **IL-12** and **IL-4**), the co-stimulators used to drive the response, and the nature of the peptide:MHC ligand all have an effect. In particular, since the decision to differentiate into T$_H$1 versus T$_H$2 cells occurs early in the immune response, the ability of pathogens to stimulate cytokine production by cells of the innate, non-adaptive immune system play an important part in shaping the subsequent adaptive response; we shall learn more about this in Chapter 9.

The consequences of inducing T$_H$1 versus T$_H$2 cells are profound; selective production of T$_H$1 cells leads to cell-mediated immunity, while production of predominantly T$_H$2 cells provides humoral immunity. A striking example of the difference this can make to the outcome of infection is seen in leprosy, a disease caused by infection with *Mycobacterium leprae*. *M.leprae*, like *M.tuberculosis*, grows in macrophage vesicles and effective host defense requires macrophage activation by T$_H$1 cells. In patients with tuberculoid leprosy, in which T$_H$1 cells are preferentially induced, few live bacteria are found, little antibody is produced and, although skin and peripheral nerves are damaged by the inflammatory responses associated with macrophage activation, the disease progresses slowly and the patient usually survives. However, when T$_H$2 cells are preferentially induced, the main response is humoral, the antibodies produced cannot reach the intracellular bacteria, and the patients develop lepromatous leprosy, in which *M. leprae* grows abundantly in macrophages, causing gross tissue destruction, which is eventually fatal.

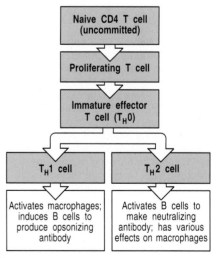

Fig. 7.23 The stages of activation of CD4 T cells. Naive CD4 T cells first respond to peptide:MHC class II complexes by making IL-2 and proliferating. These cells then differentiate into a cell type known as T$_H$0, which has some of the effector functions characteristic of T$_H$1 and T$_H$2 cells. The T$_H$0 cell has the potential to become either a T$_H$1 cell or a T$_H$2 cell. T$_H$0 cells may also have some effector actions in their own right.

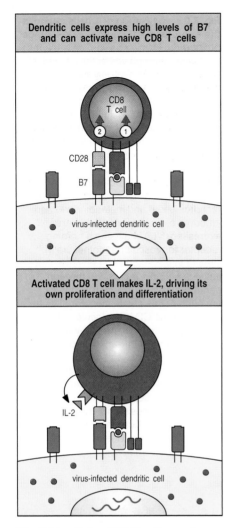

Dendritic cells express high levels of B7 and can activate naive CD8 T cells

CD8
T cell

2   1

CD28

B7

virus-infected dendritic cell

⇩

Activated CD8 T cell makes IL-2, driving its own proliferation and differentiation

IL-2

virus-infected dendritic cell

Fig. 7.24 Naive CD8 T cells can be activated directly by potent antigen-presenting cells. Naive CD8 T cells that encounter peptide:MHC class I complexes on the surface of dendritic cells, which express high levels of co-stimulatory molecules (top panel), are activated to produce IL-2 (bottom panel) and proliferate in response to it, eventually differentiating into armed cytotoxic CD8 T cells (not shown).

7-13   Naive CD8 T cells can be activated in different ways to become armed cytotoxic effector cells.

Naive CD8 T cells can differentiate only into cytotoxic cells, and perhaps because the effector actions of these cells are so destructive, they require more co-stimulatory activity to drive them to become armed effector cells than do naive CD4 T cells. This requirement can be met in two ways. The simplest is activation by antigen-presenting cells, such as dendritic cells, that have high intrinsic co-stimulatory activity. These cells can directly stimulate CD8 T cells to synthesize the IL-2 that drives their own proliferation and differentiation (Fig. 7.24). This has been exploited in the use of CD8 T cells against tumors, as we shall see in Chapter 13.

Cytotoxic T-cell responses to some viruses and tissue grafts, however, seem to require the presence of CD4 T cells during the priming of the naive CD8 T cell. In these responses, both the naive CD8 T cell and the CD4 T cell must recognize antigen on the surface of the same antigen-presenting cell. In this case, it is thought that the actions of the CD4 T cell may be necessary to compensate for inadequate co-stimulation of naive CD8 T cells by the antigen-presenting cell. This compensatory effect could occur in either of two ways. If the CD4 T cell is an armed effector cell, it may activate the antigen-presenting cell to express higher levels of co-stimulatory activity. We shall see that this is one of the actions of the specialized molecules produced by effector CD4 T cells. This would enable the antigen-presenting cell to co-stimulate the CD8 T cell directly (Fig. 7.25, left panels).

Alternatively, the CD4 T cell may be a naive or memory T cell, which secretes IL-2 in response to antigen and low levels of co-stimulatory molecules. As IL-2 receptors can be induced by receptor ligation alone, the CD8 T cell may express IL-2 receptors even though it cannot produce the IL-2 needed to drive its own proliferation. The IL-2 in this case comes instead from the adjacent responding CD4 T cell (see Fig. 7.25, right panels). It is known that adding IL-2 can eliminate the need for a co-stimulatory signal for CD8 T-cell activation in experimental situations, in keeping with the general finding that the crucial role of co-stimulation for T cells is the production of sufficient IL-2 to drive their clonal expansion, allowing them to differentiate into armed effector T cells.

Summary.

The crucial first step in adaptive immunity is the activation of naive antigen-specific T cells by professional antigen-presenting cells. The most distinctive feature of professional antigen-presenting cells is the expression of co-stimulatory activities, of which the B7.1 and B7.2 molecules are the best characterized. Naive T cells will respond to antigen only when one cell presents both specific antigen to the T-cell receptor and a B7 molecule to CD28, the receptor for B7 on the T cell. The three cell types that can serve as professional antigen-presenting cells are macrophages, dendritic cells, and B cells. Each of these cells has a distinct function in eliciting immune responses. Macrophages efficiently ingest particulate antigens and are induced by infectious agents to express MHC class II molecules and co-stimulatory activity. Dendritic cells express both MHC class II molecules and co-stimulatory activity constitutively, and may be specialized to present pathogens, such as some viruses, that do not induce co-stimulatory activity in macrophages. The unique ability of B cells to bind and internalize soluble protein antigens via their

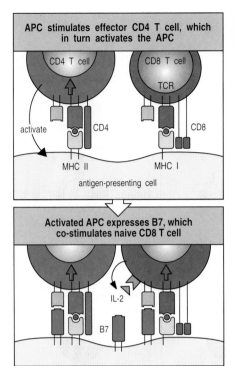

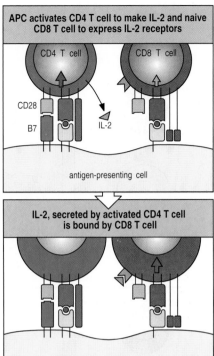

Fig. 7.25 Some CD8 T-cell responses require CD4 T cells. CD8 T cells recognizing antigen on weakly co-stimulating cells may become activated only in the presence of CD4 T cells bound to the same antigen-presenting cell (APC). There are two ways in which CD4 T cells may contribute to the activation of CD8 T cells. Left panels: an effector CD4 T cell may recognize antigen on the antigen-presenting cell and be triggered to induce increased levels of co-stimulatory activity on the antigen-presenting cell, which in turn activates the CD8 T cell to make its own IL-2. Right panels: alternatively, a naive CD4 T cell activated by the antigen-presenting cell may provide the IL-2 required for the proliferation and differentiation of the CD8 T cell. Which of these two mechanisms operates *in vivo* is not known.

receptors may be important in activating T cells to this class of antigen, provided that co-stimulatory molecules are also induced on the B cell.

The activation of T cells by professional antigen-presenting cells lead to their proliferation and the differentiation of their progeny into armed effector T cells. The proliferation and differentiation of T cells depends on the production of cytokines such as the T-cell growth factor IL-2 and its binding to a high-affinity receptor on the activated T cell. T cells whose antigen receptors are ligated in the absence of co-stimulatory signals fail to make IL-2 and instead become anergic. This dual requirement for both receptor ligation and co-stimulation helps to prevent naive T cells from responding to antigens on self-tissue cells, which lack co-stimulator activity. Proliferating T cells develop into armed effector T cells, the critical event in most adaptive immune responses. Once an expanded clone of T cells achieves effector function, its armed effector T-cell progeny can act on any target cell that displays antigen on its surface. Effector T cells can mediate a variety of functions. Their most important functions are killing of infected cells by CD8 cytotoxic T cells and the activation of macrophages by T$_H$1 cells, which together make up cell-mediated immunity, and the activation of B cells by both T$_H$2 and T$_H$1 cells to produce different types of antibody, thus driving the humoral immune response.

General properties of armed effector T cells.

All T-cell effector functions involve the interaction of an armed effector T cell with a target cell displaying specific antigen. The effector proteins released by these T cells are focused on the appropriate target cell by mechanisms that are activated by the specific recognition of antigen on

Fig. 7.26 There are three classes of effector T cells, specialized to deal with three classes of pathogens. CD8 cytotoxic cells (left panels) kill target cells that display antigenic fragments of cytosolic pathogens, most notably viruses, bound to MHC class I molecules at the cell surface. T$_H$1 cells (middle panels) and T$_H$2 cells (right panels) both express the CD4 co-receptor and recognize fragments of antigens degraded within intracellular vesicles, displayed at the cell surface by MHC class II molecules. The T$_H$1 cells, upon activation, activate macrophages, allowing them to destroy intracellular microorganisms more efficiently; they can also activate B cells to produce strongly opsonizing antibodies belonging to certain IgG subclasses (IgG1 and IgG3 in humans, and their homologs IgG2a and IgG2b in the mouse). T$_H$2 cells, on the other hand, drive B cells to differentiate and produce immunoglobulins of all other types, and are responsible for initiating B-cell responses by activating naive B cells to proliferate and secrete IgM. The various types of immunoglobulin together make up the effector molecules of the humoral immune response.

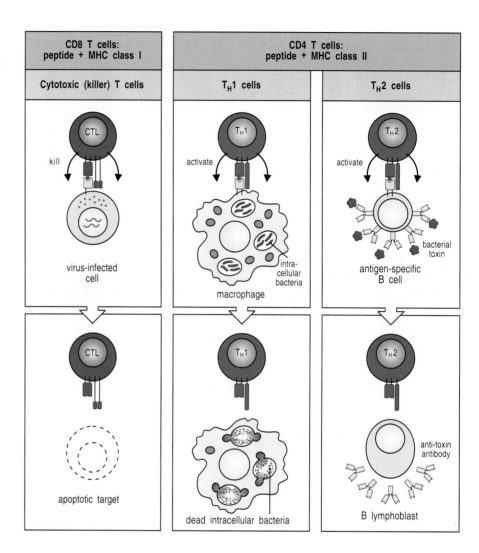

the target-cell surface. The focusing mechanism is common to all types of effector T cells, while their effector actions depend upon the array of membrane and secreted proteins they express or release upon receptor ligation; these are specific to the different effector cell types (Fig. 7.26).

7-14   Effector T-cell interactions with target cells are initiated by antigen non-specific cell-adhesion molecules.

Once an effector T cell has completed its differentiation in the lymphoid tissue it must find target cells that are displaying the specific MHC:peptide complex it recognizes. This occurs in two steps. First, the armed effector T cells emigrate from their site of activation in the lymphoid tissues and enter the blood. Second, because of the cell-surface changes that have occurred during differentiation, they then migrate into the peripheral tissues, particularly at sites of infection. They are guided to these sites by changes in the adhesion molecules expressed on the endothelium of the local blood vessels as a result of infection, and by local chemotactic factors, as we shall see in Chapter 9.

The initial binding of an effector T cell to its target, like that of a naive T cell to an antigen-presenting cell, is an antigen non-specific interaction mediated by the LFA-1 and CD2 adhesion molecules. The level of LFA-1 and of CD2 is two- to four-fold higher on armed effector T cells than on naive

Fig. 7.27 Interactions of T cells with their targets are mediated initially by non-specific adhesion molecules. The major initial interaction is between LFA-1 expressed by the T cell, illustrated here as a CD8 cytotoxic T cell, and ICAM-1 or ICAM-2 expressed by the target cell (top panel). This binding allows the T cell to remain in contact with the target cell and to scan its surface for the presence of specific peptide:MHC complexes. If the target cell does not express the specific antigen, the T cell disengages (second panel) and can scan other potential targets. If the target cell expresses the specific antigen (third panel), signaling through the T-cell receptor increases the strength of the adhesive interactions, prolonging the contact between the two cells, and stimulating the T cell to deliver its effector molecules. The T cell then disengages (bottom panel).

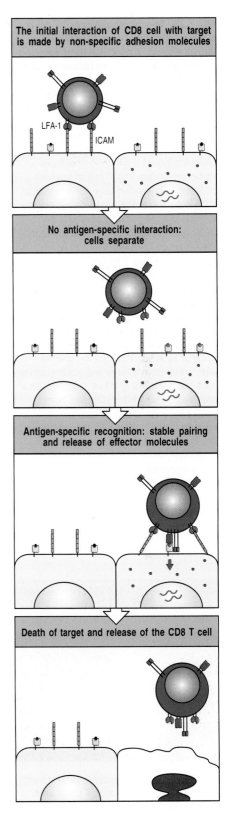

The initial interaction of CD8 cell with target is made by non-specific adhesion molecules

LFA-1   ICAM

No antigen-specific interaction: cells separate

Antigen-specific recognition: stable pairing and release of effector molecules

Death of target and release of the CD8 T cell

T cells, and so armed effector T cells can bind efficiently to target cells that have lower levels of ICAMs and LFA-3 on their surface than do professional antigen-presenting cells. This interaction is normally transient unless recognition of antigen on the target cell triggers a change in the affinity of the T-cell LFA-1 for its ligands on the target cell surface. This change causes the T cell to bind more tightly to its target, and to remain bound for long enough to release its specific effector molecules. Armed CD4 effector T cells, which activate macrophages or induce B cells to secrete antibody, must maintain contact with their targets for relatively long periods. Cytotoxic T cells, by contrast, can be observed under the microscope attaching to and dissociating from successive specific targets relatively rapidly as they kill them (Fig. 7.27). Killing of the target, or some local change in the T cell, then allows the effector T cell to detach and address new targets. How armed CD4 effector T cells disengage from their targets is not known, although current evidence suggests that CD4 binding directly to MHC class II molecules on target cells that are not displaying antigen signals the cell to detach.

7-15 The T-cell receptor complex directs the release of effector molecules and focuses them on the target cell.

The binding of the T-cell receptor to an MHC:antigen complex on a target cell not only increases the strength with which the T cell binds its target but also signals a reorganization of the cytoskeleton. This polarizes the effector cell so as to focus the release of effector molecules at the site of contact with the specific target cell (Fig. 7.28). The reorientation of the cytoskeleton is very effective at targeting the lytic granules that are preformed in cytotoxic CD8 T cells; the site of exocytosis of these granules is determined by the microtubule organizing center (MTOC), the center from which the microtubule cytoskeleton is produced.

The polarization of the cell also focuses the secretion of soluble effector molecules whose synthesis is induced by ligation of the T-cell receptor. For example the soluble cytokine IL-4, which is the principal effector molecule of T_H2 cells, is concentrated and confined to the site of contact with the target cell (see Fig. 8.5). It has recently been shown that the enhanced binding of LFA-1 to ICAM-1 creates a molecular seal surrounding the clustered T-cell receptor molecules, CD4 co-receptor, and CD28 (Fig. 7.29). The clustering of the T-cell receptor then triggers the release of effector molecules, and focuses them onto the antigen-bearing target.

Thus, the antigen-specific T-cell receptor directs the delivery of effector signals in three ways: it induces stable binding of effector cells to their specific target cells to create a tightly held narrow space in which effector molecules can be concentrated; it triggers the release and/or expression

Fig. 7.28 The polarization of T cells during specific antigen recognition allows effector molecules to be focused on the antigen-bearing target cell.
T cells, like all nucleated cells, contain several subcellular organelles such as the Golgi apparatus and the microtubule-organizing center (MTOC). Cytotoxic CD8 cells also contain specialized lysosomes called lytic granules, as shown in panel a. Binding of a T cell to its target causes the T cell to become polarized (illustrated here for a cytotoxic CD8 cell): the cytoskeleton is reoriented to align the Golgi apparatus and the microtubule-organizing center towards the target cell. Proteins stored in lytic granules are thus directed specifically onto the target cell (left panels). The photomicrograph in panel a shows a T cell, stained in green to show the presence of polymerized actin, revealing the cytoskeleton and, in red, showing the presence of granzyme A in lytic granules within the cell. In this cell the granules are clustered in a large membrane ruffle, marking the leading edge of the cell as it migrates across the substrate. Panel b shows a similar cell interacting with its specific target cell, where the granules are localized at the interface with the target cell; the electron micrograph in panel c shows the release of granules from the cytotoxic T cell. Panels a and b courtesy of G Griffiths. Panel c courtesy of E R Podack.

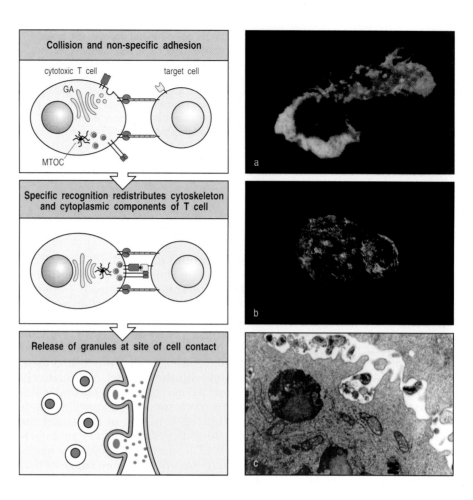

Outer ring (red)	Inner circle (green)
LFA-1: ICAM-1	TCR, CD4, CD28

Fig. 7.29   Tight junctions are formed between armed effector T cells and their targets, in this case a B cell.
The outer ring is made up of LFA-1 in the T cell and its counter-receptors on the target cell, while molecules that cluster in the center of the ring include the T-cell receptor complex, the co-receptor CD4, and CD28. Photograph courtesy of A Kupfer.

of effector molecules; and it focuses their delivery at the site of contact by inducing a reorientation of the secretory apparatus of the effector cell. All these receptor-coordinated mechanisms contribute to the selective action of effector molecules on the cells bearing specific antigen. In this way, effector T-cell activity is highly selective for those target cells that display antigen, although the effector molecules themselves are not antigen-specific.

7-16   The effector functions of T cells are determined by the array of effector molecules they produce.

The effector molecules produced by armed effector T cells fall into two broad classes: **cytotoxins**, which are stored in specialized lytic granules and released by cytotoxic CD8 T cells, and **cytokines** and related membrane-associated proteins, which are synthesized *de novo* by all effector T cells and are the principal mediators of CD4 T-cell effector actions. The cytotoxins are the principal effector molecules of cytotoxic T cells and will be discussed further in Section 7-22. It is particularly important that their release is tightly regulated because they are not specific: they can penetrate the lipid bilayer and trigger an intrinsic death program in any target cell. By contrast, the cytokines and membrane-associated proteins act by binding to specific receptors on the target cell. The main effector actions of CD4 cells are therefore directed at specialized cells expressing those receptors.

The membrane-associated effector molecules belong to the **tumor necrosis factor** (**TNF**) family of proteins, and their receptors on target cells are members of the TNF receptor (TNFR) family. TNF-α and TNF-β (lymphotoxin) are made by T$_H$1 cells and some T$_H$2 and cytotoxic T cells in soluble and membrane-associated forms, both of which are homo-trimeric. Their receptors, TNFR I and II, form homotrimers when bound to TNF. The homotrimeric structure is characteristic of all members of the TNF family, and the ligand-induced trimerization of their receptors seems to be the critical event in signaling. All three classes of effector T cells express one or more members of the TNF family upon recognizing specific antigen on the target cell. T$_H$1 and T$_H$2 cells are induced to express the TNF family member CD40 ligand, which delivers activating signals to B cells and macrophages through the receptor protein CD40. TNF-α also delivers activating signals to macrophages. The principal membrane-associated TNF-related molecule expressed by cytotoxic T cells is called **Fas ligand** (CD95L), which can trigger death in target cells bearing the receptor protein **Fas** (CD95); some T$_H$1 cells also express Fas ligand and can kill Fas-bearing cells with which they inter-act. The actions of Fas and CD40 are discussed further in Section 7-20.

The effector actions and main effector molecules of all three functional classes of effector T cells are summarized in Fig. 7.30. The cytokines are a diverse group of molecules and we shall give a brief overview of them below before discussing specifically the T-cell cytokines and their con-tributions to the effector actions of CD8 cytotoxic T cells, T$_H$1 cells, and T$_H$2 cells. As we shall see, the soluble cytokines and membrane-associated molecules often act in combination to mediate the effects of these T cells on their specific target cells.

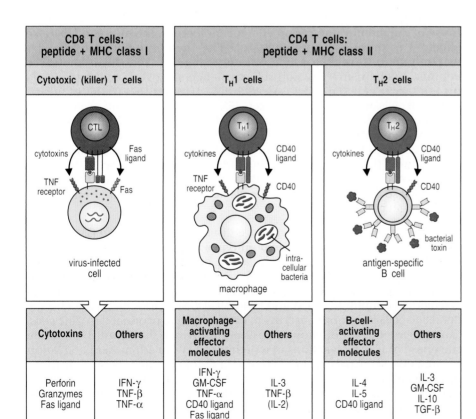

CD8 T cells: peptide + MHC class I		CD4 T cells: peptide + MHC class II			
Cytotoxic (killer) T cells		T$_H$1 cells		T$_H$2 cells	
Cytotoxins	Others	Macrophage-activating effector molecules	Others	B-cell-activating effector molecules	Others
Perforin Granzymes Fas ligand	IFN-γ TNF-β TNF-α	IFN-γ GM-CSF TNF-α CD40 ligand Fas ligand	IL-3 TNF-β (IL-2)	IL-4 IL-5 CD40 ligand	IL-3 GM-CSF IL-10 TGF-β

Fig. 7.30 The three main types of armed effector T cell produce distinct sets of effector molecules. CD8 T cells are predominantly killer T cells that recognize pathogen-derived peptides bound to MHC class I molecules. They release perforin (which creates holes in the target-cell membranes), granzymes (which are proteases), and often the cytokine IFN-γ. A membrane-bound effector molecule expressed on CD8 T cells is the ligand for Fas, a receptor whose activation induces apoptosis. CD4 T cells recognize peptides bound to MHC class II molecules and are of two functional types: T$_H$1 cells and T$_H$2 cells. T$_H$1 cells are specialized for activation of macrophages that are infected by or have ingested pathogens; they secrete IFN-γ as well as other effector molecules, and express membrane-bound CD40 ligand and/or Fas ligand. These are both members of the TNF family but CD40 ligand triggers activation, whereas Fas ligand triggers death, so their pattern of expression has a strong influence on function. T$_H$2 cells are specialized for B-cell activation; they secrete the B-cell growth factors IL-4 and IL-5. T$_H$2 cells express mainly the membrane-bound effector molecule CD40 ligand, which binds to CD40 on the B cell and induces B-cell proliferation.

7-17   Cytokines can act locally or at a distance.

Cytokines are small soluble proteins secreted by one cell that can alter the behavior or properties of the cell itself or of another cell. They are released by many cells in addition to those of the immune system. We shall discuss the cytokines released by phagocytic cells in Chapter 9 where we deal with the inflammatory reactions that play an important part in innate immunity; here we shall be concerned mainly with the cytokines that mediate the effector functions of T cells. Cytokines produced by lymphocytes are often called **lymphokines**, but this nomenclature can be confusing because some lymphokines are also secreted by non-lymphoid cells; we shall therefore use the generic term 'cytokine' for all of them. Most cytokines produced by T cells are given the name **interleukin** (**IL**) followed by a number: we have already encountered IL-2. Cytokines of immunological interest are listed in Appendix II.

Most cytokines can have a multitude of different biological effects when tested at high concentration in biological assays *in vitro* but, in recent years, targeted disruption of genes for cytokines and cytokine receptors in gene knock-out mice (see Section 2-37) has helped to clarify their physiological roles. The major actions of the cytokines produced by effector T cells are given in Fig. 7.31. As the effect of a cytokine varies depending on the target cell, the actions are listed according to the major target cell types: B cells, T cells, macrophages, hematopoietic cells, and tissue cells.

The main cytokine released by CD8 effector T cells is interferon-γ (IFN-γ), which can block viral replication or even lead to the elimination of virus from infected cells without killing them. T$_H$1 cells and T$_H$2 cells release different but overlapping sets of cytokines, which define their distinct actions in immunity; and the T$_H$0 cells from which both these functional classes derive also secrete cytokines, including IL-2, and may therefore have a distinctive effector function.

Most of the soluble cytokines have local actions that synergize with those of the membrane-bound effector molecules; the effects of all these effectors is therefore combinatorial. The membrane-bound effectors can only bind to receptors on an interacting cell, and this is therefore another mechanism by which selective effects of cytokines are focused on the target cell. T$_H$2 cells secrete IL-4, IL-5, and IL-10, all of which activate B cells, while T$_H$1 cells secrete IFN-γ, which is the main macrophage-activating cytokine, and lymphotoxin (LT or TNF-β), which is directly cytotoxic for some cells. We have already discussed in Section 7-15 how the T-cell receptor can orchestrate the polarized release of these cytokines so that they are concentrated at the site of contact with the target cell. As we shall see later, the synthesis of cytokines such as IFN-γ is also controlled so that secretion from T cells does not continue after interaction with a target cell.

Some cytokines, however, have more distant effects. IL-3 and GM-CSF, for example, which are released by both types of CD4 effector T cell, help to recruit effector cells in infection by acting on bone marrow cells to stimulate myelopoiesis, the production of macrophages and granulocytes, both of which are important non-specific effector cells in both humoral and cell-mediated immunity; IL-3 and GM-CSF also stimulate the production of dendritic cells from bone marrow precursors. IL-5, produced by T$_H$2 cells, can increase the production of eosinophils, which may contribute to the late phase of allergic reactions in which there is a predominant activation of T$_H$2 cells (see Chapter 11). Whether a cytokine effect is local or more distant is likely to reflect the amounts released, the degree to which this release is focused on the target cell, and the stability of the cytokine *in vivo* but, for most of the cytokines, in particular those with more distant effects, these factors are not yet known.

Cytokine	T-cell source	Effects on					Effect of gene knock-out
		B cells	T cells	Macrophages	Hematopoietic cells	Other somatic cells	
Interleukin-2 (IL-2)	T$_H$0, T$_H$1, some CTL	Stimulates growth and J-chain synthesis	Growth	–	Stimulates NK cell growth	–	↓ T-cell responses
Interferon-γ (IFN-γ)	T$_H$1, CTL	Differentiation IgG2a synthesis	Kills	Activation, ↑ MHC class I and class II	Activates NK cells	Antiviral ↑ MHC class I and class II	Susceptible to Mycobacteria
Lymphotoxin (LT, TNF-β)	T$_H$1, some CTL	Inhibits	Kills	Activates, induces NO production	Activates neutrophils	Kills fibroblasts and tumor cells	Absence of lymph nodes. Disorganized spleen
Interleukin-4 (IL-4)	T$_H$2	Activation, growth IgG1, IgE ↑ MHC class II induction	Growth, survival	Inhibits macrophage activation	↑ Growth of mast cells	–	No T$_H$2
Interleukin-5 (IL-5)	T$_H$2	Differentiation IgA synthesis	–	–	↑ Eosinophil growth and differentiation	–	–
Interleukin-10 (IL-10)	T$_H$2	↑ MHC class II	Inhibits T$_H$1	Inhibits cytokine release	Co-stimulates mast cell growth	–	–
Interleukin-3 (IL-3)	T$_H$1, T$_H$2, some CTL	–	–	–	Growth factor for progenitor hematopoietic cells (multi-CSF)	–	–
Tumor necrosis factor-α (TNF-α)	T$_H$1, some T$_H$2, some CTL	–	–	Activates, induces NO production	–	–	Resistance to Gram –ve sepsis
Granulocyte-macrophage colony-stimulating factor (GM-CSF)	T$_H$1, some T$_H$2, some CTL	Differentiation	Inhibits growth	Activation	↑ Production of granulocytes and macrophages (myelopoiesis) and dendritic cells	–	–
Transforming growth factor-β (TGF-β)	CD4 T cells	Inhibits growth IgA switch factor	–	Inhibits activation	Activates neutrophils	Inhibits/ stimulates cell growth	Death at ~10 weeks

Fig. 7.31 The nomenclature and functions of well-defined T-cell cytokines. The major actions are noted in boxes. Each cytokine has multiple activities on different cell types. The mixture of cytokines secreted by a given cell type produces many effects through what is called a 'cytokine network'.

Major activities of effector cytokines are highlighted in red. [↑] = increase; [↓] = decrease; CTL = cytotoxic lymphocyte; MHC = major histocompatibility complex; NK = natural killer cell; CSF = colony-stimulating factor.)

7-18   Cytokines and their receptors fall into distinct families of structurally related proteins.

Cytokines can be grouped by structure into families: these are the hematopoietins, the interferons, the chemokines, and members of the TNF family (Fig. 7.32). The latter act as trimers, most of which are membrane-bound and so are quite distinct in their properties from the other cytokines. Nevertheless, they share some important properties with the soluble T-cell cytokines, as they also are synthesized *de novo* upon antigen recognition by T cells, and affect the behavior of the target cell.

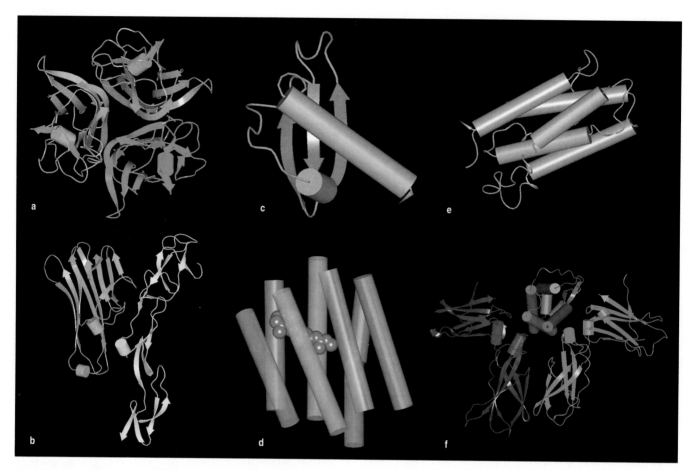

Fig. 7.32 Cytokines and their receptors belong to a small number of families of molecules. Although there are many cytokines and cytokine receptors, there are similarities between many of them that suggest that they are related members of a family of molecules. The cytokine receptors, likewise, can be grouped into families. The family of TNF-related cytokines consists of a trimeric structure as shown in (a). The receptors for these molecules are also related; the structure of the TNF-receptor is shown in (b). The chemokines are a small family of cytokines with a structure similar to that of IL-8, shown in (c). The receptor molecules for the chemokines have seven transmembrane helices and all members of this receptor family interact with G-proteins. The structure of bacteriorhodopsin is depicted in (d), showing the orientation of the seven transmembrane helices (blue) with the bound ligand, retinal (red). The structure of interferon-γ, a member of the third family of cytokines, is shown in (e). The structure of the receptor for another member of this family, human growth hormone, has been solved and is a T-shaped dimer; a model of the IL-4 receptor based on the human growth hormone structure is shown in purple and green (f), with bound IL-4 shown in red.

Cytokines act on receptors that can be grouped into equivalent families of structures with genetic, structural and functional similarity (Fig. 7.33) For instance, among the hematopoietins, IL-3, IL-5, and GM-CSF are related structurally, their genes are closely linked in the genome, and they are major cytokines produced by T_H2 cells. In addition, they bind to closely related receptors; the IL-3, IL-5, and GM-CSF receptors share a common β chain. The γ chain of the IL-2 receptor is also shared by receptors for the cytokines IL-4, IL-7, IL-9, and IL-15 and is now called the γ common chain (γc). This is also true of other groups of cytokines, suggesting that cytokines and their receptors may have diversified together in the evolution of increasingly specialized effector functions.

As mentioned above, the cytokines produced by T_H1 and T_H2 cells largely define their specific effector actions, and there is therefore considerable interest in defining more precisely their actions on specific target cells.

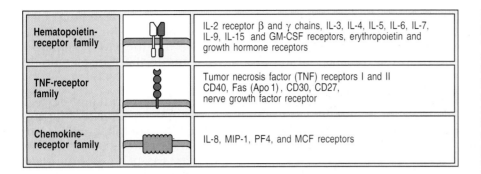

Hematopoietin-receptor family		IL-2 receptor β and γ chains, IL-3, IL-4, IL-5, IL-6, IL-7, IL-9, IL-15 and GM-CSF receptors, erythropoietin and growth hormone receptors
TNF-receptor family		Tumor necrosis factor (TNF) receptors I and II CD40, Fas (Apo 1), CD30, CD27, nerve growth factor receptor
Chemokine-receptor family		IL-8, MIP-1, PF4, and MCF receptors

Fig. 7.33 Cytokine receptors belong to families of receptor proteins, each with a distinctive structure. Some cytokine receptors are members of the hematopoietin receptor family, some are members of the tumor necrosis factor (TNF)-receptor family and some are members of the chemokine-receptor family. Each family member is a variant with a distinct specificity, performing a particular function on the cell that expresses it. In the case of the hematopoietin-receptor family, the α chain often defines the ligand specificity of the receptor, while the β or γ chain confers the intracellular signaling function. For the TNF-receptor family, the ligands may be associated with the cell membrane rather than being secreted. Of the receptors listed here, some have been mentioned already in this book, some will occur in later chapters, and some are important examples from other biological systems. The diagrams indicate the representations of these receptors that you will encounter throughout this book. MIP-1 = Macrophage inflammatory protein-1; PF4 = Platelet factor 4; MCF = Macrophage chemotactic factor.

7-19   **Binding of cytokines to their receptors triggers gene activation by activating Janus kinases, which then activate STAT proteins.**

Cytokines affect their target cells by binding to specific receptors. These receptors frequently have two or even three chains, which are often shared between several members of the receptor family, as noted above. When one of the receptor chains is activated by cytokine binding, it induces cytokine receptor aggregation, which in turn triggers the receptor to deliver signals to the cell on which it is expressed. This causes protein kinases associated with the cytoplasmic domains of cytokine receptors to become active by phosphorylating each other. These cytoplasmic kinases are all members of the **Janus** family of kinases, which is composed of a group of closely related enzymes called Jak1, Jak2, Jak3, and Tyk2. These activated kinases phosphorylate and activate members of a family of proteins that were first discovered in studies of interferon signaling. These are called **STATs**, for **S**ignal **T**ransducers and **A**ctivators of **T**ranscription, and act as gene-regulatory proteins. The way in which STAT phosphorylation leads to the transcriptional activation of specific genes is just now beginning to be unraveled.

Upon phosphorylation, a STAT protein forms a complex with other STAT proteins and unrelated cytoplasmic proteins. These complexes then enter the nucleus and bind to specific sequences in the DNA, thus activating a wide variety of genes, depending on the STAT involved. STAT-6, for instance, which is activated by IL-4 binding to the IL-4 receptor, binds to sites in the immunoglobulin heavy-chain locus whose activation is required for IL-4-induced class switching (see Chapter 8). Active STAT-6 also binds to DNA control sequences involved in the upregulation of other cell-surface proteins including MHC class II molecules. Other signaling molecules may also play a role in transducing signals from some cytokine receptors. Ras is involved in signaling from the IL-2 receptor, while the Insulin Receptor Substrate-1 (IRS-1) is involved in signaling from the IL-4 and IL-9 receptors.

Cytokine signaling is modulated by protein phosphatases, which reverse phosphorylation. The phosphatase HCP, expressed in all hematopoietic cells, is a negative regulator of cytokine signaling. A mouse mutant of HCP, called *motheaten*, has numerous abnormalities, including defects in hematopoiesis and elevated sensitivity of the B-cell receptor to signals deriving from ligand binding.

7-20   **The TNF family of cytokines are trimeric proteins, often cell-surface associated.**

Most effector T cells express members of the TNF protein family as cell-surface molecules, generally composed of three identical polypeptide chains. The most important TNF family proteins in T-cell effector function are TNF-α and TNF-β (which is also expressed as a secreted molecule), Fas ligand, and CD40 ligand, the latter two always being cell-surface associated. These molecules bind respectively to the TNF receptors I and II, to the transmembrane protein Fas, and to the transmembrane protein CD40 (all members of the TNFR family) on target cells.

Fas is expressed on many cells, especially on activated lymphocytes. Activation of Fas by the Fas ligand has profound consequences for the cell. Fas contains a 'death domain' in its cytoplasmic tail; when activated, this domain activates several cytosolic proteins that initiate a cellular suicide cascade leading to apoptosis. Fas plays an important role in maintaining lymphocyte homeostasis, as can be seen from the effects of mutations in the Fas or Fas ligand genes. Mice and humans with a mutant form of Fas develop a lymphoproliferative disease associated with severe autoimmunity. A mutation in the gene encoding the Fas ligand in another mouse strain creates a nearly identical phenotype. These mutant phenotypes represent the only examples of generalized autoimmunity caused by single-gene defects. The identification of Fas and the Fas ligand a few years ago as the pair of molecules responsible has galvanized the research community into tremendous activity in analyzing their function. Other TNFR family members, including one form of the TNF receptor itself, are also associated with death domains and can also induce programmed cell death. Thus, TNF-α and TNF-β can induce programmed cell death by binding to the TNFR.

CD40, another member of the TNFR family, is involved in macrophage and B-cell activation. The ligation of CD40 on B cells promotes growth and isotype switching, while macrophages are induced to secrete TNF-α and to become receptive to much lower concentrations of IFN-γ. The cytoplasmic tail of CD40 lacks a death domain; instead, it appears to be linked to a protein called CRAF (CD40 receptor associated factor) about which little is known. Deficiency in CD40 ligand expression is associated with immunodeficiency, as we shall learn in Chapters 8 and 10.

Summary.

Interactions between armed effector T cells and their targets are initiated by transient non-specific adhesion between the cells. T-cell effector functions are only elicited when peptide:MHC complexes on the surface of the target cell are recognized by the receptor on an armed effector T cell. This recognition event triggers the armed effector T cell to adhere more strongly to the antigen-bearing target cell and to release its effector molecules directly at the target cell, leading to the activation or death of the target. The consequences of antigen recognition by an armed effector T cell are determined largely by the set of effector molecules it produces on binding a specific target cell. CD8 killer T cells store preformed cytotoxins in specialized lytic granules whose release can be tightly focused at the site of contact with the infected target cell. Cytokines, and one or more members of the TNF family of membrane-associated effector proteins, are synthesized *de novo* by all three types of effector T cells. T_H2 cells express B-cell-activating effector molecules, while T_H1 cells express effector molecules that activate macrophages. CD8 T cells express a membrane-associated protein that induces programmed cell death; they also release IFN-γ. The membrane-associated effector molecules can only deliver signals to an interacting cell, whereas soluble cytokines can act on cytokine receptors expressed locally on the target cell, or on hematopoietic cells at a distance. The action of cytokines and membrane-associated effector molecules through their specific receptors, together with the effects of cytotoxins released by CD8 cells, account for the effector functions of T cells.

T-cell mediated cytotoxicity.

All viruses, and some bacteria, multiply in the cytoplasm of infected cells; indeed, the virus is a highly sophisticated parasite that has no bio-synthetic or metabolic apparatus of its own and, in consequence, can only replicate inside cells. Once inside cells, these pathogens are not accessible to antibodies and can be eliminated only by the destruction or modification of the infected cells on which they depend. This role in host defense is fulfilled by cytotoxic CD8 T cells. The critical role of cytotoxic T cells in limiting such infections is seen in the increased susceptibility of animals artificially depleted of these T cells, or of mice or humans that lack the MHC class I molecules that present antigen to CD8 T cells. As well as controlling infection by viruses and cytoplasmic bacteria, CD8 T cells are important in controlling some protozoan infections and are crucial, for example, in host defense against the protozoan *Toxoplasma gondii*, a vesicular parasite that exports peptides from the infected vesicles to the cytosol, from which they enter the MHC class I processing pathway. The elimination of infected cells without destruc-tion of healthy tissue requires the cytotoxic mechanisms of CD8 T cells to be both powerful and accurately targeted.

7-21 | **Cytotoxic T cells can induce target cells to undergo programmed cell death.**

Cells can die in either of two ways. Physical or chemical injury, such as the deprivation of oxygen that occurs in heart muscle during a heart attack, or membrane damage with antibody and complement, which leads to cell disintegration or **necrosis**. The dead or necrotic tissue is taken up and degraded by phagocytic cells, which eventually clear the damaged tissue and heal the wound. The other form of cell death is known as **programmed cell death** or **apoptosis**. Apoptosis is a normal cellular response that is crucial in the tissue remodeling that occurs during development and metamorphosis in all multicellular animals. As we saw in Chapter 6, most thymocytes die an apoptotic death when they fail positive selection or are negatively selected as a result of recog-nizing self antigens. The first changes seen in apoptotic cell death are fragmentation of the DNA, disruption of the nucleus, and alterations in cell morphology. The cell then destroys itself from within, shrinking by shedding membrane-bound vesicles, and degrading itself until little is left. A hallmark of this type of cell death is the fragmentation of nuclear DNA into fragments that are multiples of 200 base pairs (bp) through the activation of endogenous nucleases that cleave the DNA between nucleosomes, each of which contains about 200 bp of DNA.

There is good evidence that cytotoxic T cells kill their targets largely by programming them to undergo apoptosis. When cytotoxic T cells are mixed with target cells and rapidly brought into contact by centrifugation, they can program antigen-specific target cells to die within 5 minutes, although death may take hours to become fully evident. An early feature of T-cell killing is degradation of target cell DNA, while later effects include the loss of membrane integrity, which may also be induced by other cytotoxic mechanisms. The short period required by cytotoxic T cells to program their targets to die reflects the release of preformed effector molecules by the T cell, which activate an endogenous apoptotic pathway within the target cell (Fig. 7.34).

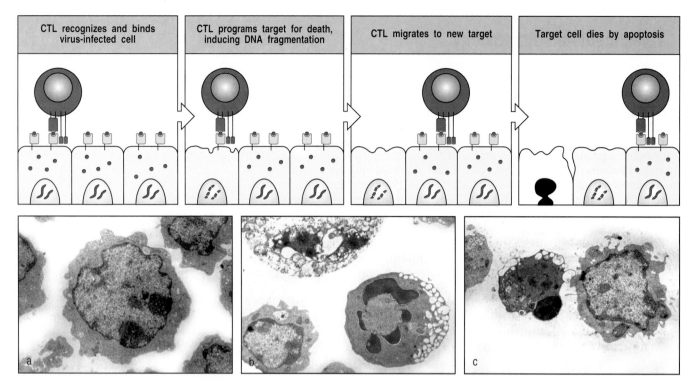

| CTL recognizes and binds virus-infected cell | CTL programs target for death, inducing DNA fragmentation | CTL migrates to new target | Target cell dies by apoptosis |

Fig. 7.34 Cytotoxic CD8 T cells can induce apoptosis (programmed cell death) in target cells. Specific recognition of peptide:MHC complexes on a target cell (top panels) by a cytotoxic CD8 T cell (CTL) leads to the death of the target cell by apoptosis. Cytotoxic T cells can recycle to kill multiple targets. Each killing requires the same series of steps, including receptor binding and directed release of cytotoxic mediators stored in lytic granules. The process of apoptosis is shown in the micrographs (bottom panels), where panel a shows a healthy cell with a regular nucleus. Early in apoptosis (panel b) the chromatin becomes condensed (shown in red at bottom right of panel) and, although the cell sheds membrane vesicles, the integrity of the cell membrane is retained, in contrast to the necrotic cell in the upper part of the same field. In late stages of apoptosis (panel c), the cell nucleus (middle cell) is very condensed, no mitochondria are visible and the cell has lost much of its cytoplasm and membrane through the shedding of vesicles. Photographs (x 3500) courtesy of R Windsor and E Hirst.

The apoptotic mechanism, as well as killing the host cell, may also act directly on cytosolic pathogens. For example, the nucleases that are activated in apoptosis to destroy cellular DNA can also degrade viral DNA. This prevents the assembly of virions and thus the release of virus and infection of nearby cells. Other enzymes activated in the course of apoptosis may destroy non-viral cytosolic pathogens. Apoptosis is therefore preferable to necrosis as a means of killing infected cells; in necrosis, intact pathogens are released from the dead cell and these can continue to infect healthy cells, or can parasitize the macrophages that ingest them.

Protein in lytic granules of cytotoxic T cells	Actions on target cells
Perforin	Polymerizes to form a pore in target membrane
Granzymes	Serine proteases, which activate apoptosis once in the cytoplasm of the target cell

Fig. 7.35 Cytotoxic proteins released by cytotoxic T cells have a role in killing target cells.

7-22   Cytotoxic proteins that trigger apoptosis are contained in the granules of CD8 cytotoxic T cells.

The principal mechanism through which cytotoxic T cells act is by the calcium-dependent release of specialized **lytic granules** upon recognition of antigen on the surface of a target cell. These granules are modified lysosomes that contain at least two distinct classes of **cytotoxins**, proteins that are expressed selectively in cytotoxic T cells and stored in the lytic granules in inactive form (Fig. 7.35). One of these, **perforin**, polymerizes to generate transmembrane pores in target cell membranes. The other class comprises at least three proteases called **granzymes**, which belong to the same family of enzymes (the serine proteases) as the

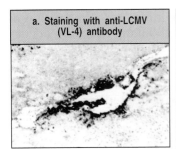	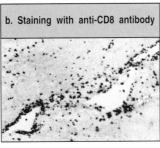	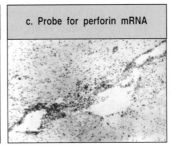	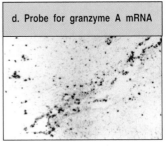
a. Staining with anti-LCMV (VL-4) antibody	b. Staining with anti-CD8 antibody	c. Probe for perforin mRNA	d. Probe for granzyme A mRNA

Fig. 7.36   CD8 T cells expressing perforin and granzymes can be seen in viral infections. In brains of mice infected with the lymphocytic choriomeningitis virus (LCMV) the presence of virus-infected cells can be demonstrated using antibodies specific for viral proteins (panel a). CD8 T cells are detected by staining with a CD8-specific antibody (panel b). These CD8 T cells are making both perforin (panel c) and granzymes (panel d) as can be revealed using radiolabeled probes for perforin and granzyme mRNAs and a photographic emulsion to show the location of the radiolabeled probes. Photographs courtesy of E Podack.

digestive enzymes trypsin and chymotrypsin. Granules that store perforin and granzymes can be seen in armed CD8 cytotoxic effector cells in tissue lesions (Fig. 7.36).

When purified granules from cytotoxic T cells are added to target cells *in vitro*, they lyse the cells by creating pores in the lipid bilayer. The pores consist of polymers of perforin, which is a major constituent of these granules. On release from the granule, perforin polymerizes into a cylindrical structure that is lipophilic on the outside and hydrophilic down a hollow center with an inner diameter of 16 nm. This structure can insert into lipid bilayers, forming a pore that allows water and salts to pass rapidly into the cell (Fig. 7.37). With the integrity of the cell membrane destroyed, the cells die rapidly. Large numbers of purified

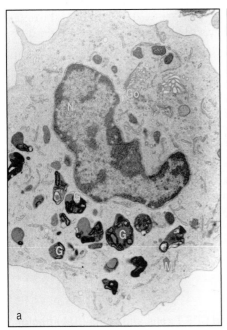

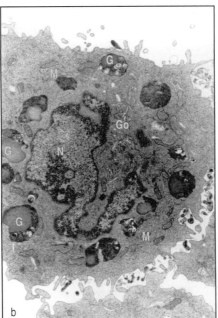

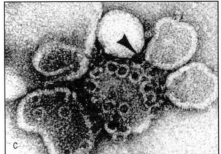

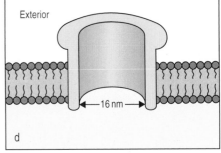

Fig. 7.37   Perforin released from the granules of cytotoxic T cells can insert into the target-cell membrane to form pores. Perforin molecules, as well as several other effector molecules, are contained in the granules of cytotoxic T cells (panel a: G = granules; N = nucleus; M = mitochondria; Go = Golgi apparatus). When a CD8 cytotoxic T cell recognizes its target, the granules are released onto the target cell (panel b, bottom right quadrant). The perforin molecules released from the granules polymerize and insert into the membrane of the target cell to form pores. The structure of these pores is best visualized when purified perforin is added to synthetic lipid vesicles (panel c: pores are seen both end on, as circles, and sideways on, arrow). The pores span the target cell membrane (panel d). Photographs courtesy of E Podack.

granules can kill target cells *in vitro* without inducing fragmentation of cellular DNA, but this lytic mechanism of cell killing probably occurs only at artificially high levels of perforin that do not reflect the physiological activity of cytotoxic T cells.

Both perforin and granzymes are required for cell killing. The separate roles of perforin and granzymes have been investigated in a cell system that relies upon similarities between the lytic granules of T cells and the granules of mast cells (see Chapter 1). Release of mast cell granules occurs upon crosslinking of the Fcε receptor (see Chapter 8), just as release of lytic granules from CD8 T cells occurs on crosslinking of the T-cell receptor, and by a similar mechanism. Both the Fcε receptor and the T-cell receptor have ITAM motifs in their cytoplasmic domains, and crosslinking leads to tyrosine phosphorylation of the ITAMs (see Chapter 3 and Section 4-27).

When a mast cell line is transfected with the gene for perforin or for granzyme, the gene products are stored in mast cell granules. When the cell is activated through its Fcε receptor the granules are released. When transfected with the gene for perforin alone, mast cells can kill other cells, but not very efficiently since large numbers of the transfected cells are needed. Mast cells transfected with the gene for granzyme B alone are unable to kill other cells. However, when perforin-transfected mast cells are also transfected with the gene encoding granzyme B, the cells or their purified granules become as effective at killing targets as granules from cytotoxic cells, and granules from both types of cell induce DNA fragmentation. This suggests that perforin makes pores through which the granzymes can move into the target cell.

The granzymes are proteases, so although they play a role in triggering apoptosis in the target cell, they cannot act directly to fragment the DNA. Rather, they must activate an enzyme, or more likely an enzyme cascade, in the target cell. Recently, it has been shown that granzyme B can cleave the ubiquitous cellular enzyme CPP-32, which is believed to play a key role in the programmed cell death of all cells.

Cells that are triggered to undergo programmed cell death are rapidly ingested by phagocytic cells in their vicinity. The phagocytes recognize some changed feature of the cell membrane, perhaps the inversion of membrane lipids. The ingested cell is then broken down into small molecules by the phagocyte without the induction of co-stimulatory proteins. Thus, apoptosis is normally an immunologically 'quiet' process; that is, apoptotic cells do not normally contribute to or stimulate immune responses.

The importance of perforin in this process is well illustrated in mice that have had their perforin gene knocked out. Such mice are severely defective in their ability to mount a cytotoxic T-cell response. Mice that are defective in the gene for granzyme B have a less profound defect, probably because there are several genes coding for granzymes, and knocking out one of them will be compensated for by synthesis of other granzymes.

7-23   Membrane proteins of activated CD8 T cells and some CD4 effector T cells can also activate apoptosis.

The release of granule contents accounts for most of the cytotoxic activity of CD8 effector T cells, as shown by the loss of most killing activity in perforin gene knock-out mice. This granule-mediated killing is strictly calcium-dependent, yet some cytotoxic actions of CD8 T cells survive calcium depletion. Moreover, some CD4 T cells are also capable of killing other cells, yet do not contain granules and make neither perforin nor granzymes. These observations implied that there must be a second independent mechanism of cytotoxicity. This mechanism involves the activation of Fas in the target cell membrane by the Fas ligand, which is expressed in the membranes of activated cytotoxic T cells and T$_H$1 cells. Activation of Fas leads to apoptosis in the target cell. As discussed in Section 7-20, the lymphoproliferative and autoimmune disorders seen in mice and humans with mutations in genes for either Fas or the Fas ligand imply that this pathway of killing is important in regulating peripheral immune responses.

7-24 Cytotoxic T cells are selective and serial killers of targets expressing specific antigen.

When cytotoxic T cells are offered a mixture of equal amounts of two target cells, one bearing specific antigen and the other not, they kill only the target cell bearing the specific antigen. The 'innocent bystander' cells and the cytotoxic T cells themselves are not killed, despite the fact that cloned cytotoxic T cells can be recognized and killed by other cytotoxic T cells just like any tissue cell. At first sight, this may seem surprising, since the effector molecules released by cytotoxic T cells lack any specificity for antigen. The explanation probably lies in the highly polar release of the effector molecules. We have seen (see Fig. 7.28) that cytotoxic T cells orient their Golgi apparatus and microtubule-organizing center to focus secretion on the point of contact with a target cell (Fig. 7.38); indeed, cytotoxic T cells attached to several different target cells reorient their secretory apparatus towards each cell in turn and kill them one by one, strongly suggesting that the mechanism whereby cytotoxic mediators are released allows attack at only one point of contact at any one time. The narrowly focused action of cytotoxic CD8 T cells allows them to kill single infected cells in a tissue without creating widespread tissue damage (Fig. 7.39) and is of critical importance in tissues where cell regeneration does not occur, as in neurons of the central nervous system, or is very limited, as in the pancreatic islets.

Cytotoxic T cells can kill their targets rapidly because they have evolved a means to store preformed cytotoxins in inactive forms. Cytotoxins are synthesized and loaded into the lytic granules on the first encounter of a naive cytotoxic precursor T cell with specific antigen. Ligation of the T-cell receptor similarly induces *de novo* synthesis of perforin and granzymes in armed effector CD8 cells, so that the supply of lytic granules is replenished. This makes it possible for a single CD8 T cell to kill many targets in succession.

Fig. 7.38 Effector molecules are released from T-cell granules in a highly polar fashion. The granules of cytotoxic T cells can be labeled with fluorescent dyes, allowing them to be seen under the microscope, and their movements followed by time-lapse photography. Here, we show a series of pictures taken during the interaction of a cytotoxic T cell with a target cell, which is eventually killed. In the top panel, at time = 0, the T cell (upper left) has just made contact with a target cell (diagonally below). At this time, the granules of the T cell, labeled with a red fluorescent dye, are distant from the point of contact. In the second panel, after 1 minute has elapsed, the granules have begun to move towards the target cell, a move that has essentially been completed in the third panel, after 4 minutes. After 40 minutes, in the last panel, the granule contents have been released into the space between the T cell and the target, which has begun to undergo apoptosis (note the fragmented nucleus). The T cell will now disengage from the target cell and can recognize and kill other targets. Photographs courtesy of G Griffiths.

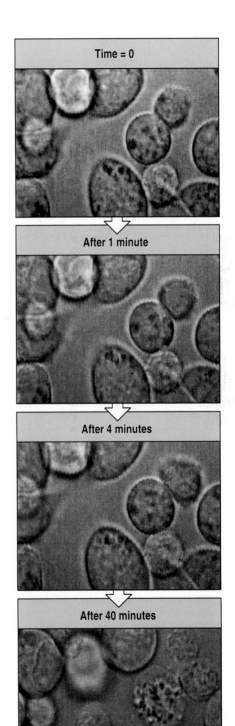

Time = 0

After 1 minute

After 4 minutes

After 40 minutes

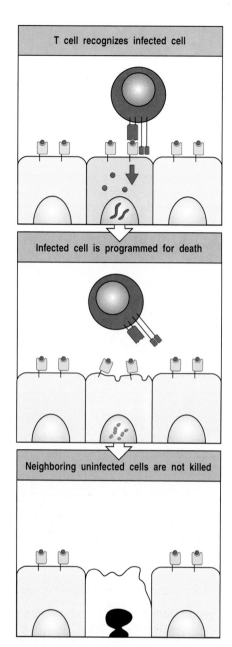

T cell recognizes infected cell

Infected cell is programmed for death

Neighboring uninfected cells are not killed

Fig. 7.39 Cytotoxic T cells kill target cells bearing specific antigen while sparing neighboring uninfected cells. All the cells in a tissue are susceptible to lysis by the cytotoxins of armed effector CD8 T cells but only infected cells are killed. Specific recognition by the T-cell receptor identifies which target cell to kill, and the polarized release of granules (not shown) ensures that neighboring cells are spared.

7-25   Cytotoxic T cells also act by releasing cytokines.

Although the secretion of perforin and granzymes is a major mechanism by which CD8 cytotoxic T cells eliminate infection, with expression of Fas ligand playing a lesser role, most cytotoxic CD8 T cells also release IFN-γ, TNF-α, and TNF-β, which contribute to host defense in several other ways. IFN-γ directly inhibits viral replication, and also induces increased expression of MHC class I and peptide transporter molecules in infected cells. This increases the chance that infected cells will be recognized as target cells for cytotoxic attack. IFN-γ also activates macrophages, recruiting them to sites of infection, both as effector cells and as antigen-presenting cells. The activation of macrophages by IFN-γ is a critical component of the host immune response to intracellular protozoan pathogens such as *Toxoplasma gondii*. IFN-γ also has a secondary role in reducing the tryptophan concentration within responsive cells and thus can kill intracellular parasites, effectively by starvation. TNF-α or TNF-β can synergize with IFN-γ in macrophage activation, and in killing some target cells through a cytokine-mediated pathway. Thus, armed cytotoxic CD8 effector T cells act in a variety of ways to limit the spread of cytosolic pathogens. The relative importance of these mechanisms remains to be determined.

Summary.

Armed CD8 cytotoxic effector T cells are essential in host defense against pathogens that live in the cytosol, the commonest of which are viruses. These cytotoxic T cells can kill any cell harboring such pathogens by recognizing foreign peptides that are transported to the cell surface bound to MHC class I molecules. CD8 cytotoxic T cells carry out their killing function by releasing two types of preformed cytotoxins: the granzymes, which seem able to induce apoptosis in any type of target cell, and the pore-forming protein perforin, which punches holes in the target-cell membrane through which the granzymes can enter. A membrane-bound molecule, the Fas ligand, expressed by CD8 and some CD4 T cells, is also capable of inducing apoptosis by binding to Fas on target cells. These properties allow the cytotoxic T cell to attack and destroy virtually any cell that is infected with a cytosolic pathogen. Cytotoxic CD8 T cells also produce IFN-γ, which is an inhibitor of viral replication and an important inducer of MHC class I expression and macrophage activation. Cytotoxic T cells kill infected targets with great precision, sparing adjacent normal cells. This precision is critical in minimizing tissue damage, while allowing the eradication of infected cells.

Macrophage activation by armed CD4 T$_H$1 cells.

Some microorganisms, such as mycobacteria, the causative agents of tuberculosis and leprosy, are intracellular pathogens that grow primarily in phagolysosomes of macrophages. There they are shielded from the effects of both antibodies and cytotoxic T cells. These microbes maintain themselves in the usually hostile environment of the phagocyte by inhibiting lysosomal fusion to the phagolysosomes in which they grow, or by preventing the acidification of these vesicles that is required to activate lysosomal proteases. Such microorganisms are eliminated when the macrophage is activated by a T$_H$1 cell. Armed T$_H$1 cells act by synthesizing membrane-associated proteins and a range of soluble cytokines whose local and distant actions coordinate the immune response to these intracellular pathogens. Armed T$_H$1 effector cells can also activate macrophages to kill recently ingested pathogens.

7-26   **Armed T$_H$1 cells have a central role in macrophage activation.**

Macrophages can recognize and ingest many types of extracellular bacteria, thereby destroying the bacteria and at the same time presenting peptides derived from them to CD4 T cells. This can lead to the generation of armed effector CD4 T cells specific for the ingested microorganism. An important function of these armed effector T cells is to act back on the macrophages themselves, enhancing their ability to kill ingested bacteria, many of which have evolved strategies for surviving and proliferating inside phagocytic cells. The induction of antimicrobial mechanisms in macrophages is known as **macrophage activation** and is the principal effector action of T$_H$1 cells. Among the extracellular pathogens that are killed when macrophages are activated is *Pneumocystis carinii*, which, because of the deficiency of CD4 T cells, is a common cause of death in people with AIDS. Macrophage activation can be measured by the ability of activated macrophages to damage a broad spectrum of microbes and certain tumor cells. This ability to act on extracellular targets extends to healthy self cells, which means that macrophages must normally be maintained in a non-activated state.

Macrophages require two signals for activation. One of these is provided by IFN-γ, while the other can be provided by a variety of means, and is required to sensitize the macrophage to respond to IFN-γ. Armed T$_H$1 cells can deliver both signals. IFN-γ is the most characteristic cytokine produced by armed T$_H$1 cells on interacting with their specific target cells, while the CD40 ligand expressed by the T$_H$1 cell delivers the sensitizing signal by contacting CD40 on the macrophage (Fig. 7.40). CD8 T cells are also an important source of IFN-γ and can activate macrophages presenting antigens derived from cytosolic proteins; mice lacking MHC class I molecules (and which therefore have no CD8 T cells) show increased susceptibility to some parasite infections. Sensitization of the macrophage can be induced by very small amounts of bacterial lipopolysaccharide, and this latter pathway may be particularly important when CD8 T cells are the primary source of the IFN-γ. It is also possible that membrane-associated TNF-α or TNF-β can substitute for CD40 ligand in macrophage activation. The cell-associated molecules apparently stimulate the macrophage to secrete TNF-α, and antibody to TNF-α can inhibit macrophage activation. T$_H$2 cells are inefficient macrophage activators because they produce IL-10, a cytokine that can deactivate macrophages, and they do not produce IFN-γ. However, they do express CD40 ligand and can deliver the contact-dependent signal required to activate macrophages to respond to IFN-γ.

7-27   **The expression of cytokines and membrane-associated molecules by armed CD4 T$_H$1 cells requires new RNA and protein synthesis.**

Within minutes of the recognition of specific antigen by armed cytotoxic effector CD8 T cells, directed exocytosis of preformed perforins and granzymes programs the target cell to die via apoptosis. In contrast, when armed T$_H$1 cells encounter their specific ligand, they must synthesize *de novo* the cytokines and cell-surface molecules that mediate their effects. This process requires hours rather than minutes, so T$_H$1 cells must adhere to their target cells for far longer than cytotoxic T cells.

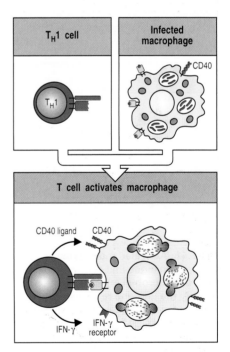

Fig. 7.40 T$_H$1 cells activate macrophages to become highly microbicidal. When a T$_H$1 cell specific for a bacterial peptide contacts an infected macrophage, the T cell is induced to secrete the macrophage-activating factor IFN-γ and to express CD40 ligand. Together, these newly synthesized T$_H$1 proteins activate the macrophage.

Recognition of its target by a T$_H$1 cell rapidly induces transcription of cytokine genes and new protein synthesis begins within one hour of receptor triggering. The newly synthesized cytokines are then delivered directly through microvesicles of the constitutive secretory pathway to the site of contact between the T-cell membrane and the macrophage. It is thought that the newly synthesized cell-surface CD40 ligand is also expressed in this polarized fashion. This means that, although all macrophages have receptors for IFN-γ, the macrophage actually displaying antigen to the armed T$_H$1 cell is far more likely to become activated by it than are neighboring uninfected macrophages.

Activated macrophages can be very destructive to host tissues. It is therefore important not only that delivery of IFN-γ be focused on the infected cells but that its production be shut off immediately the T cell loses contact with the infected macrophage. This seems to be achieved in two ways. First, the mRNA encoding IFN-γ, like that encoding a variety of other cytokines, contains a sequence (AUUUA)$_n$ in its 3' untranslated region that greatly reduces its half-life, and this serves to limit the period of cytokine production. Second, activation of the T cell appears to induce production of a new protein that promotes cytokine mRNA degradation: treatment of activated effector T cells with the protein synthesis inhibitor cycloheximide greatly increases the level of cytokine mRNA. The rapid destruction of cytokine mRNA, together with the focal delivery of IFN-γ at the point of contact between the activated T$_H$1 cell and its macrophage target, thus limits the action of the effector T cell to the infected macrophage. We shall see in Chapter 8, when we consider the activation of B cells by T$_H$2 cells, that the same mechanisms direct and limit T-cell help to the specific antigen-binding B cell.

7-28   **Activation of macrophages by armed T$_H$1 cells promotes bacterial killing and must be tightly regulated to avoid damage to host tissues.**

T$_H$1 cells activate infected macrophages through cell contact and the focal secretion of IFN-γ. This generates a series of biochemical responses that converts the macrophage into a potent antimicrobial effector cell (Fig. 7.41). Activated macrophages fuse their lysosomes more efficiently to phagosomes, exposing intracellular or recently ingested extracellular bacteria to a variety of microbicidal lysosomal enzymes. Activated macrophages make oxygen radicals and nitric oxide (NO), both of which have potent antimicrobial activity, as well as synthesizing antimicrobial peptides.

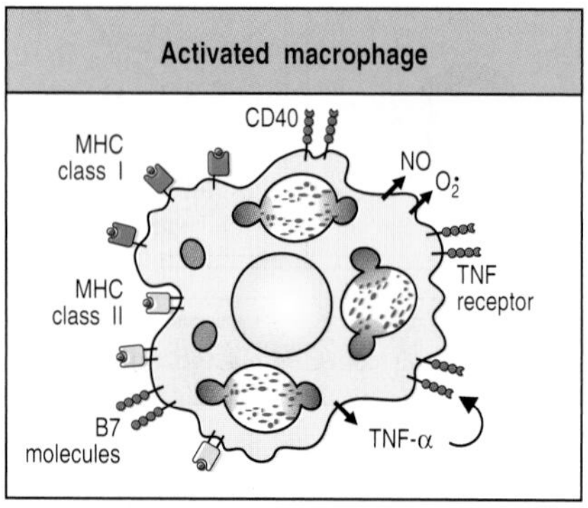

Additional changes in the activated macrophage help to amplify the immune response. The number of MHC class II molecules, B7 molecules, and CD40 and TNF receptors on the macrophage surface increases, making the cell both more effective at presenting antigen to fresh T cells, which may thereby be recruited as effector cells, and more responsive to CD40 ligand and to TNF-α. TNF-α synergizes with IFN-γ in macrophage activation, particularly in the induction of the reactive nitrogen metabolite NO, which has broad antimicrobial activity. The NO is produced by the enzyme **inducible NO synthase (iNOS)**, and mice that have had the gene for iNOS knocked out are highly susceptible to several intracellular pathogens. Activated macrophages secrete IL-12, which directs the differentiation of activated naive CD4 T cells into T$_H$1 effector cells, as we shall learn in Chapter 9. These and many other surface and secreted molecules of activated macrophages are instrumental in the effector actions of macrophages in cell-mediated as well as humoral immune responses, which we shall discuss in Chapter 8, and in recruiting other immune cells to sites of infection, a function to which we return in Chapter 9.

Fig. 7.41 Activated macrophages undergo changes that greatly increase their antimicrobial effectiveness and amplify the immune response. Activated macrophages increase their expression of CD40 and TNF receptors, and secrete TNF-α. This autocrine stimulus synergizes with IFN-γ secreted by T$_H$1 cells to increase the antimicrobial action of the macrophage, in particular by inducing the production of nitric oxide (NO) and oxygen radicals (O$_2^-$). The macrophage also upregulates its B7 proteins in response to CD40 ligand expression by the T cell, and increases its expression of class II MHC molecules, thus allowing further activation of resting CD4 T cells.

Since activated macrophages are extremely effective in destroying pathogens, one may ask why macrophages are not simply maintained in a state of constant activation. Besides the fact that macrophages consume large quantities of energy to maintain the activated state, macrophage activation *in vivo* is usually associated with localized tissue destruction that apparently results from the release of antimicrobial mediators such as oxygen radicals, NO and proteases, which are also toxic to host cells. The ability of activated macrophages to release toxic mediators is important in host defense because it enables them to attack large extracellular pathogens that they cannot ingest, such as parasitic worms. This can only be achieved, however, at the expense of tissue damage. Tight regulation of the activity of macrophages by T$_H$1 cells thus allows the specific and effective deployment of this potent means of host defense, while minimizing local tissue damage and energy consumption.

In addition to the mechanisms controlling IFN-γ synthesis already discussed, macrophage activation itself is markedly inhibited by cytokines such as transforming growth factor-β (TGF-β), IL-4, IL-10, and IL-13. Since several of these inhibitory cytokines are produced by T$_H$2 cells, the induction of CD4 T cells belonging to the T$_H$2 subset represents an important pathway for controlling the effector functions of activated macrophages.

7-29   **T$_H$1 cells coordinate the host response to intracellular pathogens.**

The activation of macrophages by IFN-γ secreted by armed T$_H$1 cells expressing CD40 ligand is central to the host response to pathogens that proliferate in macrophage vesicles. In mice in which the IFN-γ gene or the CD40 ligand gene has been destroyed by targeted gene disruption, production of antimicrobial agents by macrophages is impaired, and the animals succumb to sublethal doses of *Mycobacteria* spp., *Leishmania* spp., and vaccinia virus. Mice lacking a TNF receptor also show increased susceptibility to these pathogens. However, while IFN-γ and CD40 ligand are probably the most important effector molecules synthesized by T$_H$1 cells, the immune response to pathogens that proliferate in macrophage vesicles is complex, and other cytokines secreted by T$_H$1 cells have a crucial role in coordinating these responses (Fig. 7.42). Macrophages that are chronically infected with intracellular bacteria may lose the ability to become activated. Such cells would provide a reservoir of infection that is shielded from immune attack. Activated T$_H$1 cells can express Fas ligand and thus kill a limited range of target cells that express Fas, including macrophages, thereby destroying these infected cells.

While some intravesicular bacteria pose a hazard by incapacitating chronically infected macrophages, others, including some mycobacteria and *Listeria monocytogenes* can escape from cell vesicles and enter the cytoplasm where they are not susceptible to macrophage activation. Their presence can, however, be detected by CD8 cytotoxic T cells, which can release them by killing the cell. The pathogens released when macrophages are killed either by T$_H$1 cells or by CD8 cytotoxic T cells can be taken up by freshly recruited macrophages still capable of activation to antimicrobial activity.

Another very important function of T$_H$1 cells is recruitment of phagocytic cells to sites of infection. T$_H$1 cells recruit macrophages by two mechanisms. First, they make the hematopoietic growth factors IL-3 and GM-CSF, which stimulate the production of new phagocytic cells in the bone marrow. Second, TNF-α and TNF-β, which are secreted by T$_H$1 cells at

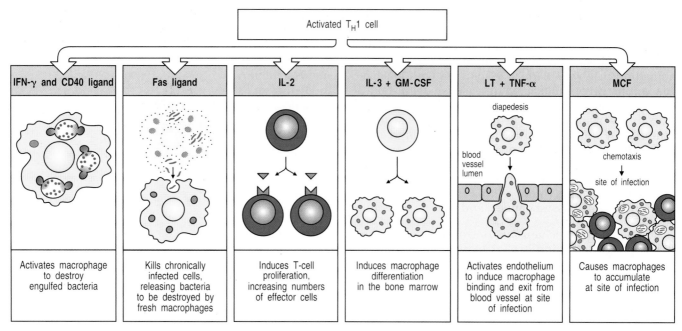

Fig. 7.42 The immune response to intracellular bacteria is coordinated by activated T$_H$1 cells. The activation of T$_H$1 cells by infected macrophages results in the synthesis of cytokines that both activate the macrophage and coordinate the immune response to intracellular pathogens. IFN-γ and CD40 ligand synergize in activating the macrophage, which allows it to kill engulfed pathogens. Chronically infected macrophages lose the ability to kill intracellular bacteria, and Fas ligand or TNF-β (LT, lymphotoxin) produced by the T$_H$1 cell can kill these macrophages, releasing the bacteria, which are taken up and killed by fresh macrophages. In this way, IFN-γ and TNF-β synergize in the removal of intracellular bacteria. IL-2 produced by T$_H$1 cells induces T-cell proliferation and potentiates the release of other cytokines. IL-3 and GM-CSF stimulate the production of new macrophages by acting on hematopoietic stem cells in the bone marrow. New macrophages are recruited to the site of infection by the action of TNF-β and TNF-α (and other cytokines) on vascular endothelium, which signal macrophages to leave the bloodstream and enter the tissues. A chemokine with macrophage chemotactic activity (MCF) signals macrophages to migrate into sites of infection and accumulate there. Thus, the T$_H$1 cell coordinates a macrophage response that is highly effective in destroying intracellular infectious agents.

sites of infection, change the surface properties of endothelial cells so that phagocytes adhere to them, while chemokines like macrophage chemotactic factor (MCF) produced by T$_H$1 cells in the inflammatory response serve to direct the migration of these phagocytic cells through the vascular endothelium to the site of the infection (see Chapter 9).

When microbes effectively resist the microbicidal effects of activated macrophages, chronic infection with inflammation can develop. Often, this has a characteristic pattern, consisting of a central area of macrophages surrounded by activated lymphocytes. This pathological pattern is called **granuloma** (Fig. 7.43). Giant cells consisting of fused macrophages usually form the center of these granulomas. This serves to 'wall-off' pathogens that resist destruction. T$_H$2 cells appear to participate in granulomas along with T$_H$1 cells, perhaps by regulating their activity and preventing widespread tissue damage. In tuberculosis, the center of the large granulomas can become isolated and the cells there die, probably from a combination of lack of oxygen and the cytotoxic effects of activated macrophages. As the dead tissue in the center resembles cheese, this process is called **caseation necrosis**. Thus, activation of inflammatory T cells can cause significant pathology. Its absence, however, leads to the more serious consequence of death from disseminated infection, which is now seen frequently in patients with AIDS and mycobacterial infection.

Fig. 7.43 Granulomas form when an intracellular pathogen or its constituents cannot be totally eliminated. When mycobacteria (red) resist the effects of macrophage activation, a characteristic localized inflammatory response called a granuloma develops. This consists of a central core of infected macrophages. The core may include multinucleated giant cells, which are fused macrophages, surrounded by large macrophages often called epithelioid cells. Mycobacteria can persist in the cells of the granuloma. The central core is surrounded by T cells, many of which are CD4-positive. The exact mechanisms by which this balance is achieved, and how it breaks down, are unknown. Granulomas, as seen in the bottom panels, also form in the lungs and elsewhere in a disease known as sarcoidosis, which may be caused by occult mycobacterial infection. Photograph courtesy of J Orrell.

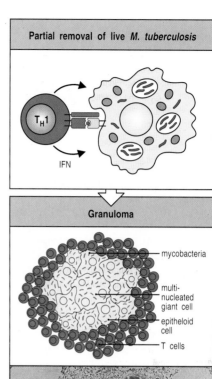

Partial removal of live *M. tuberculosis*

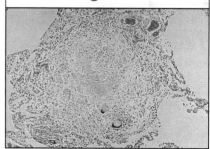

Granuloma

- mycobacteria
- multi-nucleated giant cell
- epithelioid cell
- T cells

Summary.

CD4 T cells that can activate macrophages play a critical role in host defense against those intracellular and engulfed extracellular pathogens that resist killing in non-activated macrophages. Macrophage activation is mediated both by membrane-bound signals delivered by activated T_H1 cells, as well as by their secretion of the potent macrophage-activating cytokine IFN-γ. Once activated, the macrophage can kill intracellular and ingested bacteria. Activated macrophages can also cause local tissue damage, which explains why this activity must be strictly regulated by T cells. T_H1 cells produce a range of cytokines and surface molecules that not only activate infected macrophages but can also kill chronically infected senescent macrophages, stimulate bone marrow production of new macrophages, and recruit fresh macrophages to sites of infection. Thus, T_H1 cells have a central role in controlling and coordinating host defense against certain intracellular pathogens. It is likely that the absence of this function explains the preponderance of infections with intracellular pathogens in adult AIDS patients.

Summary to Chapter 7.

Armed effector T cells play a critical role in almost all adaptive immune responses. Immune responses are initiated when naive T cells encounter specific antigen on the surface of a professional antigen-presenting cell that also expresses effective co-stimulatory molecules, usually B7.1 and B7.2. The activated T cells produce IL-2, which drives them to proliferate and differentiate into armed effector T cells. All T-cell effector functions involve cell interactions. When armed effector T cells recognize specific antigen on target cells, they release mediators that act directly on the target cell, altering its behavior. The triggering of armed effector T cells by peptide:MHC complexes is independent of co-stimulation, so that any infected target cell can be activated or destroyed by an armed effector T cell. CD8 cytotoxic T cells kill target cells infected with cytosolic pathogens, removing sites of pathogen replication. CD4 T_H1 cells activate macrophages to kill intracellular parasites. CD4 T_H2 cells are essential in the activation of B cells to secrete the antibodies that mediate humoral immune responses directed against extracellular pathogens, as will be seen in Chapter 8. Thus, effector T cells control virtually all known effector mechanisms of the adaptive immune response.

General references.

Cohen, J.J., Duke, R.C., Fadok, V.A., and Sellins, K.S.: **Apoptosis and programmed cell death in immunity.** *Ann. Rev. Immunol.* 1993, **10**:267-293.

Ihle, J.N.: **Cytokine receptor signaling.** *Nature* 1995, **377**:591–594.

Janeway, C.A., Bottomly, K.: **Signals and signs for lymphocyte responses.** *Cell* 1994, **76**:275–285.

Linsley, P.S. and Ledbetter, J.A.: **The role of the CD28 receptor during T-cell responses to antigen.** *Ann. Rev. Immunol.* 1993, **11**:191-221.

Mosmann, T.R. and Coffman, R.L.: **T$_H$1 and T$_H$2 cells: Different patterns of lymphokine secretion lead to different functional properties.** *Ann. Rev. Immunol.* 1989, **7**:145-173.

Pigott, R., and Power, C.: *The Adhesion Molecule Facts Book.* Academic Press, London, 1993.

Springer, T.A.: **Traffic signals for lymphocyte recirculation and leukocyte emigration: The multistep paradigm.** *Cell* 1994, **76**:301—314.

Stout, R.D.: **Macrophage activation by T cells: cognate and non-cognate signals.** *Curr. Opin. Immunol.* 1993, **5**:398-403

Section references.

| 7-1 | The initial interaction of naive T cells with antigen occurs in peripheral lymphoid organs. |

Picker, L.J. and Butcher, E.C.: **Physiological and molecular mechanisms of lymphocyte homing.** *Ann. Rev. Immunol.* 1993, **10**:561-591.

Tilney, N.L. and Gowans, J.L.: **The sensitization of rats by allografts transplanted to allymphatic pedicles of skin.** *J. Exp. Med.* 1971, **113**:951.

| 7-2 | Lymphocyte migration, activation, and effector function depend on cell-adhesion molecules. |

Hogg, N. and Landis, R.C.: **Adhesion molecules in cell interactions.** *Curr. Opin. Immunol.* 1993, **5**:383-390.

Picker, L.J.: **Control of lymphocyte homing.** *Curr. Opin. Immunol.* 1994, **6**:394–406.

| 7-3 | The initial interaction of T cells with antigen-presenting cells is also mediated by cell-adhesion molecules. |

Dustin, M.L. and Springer, T.A.: **T-cell receptor crosslinking transiently stimulates adhesiveness through LFA-1.** *Nature* 1989, **341**:619-624.

Hahn, W.C., Rosenstein, Y., Clavo, V., Burakoff, S.J., and Bierer, B.: **A distinct cytoplasmic domain of CD2 regulates ligand avidity and T-cell responsiveness to antigen.** *Proc. Natl. Acad. Sci. 1992,* **89**:7179-7183.

Shimizu, Y., van Seventer, G., Horgan, K.J., and Shaw, S.: **Roles of adhesion molecules in T-cell recognition: fundamental similarities between four integrins on resting human T cells (LFA-1, VLA-4, VLA-5, VLA-6) in expression, binding, and co-stimulation.** *Immunol. Rev.* 1990, **114**:109-143.

| 7-4 | Both specific ligand and co-stimulatory signals provided by a professional antigen-presenting cell are required for the clonal expansion of naive T cells. |

Liu, Y. and Janeway, C.A. Jr.: **Cells that present both specific ligand and co-stimulatory activity are the most efficient inducers of clonal expansion of normal CD4 T cells.** *Proc. Natl. Acad. Sci. 1992,* **89**:3845-3949.

Rudd, C.E.: **Upstream-Downstream: CD28 cosignaling pathways and T cell function.** *Immunity* 1996, **4**:527–534.

Sharpe, A.H.: **Analysis of lymphocyte costimulation in vivo using transgenic and 'knockout' mice.** *Curr. Opin. Immunol.* 1995, **7**:389–395.

Tivol, E.A., Borriello, F., Schweitzer, A.N., Lynch, W.P., Bluestone, J.A., and Sharpe, A.H.: **Loss of CTLA-4 leads to massive lymphoproliferation and fatal multiorgan tissue destruction, revealing a critical negative regulatory role of CTLA-4.** *Immunity* 1995, **3**:541–547.

Waterhouse, P., Penninger, J.M., Timms, E., Wakeham, A., Shahinian, A., Lee, K.P., Thompson, C.B., Griesser, H., and Mak, T.W.: **Lymphoproliferative disorders with early lethality in mice deficient in CTLA-4.** *Science* 1995, **270**:985–988.

| 7-5 | Macrophages are scavenger cells that can be induced by pathogens to present foreign antigens to naive T cells. |

Razi-Wolf, Z., Freeman, G.J., Galvin, F., Benacerraf, B., Nadler, L., and Reiser, H.: **Expression and function of the murine B7 antigen, the major co-stimulatory molecule expressed by peritoneal exudate cells.** *Proc. Natl. Acad. Sci. 1992,* **89**:4210-4214.

| 7-6 | Dendritic cells are highly efficient inducers of T-cell activation. |

Sallusto, F., Lanzavecchia, A.: **Efficient presentation of soluble antigen by cultured human dendritic cells is maintained by granulocyte/macrophage colony-stimulating factor plus interleukin-4 and downregulated by tumor necrosis factor.** *J. Exp. Med.* 1994, **179**:1109–1118

Steinman, R.M.: **The dendritic cell system and its role in immunogenicity.** *Ann. Rev. Immunol.* 1993, **9**:271-296.

| 7-7 | B cells are highly efficient at presenting antigens that bind to their surface immunoglobulin. |

Lanzavecchia, A.: **Receptor-mediated antigen uptake and its effect on antigen presentation to class II-restricted T lymphocytes.** *Ann. Rev. Immunol.* 1993, **8**:773-793.

| 7-8 | Activated T cells synthesize the T-cell growth factor interleukin-2 and its receptor. |

Jain, J., Loh, C. Rao, A.: **Transcriptional regulation of the IL-2 gene.** *Curr. Opin. Immunol.* 1995, **7**:333-342.

Minami, Y., Kono, T., Miyazaki, T., and Taniguchi, T.: **The IL-2 receptor complex: its structure, function, and target genes.** *Ann. Rev. Immunol.* 1993, **11**:245-267.

| 7-9 | The co-stimulatory signal is necessary for the synthesis and secretion of IL-2. |

Fraser, J.D., Irving, B.A., Crabtree, G.R., and Weiss, A.: **Regulation of interleukin-2 gene enhancer activity by the T-cell accessory molecule CD28.** *Science* 1991, **251**:313-316.

Lindsten, T., June, C.H., Ledbetter, J.A., Stella, G., and Thompson, C.B.: **Regulation of lymphokine messenger RNA stability by a surface-mediated T-cell activation pathway.** *Science* 1989, **244**:339-342.

| 7-10 | Antigen recognition in the absence of co-stimulation leads to T-cell tolerance. |

Fields, P.E., Gajewski, T.F., Frank, W.F.: **Blocked ras activation in anergic CD4$^+$ T cells.** *Science* 1996, **273**:1276–1278

Guerder, S., Meyerhoff, J., and Flavell, R.A.: **The role of the T cell costimulator B7.1 in autoimmunity and the induction and maintenance of tolerance to peripheral antigen.** *Immunity* 1994, **1**:155-166.

Lenschow, D.J., Walunas, J.A.: **CD28/B7 System of T cell costimulstion.** *Ann. Rev. Immunol.* 1996, **14**:233-258.

Li, W., Whaley, C.D., Mondino, A., Mueller, D.L.: **Blocked signal transduction to the ERK and JNK protein kinases in anergic CD4$^+$ T cells.** *Science* 1996, **273**:1272–1276

Mueller, D.L., Jenkins, M.K.: **Molecular mechanisms underlying functional T-cell unresponsiveness.** *Curr. Opin. Immunol.* 1995, **7**:375–381.

7-11 Proliferating T cells differentiate into armed effector T cells with altered surface properties that do not require co-stimulation to act.

Wong, S.F., Visintin, I., Wen, L, Flavell, R.A., and Janeway, C.A. Jr. **CD8 T cell clones from young NOD islets can transfer rapid onset of diabetes in NOD mice in the absence of CD4 cells.** *J. Exp. Med.* 1996, **183**:67-76.

7-12 The differentiation of CD4 T cells into T$_H$2 or T$_H$1 effector cells is the crucial event in determining whether humoral or cell-mediated immunity will predominate.

Kamogawa, Y., Minasi, L.A., Carding, S.R., Bottomly, K., and Flavell, R.A.: **The relationship of IL-4 and IFN-γ producing T cells studied by lineage ablation of IL-4-producing cells.** *Cell* 1993 **75**:985-995.

7-13 Naive CD8 T cells can be activated in different ways to become armed cytotoxic effector cells.

Azuma, M., Cayabyab, M., Buck, D., Phillips, J.H., Lanier, L.L.: **CD28 interaction with B7 co-stimulates primary allogeneic proliferative responses and cytotoxicity mediated by small, resting T lymphocytes.** *J. Exp. Med.* 1992, **175**:353-360.

7-14 Effector T-cell interactions with target cells are initiated by antigen non-specific cell-adhesion molecules.

O'Rourke, A.M. and Mescher, M.F.: **Cytotoxic T lymphocyte activation involves a cascade of signaling and adhesion events.** *Nature* 1992, **358**:253-255.

Rodrigues, M., Nussezwieg, R.S., Romero, P., and Zavala, F.: **The** *in vivo* **cytotoxic activity of CD8$^+$ T-cell clones correlates with their levels of expression of adhesion molecules.** *J. Exp. Med.* 1992, **175**:895-905.

van Seventer, G.A., Simuzi, Y., and Shaw, S.: **Roles of multiple accesory molecules in T-cell activation.** *Curr. Opin. Immunol.* 1991, **3**:294-303.

7-15 The T-cell receptor complex directs the release of effector molecules and focuses them on the target cell.

Griffiths, G.M.: **The cell biology of CTL killing.** *Curr. Opin. Immunol.* 1995, **7**:343-348.

7-16 The effector functions of T cells are determined by the array of effector molecules they produce.

Armitage, R.J., Fanslow, W.C., Strockbine, L., Sato, T.A., Cliffors, K.N., MacDuff, B.M., Anderson, D.M., Gimpel, S.D., Davis Smith, T., Maliszewski, C.R.: **Molecular and biological characterization of a murine ligand for CD40.** *Nature* 1992, **357**:80-82.

7-17 Cytokines can act locally or at a distance.

Arai, K., Lee, F., Miyajima, A., Miyatake, S., Arai, N., Yokota, T.: **Cytokines: co-ordinators of immune and inflammatory responses.** *Ann. Rev. Biochem.* 1990, **59**:783.

7-18 Cytokines and their receptors fall into distinct families of structurally related proteins.

Thompson, A.: *The cytokine Handbook.* 2nd ed. Academic Press, San Diego, 1994.

Taga, T., Kishimoto, T.: **Signaling mechanisms through cytokine receptors that share signal tranducing receptors components.** *Curr. Opin. Immunol.* 1995, **7**:17-23.

7-19 Binding of cytokines to their receptors triggers gene activation by activating *Janus* kinases which then activate STAT proteins.

Farrar, M.A., Schreiber, R.D.: **The molecular cell biology of interferon-γ and its receptor.** *Ann. Rev. Immunol.*1993, **11**:571-611.

Ihle, J., Witthuhn, B.A., Quelle, A.R., Yamanoto, K., Silvennoinen, O.: **Signaling through the hematopoietic cytokine receptors.** *Ann. Rev. Immunol.* 1995, **13**: 369-398.

Karnitz, L.M., Abraham, R.T.: **Cytokine receptor signaling mechanisms.** *Curr. Opin. Immunol.* 1995, **7**:320-326.

7-20 The TNF family of cytokines are trimeric proteins, often cell-surface associated.

Armitage, R.J.: **Tumor necrosis factor receptor superfamily members and their ligands.** *Curr. Opin. Immunol.* 1994, **6**:407-413.

7-21 Cytotoxic T cells can induce target cells to undergo programmed cell death.

Berke, G.: **Lymphocyte-triggered internal target disintegration.** *Immunol. Today* 1991, **12**:396-399.

Henkart, P.A.: **Lymphocyte-mediated cytotoxicology: two pathways and multiple effector molecules.** *Immunity* 1994, **1**:343-346.

Squier, M.K.T., Cohen, J.J.: **Cell-mediated cytotoxic mechanisms.** *Curr. Opin. Immunol.* 1994, **6**:447-452.

7-22 Cytotoxic proteins that trigger apoptosis are contained in the granules of CD8 cytotoxic T cells.

Kägi, B., Ledermann, K., Bürki, R.: **Molecular mechanisms of lympho-cyte-mediated cytotoxicity and their role in immunological protection and pathogenesis** *in vivo. Ann. Rev. Immunol.* 1994, **12**:207-232.

Shiver, J.W., Su, L., and Henkart, P.A.: **Cytotoxicity with target DNA breakdown by rat basophilic leukemia cells expressing both cytolysin and granzyme A.** *Cell* 1992, **71**:315-322.

7-23 Membrane proteins of activated CD8 T cells and some CD4 effector T cells can also activate apoptosis.

Fisher, G.H., Rosenberg, E.J., Straus, S.E., Dale, J.K., Middleton, L.A., Lin, A.Y., Strober, W., Leonardo, M.J., and Puck, J.M. **Dominant interfering Fas gene mutations impair apoptosis in a human autoimmune lymphoproliferative syndrome.** *Cell* 1995, **81**:935-946.

Suda, T., Takahashi, T., Goldstein P., and Nagata, S.: **Molecular cloning and expression of the Fas ligand, a novel member of the tumor necrosis factor family.** *Cell* 1993, **75**:1169-1178.

Watanbe F.R., Branna, C.I., Copeland, N.G., Jenkins, N.A., and Nagata, S.: **Lymphoproliferation disorder in mice explained by defects in Fas antigen that mediates apoptosis.** *Nature* 1992, **356**:314-317.

7-24 Cytotoxic T cells selectively kill targets expressing specific antigen.

Kuppers, R.C. and Henney, C.S.: **Studies on the mechanism of lymphocyte-mediated cytolysis. IX. Relationships between antigen recognition and lytic expression in killer T cells.** *J. Immunol.* 1977, **118**:71-76.

7-25 Cytotoxic T cells also act by releasing cytokines.

Ramshaw, I., Ruby, J., Ramsay, A., Ada, G., and Karupiah, G.: **Expression of cytokines by recombiant vaccinia viruses: a model for studying cytokines in virus infections** *in vivo*. *Immunol. Rev.* 1992 ,**127**:157-182.

7-26 Armed T$_H$1 cells have a central role in macrophage activation.

Munoz Fernandez, M.A., Fernandez, M.A., and Fresno, M.: **Synergism between tumor necrosis factor-alpha and interferon-gamma on macrophage activation for the killing of intracellular** *Trypanosoma crusi* **through a nitric oxide-dependent mechanism.** *Eur. J. Immunol.* 1992, **22**:301-307.

Stout, R. and Bottomly, K.: **Antigen-specific activation of effector macrophages by interferon-gamma producing (T$_H$1) T-cell clones: failure of IL-4 producing (T$_H$2) T-cell clones to activate effector functions in macrophages.** *J. Immunol.* 1989, **142**:760.

7-27 The expression of cytokines and membrane-associated molecules by armed CD4 T$_H$1 cells requires new RNA and protein synthesis.

Shaw, G., and Karmen, R.: **A conserved UAU sequence from the 3′ untranslated region of GM-CSF mRNA mediates selective mRNA degradation.** *Cell* 1986, **46**:659.

7-28 Activation of macrophages by T$_H$1 cells promotes bacterial killing and must be tightly regulated to avoid damage to host tissues.

Paulnock, D.M.: **Macrophage activation by T cells.** *Curr. Opin. Immunol.* 1992, **4**:344-349.

7-29 T$_H$1 cells coordinate the host response to intracellular bacteria and parasites.

Kindler, V., Sappino, A.-P., Grau, G.E., Piquet, P.-F., Vassali, P.: **The inducing role of tumor necrosis factor in the development of bactericidal granulomas during BCG development.** *Cell* 1989, **56**:731-740.

McInnes, A. and Rennick, D.M.: **Interleukin-4 induces cultured monocytes/ macrophages to form giant multinucleated cells.** *J. Exp. Med.* 1988, **167**:598-611.

Oppenheim, J.J., Zachariae, C.O.C., Mukaida, W., and Matsushima, K.: **Properties of the novel proinflammatory supergene intercrine cytokine family.** *Ann. Rev. Immunol.* 1991, **9**:617.

Yamamura, M., Uyemura, K., Deans, R,J., Weinberg, K., Rea, T.H., Bloom, B.R., and Modlin, R.L.: **Defining protective responses to pathogens: cytokine profiles in leprosy lesions.** *Science* 1991, **254**:277-279.

The Humoral Immune Response

8

Many of the bacteria that are most important in human infectious diseases multiply in the extracellular spaces of the body, and most intracellular pathogens must spread by moving from cell to cell through the extracellular fluids. The humoral immune response leads to the destruction of extracellular microorganisms and prevents the spread of intracellular infections. This is achieved by antibodies secreted by B lymphocytes.

There are three main ways in which antibodies contribute to immunity (Fig. 8.1). Viruses and intracellular bacteria, which need to enter cells in order to grow, spread from cell to cell by binding to specific molecules on their target cell surface. Antibodies that bind to the pathogen can prevent this and are said to **neutralize** the pathogen. Neutralization by antibodies is also important in protection from toxins. Other types of bacteria multiply outside cells, and antibodies protect against these pathogens mainly by facilitating pathogen uptake into phagocytic cells that are specialized to destroy ingested bacteria. There are two ways in which this can occur. In the first case, bound antibodies coating the pathogen are recognized by specific **Fc receptors** on the surface of phagocytic cells. Coating the surface of a pathogen to enhance phagocytosis in this way is called **opsonization**. Alternatively, antibodies binding to the surface of a pathogen may activate the proteins of the **complement** system. Complement proteins bound to the pathogen also opsonize it by binding **complement receptors** on phagocytes. Other complement components recruit phagocytic cells to the site of infection, and the terminal components of complement can lyse certain microorganisms directly by forming pores in their membranes. Which effector mechanisms are recruited in a particular response is determined by the **isotypes** of the antibodies produced.

The activation of B cells and their differentiation into antibody-secreting cells is triggered by antigen and often requires **helper T cells**. The term 'helper T cell' is often used synonymously with T_H2 cells, but a subset of T_H1 cells can also play a helping role in B-cell activation. We will therefore use the term 'helper T cell' to mean any armed effector CD4 T cell that can activate a B cell. Helper T cells also control **isotype switching** and play a role in initiating **somatic hypermutation** of antibody variable-region genes and directing the affinity maturation of antibodies that occurs during the course of a humoral immune response. In the first part of this chapter, we shall describe the interactions of B cells with helper T cells and the mechanism of affinity maturation in the specialized microenvironment of peripheral lymphoid tissues. In the rest of the chapter, we shall discuss in detail the mechanisms whereby antibodies contain and eliminate infections.

Fig. 8.1 The humoral immune response is mediated by antibody molecules that are secreted by plasma cells. Antigen that binds to the B cell antigen receptor signals B cells and is, at the same time, internalized and processed into peptides that activate armed helper T cells. Signals from the bound antigen and from the helper T cell induce the B cell to proliferate and differentiate into a plasma cell secreting specific antibody (top two panels). There are three main ways in which these antibodies protect the host from infection (bottom panels). They may inhibit the toxic effects or infectivity of pathogens by binding to them: this is termed neutralization (left panel). By coating the pathogens, they may enable accessory cells that recognize the Fc pieces of arrays of antibodies to ingest and kill the pathogen, a process called opsonization (center panel). Antibodies can also trigger the complement cascade of proteins, which strongly enhance opsonization and can directly kill some bacterial cells (right panel).

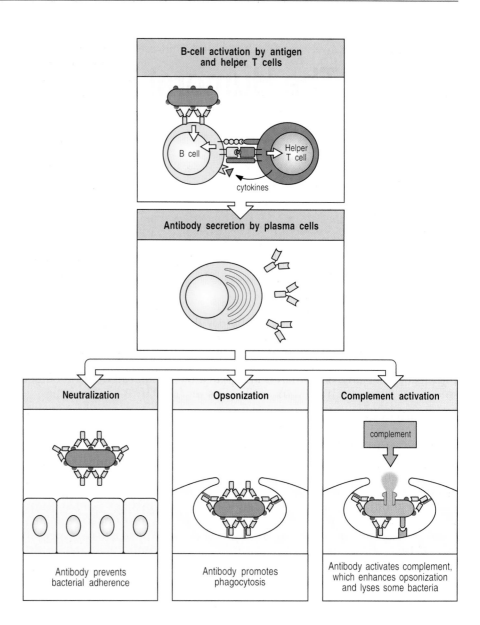

Antibody production by B lymphocytes.

The surface immunoglobulin that serves as the antigen receptor on B lymphocytes plays two roles in their activation. First, like the antigen receptor on T cells, it transmits signals directly to the cell's interior when it binds antigen (see Section 3-25). Second, it delivers the antigen to intracellular sites where it is degraded and from where it is returned to the B-cell surface as peptides bound to MHC class II molecules. The peptide:MHC class II complex can then be recognized by antigen-specific armed helper T cells, triggering them to make molecules that, in turn, cause the B cell to proliferate and its progeny to differentiate into antibody-secreting cells. Some microbial antigens can activate B cells directly in the absence of T-cell help and provide a means whereby antibodies can be produced rapidly against many important bacterial pathogens. However, the changes in the functional properties of antibody molecules that result from isotype switching, and the changes in the variable region that occur during affinity maturation, depend upon the interaction of antigen-stimulated B cells with helper T cells and other cells in the peripheral lymphoid organs. Antibodies induced by microbial antigens alone are therefore less variable and less functionally versatile than those induced with T-cell help.

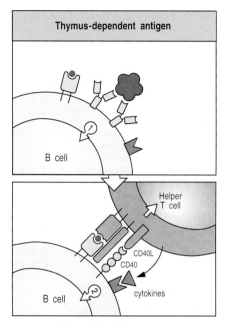

8-1 The antibody response is initiated when B cells bind antigen and are signaled by helper T cells or by certain microbial antigens.

It is a general rule in adaptive immunity that naive antigen-specific lymphocytes cannot be activated by antigen alone. Naive T cells require a co-stimulatory signal from professional antigen-presenting cells; naive B cells require accessory signals that may come either from an armed helper T cell or, in some cases, directly from microbial constituents (Fig. 8.2).

Antibody responses to protein antigens require antigen-specific T-cell help. B cells become effective targets for armed helper T cells when antigen bound by surface immunoglobulin is internalized and returned to the cell surface as peptides bound to MHC class II molecules. Helper T cells that recognize the peptide:MHC complex then deliver activating signals to the B cell. Thus, protein antigens binding to B cells provide both a specific signal to the B cell and a focus for antigen-specific T-cell help (see Fig. 8.2, top two panels). These antigens are unable to induce antibody responses in animals or humans in which the thymus fails to develop and generate peptide-specific T cells, and they are therefore known as **thymus-dependent** or **TD antigens**.

The B cell co-receptor complex of CD19:CD21:CD81 (also known as CD19:CR2:TAPA-1, see Section 3-26) can greatly enhance B-cell responsiveness to antigen. When hen egg lysozyme is coupled with three linked molecules of the complement fragment C3dg, which is a ligand for CD21/CR2 (see Section 8-27), the antigen induces antibody without added adjuvant when used to immunize mice, and at doses as much as 10 000 times smaller than unmodified hen egg lysozyme. Whether this works by increasing B-cell signaling, by inducing co-stimulatory molecules on antigen-binding B cells, or by increasing the uptake of antigen is not yet known.

Although armed helper T cells are required for B-cell responses to protein antigens, many constituents of microbes, such as bacterial polysaccharides, can directly induce B cells to produce antibody in the absence of helper T cells (see Fig. 8.2, bottom panel). These microbial antigens are known as **thymus-independent** or **TI antigens**. Thymus-independent antibody responses can be seen in individuals who lack a thymus and hence functional T lymphocytes; they provide such individuals with some protection against extracellular bacteria. We shall return at the end of this section to the special characteristics of TI antigens that enable them to activate naive B cells without engaging armed helper T cells.

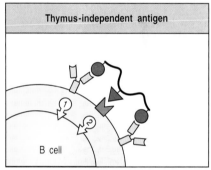

Fig. 8.2 A second signal is required for B-cell activation either by thymus-dependent or by thymus-independent antigens. The first signal required for B-cell activation is delivered through the antigen receptor (top panel). In the case of thymus-dependent antigens, the second signal is delivered by a helper T cell that recognizes degraded fragments of the antigen as peptides bound to MHC class II molecules on the B-cell surface (middle panel). In the case of thymus-independent antigens, the second signal may be delivered by the antigen itself (bottom panel), or by non-thymus-derived accessory cells (not shown). CD40L, CD40 ligand.

8-2 Armed helper T cells activate B cells that recognize the same antigen.

Thymus-dependent antibody responses require the activation of B cells by helper T cells that respond to the same antigen; this is called linked recognition. This means that before B cells can be induced to make antibody to a given pathogen in an infection, a CD4 T cell specific for peptides of the pathogen must first be activated to produce appropriate armed helper T cells. Although the epitope recognized by the armed helper T cell must therefore be linked to that recognized by the B cell, the two cells need not recognize identical epitopes. Indeed, we saw in Chapter 4 that T cells can recognize internal peptides in proteins that are quite distinct from the surface epitopes on the same molecule recognized by B cells. In the case of more complex natural antigens, such as viruses, the T cell and the B cell may not even recognize the same protein. It is, however, crucial that the peptide recognized by the T cell be a part of the antigen or antigenic complex recognized by the B cell, which can thereby produce the appropriate peptide upon internalization of antigen bound to its surface immunoglobulin.

For example, by recognizing an epitope on a viral protein coat, a B cell can internalize a complete virus particle. After internalization, the virus particle is degraded and peptides from internal viral proteins as well as coat proteins may be displayed by MHC class II molecules on the B-cell surface. Helper T cells that have been primed earlier in an infection by macrophages or dendritic cells presenting these same internal peptides can then activate the B cell to make antibodies that recognize the coat protein (Fig. 8.3).

The specific activation of the B cell by T cells sensitized to the same antigen or pathogen depends upon the ability of the antigen-specific B cell to concentrate the appropriate peptides on its surface MHC class II molecules. B cells binding a specific antigen are 10 000-fold more efficient at displaying peptide fragments of the antigen on their surface MHC class II molecules than are B cells that do not bind the antigen. Armed helper T cells will thus only help B cells whose receptors bind to the antigen containing the peptide that they recognize. As T-cell activation requires recognition of peptide:MHC class II complexes on the surface of the specific B cell, only T cells in direct contact with the antigen-binding B cell can participate. How these two cells find each other will be discussed in the next section.

The requirement for linked recognition has important consequences for the regulation and manipulation of the humoral immune response. One of these is to help ensure self tolerance, as described in Section 12-24. Another important application of linked recognition is in the design of vaccines, such as that used to immunize infants against *Haemophilus influenzae* B. This bacterial pathogen can infect the lining of the brain, called the meninges, causing meningitis and, in severe cases, neurological damage or death. Protective immunity against this pathogen is mediated by antibodies to its capsular polysaccharide. Although adults make very effective T-cell independent responses to these polysaccharide antigens, T-cell independent responses are weak in the immature immune system of the infant. To make an effective vaccine for use in infants, therefore, the polysaccharide is linked chemically to tetanus toxoid, a foreign protein to which infants are routinely and successfully vaccinated (see Fig. 1.31 and Chapter 13). B cells that bind the polysaccharide component of the vaccine can be activated by helper T cells specific for peptides of the linked toxoid (Fig. 8.4).

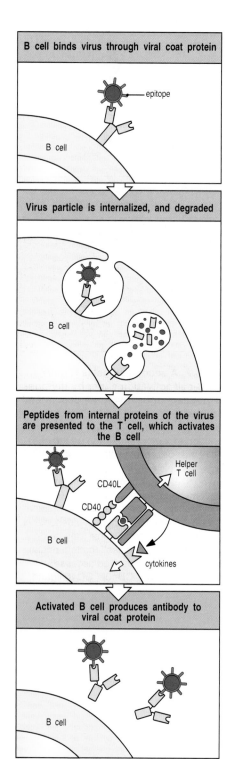

B cell binds virus through viral coat protein

epitope

B cell

Virus particle is internalized, and degraded

B cell

Peptides from internal proteins of the virus are presented to the T cell, which activates the B cell

Helper T cell

CD40L

CD40

B cell

cytokines

Activated B cell produces antibody to viral coat protein

B cell

Fig. 8.3 B cells and helper T cells must recognize epitopes of the same molecular complex in order to interact. An epitope on a viral coat protein is recognized by the surface immunoglobulin on a B cell and the virus is internalized and degraded. Peptides derived from viral proteins including internal proteins of the virus are returned to the B-cell surface bound to MHC class II molecules. Here, these complexes are recognized by helper T cells, which help to activate the B cells to produce antibody against the coat protein.

Fig. 8.4 Protein antigens attached to polysaccharide antigens allow T cells to help polysaccharide-specific B cells. *Haemophilus influenzae* B vaccine is a conjugate of bacterial polysaccharide and the tetanus toxoid protein. The B cell recognizes and binds the polysaccharide, internalizes, and degrades the toxoid protein to which it is attached, and then displays peptides derived from it on surface MHC class II molecules. Helper T cells generated in response to earlier vaccination against the toxoid recognize the complex on the B-cell surface and activate the B cell to produce antibody against the polysaccharide. This antibody can then protect against *H. influenzae* B infection.

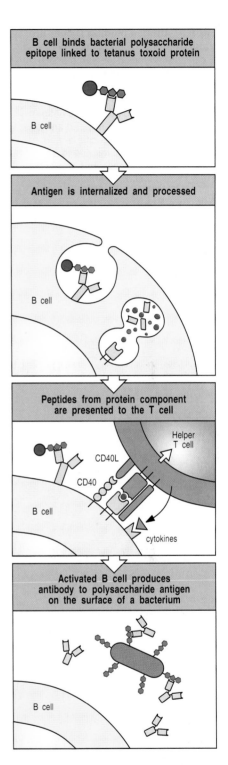

Linked recognition was originally discovered through studies on the production of antibodies to haptens, as described in Chapter 2. Haptens are small chemical groups that cannot elicit antibody responses because they cannot recruit T-cell help. When coupled to a carrier protein, however, they become immunogenic, because T cells can be primed to peptides derived from the protein. This effect is responsible for allergic responses shown by many people to the antibiotic penicillin, which reacts with host proteins to form a hapten that can stimulate an antibody response, as we shall learn in Chapter 11.

8-3   **Antigen-binding B cells are trapped in the T-cell zone of lymphoid tissues and are activated by encounter with armed helper T cells.**

One of the most puzzling features of the antibody response is the question of how an antigen-specific B cell manages to encounter an antigen-specific helper T cell. This question arises because the frequency of naive, antigen-specific cells is estimated to be between 1 in 10 000 and 1 in 1 000 000, so the chance of such a productive encounter should be between 1 in 10^8 and 1 in 10^{12}. This is a far more difficult challenge than that of getting effector T cells activated, because in that case, only one of the two cells involved has specific receptors. Moreover, T and B cells occupy quite distinct zones in peripheral lymphoid tissue (see, for example, Fig. 1.6). As in naive T-cell activation (discussed in Chapter 7), the answer appears to lie in the antigen-specific trapping of migrating lymphocytes.

When an antigen is introduced into mice, it is captured and processed by professional antigen-presenting cells, especially the dendritic cells (interdigitating reticular cells) that migrate to the T-cell zones of local lymph nodes. Recirculating naive T cells pass by such cells continuously and those rare T cells whose receptors bind peptides derived from the antigen are trapped very efficiently. This trapping clearly involves the specific antigen receptor on the T cell, although it is stabilized by activation of adhesion molecules as we learned in Section 7-3. Ingenious experiments with mice transgenic for specific rearranged immunoglobulin genes show that, in the presence of antigen, B cells with antigen-specific receptors are also trapped in the T-cell zones of lymphoid tissue. It is not known whether this unusual arrest of migrating antigen-binding B cells occurs by a similar mechanism to that of T cells—the activation of adhesion molecules by antigen encounter—but this seems likely.

Trapping of B cells in the T-cell zones, which are also the sites of helper T-cell activation, provides an elegant solution to the problem posed at the beginning of this section. T cells are trapped and activated in the T-cell zones; as B cells migrate through high endothelial venules they first enter these same T-cell zones. Those rare B cells that are specific

Fig. 8.5 Antigen binding B cells are trapped in the T-cell zone. T cells and B cells are sorted at the same site in lymphoid tissue. T cells stay in the T-cell zone provided they encounter antigen. B cells normally move rapidly through this area, unless they bind specific antigen, in which case they are trapped and can interact with antigen-specific armed helper T cells. This gives rise to a primary focus of B cells and T cells.

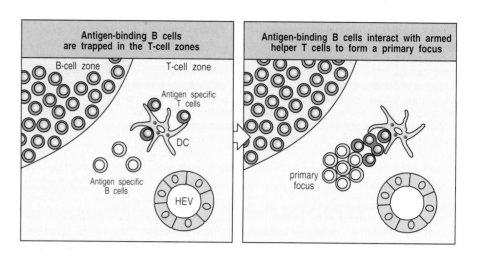

for the same antigen are trapped, while most B cells quickly move through the T-cell zone into the B-cell zone. Thus, antigen-specific B cells are trapped in precisely the correct location to establish primary foci (Fig. 8.5), to which we now turn.

8-4   **Peptide:MHC class II complexes on a B cell trigger armed helper T cells to make membrane-bound and secreted molecules, which activate the B cell.**

Armed helper T cells activate B cells when they recognize the appropriate peptide:MHC class II complex on the B-cell surface. As with armed T$_H$1 cells acting on macrophages, specific recognition of peptide:MHC class II complexes on B cells triggers armed helper T cells to synthesize both cell-bound and secreted effector molecules that synergize in B-cell activation. One particularly important effector molecule, which has a role in directing all phases of the B-cell response, is a T-cell surface molecule of the tumor necrosis factor (TNF) family, known as the **CD40 ligand (CD40L)** because it binds to the B-cell surface molecule CD40. **CD40** is a member of the TNF-receptor family of cytokine receptors and is analogous to the TNF receptor on macrophages and Fas on cytotoxic T-cell targets. Binding of CD40 by CD40 ligand helps to drive the resting B cell into the cell cycle and is essential for B-cell responses to thymus-dependent antigens; people and mice with mutations that affect CD40 ligand make very weak and ineffective antibody responses and suffer from severe humoral immunodeficiency, as we shall see in Chapter 10.

B cells are stimulated to proliferate *in vitro* when they are exposed to a mixture of artificially synthesized CD40 ligand and the cytokine IL-4. IL-4 is also made by armed T$_H$2 cells when they recognize their specific ligand on the B-cell surface, and IL-4 and CD40 ligand are thought to synergize in driving the clonal expansion that precedes antibody production *in vivo*. IL-4 is secreted in a polar fashion by the T$_H$2 cell and is directed at the site of contact with the B cell (Fig. 8.6) so that it acts selectively on the antigen-specific target B cell.

The initial steps in the activation of B cells by helper T cells are strikingly analogous to those of the activation of macrophages by T$_H$1 cells. However, while the activation of infected macrophages leads directly to the destruction of the pathogen, naive B cells, like naive T cells, must

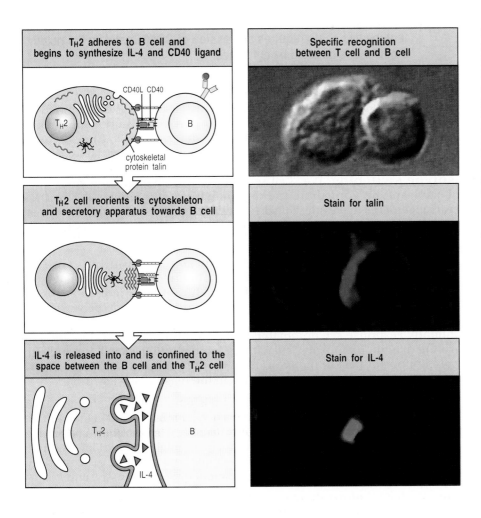

TH2 adheres to B cell and begins to synthesize IL-4 and CD40 ligand	Specific recognition between T cell and B cell
TH2 cell reorients its cytoskeleton and secretory apparatus towards B cell	Stain for talin
IL-4 is released into and is confined to the space between the B cell and the TH2 cell	Stain for IL-4

Fig. 8.6 When an armed helper T cell encounters an antigen-binding B cell, it is triggered to express CD40 ligand (CD40L) and to secrete IL-4 and other cytokines. Cytokines are released at the point of contact with the antigen-binding B cell, as shown by staining for IL-4 (bottom right panel), which shows the IL-4 confined to the space between the B cell and the helper T cell. In the center right panel, the helper T cell is stained for the cytoskeletal protein talin, showing that the cytoskeleton in the helper T cell is polarized, directing the secretion of the IL-4 to the point of contact between the cells. Photographs courtesy of A Kupfer.

undergo clonal expansion before they can differentiate into effector cells. The immediate effect of activation by helper T cells is therefore to trigger **primary foci** of B-cell proliferation. Some of these B cells then differentiate into antibody-secreting plasma cells (Fig. 8.7). Two additional cytokines, IL-5 and IL-6, both secreted by helper T cells, contribute to these later stages in B-cell activation.

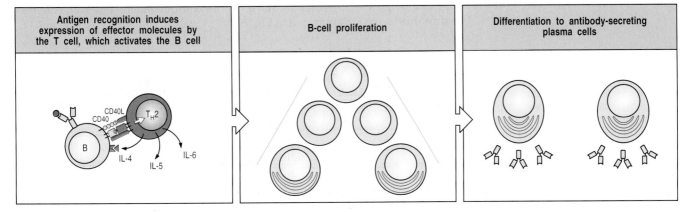

| Antigen recognition induces expression of effector molecules by the T cell, which activates the B cell | B-cell proliferation | Differentiation to antibody-secreting plasma cells |

Fig. 8.7 Armed helper T cells stimulate the proliferation and then the differentiation of antigen-binding B cells. The specific interaction of an antigen-binding B cell with an armed helper T cell leads to the expression of the B-cell stimulatory molecule CD40 ligand (CD40L) on the helper T-cell surface and to the secretion of the B-cell stimulatory cytokines, IL-4, IL-5, and IL-6, which drive the proliferation and differentiation of the B cell into antibody-secreting plasma cells.

| 8-5 | Isotype switching requires expression of CD40 ligand by the helper T cell and is directed by cytokines. |

Antibodies are remarkable, as we saw in Chapter 3, not only for the diversity of their antigen-binding sites but also for their versatility as effector molecules. The specificity of an antibody response is determined by the antigen-binding site, comprising the two variable domains; however, the effector action of the antibody is determined by the isotype of its heavy-chain constant domains. A given heavy-chain variable domain can become associated with the constant region of any isotype through **isotype switching**. We shall see later in this chapter how antibodies of each isotype contribute to the elimination of pathogens. The DNA rearrangements that underlie isotype switching and confer this functional diversity on the humoral immune response are directed by cytokines, especially those released by armed CD4 effector T cells.

All mature naive B cells express cell-surface IgM and IgD, yet IgM comprises less than 10% of the immunoglobulin found in plasma, where the most abundant isotype is IgG. Much of the antibody in plasma, therefore, has been produced by B cells that have undergone isotype switching. Little IgD antibody is produced at any time, so the early stages of the antibody response are dominated by IgM antibodies. Later, IgG and IgA are the predominant isotypes, with IgE contributing a small but biologically important part of the response. The overall predominance of IgG results, in part, from its longer lifetime in the plasma (see Fig. 3.20).

These changes do not occur in individuals who lack a functional CD40 ligand, which is necessary for interactions between B cells and helper T cells; such individuals make only small amounts of IgM antibodies in response to T-dependent antigens and have abnormally high levels of IgM in their plasma, perhaps induced by thymus-independent antigens expressed by pathogens that chronically infect these patients (see Sections 8-9 and 8-10).

Most of what is known about the regulation of isotype switching by helper T cells has come from experiments in which mouse B cells are stimulated with LPS and purified cytokines *in vitro*. These experiments show that different cytokines preferentially induce switching to different isotypes. Some of these cytokines are the same as those that drive B-cell proliferation in the initiation of a B-cell response. In the mouse, IL-4 preferentially induces switching to IgG1 and IgE, while TGF-β induces switching to IgG2b and IgA. T_H2 cells make both of these cytokines as well as IL-5, which induces IgA secretion by cells that have already undergone switching. Although T_H1 cells are poor initiators of antibody responses, they participate in isotype switching by releasing IFN-γ, which preferentially induces switching to IgG2a and IgG3. The cytokines that direct B cells to make the different isotypes of antibody are summarized in Fig. 8.8.

Fig. 8.8 Different cytokines induce switching to different isotypes. The individual cytokines induce (purple) or inhibit (red) production of certain isotypes. Much of the inhibitory effect is probably the result of directing switching to a different isotype. These data are drawn from experiments with mouse cells.

Role of cytokines in regulating Ig isotype expression							
Cytokines	IgM	IgG3	IgG1	IgG2b	IgG2a	IgA	IgE
IL-4	Inhibits	Inhibits	Induces		Inhibits		Induces
IL-5						Augments production	
IFN-γ	Inhibits	Induces	Inhibits		Induces		Inhibits
TGF-β	Inhibits	Inhibits		Induces		Induces	

Cytokines induce isotype switching by stimulating the formation and splicing of mRNA transcribed from the switch recombination sites that lie 5' to each C$_H$ gene (see Fig. 3.26). When activated B cells are exposed to IL-4, for example, transcription from a site upstream of the switch regions of C$_{\gamma 1}$ and C$_\varepsilon$ can be detected a day or two before switching occurs (Fig. 8.9). Recent data suggest that the production of a spliced switch transcript plays a role in directing switching but the mechanism is not yet clear. Each of the cytokines that induces switching appears to induce transcription from the switch regions of two different C$_H$ genes, promoting specific recombination to one or other of these genes only. Such a directed mechanism is supported by the observation that individual B cells frequently undergo switching to the same C$_H$ gene on both chromosomes, even though only one of the chromosomes is producing the expressed antibody. Thus, helper T cells regulate both the production of antibody by B cells and the isotype that determines the effector function of the antibody that is ultimately produced. How the balance between different isotypes is regulated in the humoral immune response to a given pathogen is not understood.

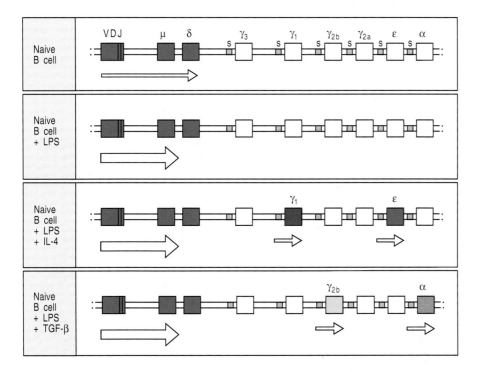

Fig. 8.9 Isotype switching is preceded by transcriptional activation of C$_H$ genes. Resting naive B cells transcribe the μ and δ loci at a low rate, giving rise to surface IgM and IgD. Bacterial lipopolysaccharide (LPS), which can activate B cells independently of antigen (see Section 8-10), induces IgM secretion. In the presence of IL-4, however, C$_{\gamma 1}$ and C$_\varepsilon$ are transcribed at a low rate, presaging switches to IgG1 and IgE production. The transcripts originate 5' of the region to which switching occurs, and do not code for protein. Similarly, TGF-β gives rise to C$_{\gamma 2b}$ and C$_\alpha$ transcripts, and drives switching to IgG2b and IgA. It is not known what determines which of the two transcriptionally activated C$_H$ gene segments undergoes switching. Arrows indicate transcription.

8-6   **Activated B cells proliferate extensively in the specialized microenvironment of the germinal center.**

In cultures of suspensions of lymphocytes, the interaction of naive antigen-binding B cells and specific armed helper T cells can lead to the production of antibody of all isotypes. However, although B-cell proliferation and differentiation (including isotype switching) can all be induced in this way *in vitro*, interactions with T cells in suspension culture cannot reproduce, either in magnitude or in complexity, the responses obtained using the same cells cultured with fragments of spleen, or the antibody response achieved *in vivo*. In particular, the gradual increase in the affinity of antibodies for the inducing antigen that is seen in the course of an antibody response requires specialized features of lymphoid tissue. This phenomenon, which is known as **affinity maturation**, is the consequence of somatic hypermutation of the immunoglobulin genes coupled with selection of B cells with high-affinity surface immunoglobulin, and depends upon the interaction of activated B cells with cells in the specialized microenvironment of the **germinal center**, which forms after antigen stimulation and which has already been mentioned in Chapter 5 as a site of intense B-cell proliferation in the lymph nodes and spleen.

Germinal centers are formed a week or so after antigen stimulation. B cells that have been activated by helper T cells in the T-cell zones of lymphoid tissues can follow either of two fates: some migrate to the medullary cords and differentiate into short-lived plasma cells secreting IgM or IgG, thus providing an early source of circulating antibodies (discussed in Chapter 9); however, others migrate along with the T cells that activated them into the **primary follicles** and form germinal centers (Fig. 8.10). Primary follicles contain resting B cells clustered around a dense network of processes extending from a specialized cell type, the **follicular dendritic cell** (**FDC**), which is thought to make a central contribution to the selective events that underlie the antibody response.

The cellular origins of follicular dendritic cells are obscure; they are unrelated to the dendritic cells that activate T cells. They lack MHC class II expression and are not derived from hematopoietic stem cells; indeed their only similarity to dendritic cells is their branched morphology (dendritic means 'branched'). Their role in driving the maturation of the

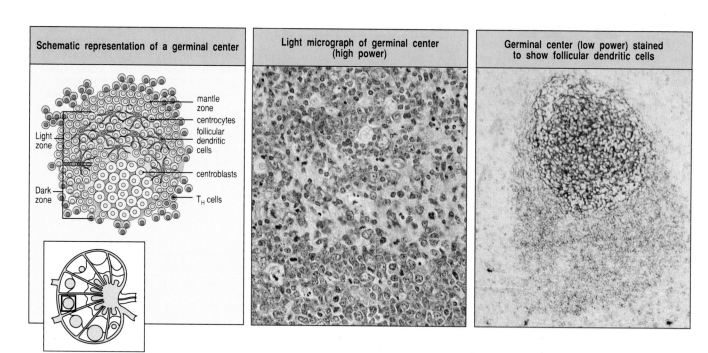

| Schematic representation of a germinal center | Light micrograph of germinal center (high power) | Germinal center (low power) stained to show follicular dendritic cells |

Fig. 8.10 Germinal centers are formed when activated B cells enter lymphoid follicles. The germinal center is a specialized microenvironment in which B-cell proliferation, somatic hypermutation, and selection for antigen binding all occur. Rapidly proliferating B cells in germinal centers are called centroblasts. Closely packed centroblasts form the so-called 'dark zone' of the germinal center, as can be seen in the lower part of the center panel, which shows a section through a germinal center. As these cells mature, they stop dividing and become small centrocytes, moving out into an area of the germinal center called the 'light zone' (the upper part of the center panel), where the centrocytes make contact with a dense network of follicular dendritic cell processes. The follicular dendritic cells are not stained in the center panel but can be seen clearly in the right panel where both follicular dendritic cells (stained blue with an antibody to Bu10, a marker specific for follicular dendritic cells) in the germinal center as well as the mature B cells in the mantle zone (stained brown with an antibody to IgD) can be seen. The plane of this section reveals mostly the dense network of follicular dendritic cells in the light zone, although the less-dense network in the dark zone can just be seen at the bottom of the figure. Photographs courtesy of I MacLennan.

humoral immune response depends chiefly on their ability to hold intact antigens on their surfaces for long periods, ranging from months to years in some cases. Follicular dendritic cells express the complement receptors CR1, CR2, and CR3 (see Section 8-27) and receptors for the Fc piece of immunoglobulin; these may be involved in holding antibody and complement-associated antigen in this site (see Section 8-16). Other specialized properties of follicular dendritic cells, for example the ability to attract B cells to the follicles, are poorly characterized because this cell type is difficult to study outside an intact lymphoid organ.

When activated B cells enter the primary lymphoid follicle, they start dividing to form germinal centers. The proliferating B cells in germinal centers divide about once every 6 hours and can be distinguished by their morphological characteristics, which are typical of blast cells (see Fig. 1.17): thus they are large cells with an expanded cytoplasm, which stains intensely for RNA, and diffuse chromatin in the nucleus. These B-cell blasts are called **centroblasts**. The visible focus of centroblasts that forms in a few days within a primary lymphoid follicle is called the dark zone of the germinal center. The centroblasts give rise to **centrocytes** which enter the follicular dendritic cell network in the light zone (see Fig. 8.10). The helper T cells that migrate to the primary follicle along with the activated B cells also undergo some clonal expansion and can be seen intermingled with the centrocytes in the light zone. The remaining B cells that are not specific for antigen are pushed to the outside to form the **mantle zone**.

The rapid proliferation of cells in the germinal center greatly increases the number of B cells specific for the pathogen that initiated the antibody response. By dissecting out individual germinal centers and even individual B cells, and using the polymerase chain reaction (see Section 2-27) to analyze the DNA encoding expressed immunoglobulin chains, it has been possible to demonstrate that the B cells in each germinal center rapidly proliferate, so that after a few days, most germinal center B cells are derived from only one or a few founder cells. This technique has also revealed that the germinal centers are the site of somatic hypermutation of immunoglobulin variable-domain genes.

| 8-7 | **Somatic hypermutation occurs in the rapidly dividing centroblasts in the germinal center.** |

Affinity maturation in the course of an immune response can be viewed as a Darwinian process, requiring first the generation of variability in B-cell receptors and then selection for those with the highest affinity for antigen. The variability is generated by somatic hypermutation of the immunoglobulin variable-domain genes; selection of cells bearing these mutated receptors by antigen occurs on the surface of the follicular dendritic cell.

Somatic hypermutation is believed to take place in dividing centroblasts, whose rearranged immunoglobulin variable-region genes accumulate mutations at a rate of about one base pair per 10^3 per cell division. (The mutation rate of all other known somatic cell DNA is one base pair per 10^{10} per cell division). As there are about 360 base pairs encoding each of the expressed heavy- and light-chain variable-region genes in a B cell, and about three out of every four base changes results in an altered amino acid, every second cell will acquire a mutation in its receptor at each division.

Somatic hypermutation affects all the rearranged variable-region genes in a B cell, whether they are expressed in immunoglobulin chains or not. These mutations also affect some DNA flanking the rearranged V gene but they generally do not extend into the constant-region exons. Thus, the rearranged variable-region genes in a B cell are somehow targeted for the introduction of random somatic point mutations. The resulting mutant receptors are expressed on the progeny of the rapidly dividing centroblasts, which are small cells called centrocytes, all derived from the few antigen-specific progenitors that persist in the germinal center. As the number of centrocytes increases in the germinal center, two distinct regions begin to be distinguished; the dark zone, where proliferating centroblasts are packed closely together and where there are few follicular dendritic cells, and the light zone, where less densely packed centrocytes make contact with the numerous cells of the follicular dendritic cell network (see Fig. 8.10). The centrocytes eventually give rise to memory B cells and antibody-secreting plasma cells.

8-8   Non-dividing centrocytes with the best antigen-binding receptors are selected for survival.

Centrocytes are programmed to die within a fixed period unless their surface immunoglobulin is bound to antigen and they are subsequently contacted by a helper T cell bearing CD40 ligand. After somatic hypermutation, the surface immunoglobulin on the centrocytes derived from a single progenitor B cell may bind antigen either better or worse than the immunoglobulin expressed on its precursor. Some will inevitably lose the ability to bind antigen at all and centrocytes bearing these mutations die: a characteristic feature of germinal centers is the presence of **tingible body macrophages**, which are phagocytes engulfing apoptotic cells. If, on the other hand, the mutant surface immunoglobulin of the centrocyte binds antigen well, the cell is induced to express the $bcl-x_L$ gene, whose product inhibits apoptotic cell death, and the cell is rescued. Fig. 8.11 illustrates the alternative fates of B cells with receptors of lower and higher affinity for an antigen after somatic hypermutation. Those B cells whose receptors now have a lower affinity for antigen will have to compete with cells having higher affinity. Hence, affinity maturation occurs in the primary response as well as in secondary and subsequent responses, as we shall see in Chapter 9.

Centrocyte selection seems to involve two stages. First, the centrocytes enter the dense follicular dendritic cell network of the light zone, where they have the opportunity to bind and take up antigen from follicular dendritic cells. Centrocytes with the highest affinity receptors for antigen are the most likely to succeed. If a centrocyte binds and internalizes the antigen, it then moves to the outer edge of the light zone where helper T cells expressing CD40 ligand are concentrated. Centrocytes that fail to take up antigen from follicular dendritic cells die and are phagocytozed by local macrophages; cell death in the germinal center is seen to occur in the area of the light zone rich in follicular dendritic cells.

In the second stage of centrocyte selection, centrocytes that have successfully taken up and processed antigen from follicular dendritic cells engage in an antigen-specific interaction with the helper T cells at the edge of the light zone, exchanging signals that induce further proliferation of the participating T and B cells, and differentiation of the latter, either to memory B cells or to plasma cells. The involvement of T cells in the selective process serves to prevent centrocytes that have acquired specificity for self antigens from being selected. Evidence both *in vivo* and *in vitro* indicates that CD40 ligation during centrocyte interaction with helper T cells is necessary but insufficient for memory B-cell formation.

As the centrocytes are selected in this way for antigen binding, the mutations in the expressed immunoglobulin genes of the surviving cells

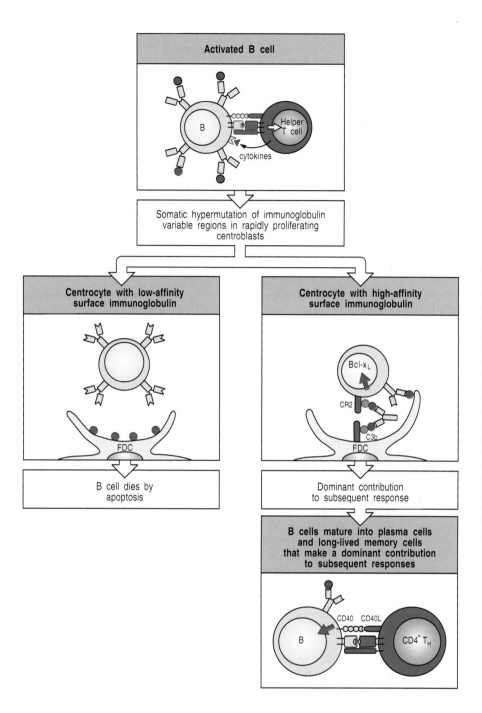

Fig. 8.11 After somatic hypermutation, B cells with high-affinity receptors for antigen are rescued from apoptosis by binding antigen on the surface of follicular dendritic cells and receiving signals from specific helper cells. Somatic hypermutation occurs during the proliferation of centroblasts in germinal centers. The centroblasts give rise to small, non-dividing centrocytes. These interact with follicular dendritic cells (FDCs) that display antigen in a complex with antibody and complement on their surface. Centrocytes whose receptors no longer bind antigen die by apoptosis, while centrocytes with receptors that bind well are induced to express Bcl-x_L and survive. It is not known if Bcl-x_L is induced by the B-cell receptor binding to antigen, as shown here, or by making contact with helper T cells, as shown in the bottom panel. The higher the affinity of the receptor for antigen, the better the centrocyte will compete with other centrocytes. Binding of the B-cell co-receptor complex (CR2:CD19) to complement displayed together with antigen on the follicular dendritic cell surface is thought to amplify the signal from the antigen receptor. This process allows selection of B cells of progressively higher affinity to contribute to the response. A B cell that binds antigen can then present fragments of the antigen to antigen-specific helper T cells that surround the germinal center (see Fig. 8.10). These further stimulate the B cells to enter the memory B-cell pool or to become plasma cells.

have altered amino acids, mainly in the complementarity determining regions (CDRs), while mutations in sequences encoding framework residues, which might affect the stability of the variable domain, tend to be silent, as we saw in Chapter 3. In addition, it appears that CDRs have been selected to be particularly susceptible to somatic hypermutation by using particular codons that are more readily altered by this process.

The selection of centrocytes in germinal centers resembles, in some respects, the positive selection of thymocytes. However, B cells are selected during the response to foreign antigen instead of during ontogeny, and the selecting antigen is the foreign antigen itself, providing a direct check on the ability of each cell to produce antibodies that can bind the invading pathogen at the time when they are needed.

Fig. 8.12 Plasma cells secrete antibody at a high rate but can no longer respond to antigen or helper T cells. B cells can take up antigen and present it to helper T cells, which induce them to grow, switch isotype, or undergo somatic hypermutation; however, they do not secrete significant amounts of antibody. Plasma cells are terminally differentiated B cells with a finite lifespan and they secrete antibodies. They can no longer interact with helper T cells because they lack surface immunoglobulin receptors and MHC class II molecules. They have also lost the ability to change isotype or undergo somatic hypermutation.

	Property					
	Intrinsic			Inducible		
B-lineage cell	Surface Ig	Surface MHC class II	High-rate Ig secretion	Growth	Somatic hyper-mutation	Isotype switch
Resting B cell	Yes	Yes	No	Yes	Yes	Yes
Plasma cell	No	No	Yes	No	No	No

B cells that have successfully bound antigen and survived selection leave the germinal center to become either memory B cells or antibody-secreting plasma cells. The differentiation of a B cell into a plasma cell is accompanied by many morphological changes that reflect its commitment to the production of large amounts of secreted antibody (Fig. 8.12). Plasma cells have abundant cytoplasm that is dominated by multiple layers of rough endoplasmic reticulum (see Fig. 1.17). The nucleus shows a characteristic pattern of peripheral chromatin condensation, a prominent perinuclear Golgi apparatus is visible, and the cisternae of the endoplasmic reticulum are rich in immunoglobulin, which makes up 10–20% of all the protein synthesized. Surface immunoglobulin and MHC class II molecules are low or absent, so plasma cells can no longer interact with antigen or helper T cells and antibody secretion is independent of both antigen and T-cell regulation. Plasma cells have a lifespan of about 4 weeks in bone marrow or the lamina propria of epithelial surfaces after their final differentiation, and this helps to limit the duration of antibody responses.

The alternative fate of B cells leaving the germinal center is to become memory B cells that do not secrete antibody in the primary response but can be rapidly activated upon subsequent challenge with the same antigen. It is not known exactly what signals determine whether a given B cell will become a memory B cell or a plasma cell.

8-9 **B-cell responses to bacterial antigens with intrinsic B-cell activating ability do not require T-cell help.**

Although antibody responses to protein antigens are dependent on helper T cells, people and mice with T-cell deficiencies nevertheless make antibodies to many bacteria. This is because the special properties of some bacterial polysaccharides, polymeric proteins, and lipopolysaccharides enables them to stimulate naive B cells in the absence of T-cell help. These antigens are known as thymus-independent antigens (TI antigens) because they stimulate strong antibody responses in athymic animals or individuals. In normal individuals, these bacterial products induce antibody responses in the absence of T-cell responses, which cannot be induced by these non-protein antigens since they are mediated by T cells that recognize antigen mainly as peptides bound to MHC molecules. However B-cell responses to these TI antigens may receive help from T cells which recognize non-protein antigens and which can develop outside of the thymus, as they are greatly diminished in animals that have no T cells at all.

Thymus-independent antigens fall into two classes, which activate B cells by different mechanisms. Antigens in the first class, the **TI-1 antigens**, contain an intrinsic activity that can directly induce the proliferation of B cells. At high concentration, these molecules cause the proliferation and differentiation of most B cells, regardless of their antigen specificity; this is known as **polyclonal activation** (Fig. 8.13, top two panels). As a result of their ability to stimulate most B cells to divide, TI-1 antigens are often called **B-cell mitogens**, a mitogen being a substance that induces cells to undergo mitosis. When B cells are exposed to concentrations of TI-1 antigens that are 10^3–10^5 times lower than those used for polyclonal activation, only those B cells whose immunoglobulin receptors bind these TI-1 molecules become activated, because only by binding to antigenic determinants on the molecule are they able to concentrate sufficient TI-1 molecules on the cell surface to be activated (see Fig. 8.13, bottom two panels). In the presence of large amounts of the TI-1 antigen, this concentrating effect is not required and all B cells can be stimulated.

It is likely that during normal infections *in vivo*, concentrations of TI-1 antigens are low; thus, only antigen-specific B cells are likely to be activated and these will produce antibodies specific for TI-1 antigens. Such responses play an important role in specific defense against several extracellular pathogens, as they arise earlier than T-dependent responses because they do not require prior priming and clonal expansion of helper T cells. However, TI-1 antigens are inefficient inducers of isotype switching, affinity maturation, or memory B cells, all of which require specific T-cell help.

8-10 | B-cell responses to bacterial polysaccharides do not require specific T-cell help.

The second class of thymus-independent antigens consist of molecules such as bacterial cell wall polysaccharides that have highly repetitive structures. These thymus-independent antigens, called **TI-2 antigens**, contain no intrinsic B-cell stimulating activity. Whereas TI-1 antigens can activate both immature and mature B cells, TI-2 antigens can only activate mature B cells; immature B cells, as we saw in Chapter 5, are inactivated by repetitive epitopes. This may be why infants do not make antibodies to polysaccharide antigens efficiently; most of their B cells are immature. Responses to several TI-2 antigens are prominent among B-1 B cells (also known as CD5 B cells), which comprise an autonomous subpopulation of B cells (see Chapter 5). These may be rather late in developing their full function, which occurs in the human at around 5 years of age.

TI-2 antigens most probably act by extensively crosslinking the cell-surface immunoglobulin of specific mature B cells (Fig. 8.14, left panels). Excessive crosslinking of receptors, however, renders mature B cells unresponsive, just as it does immature B cells. Thus, epitope density seems to be critical in the activation of B cells by TI-2 antigens: too low a density and the level of receptor crosslinking is insufficient to activate the cell; too high a density and the cell becomes anergic.

Although responses to TI-2 antigens can be seen in nude mice that lack a thymus, depletion of all T cells by knocking out the T-cell receptor β and δ loci eliminates responses to TI-2 antigens. Moreover, responses to TI-2 antigens can be augmented *in vivo* by transferring small numbers of T cells to such T-cell deficient mice. How T cells contribute to TI-2 responses is not clear. One possibility is that T cells can recognize and become activated by TI-2 antigens through cell-surface triggering

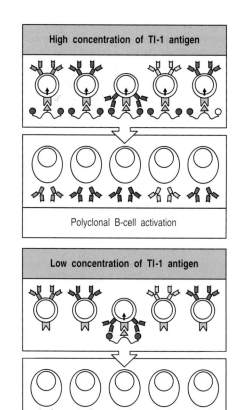

High concentration of TI-1 antigen

Polyclonal B-cell activation

Low concentration of TI-1 antigen

TI-1 antigen-specific antibody response

Fig. 8.13 T-cell independent type I antigens (TI-1 antigens) are polyclonal B-cell activators at high concentrations. At high concentrations, the signal delivered by the B-cell activating moiety on TI-1 antigens is sufficient to induce proliferation and antibody secretion by B cells in the absence of specific antigen binding to surface immunoglobulin, so all B cells respond (top two panels). At low concentrations, only specific antigen-binding B cells bind enough of the TI-1 antigen to focus its B-cell activating properties on the B cell; this gives a specific antibody response to epitopes on the TI-1 antigen (bottom two panels).

Fig. 8.14 B-cell activation by TI-2 antigens requires, or is greatly enhanced by cytokines. Multiple crosslinking of the B-cell receptor by TI-2 antigens can lead to antibody production (left panels), but there is evidence that helper T cells greatly augment these responses and lead to isotype switching as well (right panels). It is not clear how T cells are activated in this case, since polysaccharide antigens cannot produce peptide fragments that might be recognized by T cells on the B-cell surface. One possibility is that a component of the antigen binds to a cell-surface molecule common to T cells of all specificities as shown in the figure; an alternative is that some minor population, such as γ:δ T cells or double-negative α:β T cells, can recognize polysaccharide antigens bound to unconventional MHC class I or class I-like molecules. However, these mechanisms are speculative.

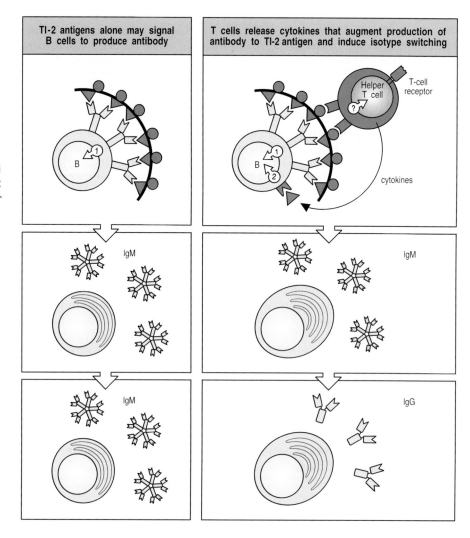

molecules shared by all T cells (see Fig. 8.14, right panels). Alternatively, the help may come from γ:δ T cells or from CD4, CD8 double-negative α:β T cells that can recognize, through their receptors, certain polysaccharides bound to unconventional MHC class I or class I-like molecules such as CD1. Such T cells can develop outside of the thymus, principally in the gut.

B-cell responses to TI-2 antigens provide a prompt and specific response to an important class of pathogens. Most extracellular bacterial pathogens have cell-wall polysaccharides that enable them to resist ingestion by phagocytes. This allows them not only to escape direct destruction by phagocytes but also to avoid stimulating T-cell responses through the presentation of bacterial peptides by macrophages. Antibody that is produced rapidly in response to this polysaccharide capsule without the help of peptide-specific T cells can coat such encapsulated **pyogenic bacteria**, promoting their ingestion and hence destruction, and is likely to be an important part of the humoral immune response in many bacterial infections. We mentioned earlier the importance of antibodies to the capsular polysaccharide of *Haemophilus influenzae* B, a TI-2 antigen, in protective immunity to this bacterium. A further example of the importance of TI-2 responses can be seen in patients with an immunodeficiency disease known as the **Wiskott-Aldrich syndrome**. These patients can respond, although poorly, to protein antigens but fail to make antibody to polysaccharide antigens and are highly susceptible to infection with extracellular bacteria that have polysaccharide capsules.

	TD antigen	TI-1 antigen	TI-2 antigen
Antibody response in infants	Yes	Yes	No
Antibody production in congenitally athymic individual	No	Yes	Yes
Antibody response in absence of T cells	No	Yes	No
Primes T cells	Yes	No	No
Polyclonal B-cell activation	No	Yes	No
Requires repeating epitopes	No	No	Yes
Examples of antigen	Diphtheria toxin Viral hemagglutinin Purified protein derivative (PPD) of *Mycobacterium tuberculosis*	Bacterial lipopoly-saccharide *Brucella abortus*	Pneumococcal poly-saccharide Salmonella-polymerized flagellin Dextran Hapten-conjugated ficoll (polysucrose)

Fig. 8.15 Properties of different classes of antigens that elicit antibody responses.

Thus, the TI responses are important components of the humoral immune response to non-protein antigens that are unable to recruit peptide-specific T-cell help; the distinguishing features of thymus-dependent, TI-1 and TI-2 antibody responses are summarized in Fig. 8.15.

Summary.

B-cell activation by many antigens, especially monomeric proteins, requires binding of the antigen by the B-cell surface immunoglobulin and interaction of the B cell with antigen-specific helper T cells. These helper T cells induce a phase of vigorous B-cell proliferation, after which the clonally expanded progeny of the naive B cells differentiate into either antibody-secreting plasma cells or memory B cells. During the differentiation of activated B cells, several changes can occur in the antibodies produced. First, the antibody isotype may change. Second, the antigen-binding properties of the antibody may change by somatic hypermutation of variable-region genes. Somatic hypermutation can lead to the loss of antigen binding and the death of the B cell, or to increased affinity of the antibody for the eliciting antigen and further selective expansion. Somatic hypermutation and selection for high-affinity binding occur in germinal centers formed by proliferating B cells in the lymphoid follicles, where antigen is displayed on the surface of follicular dendritic cells. Helper T cells control these processes by selectively activating cells displaying antigenic peptides, by secreting cytokines that induce isotype switching, and by inducing proliferation and differentiation into plasma cells and memory B cells. Some non-protein antigens stimulate B cells in the absence of specific helper T cells; these thymus-independent antigens do not induce either isotype switching or memory B cells but may play a critical role in host defense against pathogens whose surface antigens cannot elicit T-cell responses.

The distribution and functions of immunoglobulin isotypes.

Extracellular pathogens may find their way to most sites in the body and antibodies must be equally widely distributed to combat them. Most are distributed by diffusion from their site of synthesis but specialized transport mechanisms are required to deliver them to internal epithelial surfaces, such as those of the lung and intestine. The location of antibodies is determined by their isotype, which can limit their diffusion or enable them to engage specific transporters that deliver them across various epithelia. In this part of the chapter, we shall describe the mechanisms whereby antibodies of different isotypes are directed to the compartments of the body in which their distinct effector functions are appropriate, and discuss the protective functions of antibodies that result solely from their binding to pathogens. In the last two parts of the chapter, we shall discuss the effector cells and molecules that are specifically engaged by antibodies of the different isotypes.

8-11 | Antibodies of different isotypes operate in distinct places and have distinct effector functions.

Pathogens most commonly enter the body across epithelial barriers presented by the mucosa of the respiratory, digestive, and urogenital tracts, or through damaged skin. Pathogens entering in this way can then establish infections in the tissues. Less often, insects, wounds, or hypodermic needles introduce microbes directly into the blood. The body's mucosal surfaces, tissues, and blood all need to be protected by antibodies from such infections, and antibodies of different isotypes are adapted to function in different compartments. Since a given variable region can become associated with any constant region through isotype switching, B cells can produce antibodies, all specific for the same eliciting antigen, which provide all of the protective functions appropriate for each body compartment.

The first antibodies to be produced in a humoral immune response are always IgM, because VDJ joining occurs just 5′ to the C_μ gene exons (see Figs. 8.9 and 3.17). These early IgM antibodies are produced before B cells have undergone somatic hypermutation and therefore tend to be of low affinity. IgM molecules, however, form pentamers whose 10 antigen-binding sites can bind simultaneously to multivalent antigens, such as bacterial cell-wall polysaccharides, compensating for the relatively low affinity of the monomers by multipoint binding that confers high avidity. As a result of the large size of the pentamers, IgM is usually thought to be confined to the blood, although some studies in rats show it can enter tissues rapidly as well. Their pentameric structure also makes IgM antibodies especially potent in activating the complement system, as we shall see later. Infection of the bloodstream has serious consequences unless it is controlled quickly, and the rapid production of IgM and its efficient activation of the complement system are important in controlling such infections. IgM is also produced in secondary and subsequent responses, and after somatic hypermutation, although other isotypes dominate the later phases of a response.

Antibodies of the other isotypes, IgG, IgA, and IgE, are smaller and diffuse easily out of the blood into the tissues. Although most IgA, as we saw in Chapter 3, forms dimers, IgG and IgE are always monomeric, as is some percentage of IgA. The affinity of the individual antigen-binding sites for antigen is therefore critical for the effectiveness of antibodies of all three of these isotypes, and B cells are selected for increased affinity in the germinal centers, mainly after they have undergone switching to these isotypes. IgG is the principal isotype in the blood and extracellular fluid, while IgA is the principal isotype in secretions, the most important being those of the mucous epithelium of the intestinal and respiratory tracts. While IgG efficiently opsonizes pathogens for engulfment by phagocytes and activates the complement system, IgA is a poor opsonin and a weak activator of complement. This distinction is not surprising, as IgG operates mainly in the body tissues where accessory cells and molecules are available, while IgA operates mainly on body surfaces where complement and phagocytes are not normally present, and therefore functions chiefly as a neutralizing antibody. Finally, IgE antibody is present only at very low levels in blood or extracellular fluid, but is bound avidly by receptors on mast cells that are found just beneath the skin and mucosa, and along blood vessels in connective tissue. Antigen binding to this IgE triggers mast cells to release powerful chemical mediators that induce reactions, such as coughing, sneezing, and vomiting, that can expel infectious agents. The distribution and main functions of antibodies of the different isotypes are summarized in Fig. 8.16.

Functional activity	IgM	IgD	IgG1	IgG2	IgG3	IgG4	IgA	IgE
Neutralization	+	−	++	++	++	++	++	−
Opsonizaton	−	−	+++	−	++	+	+	−
Sensitization for killing by natural killer cells	−	−	++	−	++	−	−	−
Sensitization of mast cells	−	−	−	−	−	−	−	++++
Activates complement system	++++	−	++	+	++	−	+	−

Distribution	IgM	IgD	IgG1	IgG2	IgG3	IgG4	IgA	IgE
Transport across epithelium	+	−	−	−	−	−	+++ (dimer)	−
Transport across placenta	−	−	+++	+++	+++	+++	−	−
Diffusion into extravascular sites	+/−	−	+++	+++	+++	+++	++ (monomer)	+
Mean serum level (mg ml^{-1})	1.5	0.04	9	3	1	0.5	2.1	3×10^{-5}

Fig. 8.16 Each human Ig isotype has specialized functions and a unique distribution. The dominant effector functions of each isotype (++++) are shaded in dark red, the major functions (+++) are shown in light red, while lesser functions (++) are shown in dark pink, and very minor functions (+) in pale pink. The distributions are similarly marked, with actual average levels in serum shown in the bottom row.

8-12 **Transport proteins that bind to the Fc domain of antibodies carry specific isotypes across epithelial barriers.**

The primary site of synthesis of IgA antibodies, and their main loci of action, are at the epithelial surfaces of the body. IgA-secreting plasma cells are found predominantly in the connective tissue called lamina propria, which lies immediately below the basement membrane of many surface epithelia. From there, the IgA antibodies must be transported across the epithelium to its external surface, for example to the lumen of the gut or the bronchi. The IgA antibody synthesized in the lamina propria is secreted as an IgA dimeric molecule associated with a single J chain (see Fig. 3.22). This polymeric form of IgA binds specifically to a molecule called the poly-Ig receptor expressed on the basolateral surfaces of the overlying epithelial cells (Fig. 8.17). When the poly-Ig receptor has bound a molecule of dimeric IgA, the complex is internalized and carried through the cytoplasm of the epithelial cell in a transport vesicle to its apical surface. This process is called **transcytosis**. At the apical surface of the epithelial cell, the poly-Ig receptor is cleaved enzymatically, releasing the extracellular portion of the receptor still attached to the Fc piece of the dimeric IgA. This fragment of the receptor, called the **secretory component**, may help to protect the dimeric IgA from proteolytic cleavage. Those molecules of dimeric IgA that diffuse from the lamina propria into the bloodstream are excreted into the gut via the bile. Therefore, it is not surprising that patients with obstructive jaundice, a condition in which bile is not excreted, show a marked increase in dimeric IgA in the plasma.

The principal sites of IgA synthesis and secretion are the gut, the respiratory epithelium, the lactating breast, and various other exocrine glands such as the salivary and tear glands. It is believed that the primary functional role of IgA antibodies is to protect epithelial surfaces from infectious agents, as IgG antibodies protect the extracellular spaces of the internal milieu. IgA antibodies prevent the attachment of bacteria or toxins to epithelial cells or the absorption of foreign substances, and provide the first line of defense against a wide variety of pathogens. Newborn infants are especially vulnerable to infection, having had no prior exposure to the microbes in the environment they enter at birth. IgA antibodies are secreted in breast milk and thereby transferred to the gut of the newborn infant where they provide protection from newly encountered bacteria until the infant can synthesize its own protective antibody.

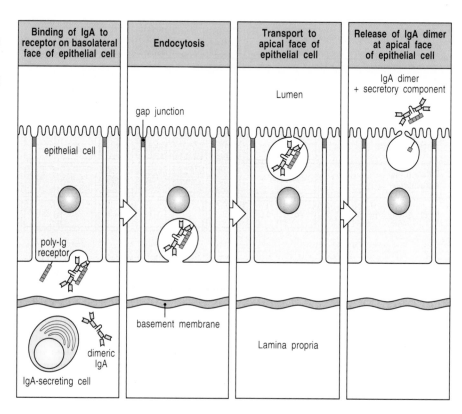

Fig. 8.17 Transcytosis of IgA antibody across epithelia is mediated by the poly-Ig receptor, a specialized transport protein. Most IgA antibody is synthesized in plasma cells lying just beneath epithelial basement membranes of the gut, respiratory epithelia, tear and salivary glands, and the lactating mammary gland. The IgA dimer bound to a J chain diffuses across the basement membrane and is bound by the poly-Ig receptor on the basolateral surface of the epithelial cell. The bound complex undergoes transcytosis in which it is transported in a vesicle across the cell to the apical surface, where the poly-Ig receptor is cleaved to leave the extracellular, IgA-binding component bound to the IgA molecule as the so-called secretory component. The residual piece of the poly-Ig receptor is non-functional and is degraded. In this way, IgA is transported across epithelia into the lumen of several organs that are in contact with the external environment.

| Binding of IgA to receptor on basolateral face of epithelial cell | Endocytosis | Transport to apical face of epithelial cell | Release of IgA dimer at apical face of epithelial cell |

Fig. 8.18 FcRn binds to the Fc piece of IgG. The structure of a molecule of FcRn (white) bound to the Fc piece of IgG (blue) is shown. FcRn transports IgG molecules across the placenta in humans and across the gut in rats and mice. Photograph courtesy of P Bjorkman.

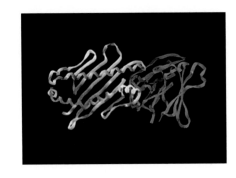

IgA is not the only protective antibody conferred on the infant by its mother. Maternal IgG is transported across the placenta directly into the bloodstream of the fetus during intrauterine life; human babies at birth have as high a level of plasma IgG as their mothers, and with the same range of specificities. The selective transport of IgG from mother to fetus results from a specific IgG transport protein in the placenta, FcRn, which is closely related in structure to MHC class I molecules. Despite this similarity, FcRn binds IgG quite differently from the binding of peptide in MHC class I, as its peptide-binding groove is occluded. It binds to the Fc portion of IgG molecules (Fig. 8.18). Two molecules of FcRn bind one molecule of IgG, bearing it across the placenta.

In some rodents, FcRn also delivers IgG to the circulation of the neonate from the gut lumen. Maternal IgG is ingested by the newborn animals in colostrum, the protein-rich fluid in the postnatal mammary gland. In this case, transport is from the lumen of the gut into the blood and tissues. This receptor is found only in fetal and early postnatal life and seems to have as its counterpart in humans the transplacental FcRn.

By means of these specialized transport systems, mammals of various species are supplied from birth with antibodies against pathogens common in their environments. As they mature and make their own antibodies of all isotypes, these are distributed selectively to different sites in the body (Fig. 8.19). Thus, throughout life, isotype switching and the distribution of isotypes through the body provides effective protection against infection in extracellular spaces.

8-13   High-affinity IgG and IgA antibodies can neutralize bacterial toxins.

Many bacteria cause disease by secreting molecules, called bacterial toxins, that damage or disrupt the function of somatic cells (Fig. 8.20). To have an effect, the toxins must interact with a specific molecule that serves as a receptor on the surface of the target cell. In many toxins, the receptor-binding domain is carried on one polypeptide chain, while the toxic function is carried by a second chain. Antibodies that bind to the receptor-binding site on the toxin molecule can prevent the toxin from binding to the cell and thus protect the cell from toxic attack (Fig. 8.21). This protective effect of antibodies, as we have already mentioned, is called **neutralization**, and antibodies acting in this way are referred to as **neutralizing antibodies**.

Most toxins are active at nanomolar concentrations: a single molecule of diphtheria toxin can kill a cell. To neutralize toxins, therefore, antibodies must be able to diffuse into the tissues and bind the toxin rapidly and with high affinity. The diffusibility of IgG antibodies in the extracellular fluids and their high affinity make these the principal neutralizing antibodies for toxins found at this site. IgA antibodies similarly neutralize toxins at the mucosal surfaces of the body.

Diphtheria and tetanus toxins are among the bacterial toxins in which the toxic and the receptor-binding functions of the molecule are on two separate chains. It is therefore possible to immunize individuals, usually infants, with modified toxin molecules in which the toxic chain has been

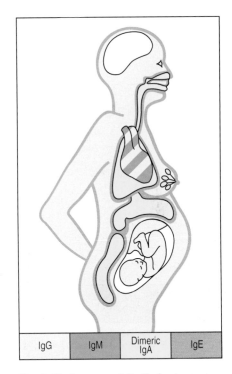

| IgG | IgM | Dimeric IgA | IgE |

Fig. 8.19 Immunoglobulin isotypes are selectively distributed in the body. IgG and IgM predominate in plasma, while IgG, along with some IgM and monomeric IgA, are the major isotypes in extracellular fluid within the body. Polymeric IgA predominates in secretions across epithelia, including breast milk. The fetus receives IgG from the mother by transplacental transport. IgE is found mainly as mast-cell-associated antibody just beneath epithelial surfaces (especially the respiratory tract, gastrointestinal tract, and skin). The brain is normally devoid of immunoglobulin.

Fig. 8.20 Many common diseases are caused by bacterial toxins. Several examples are shown here. These are all exotoxins, or secreted proteins of bacteria. Bacteria also have endotoxins, or non-secreted toxins that are released when the bacterium dies. The endotoxins are also important in the pathogenesis of disease but here the host response is more complex (see Chapter 9).

Disease	Organism	Toxin	Effects *in vivo*
Tetanus	*Clostridium tetani*	Tetanus toxin	Blocks inhibitory neuron action leading to chronic muscle contraction
Diphtheria	*Corynebacterium diphtheriae*	Diphtheria toxin	Inhibits protein synthesis leading to epithelial cell damage and myocarditis
Gas gangrene	*Clostridium perfringens*	Clostridial-α toxin	Phospholipase activation leading to cell death
Cholera	*Vibrio cholerae*	Cholera toxin	Activates adenylate cyclase, elevates cAMP in cells, leading to changes in intestinal epithelial cells that cause loss of water and electrolytes
Anthrax	*Bacillus anthracis*	Anthrax toxic complex	Increases vascular permeability leading to edema, hemorrhage and circulatory collapse
Botulism	*Clostridium botulinum*	Botulinus toxin	Blocks release of acetylcholine leading to paralysis
Whooping cough	*Bordetella pertussis*	Pertussis toxin	ADP-ribosylation of G proteins leading to lymphocytosis
		Tracheal cytotoxin	Inhibits cilia and causes epithelial cell loss
Scarlet fever	*Streptococcus pyogenes*	Erythrogenic toxin	Vasodilation leading to scarlet fever rash
		Leukocidin Streptolysins	Kills phagocytes, allowing bacterial survival
Food poisoning	*Staphylococcus aureus*	Staphylococcal enterotoxin	Acts on intestinal neurons to induce vomiting. Also a potent T-cell mitogen (SE superantigen)
Toxic-shock syndrome	*Staphylococcus aureus*	Toxic-shock syndrome toxin	Causes hypotension and skin loss. Also a potent T-cell mitogen (TSST-1 superantigen)

denatured. These modified toxin molecules, which are called toxoids, lack toxic activity but retain the receptor-binding site, so that immunization with the toxoid induces neutralizing antibodies effective in protecting against the native toxin.

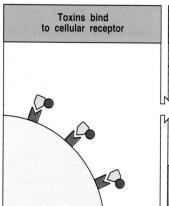 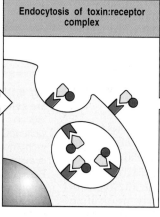 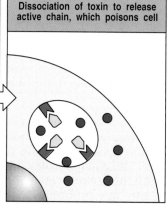 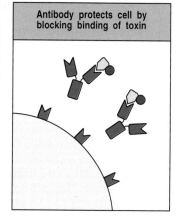

| Toxins bind to cellular receptor | Endocytosis of toxin:receptor complex | Dissociation of toxin to release active chain, which poisons cell | Antibody protects cell by blocking binding of toxin |

Fig. 8.21 Neutralization by IgG antibodies protects cells from toxin action. Many bacteria (as well as venomous insects and snakes) mediate their effects by elaborating cellular poisons or toxins (see Fig. 8.20). These toxins usually contain several distinct moieties. One piece of the toxin must bind a cellular receptor, which allows the molecule to be internalized. A second part of the toxin molecule then enters the cytoplasm and poisons the cell. In some cases, a single molecule of toxin can kill a cell. Antibodies that inhibit toxin binding can prevent, or neutralize, these effects.

In the case of some insect or animal venoms, where toxicity is such that a single exposure is capable of causing severe tissue damage or death, the adaptive immune response is too slow to generate neutralizing antibodies. Exposure to these venoms is a rare event and protective vaccines have not been developed for use in humans. Instead, for these toxins, neutralizing antibodies are generated by immunizing other species, such as horses, with insect and snake venoms to produce anti-venins for use in protecting humans. Transfer of antibodies in this way is known as **passive immunization** (see Section 2-29).

8-14 High-affinity IgG and IgA antibodies can inhibit the infectivity of viruses.

When animal viruses infect cells, they must first bind to a specific cell-surface protein, often a cell-type-specific protein that determines which cells they can infect. For example, the influenza virus carries a surface protein called **influenza hemagglutinin**, which binds to terminal sialic acid residues of the carbohydrate moieties found on certain glycoproteins expressed by epithelial cells of the respiratory tract. It is known as hemagglutinin because it recognizes similar sialic acid residues on chicken red blood cells and can agglutinate such cells by binding to these sites. Antibodies to the hemagglutinin can inhibit infection by the influenza virus. Such antibodies are called virus-neutralizing antibodies and, as with the neutralization of toxins, and for the same reasons, high-affinity IgA and IgG antibodies are particularly important in virus neutralization.

Many antibodies that neutralize viruses do so by directly blocking viral binding to surface receptors (Fig. 8.22). However, viruses are sometimes successfully neutralized when only a single molecule of antibody is bound to a virus particle that has many receptor-binding proteins on its surface. In these cases, the antibody must cause some change in the virus that disrupts its structure and either prevents it from interacting with its receptors or interferes with the fusion of the virus membrane with the cell surface after the virus has engaged its surface receptor. The viral nucleic acids thus cannot enter the cell and replicate there.

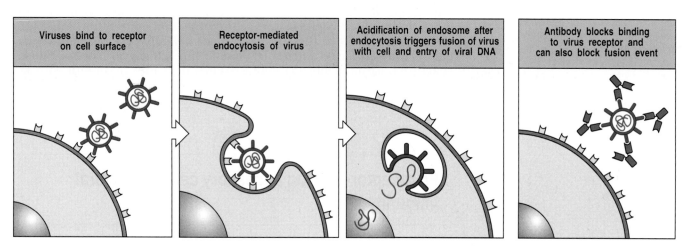

| Viruses bind to receptor on cell surface | Receptor-mediated endocytosis of virus | Acidification of endosome after endocytosis triggers fusion of virus with cell and entry of viral DNA | Antibody blocks binding to virus receptor and can also block fusion event |

Fig. 8.22 Viral infection of cells can be blocked by neutralizing antibodies. For a virus to infect a cell, it must insert its genes into the cytoplasm. For enveloped viruses, as shown in the figure, this requires binding of the virus to the cell surface and fusion of viral and cell membranes. For some viruses, this fusion event takes place on the cell surface (not shown); for others it can only occur within the more acidic environment of endosomes as shown here. Non-enveloped viruses must also bind to receptors on cell surfaces but they enter the cytoplasm by disrupting endosomes. Antibodies binding to viral surface proteins can inhibit either the initial binding of virus or its subsequent entry into the cell.

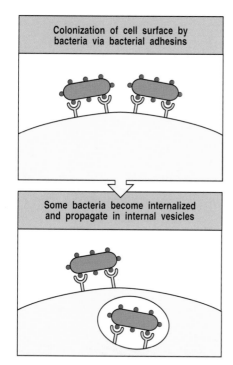

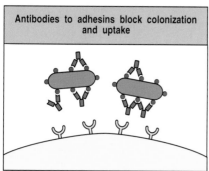

Fig. 8.23 Antibodies can prevent attachment of bacteria to cell surfaces. Many bacterial infections require an interaction between the bacterium and a cell surface. This is particularly true for infections of mucosal surfaces. The attachment process involves very specific molecular interactions between bacterial adhesins and their ligands on host cells; antibodies to bacterial adhesins can block such infections.

<table>
<tr><td>8-15</td><td>**Antibodies can block the adherence of bacteria to host cells.**</td></tr>
</table>

Many bacteria have specific cell-surface molecules called adhesins which allow them to bind to the surface of host cells. This adherence reaction is critical to the infectivity of these bacteria, whether they enter the cell, as occurs with some pathogens such as *Salmonella* spp., or remain attached to the cell surface as extracellular pathogens (Fig. 8.23). For example, the bacterium *Neisseria gonorrhoeae*, the causative agent of the sexually transmitted disease gonorrhea, has a cell-surface protein known as pilin. Pilin allows the bacterium to adhere to the epithelial cells of the urinary and reproductive tracts and is essential to its infectivity. Antibodies to pilin can inhibit this adhesive reaction and prevent infection.

IgA antibodies secreted onto the mucosal surfaces of the intestinal, respiratory, and reproductive tracts are particularly important in preventing the adhesion of bacteria, viruses, or other pathogens to the epithelial cells, that usually precedes infection by this route. The adhesion of bacteria to cells within the body can also contribute to pathogenesis, and IgG antibodies to adhesins can protect from damage in this way.

<table>
<tr><td></td><td>**Summary.**</td></tr>
</table>

The antibody response begins with antigen binding to IgM-expressing B cells and can then lead to the production of antibody of the same specificity in all different isotypes. Each isotype is specialized both in its localization in the body and in the functions it can perform. IgM antibodies are synthesized early in a response and are found mainly in blood. They are pentameric in structure and specialized to activate complement efficiently upon binding antigen. IgG antibodies are synthesized later in the response, are usually of higher affinity, and are found in blood and in extracellular fluid where they can neutralize toxins, viruses, and bacteria, opsonize them for phagocytosis, and activate the complement system. IgA antibodies are synthesized as monomers, which enter blood and extracellular fluids, or in lamina propria as dimeric molecules that are selectively transported across epithelia into sites such as the lumen of the gut, where they neutralize toxins and viruses, and block the entry of bacteria across the intestinal epithelium. Most IgE antibody is bound to the surface of mast cells that reside mainly just below body surfaces; antigen binding to this IgE triggers local defense reactions. Thus, each of these isotypes occupies a specific site in the body and has a specific role to play in defending the body against extracellular pathogens and their toxic products.

Fc receptor-bearing accessory cells in humoral immunity.

The ability of high-affinity antibodies to neutralize toxins, viruses, or bacteria can protect against infection but does not, on its own, solve the problem of how to remove the pathogens and their products from the body. Moreover, many pathogens are not neutralized by antibody and must be destroyed by other means. To dispose of neutralized microorganisms and to attack resistant extracellular pathogens, antibodies can activate a variety of **accessory effector cells** bearing receptors, the **Fc receptors**, specific for the Fc piece of antibodies of a particular isotype. These accessory cells include the phagocytic cells (macrophages and polymorphonuclear neutrophilic leukocytes), which ingest antibody-coated bacteria and kill them, and other cells—natural killer cells, eosinophils, and mast cells (see Fig. 1.4)—which are triggered to secrete stored mediators when their Fc receptors are engaged. These accessory cells are activated when their Fc receptors are aggregated by binding to the multiple immunoglobulin Fc pieces of antibody molecules bound to a pathogen.

| 8-16 | **The Fc receptors of accessory cells are signaling receptors specific for immunoglobulins of different isotypes.** |

The Fc receptors comprise a family of molecules that bind to the Fc portion of immunoglobulin molecules. Each member of the family recognizes immunoglobulin of one or a few closely related isotypes through a recognition domain on the α chain of the Fc receptor. Fc receptors are themselves members of the immunoglobulin gene superfamily of proteins. Different accessory cells bear Fc receptors for antibodies of different isotypes, and the isotype of the antibody thus determines which accessory cell will be engaged in a given response. The different Fc receptors, the cells that express them, and their isotype specificity, are shown in Fig. 8.24.

Fc receptors, like the T-cell receptor, function as part of a multi-subunit complex. Only the α chain is required for specific recognition; the other chains are required for transport to the cell surface and for signal transduction when Fc is bound. Indeed, signal transduction by most Fc receptors is mediated by a chain called the γ chain that is closely related to the T-cell receptor ζ chain. This is the case for some Fcγ receptors and for the high-affinity receptor for IgE; an exception is human FcγRII-A, in which the cytoplasmic domain of the α chain replaces the function of the γ chain. In the case of the FcγRII-B receptor, alternative splicing of

Receptor	FcγRI (CD64)	FcγRII-A (CD32)	FcγRII-B2	FcγRII-B1	FcγRIII (CD16)	FcεRI
Structure	α 74 kDa γ	α 40 kDa γ-like domain			α 50–70 kDa γ or ζ or	α 45 kDa β 33 kDa γ 9 kDa
Binding	IgG1 10^8 M^{-1}	IgG1 2×10^6 M^{-1}	IgG1 2×10^6 M^{-1}	IgG1 2×10^6 M^{-1}	IgG1 5×10^5 M^{-1}	IgE 10^{10} M^{-1}
Order of affinity	1) IgG1 2) IgG3=IgG4 3) IgG2	1) IgG1 2) IgG3=IgG4 3) IgG2	1) IgG1 2) IgG3=IgG4 3) IgG2	1) IgG1 2) IgG3=IgG4 3) IgG2	IgG1=IgG3	
Cell type	Macrophages Neutrophils Eosinophils	Macrophages Neutrophils Eosinophils Platelets	Macrophages Neutrophils Eosinophils Platelets Langerhans' cells	B cells	NK cells Eosinophils Macrophages Neutrophils Langerhans' cells	Mast cells Eosinophils Basophils
Effect of ligation	Uptake	Uptake Granule release (eosinophils)	Uptake Granule release (eosinophils)	Inhibition of stimulation —no uptake	Induction of killing (NK cells)	Secretion of granules

Fig. 8.24 Distinct receptors for the Fc region of the different immunoglobulin isotypes are expressed on different accessory cells. The subunit structure, binding properties, and cell type expressing these receptors are shown. The complete multimolecular structure of most receptors is not yet known but they may all be multichain molecular complexes similar to the Fcε receptor I (FcεRI). The exact chain composition of any receptor may vary from one cell type to another. For example, FcγRIII in neutrophils is expressed as a molecule with a glycophosphoinositol membrane anchor and without γ chains, while in NK cells it is a transmembrane molecule associated with γ chains as shown. The binding affinities are taken from data on human receptors.

the α chain in different cell types produces two isoforms, which differ in their ability to cause endocytosis of bound immune complexes. The isoform found in macrophages, called FcγRII-B2, is endocytosed very efficiently whereas, in B cells, alternative splicing gives rise to the B1 isoform, which has an insertion in its cytoplasmic tail that blocks endocytosis. Instead, the cytoplasmic tail of FcγRII-B1 binds the phosphatase PTP1C and functions as part of a regulatory mechanism that inhibits the activation of naive B cells (see Section 9-29).

Although the most prominent function of Fc receptors is the activation of accessory cells against pathogens, they may also contribute in other ways to immune responses. For example, the Fc receptor on B cells negatively regulates some B-cell responses, while the Fc receptors expressed by the Langerhans' cells of the skin enable them to ingest antigen:antibody complexes and present peptides to T cells. The stable binding of such complexes to the Fc receptors on the follicular dendritic cell surface enables them to drive the maturation of humoral immune responses.

8-17   Fc receptors on phagocytes are activated by antibodies bound to the surface of pathogens.

Phagocytes are activated by IgG antibodies, especially IgG1 and IgG3, which bind to specific Fcγ receptors on the phagocyte surface (see Fig. 8.24). As phagocyte activation can initiate an inflammatory response and cause tissue damage, it is essential that the Fc receptors on phagocytes be able to distinguish antibody molecules bound to a pathogen from the majority of free antibody molecules that are not bound to anything. This condition is met by the aggregation or multimerization of antibodies that occurs when antibodies bind to multimeric antigens or antigenic particles, such as viruses and bacteria.

If Fc receptors on the surface of an accessory cell bind an immunoglobulin monomer with low affinity, they will bind such antibody-coated particles with high avidity, and this is probably the principal mechanism by which bound antibodies are distinguished from free immunoglobulin. However, mutations in the hinge region of some antibodies affect the ability of aggregates to bind to the Fc receptor, although they have no effect on monomer binding. This suggests that subtle conformational changes in antibody molecules that accompany binding to antigen may also be important in allowing Fc receptors to distinguish bound from free antibody (Fig. 8.25).

Fig. 8.25 Bound antibody is distinguishable from free immunoglobulin by its state of aggregation and/or by conformational change. Free immunoglobulin molecules cannot bind Fc receptors. Antigen-bound immunoglobulin, however, can bind because several antibody molecules that are bound to the same surface bind to Fc receptors with high avidity. Some studies also suggest that antigen binding and aggregation induce a conformational change in the Fc portion of the immunoglobulin molecule, increasing its affinity for the Fc receptor. Both effects probably contribute to discrimination by Fc receptors between free and bound antibody.

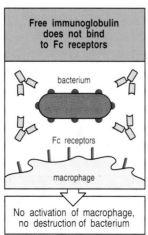
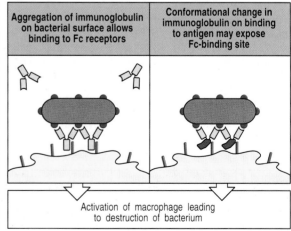

The result is that Fc receptors enable accessory cells to detect pathogens through bound antibody molecules. Thus, specific antibody and Fc receptors provide the means by which accessory cells that lack intrinsic specificity can identify and remove pathogens and their products from the extracellular spaces of the body.

8-18 Fc receptors on phagocytes allow them to ingest and destroy opsonized extracellular pathogens.

The most important accessory cells in humoral immune responses are the phagocytic cells of the monocytic and myelocytic lineages, particularly the macrophages and the polymorphonuclear neutrophilic leukocytes or **neutrophils**. Phagocytosis is the ingestion of particles by cells and involves binding of the particle to the surface of the phagocyte, followed by its internalization and destruction.

Many bacteria are directly recognized, ingested, and destroyed by phagocytes, and these bacteria are not pathogenic in normal individuals (see Chapter 9). Bacterial pathogens, however, often have polysaccharide capsules that allow them to resist direct engulfment by phagocytes. These bacteria become susceptible to phagocytosis only when they are coated with antibody that engages the Fcγ receptors on phagocytic cells, triggering their uptake and destruction (Fig. 8.26). Coating a microorganism with molecules that allow its destruction by phagocytes is known as opsonization. Bacterial polysaccharides, as we have seen, belong to the TI-2 class of T-cell independent antigens, and opsonization by thymus-independent antibodies produced in response to bacterial polysaccharides early in an immune response is important in ensuring the prompt destruction of many encapsulated bacteria.

Both the internalization and the destruction of microorganisms are greatly enhanced by interactions between the molecules coating an opsonized microorganism and their specific receptors on the phagocyte surface. When an antibody-coated pathogen binds to Fcγ receptors on the surface of a phagocytic cell, for example, the cell surface extends around the surface of the particle through successive binding of cellular Fcγ receptors to bound antibody Fc domains on the pathogen surface.

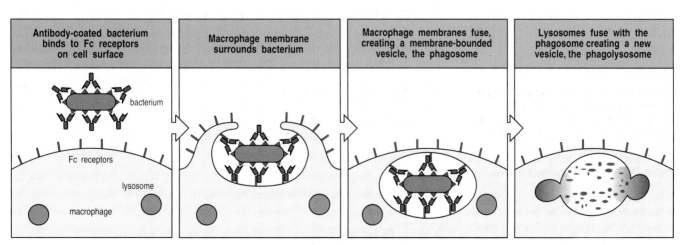

| Antibody-coated bacterium binds to Fc receptors on cell surface | Macrophage membrane surrounds bacterium | Macrophage membranes fuse, creating a membrane-bounded vesicle, the phagosome | Lysosomes fuse with the phagosome creating a new vesicle, the phagolysosome |

Fig. 8.26 A major function of Fc receptors on phagocytes is to trigger the uptake and degradation of antibody-coated bacteria. Many bacteria resist phagocytosis by macrophages and polymorphonuclear leukocytes. Antibodies binding to these bacteria, however, allow them to be ingested and degraded through interaction of the multiple Fc domains arrayed on the bacterial surface with Fc receptors on the phagocyte surface. Fc-receptor binding also signals the phagocyte to increase the rate of phagocytosis, fuse lysosomes with phagosomes, and increase its bactericidal activity (see Fig. 8.27).

Fig. 8.27 Ingestion of antibody-coated bacteria triggers production or release of many bactericidal agents in phagocytic cells. Most of these agents are found in both macrophages and polymorphonuclear neutrophilic leukocytes. Some of them are toxic; others, such as lactoferrin, work by binding essential nutrients and preventing their uptake by the bacteria. The same agents can be released by phagocytes interacting with large, antibody-coated surfaces such as parasitic worms or host tissues. As these mediators are also toxic to host cells, phagocyte activation can cause extensive tissue damage in infection.

Class of mechanism	Specific products
Acidification	pH=~3.5–4.0, bacteriostatic or bactericidal
Toxic oxygen-derived products	Superoxide O_2^-, hydrogen peroxide H_2O_2, singlet oxygen $^1O_2^{\bullet}$, hydroxyl radical $OH^{\bullet}$, hypohalite OCl^-
Toxic nitrogen oxides	Nitric oxide NO
Antimicrobial peptides	Defensins, cationic proteins
Enzymes	Lysozyme—dissolves cell walls of some Gram-positive bacteria. Acid hydrolases—further digest bacteria
Competitors	Lactoferrin—binds Fe, vitamin B12 binding protein

This is an active process that is triggered by the binding of Fcγ receptors. Endocytosis of the particle leads to its enclosure in an acidified cytoplasmic vesicle called a phagosome. The phagosome then fuses with one or more lysosomes to generate a phagolysosome, releasing the lysosomal enzymes into the phagosome interior where they destroy the bacterium (see Fig. 8.26).

Phagocytes can also damage bacteria through the generation of a variety of toxic products. The most important of these are hydrogen peroxide (H_2O_2), the superoxide anion (O_2^-), and nitric oxide (NO), which are directly toxic to the bacterium. They are generated in a process known as the **respiratory burst**. Production of these metabolites is induced by the binding of aggregated antibodies to Fcγ receptors. The microbicidal products of activated phagocytes can also damage host cells, and a series of enzymes, including catalase (which degrades hydrogen peroxide) and superoxide dismutase (which converts the superoxide anion into hydrogen peroxide), are also produced during phagocytosis. These control the action of these products so that they act primarily on pathogens within phagolysosomes. The agents whereby phagocytic cells damage and destroy ingested bacteria are summarized in Fig. 8.27.

Some particles are too large for a phagocyte to ingest: parasitic worms are one example. In this case, the phagocyte attaches to the surface of the parasite via its Fcγ or Fcε receptors, and the lysosomes fuse with the attached surface membrane (Fig. 8.28). This reaction discharges the contents of the lysosome onto the surface of the antibody-coated parasite, damaging it directly in the extracellular space. Whereas the principal phagocytes in the destruction of bacteria are macrophages and neutrophils, large parasites such as helminths are more usually attacked by eosinophils. Thus, Fcγ receptors can trigger the internalization of external particles by phagocytosis, or the externalization of internal vesicles by exocytosis. The latter process is usually mediated by antigen crosslinking of IgE bound to the high-affinity Fcε receptor I. We shall see in the next three sections that natural killer cells and mast cells also release mediators stored in their vesicles when their Fc receptors are aggregated.

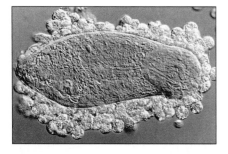

Fig. 8.28 Eosinophils attack a schistosome larva in the presence of serum from an infected patient. Large parasites, such as worms, cannot be ingested; however, when the worm is coated with antibody, especially IgE, eosinophils can attack it via the high-affinity Fcε receptor I. Similar attacks can be mounted by other Fc receptor-bearing cells on various larger targets. Photograph courtesy of A Butterworth.

8-19 **Fc receptors activate natural killer cells to destroy antibody-coated targets.**

Infected cells are usually destroyed by T cells alerted by foreign peptides bound to cell-surface MHC molecules. However, virus-infected cells may also signal the presence of intracellular infection by expressing on

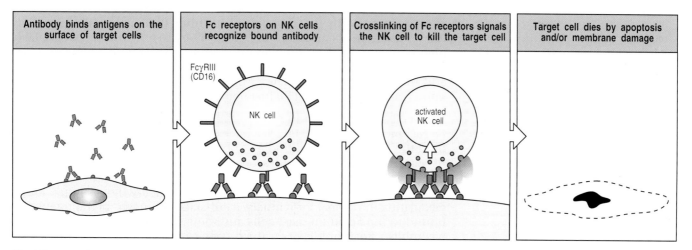

Fig. 8.29 Antibody-coated target cells can be killed by natural killer cells (NK cells) in antibody-dependent cell-mediated cytotoxicity (ADCC). NK cells are large granular non-T, non-B lymphoid cells that have FcγRIII receptors (CD16) on their surface. When these cells encounter cells coated with IgG antibody, they rapidly kill the target cell. The importance of ADCC in host defense or tissue damage is still controversial.

their surfaces viral proteins that can be recognized by antibodies. Cells bound by such antibodies can then be killed by a specialized non-T, non-B lymphoid cell called a **natural killer (NK) cell**.

Natural killer cells are large lymphoid cells with prominent intracellular granules; they make up a small fraction of peripheral blood lymphoid cells. These cells bear no known antigen-specific receptors but are able to recognize and kill a limited range of abnormal cells. They were first discovered because of their ability to kill some tumor cells but are now known to play an important part in innate immunity, as will be discussed in Chapter 9.

The destruction of antibody-coated target cells by NK cells is called **antibody-dependent cell-mediated cytotoxicity (ADCC)** and is triggered when antibody bound to the surface of a cell interacts with Fc receptors on the NK cell (Fig. 8.29). NK cells express the Fc receptor FcγRIII (CD16). FcγRIII recognizes the IgG1 and IgG3 subclasses and triggers cytotoxic attack by the NK cell on antibody-coated target cells by mechanisms exactly analogous to those we have encountered in cytotoxic T cells, involving the release of cytoplasmic granules containing perforin and granzymes. The importance of ADCC in defense against infection with bacteria or viruses has not yet been fully established. However, ADCC represents yet another mechanism by which, through engaging an Fc receptor, antibodies can direct an antigen-specific attack by an effector cell lacking specificity for antigen.

8-20 **Mast cells, basophils, and activated eosinophils bind IgE antibody with high affinity.**

When pathogens cross epithelial barriers and establish a local focus of infection, the host must mobilize its defenses and direct them to the site of pathogen growth. One mechanism by which this is achieved is to activate a specialized cell type known as a **mast cell**. Mast cells are large cells containing distinctive cytoplasmic granules that contain a mixture of molecules including **histamine**, which act rapidly to make local blood vessels more permeable. Mast cells have a distinct appearance after staining with the dye toluidine blue that makes them readily iden- tifiable in tissues (see Fig. 1.4). They are found in particularly high concentrations in the submucosal tissues lying just beneath body surfaces, including those of the gastrointestinal and respiratory tracts, and in connective tissues along blood vessels—especially those layers known as the dermis that lie just below the epidermis of the skin.

Mast cells are activated to release their granules via antibody bound to Fc receptors specific for IgE. We have seen earlier that other Fc receptors bind the Fc region of antibodies only when these are bound to antigen. By contrast, the Fc receptors on mast cells bind monomeric IgE antibodies with a very high affinity, measured at approximately $10^{10}M^{-1}$. These Fc receptors are called FcεRI. Thus, even at the low levels of IgE found circulating in normal individuals, a substantial portion of the total IgE is bound to the FcεRI on mast cells and their circulating counterparts, the basophils. Eosinophils are a third type of granulocytic cell that can be triggered to degranulate via Fcε receptors, but they express these only when activated and recruited to an inflammatory site.

Although mast cells are thus usually stably associated with bound IgE, they are not activated simply by the binding of monomeric antigens to cell-surface IgE. Mast-cell activation occurs when the bound IgE is crosslinked by binding multivalent antigen. Signaling in this way activates the mast cell to release the contents of its prominent granules and initiates a local inflammatory response. The immediate consequence of antigen crosslinking of the IgE displayed on the mast-cell surface is degranulation, which occurs within seconds (Fig. 8.30). This releases

Fig. 8.30 IgE antibody crosslinking on mast-cell surfaces leads to rapid mast-cell release of inflammatory mediators. Mast cells are large cells found in connective tissue that can be distinguished by secretory granules containing many inflammatory mediators. They bind stably to monomeric IgE antibodies through the very high-affinity Fcε receptor I. Antigen crosslinking of the bound IgE antibody molecules triggers rapid degranulation, releasing inflammatory mediators into the surrounding tissue. These mediators trigger local inflammation, which recruits cells and proteins required for host defense to sites of infection. Mast-cell degranulation is also the basis of the acute allergic reaction causing asthma, hayfever and the life-threatening response known as systemic anaphylaxis (see Chapter 11). Photographs courtesy of A M Dvorak.

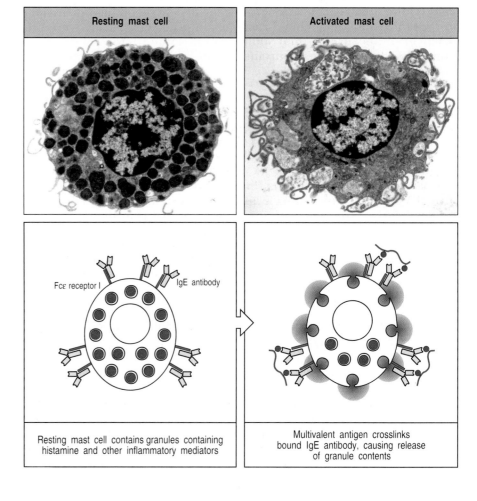

Resting mast cell

Activated mast cell

Fcε receptor I   IgE antibody

Resting mast cell contains granules containing histamine and other inflammatory mediators

Multivalent antigen crosslinks bound IgE antibody, causing release of granule contents

the stored histamine, causing a local increase in blood flow and vascular permeability that quickly leads to fluid accumulation in the surrounding tissue and an influx of blood-borne cells such as polymorphonuclear leukocytes. Such local inflammatory responses serve to bring increased antibody and increased numbers of phagocytes, effector lymphocytes, and eosinophils to a site of infection in a period of a few minutes to a few hours. Thus, mast cells form a part of the front line of host defenses against pathogens that enter the body across epithelial barriers.

| 8-21 | **Mast-cell activation by specific IgE antibody plays an important role in resistance to parasite infection.** |

Mast cells are thought to serve at least three important functions in host defense. First, their location near body surfaces allows them to recruit both specific and non-specific effector elements to sites where infectious agents are most likely to enter the internal milieu. Second, they also increase the flow of lymph from sites of antigen deposition to the regional lymph nodes, where naive lymphocytes are first activated. Third, their ability to trigger muscular contraction can lead to the physical expulsion of pathogens from the lungs or the gut. There is increasing evidence that such IgE-mediated responses are crucial to defense against parasitic infestation.

Evidence for the role of IgE antibody, mast cells, and other Fcε-expressing leukocytes such as eosinophils in host defense against parasites comes from several sources. First, intestinal mastocytosis is a feature of helminth infection; a special mouse strain called W/W^V, which has a mast-cell deficiency caused by a defect in c-kit, shows impaired clearance of the intestinal nematodes *Trichinella spiralis* and *Nippostrongylus brasiliensis*. Resistance to these pathogens is restored by bone marrow transplantation from normal congenic mice. Second, the production of IgE antibodies and the presence of blood eosinophilia is strongly associated with infections by certain classes of parasites, particularly helminths. Third, depletion of eosinophils using polyclonal anti-eosinophil antisera causes increased severity of experimental schistosomal infection in mice. Fourth, examination of tissues infected by parasites shows degranulated eosinophils adherent to helminths, and experiments *in vitro* have shown that eosinophils can kill the parasitic helminth *Schistosoma mansoni* in the presence of specific IgE (see Fig. 8.28) or IgG anti-schistosome antibodies. This killing is enhanced by binding of complement component C3b to the parasite, which ligates C3b receptors on eosinophils.

The role of IgE, mast cells, basophils, and eosinophils can also be seen in resistance to the feeding of blood-sucking ixodid ticks. Normal skin at the site of a tick bite shows an accumulation of mast cells, basophils, and eosinophils, some of which are degranulated, indicative of recent activation. Resistance to subsequent feeding by these ticks develops after the first exposure, suggesting a specific immunological mechanism. Mast cell-deficient mice show no such acquired resistance, and depletion of either basophils or eosinophils using specific polyclonal antibodies also reduces resistance to tick feeding. Finally, recent experiments have shown that tick resistance is mediated by specific IgE antibody.

Thus, much data from both clinical studies and experiments support a role for this system of IgE binding to the high-affinity FcεRI in host resistance to pathogens that enter across epithelia. We shall see later, in Chapter 11, that this same system accounts for many of the symptoms in allergic diseases such as asthma.

Summary.

Antibody-coated pathogens are recognized by Fc receptors on the surfaces of various cells that bind to the constant-region domains of the bound antibodies and trigger the destruction of the pathogen. Fc receptors comprise a family of molecules each of which recognizes immunoglobulins of specific isotypes. Fc receptors on macrophages and neutrophils recognize the constant regions of IgG antibodies bound to the surface of a pathogen and trigger the engulfment and destruction of IgG-coated bacteria by these phagocytic cells. Binding to the Fc receptor also induces the production of microbicidal agents in the intracellular vesicles of the phagocyte. Eosinophils are important in the elimination of parasites too large to be engulfed; they bear Fc receptors specific for the constant region of IgG, as well as high-affinity receptors for IgE; aggregation of these receptors triggers the release of toxic substances onto the surface of the parasite. NK cells and mast cells also release their granule contents when their Fc receptors are engaged. Mast cells also act as accessory cells in humoral immune responses but the high-affinity receptor for IgE is expressed constitutively by mast cells and differs from other Fc receptors in that it can bind free monomeric antibody, thereby allowing an immediate response to pathogens at the site of entry into the tissues. When the IgE on the surface of a mast cell is aggregated by binding to antigen, it triggers the mast cell to release histamine that increases the blood flow to sites of infection and thereby recruits antibodies and effector cells. Mast cells are found principally below epithelial surfaces of the skin and the digestive and respiratory tracts and their activation by innocuous substances is responsible for many of the symptoms of acute allergic reactions.

The complement system in humoral immunity.

Complement was discovered many years ago as a heat-labile component of normal plasma that augments opsonization of bacteria by antibodies and allows some antibodies to kill bacteria. This activity was said to 'complement' the antibacterial activity of antibody, hence the name complement. The complement system is made up of a large number of distinct plasma proteins; one is activated directly by bound antibody to trigger a cascade of reactions each of which results in the activation of another complement component. Some activated complement proteins bind covalently to bacteria, opsonizing them for engulfment by phagocytes bearing **complement receptors**. Small fragments of some complement proteins act as chemoattractants to recruit phagocytes to the site of complement activation and activate them. The **terminal complement components** damage certain bacteria by creating pores in the bacterial membrane.

The effector functions of complement can be activated through three pathways (Fig. 8.31). The **classical pathway** is activated by antibody binding to antigen. The **lectin pathway** is initiated by binding of a serum lectin, the mannan-binding lectin, to mannose-containing proteins or to carbohydrates on bacteria or viruses. Finally, the **alternative pathway** can be initiated when a spontaneously activated complement component binds to the surface of a pathogen. It provides an amplification loop for the classical pathway of complement activation because one of the activated components of the classical pathway can also initiate the alternative pathway. Complement thus appears to be an important

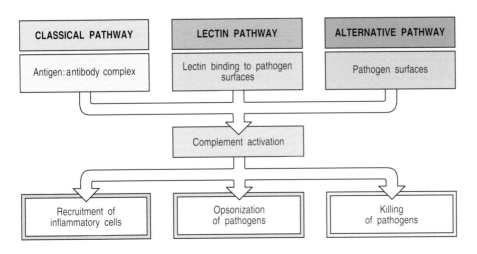

Fig. 8.31 Schematic overview of the complement cascade. There are three pathways of complement activation: the classical pathway, which is triggered by antibody; the lectin-mediated pathway, which is triggered by normal serum proteins that bind some encapsulated bacteria; and the alternative pathway, which is triggered directly on pathogen surfaces. They all generate a crucial enzymatic activity that, in turn, generates the effector activities of complement. The three main consequences of complement activation are opsonization of pathogens, the recruitment of inflammatory cells, and direct killing of pathogens.

part of innate humoral immunity that has been harnessed by the adaptive humoral response. We shall focus here on the classical pathway, touching on the alternative pathway in its role in amplifying the classical pathway but leaving the details of how the lectin and alternative pathways can be initiated in the absence of antibody for Chapter 9, where we discuss innate mechanisms of immunity.

8-22   Complement is a system of plasma proteins that interact with bound antibodies and surface receptors to aid in the elimination of pathogens.

In the humoral immune response, binding of either IgM or most classes of IgG to a pathogen activates the complement cascade. The events of the complement cascade can be divided into two sequences of reactions, which we shall call 'early' and 'late' events. The early events consist of a series of proteolytic steps in which an inactive precursor protein is cleaved to yield a large active fragment, which binds to the surface of a pathogen and contributes to the next cleavage, and a small peptide fragment that is released from the cell and often mediates inflammatory responses. The early events end with the production of a protease called a **C3 convertase**, which binds covalently to the pathogen surface. Here it generates the two main effector molecules of the complement system: an opsonin that binds covalently to pathogen surfaces, and a small peptide mediator of inflammation. The C3 convertase also generates a C5 convertase that initiates the late events of complement activation. These comprise a sequence of polymerization reactions in which the terminal complement components interact to form a **membrane-attack complex**, which creates a pore in membranes of certain pathogens that can lead to their death.

The C3 convertase thus occupies a central position in the complement cascade (Fig. 8.32). The reactions triggered by bound antibody molecules are called the classical pathway of complement activation because this pathway was discovered first. However, the alternative pathway of complement activation, in which the early events are triggered in the absence of antibody, probably arose first in evolution. The related lectin-dependent pathway may be an evolutionary intermediate (see Chapter 9). Each pathway generates a C3 convertase by a different route but two of the three convertases are identical and all are homologous and have the same activity, so the principal effector molecules and the late events are the same for all three pathways.

Fig. 8.32 Overview of the main components and effector actions of complement. The early events of all three pathways of complement activation involve a series of cleavage reactions culminating in the formation of an enzymatic activity called a C3 convertase, which cleaves complement component C3. This is the point at which the three pathways converge and the effector functions of complement are generated. The larger cleavage fragment of C3 (C3b) binds to the membrane and opsonizes bacteria, allowing phagocytes to internalize them. The small fragments of C5 and C3, called C5a and C3a, are peptide mediators of local inflammation. C4a, marked with a *, is generated by cleavage of C4 during the early events of the classical pathway (and not by the action of C3 or C5 convertase); it is also a peptide mediator of inflammation but its effects are relatively weak. Similarly, the large cleavage fragment of C4, C4b, is a weak opsonin (not shown). Finally, the C3b bound to the C3 convertase binds C5, allowing the C3 convertase to generate C5b, which associates with the bacterial membrane and triggers the late events, in which the terminal components of complement assemble into a membrane-attack complex that can damage the membrane of certain pathogens.

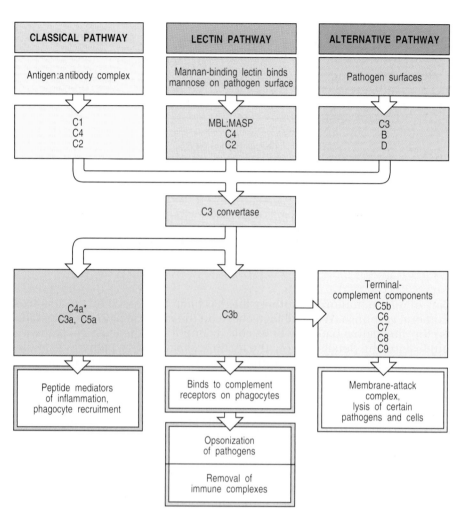

The nomenclature of complement proteins is often a significant obstacle to understanding this system. The following conventional definitions will be used here. All components of the classical complement pathway are designated by the letter C followed by a number, and the native components have a simple number designation, for example C1 and C2. Unfortunately, the components were numbered in the order of their discovery, and not the sequence of reactions, which is C1, C4, C2, C3, C5, C6, C7, C8, and C9. The products of the cleavage reactions are designated by added lower-case letters, the larger fragment being designated b and the smaller a; thus for example C4 is cleaved to C4b and C4a. The components of the alternative pathway, instead of being numbered, are designated by different capital letters, for example B and D. As with the classical pathway, their cleavage products are designated by the addition of lowercase a and b: thus, the large fragment of B is called Bb and the small fragment Ba. Activated complement components are often designated by a horizontal line, for example C2b; however, we shall not use this convention. It is also useful to be aware that the large active fragment of C2 was originally designated C2a, and is still called that in some texts and research papers. Here, for consistency, we will call all large fragments of complement b, so the large active fragment of C2 will be designated C2b.

An overview of the complement system is shown in Fig. 8.32. The generation of the C3 convertase, so called because it is specific for the cleavage of complement component C3, results in the rapid cleavage of many molecules of C3 to produce C3b, which binds covalently to the pathogen surface. The cleavage of C3 and the binding of large numbers of C3b molecules to the surface of the pathogen is a pivotal event in complement activation. At this point the pathways of complement activation converge, the main effector activities of complement are generated, and the late events begin, with C3b playing a central part. Bound C3b and its derivative fragments are the major opsonins of the complement system, binding to **complement receptors** on phagocytes and facilitating engulfment of the pathogen. C3b also binds C5, allowing it to be cleaved by the C2b component of the C4b,2b,3b C5 convertase to initiate the assembly of the membrane-attack complex. C5a and C3a mediate local inflammatory responses, recruiting fluid, cells, and proteins to the site of infection. Finally, the binding of C3b initiates the alternative pathway, thereby amplifying complement activation.

It is clear that a pathway leading to such potent inflammatory and destructive effects, and which, moreover, has a built-in amplification step, is potentially dangerous and must be subject to tight regulation. One important safeguard is that key activated complement components are rapidly inactivated unless they bind to the pathogen surface on which their activation is initiated. There are also several points on the pathway where regulatory proteins act on complement components to prevent the inadvertent activation of complement on host cells and hence accidental damage to them. We shall return to these regulatory mechanisms at the end of this part of the chapter.

We have now met all the relevant components of complement, albeit in a superficial manner, and we are ready for a more detailed account of their functions. To help distinguish the different components according to their functions, we shall use a color code in figures in this section that list the various components and their activities: this is introduced in Fig. 8.33, where all the components of complement are grouped by function.

Functional protein classes in the complement system	
Binding to antigen: antibody complexes	C1q
Activating enzymes	C1r C1s C2b Bb D
Membrane-binding proteins and opsonins	C4b C3b
Peptide mediators of inflammation	C5a C3a C4a
Membrane-attack proteins	C5b C6 C7 C8 C9
Complement receptors	CR1 CR2 CR3 CR4 C1qR
Complement-regulatory proteins	C1INH C4bp CR1 MCP DAF H I P CD59

Fig. 8.33 Functional protein classes in the complement system.

| 8-23 | **The C1q molecule binds to antibody molecules to trigger the classical pathway of complement activation.** |

The first component of the classical pathway of complement activation is C1, which is a complex of three proteins called C1q, C1r, and C1s, two molecules each of C1r and C1s being bound to each molecule of C1q (Fig. 8.34). Complement activation is initiated when antibodies attached to the surface of a pathogen bind C1q. C1q can be bound by either IgM or IgG antibodies (see Fig. 8.16) but, because of the structural requirements of binding to C1q, neither of these antibody isotypes can activate complement in solution; the cascade is initiated only when they are bound to multiple sites on a cell surface, normally that of a pathogen.

The C1q molecule has six globular heads joined to a common stem by long, filamentous domains that resemble collagen molecules; the whole C1q complex has been likened to a bunch of six tulips held together by the stems. Each globular head can bind to one Fc domain, and binding of two or more globular heads activates the C1q molecule. In plasma, the

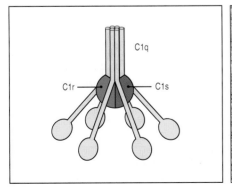
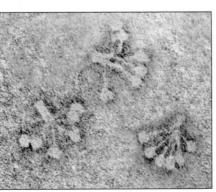

Fig. 8.34 The first protein in the classical pathway of complement activation is C1, which is a complex of C1q, C1r, and C1s. C1q is composed of six identical subunits with globular heads and long, collagen-like tails. The tails bind to two molecules each of C1r and C1s; the heads bind to the Fc domains of immunoglobulin molecules. Photograph (x 500 000) courtesy of K B M Reid.

Fig. 8.35 The two conformations of IgM. The left panel shows the planar conformation of soluble IgM while the right panel shows the staple conformation of IgM bound to a bacterial flagellum. Photographs (x 760 000) courtesy of K H Roux.

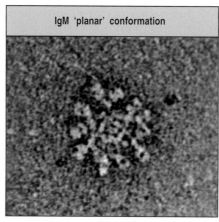

IgM 'planar' conformation

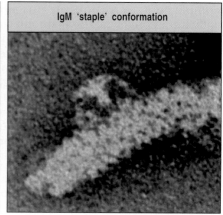

IgM 'staple' conformation

pentameric IgM molecule has a planar conformation that does not bind C1q (Fig. 8.35, left panel); however, binding to the surface of a pathogen deforms the IgM pentamer so that it looks like a staple (see Fig. 8.35, right panel), and this distortion exposes binding sites for the C1q heads. Although C1q binds with low affinity to some subclasses of IgG in solution, the binding energy required for C1q activation is achieved only when a single molecule of C1q can bind two or more IgG molecules bound within 30–40 nm of each other. This requires the random binding of many IgG molecules to a single pathogen. For this reason, IgM is much more efficient in activating complement than IgG.

The binding of C1q to a single bound IgM molecule, or to two or more bound IgG molecules, leads to the activation of an enzymatic activity in C1r; the active form of C1r then cleaves its associated C1s to generate an active serine protease (Fig. 8.36). The activation of C1s completes the first step in the classical pathway of complement activation.

Fig. 8.36 The classical pathway of complement activation is initiated by binding of C1q to antibody on a bacterial surface. In the left panels, one molecule of IgM, bent into the 'staple' conformation by binding several identical epitopes on a pathogen surface, allows the globular heads of C1q to bind to its Fc pieces on the surface of the pathogen. In the right panels, multiple molecules of IgG bound on the surface of a pathogen allow binding of a single molecule of C1q to two or more Fc pieces. In both cases, binding of C1q activates the associated C1r, which becomes an active enzyme that cleaves the proenzyme C1s, generating a serine protease that initiates the classical complement cascade.

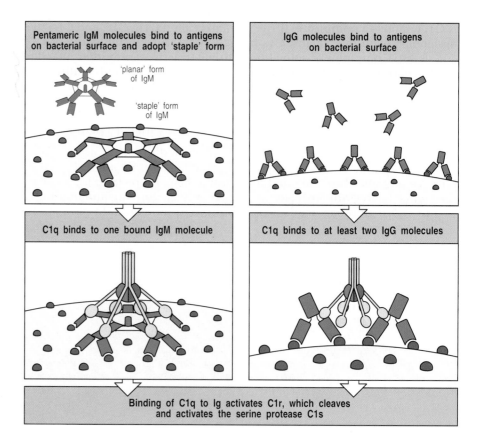

Pentameric IgM molecules bind to antigens on bacterial surface and adopt 'staple' form

'planar' form of IgM

'staple' form of IgM

IgG molecules bind to antigens on bacterial surface

C1q binds to one bound IgM molecule

C1q binds to at least two IgG molecules

Binding of C1q to Ig activates C1r, which cleaves and activates the serine protease C1s

8-24	**The classical pathway of complement activation generates a C3 convertase bound to the pathogen surface.**

Once bound antibody has activated C1s, the C1s enzyme acts on the next two components of the classical pathway, cleaving C4 and then C2 to generate two large fragments, C4b and C2b, which together form the C3 convertase of the classical pathway. In the first step, C1s cleaves the plasma protein C4 to produce C4b, which binds covalently to the surface of the pathogen. The covalently attached C4b then binds one molecule of C2, making it susceptible, in turn, to cleavage by C1s. C1s cleaves C2 to produce the large fragment C2b, which is itself a serine protease. The complex of C4b with the active serine protease C2b remains on the surface of the pathogen as the C3 convertase of the classical pathway. Its most important activity is to cleave large numbers of C3 molecules to C3b, some of which bind to the pathogen surface, and C3a, which initiates a local inflammatory response. These reactions, which comprise the classical pathway of complement activation, are shown in schematic form in Fig. 8.37.

It is important that the C3 convertase is attached firmly to the pathogen so that C3 activation occurs there and not on host-cell surfaces. This is achieved principally by the covalent binding of C4b to the pathogen surface. Cleavage of C4 exposes a highly reactive thioester bond on the C4b molecule that allows it to bind covalently to molecules in the immediate vicinity of its site of activation: this may be the bound antibody molecule that activated the classical pathway, or any adjacent protein on the pathogen surface. If C4b does not rapidly form this bond, the thioester bond is cleaved by reacting with water (hydrolysis), irreversibly inactivating C4b (Fig. 8.38). This helps to prevent C4b from diffusing from its site of activation on the microbial surface to become coupled to host cells.

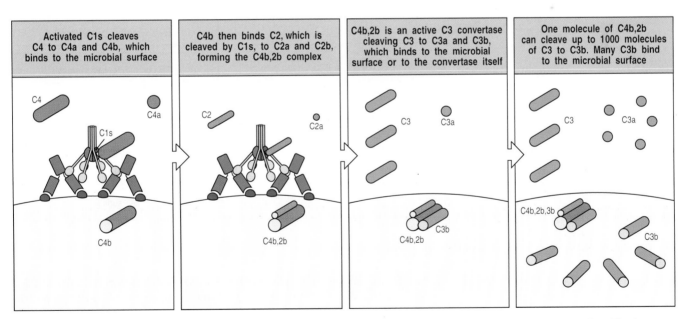

Fig. 8.37 The classical pathway of complement activation generates a C3 convertase that deposits large numbers of C3b molecules on the pathogen. The steps in the reaction are outlined here and detailed in the text. The cleavage of C4 by C1s exposes a reactive group on C4b that allows it to bind covalently to the pathogen surface (see Fig. 8.38). C4b then binds C2, making it susceptible to cleavage by C1s. The larger C2b fragment is the active protease component of the C3 convertase, which cleaves many molecules of C3 to produce C3b, which binds to the pathogen surface, and C3a, an inflammatory mediator. The C4b,2b,3b complex forms the classical pathway C5 convertase.

Fig. 8.38 Cleavage of C4 exposes an active thioester bond that causes the large fragment, C4b, to bind covalently to nearby molecules on the bacterial cell surface. Intact C4 consists of an α, β and γ chain with a shielded thioester bond on the α chain that is exposed when the α chain is cleaved by C1s to produce C4b. The thioester bond (arrowed in the third panel) is rapidly hydrolyzed by water, inactivating C4b unless it reacts with hydroxyl or amino groups to form a covalent linkage with molecules on the pathogen surface. The homologous protein C3 has an identical reactive thioester bond that is also exposed on the C3b fragment when C3 is cleaved by C2b. The covalent attachment of C3b and C4b enables these molecules to act as opsonins and is important in confining complement activation to the pathogen surface.

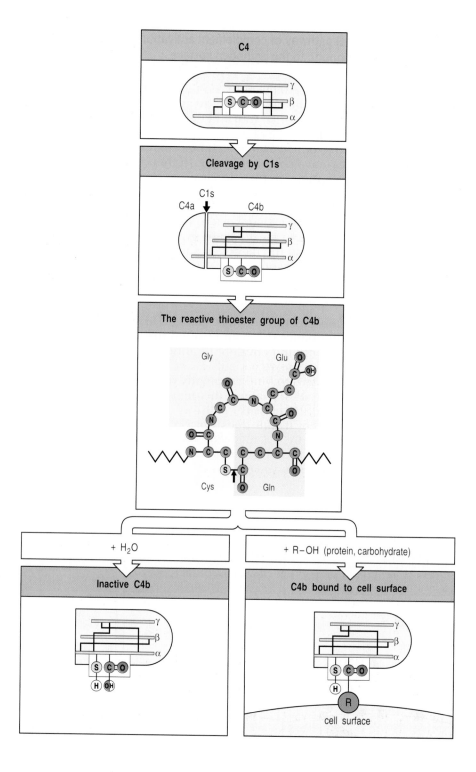

C2 becomes susceptible to cleavage by C1s only when it is bound by C4b, and the C2b serine protease is thereby also confined to the pathogen surface where it remains associated with C4b, providing the enzymatic activity of the C3 convertase of the classical pathway. The activation of C3 molecules thus also occurs at the surface of the pathogen, and the C3b cleavage product of C3 binds covalently by the same mechanism as C4b, as we shall see below. The proteins of the classical pathway of complement activation and their active forms are listed in Fig. 8.39.

Proteins of the classical pathway of complement activation		
Native component	Active form	Function of the active form
C1 (C1q: C1r$_2$:C1s$_2$)	C1q	Binds to antibody that has bound antigen, activates C1r
	C1r	Cleaves C1s to active protease
	C1s	Cleaves C4 and C2
C4	C4b	Covalently binds to pathogen and opsonizes it. Binds C2 for cleavage by C1s
	C4a	Peptide mediator of inflammation (weak)
C2	C2b	Active enzyme of classical pathway C3/C5 convertase: cleaves C3 and C5
	C2a	Precursor of vasoactive C2 kinin
C3	C3b	Many molecules bind pathogen surface and act as opsonins. Initiates amplification via the alternative pathway. Binds C5 for cleavage by C2b
	C3a	Peptide mediator of inflammation (intermediate)

Fig. 8.39 The proteins of the classical pathway of complement activation.

8-25 The cell-bound C3 convertase deposits large numbers of C3b molecules on the pathogen surface.

The C3 convertase of the classical pathway, consisting of the complex C4b,2b, cleaves C3 into C3b and C3a. C3 is structurally and functionally homologous to C4, and C3b, like C4b has a reactive thioester bond that is exposed by cleavage. This allows C3b to bind covalently to adjacent molecules on the pathogen surface; otherwise it is inactivated by hydrolysis. Complement component C3 is the most abundant complement protein in plasma, existing at a concentration of 1.2 mg ml^{-1}, and up to 1000 molecules of C3b can bind in the vicinity of a single active C3 convertase (see Fig. 8.37). Thus, the main effect of complement activation is to deposit large quantities of C3b on the surface of the initiating pathogen where it forms a covalently bonded coat that, as we shall see, can signal the ultimate destruction of the pathogen by phagocytes.

The next step in the cascade is the generation of the C5 convertase by the binding of C3b to C4b,2b to yield C4b,2b,3b. This complex binds C5 and makes C5 susceptible to cleavage by the serine protease activity of C2b, initiating the generation of the membrane-attack complex. This reaction is much more limited than cleavage of C3, as C5 can be cleaved only if it binds C3b that is part of the C4b,2b,3b,C5 convertase complex. Thus, the end result of the early events of complement activation by the classical pathway is the binding of large numbers of C3b molecules on the surface of the pathogen, with the generation of a more limited number of C5b molecules, and the release of C3a and C5a.

The many C3b molecules deposited on the pathogen surface can be recognized by complement receptors on phagocytic cells, stimulating them to engulf the pathogen. The small peptides C4a, C3a, and especially C5a, which are generated by the cleavage of C4, C3, and C5, are local inflammatory mediators of increasing potency. Finally, as already mentioned, the generation of C5b leads to the formation of the membrane-attack complex. Before discussing these effector functions of complement in greater detail, we will see how bound C3b can amplify the effects of the classical pathway by initiating activation of the alternative pathway.

8-26 Bound C3b initiates the alternative pathway of complement activation to amplify the effects of the classical pathway.

Apart from the initiating step, the events of the alternative pathway of complement activation are exactly analogous to those of the classical pathway and involve homologous activated components. Thus, in each case, a large active fragment is deposited on the surface of the pathogen where it binds a second component and renders it susceptible to cleavage by an activating protease to generate the active protease component of the resulting C3 convertase (Fig. 8.40).

In the classical pathway, the first covalently bound fragment is C4b, generated by the cleavage of C4 by activated C1s. In the alternative pathway, the first covalently bound fragment is C3b, and the alternative pathway is activated by the covalent binding of C3b to the pathogen surface. We have already seen that C3b is structurally and functionally homologous to C4b, the first active fragment to bind to the pathogen surface in the classical pathway. In the second step of the alternative pathway, C3b binds to factor B, which is structurally and functionally homologous to C2.

Binding of factor B to C3b makes it susceptible to cleavage by the plasma protease factor D. This cleavage yields a small fragment Ba and an active protease Bb, which remains bound to C3b to make the complex C3b,Bb, which is the C3 convertase of the alternative pathway of complement activation. Note that C3b,Bb is the exact structural and functional homolog of C4b,2b, the C3 convertase of the classical pathway, and that the homologous components C2 of the classical pathway and factor B of the alternative pathway are encoded in adjacent genes in the class III region of the MHC (see Fig. 4.17). The components of the alternative pathway of complement activation are summarized in Fig. 8.41.

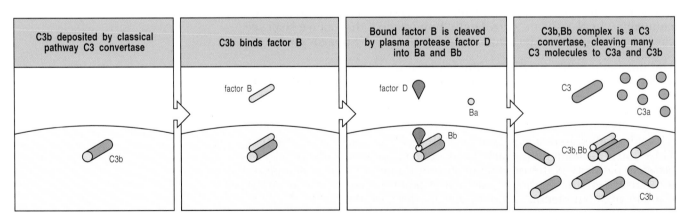

| C3b deposited by classical pathway C3 convertase | C3b binds factor B | Bound factor B is cleaved by plasma protease factor D into Ba and Bb | C3b,Bb complex is a C3 convertase, cleaving many C3 molecules to C3a and C3b |

Fig. 8.40 The alternative pathway of complement activation can amplify the classical pathway by depositing more C3b molecules on the pathogen. C3b deposited by the classical pathway can bind factor B, making it susceptible to cleavage by factor D. The C3b,Bb complex is the C3 convertase of the alternative pathway of complement activation and its action, like that of C4b,2b, results in the deposition of many molecules of C3b on the pathogen surface.

Proteins of the alternative pathway of complement activation		
Native component	Active fragments	Function
C3	C3b	Binds to pathogen surface, binds B for cleavage by D, C3b,Bb is C3 convertase and C3b$_2$Bb is C5 convertase
Factor B (B)	Ba	Small fragment of B, unknown function
	Bb	Bb is active enzyme of the C3 convertase C3b,Bb and C5 convertase C3b$_2$Bb
Factor D (D)	D	Plasma serine protease, cleaves B when it is bound to C3b to Ba and Bb

Fig. 8.41 The proteins of the alternative pathway of complement activation.

The C3 convertase of the alternative pathway, like that of the classical pathway, can cleave many molecules of C3 to generate yet more active C3b on the surface of the pathogen (see Fig. 8.40). The net result of activation of the classical pathway and its amplification via the alternative pathway is the rapid saturation of the surface of a pathogen with C3b, with the release of the small inflammatory mediator C3a. Some of the bound C3b binds to pre-existing C3 convertase, yielding C3b$_2$Bb, the alternative pathway C5 convertase. C3b$_2$Bb can cleave C5 into C5b, which initiates the generation of the membrane-attack complex, and C5a, a potent inflammatory mediator. We now return to the effector actions initiated by C3b.

8-27 | Some complement components bind to specific receptors on phagocytes and help to stimulate their activation.

The most important action of complement is to facilitate the uptake and destruction of pathogens by phagocytic cells. This occurs by specific recognition of bound complement components by **complement receptors (CRs)** on phagocytes. Similar receptors on red blood cells play a role in the clearance of soluble antigen:antibody complexes from the circulation, as we shall see in the next section. The complement receptors expressed on phagocytic cells bind pathogens opsonized with bound complement components: opsonization of pathogens is a major function of C3b and its proteolytic derivatives. C4b, the functional homolog of C3b, also acts as an opsonin but plays a relatively minor role, largely because so much more C3b is generated than C4b.

The five known types of receptors for bound complement components are listed, with their functions and distribution, in Fig. 8.42. The best characterized of these receptors is the C3b receptor **CR1**, which is expressed on both macrophages and polymorphonuclear leukocytes. C3b alone cannot stimulate phagocytosis via CR1, but it can enhance phagocytosis and microbicidal activity induced either by the binding of IgG to the Fcγ receptor (Fig. 8.43) or by other immune mediators, such as the T cell-derived cytokine IFN-γ. The small complement fragment C5a can also activate macrophages to ingest bacteria coated with complement alone by binding to a specific receptor, the **C5a receptor**, which has seven membrane-spanning domains. Receptors of this type typically couple with guanine nucleotide-binding proteins called G proteins, and the C5a receptor signals cells in this way. It is particularly important in the destruction of pathogens coated with complement

Fig. 8.42 Distribution and function of receptors for complement proteins on the surfaces of cells. There are several different receptors specific for different bound complement components. CR1 and CR3 are especially important in inducing phagocytosis of bacteria bearing complement components. CR1 on erythrocytes also plays an important role in clearing immune complexes from the circulation (see Fig. 8.45). CR2 is found mainly on B cells, where it is also part of the B cell co-receptor complex and the receptor by which the Epstein-Barr virus selectively infects B cells, causing infectious mononucleosis.

Receptor	Specificity	Functions	Cell types
CR1	C3b, C4b	Promotes C3b and C4b decay, Stimulates phagocytosis, Erythrocyte transport of immune complexes	Erythrocytes, macrophages, monocytes, polymorphonuclear leukocytes, B cells, FDC
CR2 (CD21)	C3d, C3dg, C3bi Epstein-Barr virus	Part of B-cell co-receptor, Epstein-Barr virus receptor	B cells, FDC
CR3 (CD11b/CD18)	C3bi	Stimulates phagocytosis	Macrophages, monocytes, polymorphonuclear leukocytes, FDC
CR4 (gp150,95) (CD11c/CD18)	C3bi	Stimulates phagocytosis	Macrophages, monocytes, polymorphonuclear leukocytes
C1q receptor	C1q (collagen region)	Binding of immune complexes to phagocytes	B cells, macrophages, monocytes, platelets, endothelial cells

and IgM, since phagocytes do not have Fc receptors for IgM (Fig. 8.44). A further contribution to activation can be made by binding of the phagocyte to extracellular matrix-associated proteins like fibronectin, encountered when phagocytes are recruited to connective tissue and activated there.

Three other complement receptors, CR2 (also known as CD21), CR3, and CR4, bind to inactivated forms of C3b that remain attached to the pathogen surface. Like several other key components of complement, C3b is subject to the action of regulatory mechanisms that can cleave C3b into inactive derivatives (see Section 8-31). One of the inactive derivatives of C3b, known as C3bi, remains attached to the pathogen and acts as an opsonin in its own right when bound by the complement receptors CR2 or CR3. Unlike the binding of C3b to CR1, binding of C3bi to CR3 is sufficient on its own to stimulate phagocytosis. A second breakdown product of C3b, called C3dg, binds only to CR2.

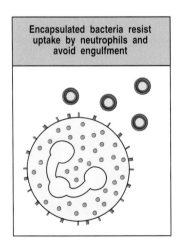

Encapsulated bacteria resist uptake by neutrophils and avoid engulfment

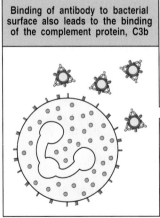

Binding of antibody to bacterial surface also leads to the binding of the complement protein, C3b

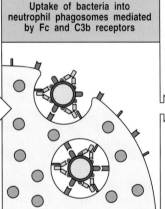

Uptake of bacteria into neutrophil phagosomes mediated by Fc and C3b receptors

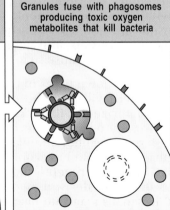

Granules fuse with phagosomes producing toxic oxygen metabolites that kill bacteria

Fig. 8.43 Encapsulated bacteria are more efficiently engulfed by phagocytes when they are also coated with complement. The phagocytes shown here are polymorphonuclear neutrophilic leukocytes (neutrophils); macrophages also bear complement receptors that act in the same way. Here, the neutrophil binds the bacterium by both Fc receptors and complement receptors, which synergize in inducing pathogen uptake and neutrophil activation.

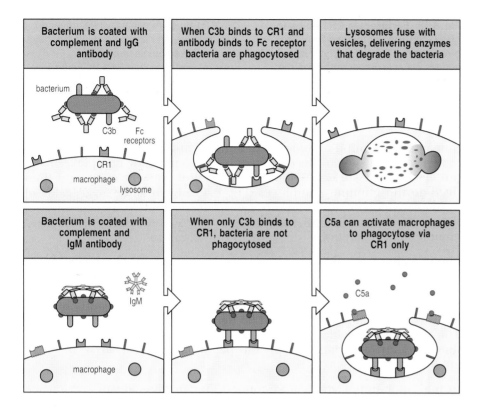

| Bacterium is coated with complement and IgG antibody | When C3b binds to CR1 and antibody binds to Fc receptor bacteria are phagocytosed | Lysosomes fuse with vesicles, delivering enzymes that degrade the bacteria |
| Bacterium is coated with complement and IgM antibody | When only C3b binds to CR1, bacteria are not phagocytosed | C5a can activate macrophages to phagocytose via CR1 only |

Fig. 8.44 Complement CR1 receptors require ancillary activating signals to participate in phagocytosis.
Fc receptors and complement receptors synergize in inducing phagocytosis, and bacteria coated with IgG antibody and complement are therefore more readily ingested than those coated with IgG alone (upper panels). When bacteria are coated with IgM antibody and complement, however, they cannot be ingested unless the phagocyte is pre-activated, for example by T cells or by C5a, as phagocytes do not have Fc-receptors for IgM (lower panels).

The complement receptor CR2, which recognizes C3bi and C3dg, is an important part of the B-cell co-receptor complex. It is believed that binding of C3bi and/or C3dg to CR2 plays a critical role in B-cell responses by providing a link between the B-cell antigen receptor and its co-receptor, making the B cell 100- to 10 000-fold more sensitive to antigen. CR2 also makes B cells susceptible to the **Epstein-Barr virus (EBV)**, which binds specifically to CR2 and is the cause of **infectious mononucleosis**. CR3 and CR4 are members of the CD11/CD18 leukocyte integrin family, of which LFA-1 is the third member. Their roles as complement receptors are less well understood, as is the role of the C1q receptor.

The central role of opsonization by C3b and its inactive fragments in the destruction of extracellular pathogens can be seen in the effects of various complement deficiency diseases. Whereas individuals deficient in any of the late components of complement are relatively unaffected, individuals deficient in C3 or in molecules that catalyze C3b deposition show increased susceptibility to infection by a wide range of extracellular bacteria, as we shall see in Chapter 10.

8-28   **Complement receptors are important in the removal of immune complexes from the circulation.**

Many small soluble antigens form antibody:antigen complexes that contain too few molecules of IgG to be readily bound to Fcγ receptors. These include toxins bound by neutralizing antibodies and debris from dead microorganisms. Such **immune complexes** are found following most infections and antibody responses, and they are removed from the circulation through the action of complement. The soluble immune complexes trigger their own removal by directly activating complement, so that the activated components C4b and C3b bind covalently to the complex, which is then cleared from the circulation by the binding of C4b and C3b to CR1 on the surface of erythrocytes. The erythrocytes

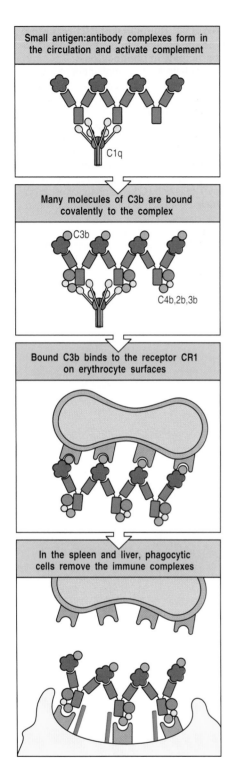

Small antigen:antibody complexes form in the circulation and activate complement

C1q

Many molecules of C3b are bound covalently to the complex

C3b

C4b,2b,3b

Bound C3b binds to the receptor CR1 on erythrocyte surfaces

In the spleen and liver, phagocytic cells remove the immune complexes

Fig. 8.45 Erythrocyte CR1 helps to clear immune complexes from the circulation. CR1 on the erythrocyte surface plays an important role in the clearance of immune complexes from the circulation. Immune complexes bind to CR1 on erythrocytes, which transport them to the liver and spleen, where they are removed by macrophages expressing receptors for both Fc and bound complement components.

transport the bound complexes of antigen, antibody, and complement to the liver and spleen. Here, macrophages remove the complexes from the erythrocyte surface without destroying the erythrocyte, and then degrade the immune complexes (Fig. 8.45). Even larger aggregates of particulate antigen and antibody can be made soluble by activation of the classical complement pathway, and then removed by binding to complement receptors.

Immune complexes that are not removed tend to deposit in the basement membranes of small blood vessels, most notably those of the renal glomerulus where the blood is filtered to form urine. Immune complexes that pass through the basement membrane of the glomerulus bind to CR1 on the renal podocytes that lie beneath the basement membrane. The functional significance of these receptors is unknown; however, they play an important part in the pathology that can arise in some autoimmune diseases.

In the autoimmune disease systemic lupus erythematosus, which we describe in Chapter 12, excessive levels of circulating immune complexes cause huge deposits of antigen, antibody, and complement on the podocytes, damaging the glomerulus; kidney failure is the principal danger in this disease. Immune complexes can also be a cause of pathology in patients with deficiencies in the early components of complement. Such patients do not clear immune complexes effectively and they also suffer tissue damage, especially kidney damage, in a similar way.

8-29   Small peptide fragments released during complement activation trigger a local response to infection.

Many molecules released during immune responses induce a local inflammatory response. We have seen earlier in this chapter how mast cells can be triggered to release local inflammatory mediators, and we shall see in Chapter 9 that similar reactions can be produced by activated phagocytes.

The small complement fragments C3a, C4a, and C5a act on specific receptors to produce similar local inflammatory responses and are therefore often referred to as **anaphylatoxins** (anaphylaxis is an acute systemic inflammatory response; see Section 11-10). Of the three, C5a is the most stable, has the highest specific biological activity, and acts on the best defined receptor. All three induce smooth muscle contraction and increase vascular permeability, and C3a and C5a can activate mast cells to release mediators that cause similar effects. These changes recruit antibody, complement, and phagocytic cells to the site of an infection, and the increased fluid in the tissues hastens the movement of pathogen-containing antigen-presenting cells to the local lymph nodes, contributing to the prompt initiation of the adaptive immune response.

C5a also acts directly on neutrophils and monocytes to increase their adherence to vessel walls, their migration toward sites of antigen deposition, and their ability to ingest particles, as well as increasing the

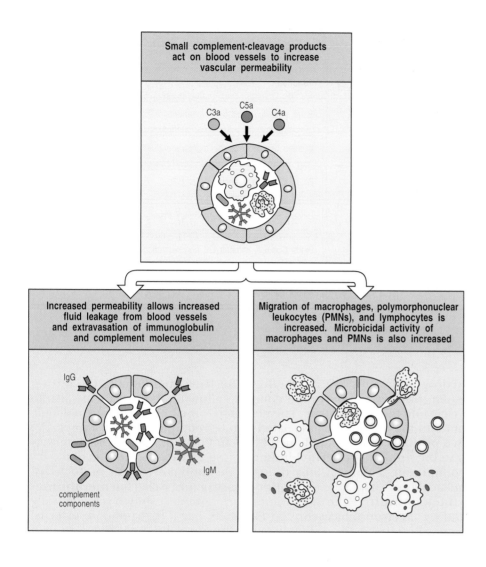

Fig. 8.46 Local inflammatory responses can be induced by small complement fragments, especially C5a. The small complement fragments are differentially active, C5a being more active than C3a, which is more active than C4a. They cause local inflammatory responses by acting directly on local blood vessels and C5a also acts indirectly by activating mast cells. Like mast-cell activation by IgE, these small complement fragments stimulate local increases in blood flow, increased binding of phagocytes to local endothelial cells, and increased local vascular permeability leading to the accumulation of fluid, protein, and cells in the local tissues. The fluid increases lymphatic drainage, bringing antigen to local lymph nodes. The antibodies, complement, and cells thus recruited participate in pathogen clearance by enhancing phagocytosis. The small complement fragments also directly increase the activity of the phagocytes.

expression of CR1 and CR3 on the surfaces of these cells. In this way C5a and, to a lesser extent, C3a and C4a, act in concert with other complement components to hasten the destruction of pathogens by phagocytes (Fig. 8.46).

8-30 | The terminal complement proteins polymerize to form pores in membranes that can kill pathogens.

The most dramatic effect of complement activation is the assembly of the terminal components of complement (Fig. 8.47) to form a membrane-attack complex. The reactions leading to the formation of this complex are shown schematically in Figs. 8.48 and 8.49. The end result is a pore in the lipid bilayer membrane that destroys membrane integrity. This is thought to kill the pathogen by destroying the proton gradient across the pathogen cell membrane.

The first step in the formation of the membrane-attack complex is the cleavage of C5 by a C5 convertase (see Fig. 8.48). One molecule of C5b binds one molecule of C6, and the C5b,6 complex then binds one molecule of C7. This reaction leads to a conformational change in the constituent molecules, with the exposure of a hydrophobic site on C7. This hydrophobic domain of C7 inserts into the lipid bilayer; similar

Fig. 8.47 The terminal complement components that assemble to form the membrane-attack complex.

The terminal complement components that form the membrane-attack complex		
Native protein	Active component	Function
C5	C5a	Small peptide mediator of inflammation
	C5b	Initiates assembly of the membrane-attack system
C6	C6	Binds C5b, forms acceptor for C7
C7	C7	Binds C5b,6, amphiphilic complex inserts in lipid bilayer
C8	C8	Binds C5b,6,7, initiates C9 polymerization
C9	C9n	Polymerizes to C5b,6,7,8 to form a membrane-spanning channel, lysing membrane

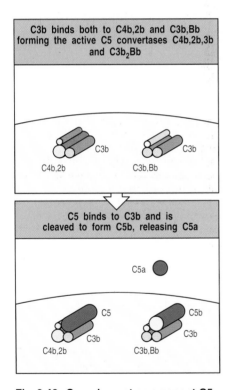

Fig. 8.48 Complement component C5 is activated by a C5 convertase when C5 is complexed to C3b. Top panel: C5 convertases are formed when C3b binds either the classical pathway C3 convertase, C4b,2b to form C4b,2b,C3b, or the alternative pathway C3 convertase, C3b,Bb to form C3b₂Bb. Bottom panel: C5 binds to the C3b in these complexes and is cleaved by the active enzyme C2b or Bb to form C5b and the inflammatory mediator C5a. The production of C5b initiates the assembly of the terminal complement components.

hydrophobic sites are exposed on the later components C8 and C9 when they are bound to the complex, allowing these proteins also to insert into the lipid bilayer. The next step is the binding of one molecule of C8 to the membrane-associated C5b,6,7 complex. C8 is a complex of two proteins, called C8β, which binds to C5b, and C8α-γ, which inserts into the lipid bilayer. The binding of C8β allows the binding of the α-γ component. Finally, C8α-γ induces the polymerization of 10 to 16 molecules of C9 into the annular or ring structure called the **membrane-attack complex**. The membrane-attack complex, shown schematically and by electron microscopy in Fig. 8.49, has a hydrophobic external face, allowing it to associate with the lipid bilayer, but a hydrophilic internal channel. The diameter of this channel is about 100Å, allowing free passage of solute and water across the lipid bilayer. The disruption of the lipid bilayer leads to the loss of cellular homeostasis, the disruption of the proton gradient across the membrane, the penetration of enzymes such as lysozyme into the cell, and the eventual destruction of the pathogen.

The membrane-attack complex is strikingly similar to the perforin pores generated by cytotoxic T cells and NK cells, and the main components of these two structures, C9 and perforin 1, are products of closely related genes. The diameter of the membrane-attack complex inner channel is smaller than that of the perforin ring, which has an inner diameter of about 160Å. The larger perforin pore may be required to allow ready access of granzymes to the interior of the target cell to initiate apoptosis.

Although the effect of the membrane-attack complex is very dramatic (see Fig. 8.49, lower panels), particularly in experimental demonstrations when antibodies to red blood cell membranes are used to trigger the complement cascade, the significance of these components in host defense seems to be quite limited. To date, deficiencies in complement components C5–C9 have been associated with susceptibility only to *Neisseria* spp., the bacteria that cause the sexually transmitted disease gonorrhea and a common form of bacterial meningitis. The opsonizing and inflammatory actions of the earlier components of the complement cascade thus appear to be most important for host defense against infection.

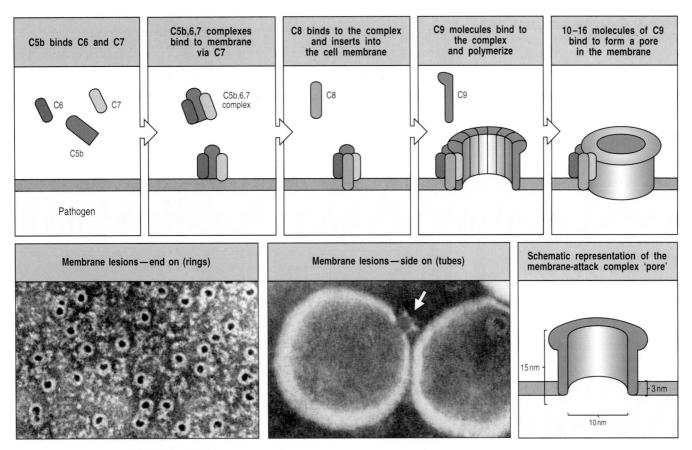

Fig. 8.49 The membrane-attack complex assembles to generate a pore in the lipid bilayer membrane. The sequence of steps and their approximate appearance is shown here in schematic form. C5b, generated by cleavage of C5 bound to C3b by the convertase C4b,2b,3b (or, in the alternative pathway, C3b₂Bb), triggers the assembly of one molecule each of C6, C7 and C8, in that order. C7 and C8 undergo conformational changes that expose hydrophobic domains that insert into the membrane. This complex causes moderate membrane damage in its own right, and also serves to induce polymerization of C9, again with exposure of a hydrophobic site. Up to 16 molecules of C9 are then added to the assembly to generate a channel of 100Å diameter in the membrane. This channel disrupts the bacterial outer membrane, killing the bacterium. The electron micrographs show erythrocyte membranes with membrane-attack complexes in two orientations, end on and side on. Note the resemblance of these complexes to pores caused by perforin. C9 and perforin 1, the major components of these two membrane lesions, are products of related genes. Photographs courtesy of S Bhakdi and J Tranum-Jensen.

8-31 | **Complement regulatory proteins serve to protect host cells from the effects of complement activation.**

When the components of complement are activated, as we have seen, they usually bind immediately to molecules on the pathogen surface and are thereby confined to the microbe on which their activation was initiated. However, activated complement components can sometimes escape to bind proteins on host cells; and all components of complement are activated spontaneously at a low rate in plasma. These activated complement components have the potential to destroy any cells to which they bind. Host cells are protected from such inadvertent damage by a series of complement regulatory proteins, summarized in Fig. 8.50. Some of these proteins are associated with the host cell surface, and similar proteins protect host cells from accidental triggering of the alternative pathway of complement activation, thereby confining these reactions to the surfaces of pathogens.

Fig. 8.50 The proteins that regulate the activity of complement.

Control proteins of the classical and alternative pathways	
Name (symbol)	**Role in the regulation of the complement activation**
C1 inhibitor (C1INH)	Binds to activated C1r, C1s, removing it from C1q
C4-binding protein (C4BP)	Binds to C4b displacing C2b; co-factor for C4b cleavage by I
Complement-receptor 1 (CR1)	Binds C4b displacing C2b, or C3b displacing Bb; co-factor for I
Factor H (H)	Binds C3b displacing Bb; co-factor for I
Factor I (I)	Serine protease that cleaves C3b and C4b; aided by H, MCP, C4BP or CR1
Decay-accelerating factor (DAF)	Membrane protein that displaces Bb from C3b and C2b from C4b
Membrane co-factor protein (MCP)	Membrane protein that promotes C3b and C4b inactivation by I
CD59 (protectin)	Prevents formation of MAC on homologous cells. Widely expressed on membranes

The regulatory reactions are shown in Fig. 8.51. The activation of C1 is controlled by a plasma protein, the **C1 inhibitor** (**C1INH**), which binds the active enzyme moiety, C1r:C1s, and causes it to dissociate from C1q, which remains bound to antibody on the pathogen (see Fig. 8.51, top row). In this way, C1INH limits the time during which active C1s is able to cleave C4 and C2. In the same way, C1INH serves to limit the spontaneous activation of C1 in the plasma. Its importance can be seen in the C1INH deficiency disease **hereditary angioneurotic edema**, in which chronic spontaneous complement activation leads to the production of excess cleaved fragments of C4 and C2. The small fragment of C2, C2a is further cleaved into a peptide, the C2 kinin, that causes extensive swelling, the most dangerous being local swelling in the trachea, which can lead to suffocation. Bradykinin, which has similar actions to C2 kinin, is also produced in an uncontrolled fashion in this disease, as a result of the lack of inhibition of another plasma protease regulated by C1INH. This disease is fully corrected by replacing C1INH. The large activated fragments of C4 and C2, which normally combine to form the C3 convertase, do not damage host cells in such patients because C4b is rapidly inactivated in plasma (see Fig. 8.38) and the convertase does not form. Any convertase that accidentally forms on a host cell, however, is inactivated by further control mechanisms.

First, C2b can be displaced from the complex by either of two proteins—a serum protein called C4-binding protein (C4BP), or a cell-surface protein called decay-accelerating factor (DAF) (see Fig. 8.51, second row). These compete with C2b for binding to C4b. When C4BP binds to C4b, C4b becomes highly susceptible to cleavage by a plasma protein called factor I. Factor I inactivates C4b by cleaving it into the subfragments C4c and C4d. An essentially analogous mechanism operates to inactivate C3b. In this case, either the complement receptor CR1 or a plasma protein called factor H bind to C3b, displacing C2b and making C3b susceptible to cleavage by factor I (see Fig. 8.51, third row). Factor H also has a binding site for sialic acid, which is abundant on mammalian cells but is absent in most bacteria. A second membrane-associated protein, called membrane co-factor protein (MCP) can bind to membrane-associated C3b and catalyze its destruction by factor I. All of the proteins

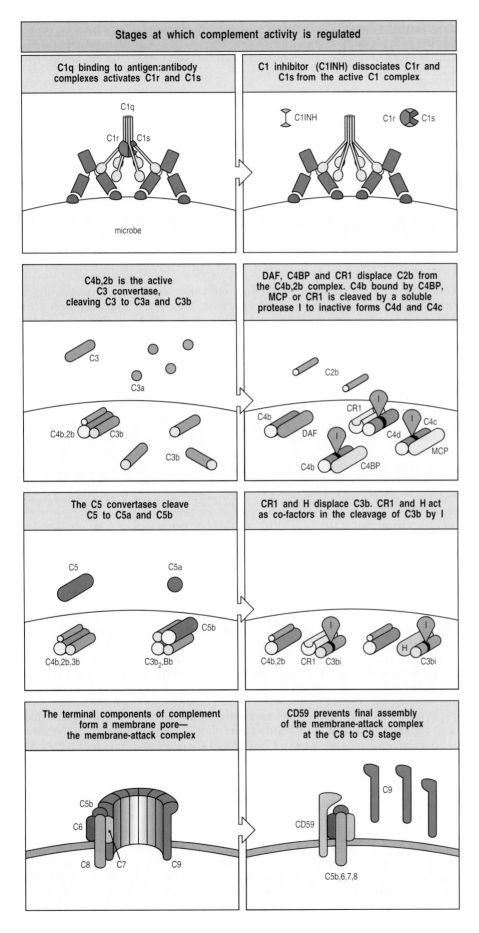

Fig. 8.51 Complement activation is regulated by a series of proteins that serve to protect host cells from accidental damage. These act on different stages of the complement cascade, dissociating complexes or catalyzing the enzymatic degradation of covalently bound complement proteins. Stages in the complement cascade are shown schematically down the left side of the figure, with the control reactions on the right.

Stages at which complement activity is regulated

C1q binding to antigen:antibody complexes activates C1r and C1s

C1 inhibitor (C1INH) dissociates C1r and C1s from the active C1 complex

C4b,2b is the active C3 convertase, cleaving C3 to C3a and C3b

DAF, C4BP and CR1 displace C2b from the C4b,2b complex. C4b bound by C4BP, MCP or CR1 is cleaved by a soluble protease I to inactive forms C4d and C4c

The C5 convertases cleave C5 to C5a and C5b

CR1 and H displace C3b. CR1 and H act as co-factors in the cleavage of C3b by I

The terminal components of complement form a membrane pore— the membrane-attack complex

CD59 prevents final assembly of the membrane-attack complex at the C8 to C9 stage

that bind the homologous C4b and C3b molecules share one or more copies of a structural element called the short consensus repeat (SCR), complement control protein (CCP) repeat, or (especially in Japan) the Sushi domain.

The activity of the terminal complement components is also regulated by cell-surface proteins; the best known is protectin or CD59 (see Fig. 8.51, bottom row). CD59 and DAF are both linked to the cell surface by a phosphoinositol glycolipid tail, like many other membrane proteins. The disease **paroxysmal nocturnal hemoglobinuria**, characterized by episodes of intravascular red blood cell lysis by complement, is most often caused by deficiencies of both CD59 and DAF in patients who fail to generate the phosphoinositol glycolipid linkage. Cells that lack CD59 only are also susceptible to destruction from spontaneous activation of the complement cascade.

Summary.

The complement system is one of the major mechanisms whereby antigen recognition is converted into an effective defense against infection and is particularly important in defense against extracellular bacteria. Complement is a system of plasma proteins that can be activated by antibody, leading to a cascade of reactions that occurs on the surface of pathogens and generates active components with various effector functions. There are three pathways of complement activation: the classical pathway, which is triggered by antibody; the lectin-activated pathway; and the alternative pathway, which provides an amplification loop for the classical pathway. Both the lectin-activated pathway and the alternative pathway are initiated independently of antibody as part of innate immunity. The early events in all pathways consist of a sequence of cleavage reactions in which the larger cleavage product binds covalently to the pathogen surface or antigen:antibody complex and contributes to the activation of the next component. The pathways converge with the formation of a C3 convertase enzyme, which cleaves C3 to produce the active complement component C3b. The binding of large numbers of C3b molecules to the pathogen is the central event in complement activation. Bound complement components, especially bound C3b and its inactive fragments, are recognized by specific complement receptors on phagocytic cells, which engulf pathogens opsonized by C3b and its inactive fragments. Erythrocytes also express a complement receptor specific for C3b, which allows them to bind and transport soluble immune complexes, leading to their clearance by Fc-receptor-expressing phagocytes in the spleen. The complement system also plays a major role in enhancing adaptive humoral immunity; C3b, C3bi and C3dg bound to antigen lower the threshold for activation of B cells. These same C3 fragments similarly play an important role in immunological memory by enhancing the binding of antigen complexed with antibody to follicular dendritic cells in germinal centers, which act as a long-lasting antigen depot. The small cleavage fragments of C3, C4, and especially C5, recruit phagocytes to sites of infection and activate them by binding to specific receptors having seven membrane-spanning domains. Together, these activities promote the uptake and destruction of pathogens by phagocytes. The molecules of C3b that bind the C3 convertase itself initiate the late events, binding C5 to make it susceptible to cleavage by C2b or Bb. The larger C5b fragment triggers the assembly of a membrane-attack complex, which can result in the lysis of certain pathogens. These effects seem to be important only for the killing of a few pathogens but may play a major role in immunopathology. The activity of complement components is modulated by a system of regulatory proteins that prevent tissue damage as a result of inadvertent binding of activated complement components to host cells or spontaneous activation of complement components in plasma.

Summary to Chapter 8.

The humoral immune response to infection involves the production of antibody by B lymphocytes, the binding of this antibody to the pathogen, and the elimination of the pathogen by accessory cells and molecules of the humoral immune system. The production of antibody usually requires the action of helper T cells specific for a peptide fragment of the antigen recognized by the B cell. The B cell then proliferates and differentiates in the specialized microenvironment of lymphoid tissues, where somatic hypermutation generates diversity in the surface immunoglobulin of the B cell. The B cells that bind antigen most avidly are selected for further differentiation by contact with antigen on the surface of follicular dendritic cells and interactions with antigen-specific germinal center helper T cells. These events allow the affinity of antibodies to increase over the course of an antibody response, especially in repeated responses to the same antigen. Helper T cells also direct isotype switching, leading to the production of antibody of various isotypes that can be distributed to various body compartments. IgM is produced early in the response and plays a major role in protecting against infection in the bloodstream, while more mature isotypes such as IgG diffuse into the tissues. Multimeric IgA is produced in lamina propria and transported across epithelial surfaces, while IgE is made in small amounts and binds avidly to the surface of mast cells. Antibodies that bind with high affinity to critical sites on toxins, viruses, and bacteria can neutralize them. However, pathogens and their products are destroyed and removed from the body largely through uptake into phagocytes and degradation inside these cells. Antibodies that coat pathogens bind to Fc receptors on phagocytes, which are thereby triggered to engulf and destroy them. Fc receptors on other cells lead to exocytosis of stored mediators, and this is particularly important in allergic reactions, where mast cells are triggered by antigen binding to IgE antibody to release inflammatory mediator molecules, as we shall learn in Chapter 11. Antibodies can also initiate pathogen destruction by activating the complement system of plasma proteins. Components of complement can opsonize pathogens for uptake by phagocytes, can recruit phagocytes to sites of infection, and can directly destroy pathogens by creating membrane pores in their surfaces. Thus, the humoral immune response is targeted to specific pathogens through production of specific antibody; however, the effector actions of that antibody are determined by the isotype of the antibody and are the same for all pathogens bound by antibody of a particular isotype.

General references.

Cambier, J.C., Pleissen, C.M. and Clack M.E.: **Signal transduction by B-cell antigen receptors and its conceptions.** *Ann. Rev. Immunol.* 1994. **12**:458-486.

Law, S.K.A. and Reid, K.B.M.: *Complement.*, 1st edn. Oxford, IRL Press, 1988.

Metzger, H. (ed.): *Fc receptors and the action of antibodies*, 1st edn. Washington, DC, American Society for Microbiology, 1990.

Moller, G. (ed.): **The B-cell antigen receptor complex.** *Immunol. Rev.* 1993, **132**:1-206.

Rajewsky, K.: **Clonal selection and learning in the antibody system.** *Nature* 1996, **381**:751-758.

Ross, G.D. (ed.): *Immunobiology of the complement system*, 1st edn. Orlando, Academic Press, 1986.

Section references.

8-1 The antibody response is initiated when B cells bind antigen and are signaled by helper T cells or by certain microbial antigens.

DeFranco, A.L.: **Molecular aspects of B-lymphocyte activation.** *Ann. Rev. Cell Biol.* 1987, **3**:143-178.

8-2 Armed helper T cells activate B cells that recognize the same antigen.

Parker, D.C.: **T cell-dependent B-cell activation.** *Ann. Rev. Immunol.* 1993, **11**:331-340.

8-3 Antigen-binding B cells are trapped in the T-cell zone of lymphoid tissues and are activated by encounter with armed helper T cells.

Cyster, J.G., Hartley, S.B., Goodnow, C.C.: **Competition for follicular niches excludes self-reactive cells from the recirculating B-cell repertoire.** *Nature* 1994, **371**:389-395.

8-4 Peptide:MHC class II complexes on a B cell trigger armed helper T cells to make membrane-bound and secreted molecules, which activate the B cell.

Banchereau, J., Bazan, F., Blanchard, D., Briere, F., Galizzi, J.P., Vankooten, C., Liu, Y.J., Rousset, F., and Saeland, S. **The CD40 antigen and its ligand.** *Ann. Rev. Immunol.* 1994, **12**: 881-922.

Foy, T. M. , Aruffo, A., Bajorath, J., Buhlmann, JE., Noelle,R.J.: **Immune regulation by CD40 and its ligand GP39.** *Ann.Rev.Immunol.* 1996, **14**:591-617.

8-5 Isotype switching requires expression of CD40 ligand by the helper T cell and is directed by cytokines.

Aruffo, A., Farrington, M., Hollenbaugh, D., Li, X., Milatovich, A., Nonoyama, S., Bajorath, J., Grosmaire, L.S., Stenkamp, R., Neubauer, M, Roberts, R.L., Noelle, R.J., Ledbetter, J.A., Francke, U., and Ochs, H.D.: **The CD40 ligand, gp39, is defective in activated T cells from patients with X-linked hyper-IgM syndrome.** *Cell* 1993, **72**:291-300.

Lorenz, M., Jung, S., Radbruch, A.: **Switch transcripts in immunoglobulin class switching.** *Science* **267**:1825-1828.

Stavnezer, J.: **Immunoglobulin class switching.** *Curr. Opin. Immunol.* 1996, **8**:199-205.

8-6 Activated B cells proliferate extensively in the specialized microenvironment of the germinal center.

Kelsoe,G.: **Life and death in germinal centers (Redux).** *Immunity* 1996, **4**:107-111.

MacLennan, I.C.M.: **Germinal centres.** *Ann. Rev. Immunol. 1994*, **12**: 117-139.

8-7 Somatic hypermutation occurs in the rapidly dividing centroblasts in the germinal center.

Han, S.H., Hathcock, K., Zheng, B., Kelper, T.B., Hodes, R., Kelso, G.: **Cellular interaction in germinal centers: roles of CD40-ligand and B7-1 and B7-2 in established germinal centres.** *J. Immunol.* 1995, **155**:556-567.

Han, S.H., Zheng, B., Dal Porto, J., Kelsoe, G.: **In situ studies of the primary immune response to (4-Hydroxy-3-Nitrophenyl) Acetyl IV. Affinity-dependent, antigen-driven B cell apoptosis in germinal centers as a mechanism for maintaining self-tolerence.** *J. Exp. Med.* 1995, **182**:1635-1644.

Küppers, R., Zhao, M., Hansmann, M.L., Rajewsky,K.:**Tracing B cell development in human germinal centres by molecular analysis of single cells picked from histological sections.***EMBO J.* 1993, **12**:4955-4967

Wagner, S. D., .Neuberger, M.S.: **Somatic hypermutation of immunoglobulin genes.** *Ann. Rev. Immunol.* 1996, **14**:441-457.

8-8 Non-dividing centrocytes with the best antigen-binding receptors are selected for survival.

Casamayor-Palleja, M., Feuillard, J., Ball, J., Drew, M., MacLennan, I.C.M.: **Centrocytes rapidly adopt a memory B cell phenotype on co-culture with autologous germinal centre T cell-enriched preparations.** *Intl. Immunol.* 1995, **8**:737-744.

Humphrey, J.H., Grennan, D., and Sundaram, V.: **The origin of follicular dendritic cells in the mouse and the mechanism of trapping of immune complexes on them.** *Eur. J. Immunol.* 1984, **14**:1859.

Kosco, M.H., Szakal, A.K., Tew, J.G.: *In vivo*- **obtained antigen presented by germinal center B cells to T cells** *in vitro*. *J. Immunol.* 1988, **140**:354-360.

Tew, J.G., DiLosa, R.M., Burton, G.F., Kosco, M.H., Kupp, L.I., Masuda, A., Szakal, A.K.: **Germinal centers and antibody production in bone marrow.** *Immunol. Rev.* 1992, **126**:99-112.

8-9 B-cell responses to bacterial antigens with intrinsic B-cell activating ability do not require T-cell help.

Anderson, J., Coutinho, A., Lernhardt, W., and Melchers, F.: **Clonal growth and maturation to immunoglobulin secretion** *in vitro* **of every growth-inducible B lymphocyte.** *Cell* 1977, **10**:27-34.

Coutinho, A.: **The theory of the one non-specific model for B-cell activation.** *Transplant. Rev.* 1975, **23**:49.

8-10 B-cell responses to bacterial polysaccharides do not require specific T-cell help.

Mond, J.J., Lees, A., Snapper, C.M.: **T cell-independent antigens type 2.** *Ann. Rev. Immunol.* 1995, **13**:655-692.

8-11 Antibodies of different isotypes operate in distinct places and have distinct effector functions.

Janeway, C.A., Rosen, F.S., Merler, E., and Alper, C.A.: *The gamma globulins,* 2nd edn. Boston, Little Brown and Co., 1967.

8-12 Transport proteins that bind to the Fc domain of antibodies carry specific isotypes across epithelial barriers.

Simister, N.E. and Mostov, K.E.: **An Fc receptor structurally related to MHC class I antigens.** *Nature* 1989, **337**:184-187.

Mostov, K.E.: **Transepithelial transport of Immunoglobulins.** *Ann. Rev. Immunol.* 1994. **12**: 63-84.

Burmeister, W.P., Gastinel, L.N., Simister, N.E., Blum, M.L., Bjorkman, P.J.: **Crystal structure at 2.2 Å resolution of the MHC-related neonatal Fc receptor.** *Nature* 1994. **372**: 336-343.

8-13 High-affinity IgG and IgA antibodies can neutralize bacterial toxins.

Robbins, F.C., Robbins, J.B.: **Current status and prospects for some improved and new bacterial vaccines.** *Am. J. Pub. Health* 1986. **7**:105-125.

8-14 High-affinity IgG and IgA antibodies can inhibit the infectivity of viruses.

Mandel, B.: **Neutralization of polio virus: a hypothesis to explain the mechanism and the one hit character of the neutralization reaction.** *Virology* 1976, **69**:500-510.

Possee, R.D., Schild, G.C., and Dimmock, N.J.: **Studies on the mechanism of neutralization of influenza virus by antibody: evidence that neutralizing antibody (anti-hemaglutanin) inactivates influenza virus** *in vivo* **by inhibiting virion transcriptase activity.** *J. Gen. Virol.* 1982, **58**:373-386.

8-15 Antibodies can block the adherence of bacteria to host cells.

Fischetti, V.A. and Bessen, D.: **Effect of mucosal antibodies to M protein in colonization by group A streptococci.** In Switalski L., Hook, M., and Beachery, E. (eds.): *Molecular mechanisms of microbial adhesion.* New York, Springer, 1989, pp.128-142.

8-16 The Fc receptors of accessory cells are signaling receptors specific for immunoglobulins of different isotypes.

Ravetch, J.V. and Kinet, J.: **Fc receptors.** *Ann. Rev. Immunol.* 1993, **9**:457-492.

Takai, T., Li, M., Sylvestre, D., Clynes, R., and Ravetch, J.V.: **FcRγ chain deletion results in pleiotrophic effector-cell defects.** *Cell* 1994, **76**:519-529.

8-17 Fc receptors on phagocytes are activated by antibodies bound to the surface of pathogens.

Burton, D.R.: **The conformation of antibodies.** In Metzger, H. (ed.): *Fc receptors and the action of antibodies*, 1st edn. Washington, DC, Raven Press, 1990, 31-54.

8-18 Fc receptors on phagocytes allow them to ingest and destroy opsonized extracellular pathogens.

Gounni, A.S., Lamkhioued, B., Ochiai, K., Tanaka, Y., Delaporte, E., Capron A., Kinet, J-P. and Capron, M.: **High-affinity IgE receptor on eosinophils is involved in defence against parasites.** *Nature*, 1994 **367**:183-186.

Karakawa, W.W., Sutton, A., Schneerson, R., Karpas, A., and Vann, W.F.: **Capsular antibodies induce type-specific phagocytosis of capsulated** *Staphylococcus aureus* **by human polymorphonuclear leukocytes.** *Infect. Immun.* 1986, **56**:1090-1095.

8-19 Fc receptors activate natural killer cells to destroy antibody-coated targets.

Lanier, L.L. and Phillips, J.H.: **Evidence for three types of human cytotoxic lymphocyte.** *Immunol. Today* 1986, **7**:132.

Lanier, L.L., Ruitenberg, J.J., and Phillips, J.H.: **Functional and biochemical analysis of CD16 antigen on natural killer cells and granulocytes.** *J. Immunol.* 1988, **141**:3487-3485.

8-20 Mast cells, basophils, and activated eosinophils bind IgE antibody with high affinity.

Beaven, M.A. and Metzger, H.: **Signal transduction by Fc receptors: the FcεRI case.** *Immunol. Today* 1993, **14**:222-226.

Sutton, B.J. and Gould, H.J.: **The human IgE network.** *Nature* 1993, **366**:421-428.

8-21 Mast cell activation by specific IgE antibody plays an important role in resistance to parasite infection.

Capron, A. and Dessaint, J.P.: **Immunologic aspects of schistosomiasis.** *Ann. Rev. Med.* 1992, **43**:209-218.

Galli, S.J., Tsai, M., and Wershil, B.K.: **The c-kit receptor, stem cell factor, and mast cells. What each is teaching us about the others.** *Am. J. Path.* 1993, **142**:965-974.

Gounni, A.S., Lamkhioued, B., Ochiai, K., Tanaka, Y., Delaporte, E., Capron, A., Kinet, J.P., and Capron, M.: **High-affinity IgE receptor on eosinophils is involved in defence against parasites.** *Nature* 1994, **367**:183-186.

Grencis, R.K., Else, K.J., Huntley, J.F., and Nishikawa, S.I.: **The** *in vivo* **role of stem cell factor (c-kit ligand) on mastocytosis and host protective immunity to the intestinal nematode** *Trichinella spiralis* **in mice.** *Parasite Immunol.* 1993, **15**:55-59.

Ishikawa, N., Horii, Y., and Nawa, Y.: **Reconstitution by bone marrow grafting of the defective protective capacity at the migratory phase but not at the intestinal phase of** *Nippostrongylus brasiliensis* **infection in W/Wv mice.** *Parasite Immunol.* 1994, **16**:181-186.

Kasugai, T., Tei, H., Okada, M., Hirota, S., Morimoto, M., Yamada, M., Nakama, A., Arizono, N., and Kitamura, Y.: **Infection with** *Nippostrongylus brasiliensis* **induces invasion of mast cell precursors from peripheral blood to small intestine.** *Blood* 1995, **85**:1334-1340.

Ushio, H., Watanabe, N., Kiso, Y., Higuchi, S., and Matsuda, H.: **Protective immunity and mast cell and eosinophil responses in mice infested with larval** *Haemaphysalis longicornis* **ticks.** *Parasite Immunol.* 1993, **15**:209-214.

8-22 Complement is a system of plasma proteins that interacts with bound antibodies and surface receptors to aid in the elimination of pathogens.

Tomlinson, S.: **Complement defense mechanisms.** *Curr. Opin. Immunol.* 1993, **5**:83-89.

8-23 The C1q molecule binds to antibody molecules to trigger the classical pathway of complement activation.

Cooper, N.R.: **The classical complement pathway. Activation and regulation of the first complement component.** *Adv. Immunol.* 1985, **37**:151-216.

Perkins, S.J. and Nealis, A.S.: **The quaternary structure in solution of human complement subcomponent C1r2Cls2.** *Biochem. J.* 1989, **263**:463-469.

8-24 The classical pathway of complement activation generates a C3 convertase bound to the pathogen surface.

Chan, A.R., Karp, D.R., Shreffler, D.C., and Atkinson, J.P.: **The 20 faces of the fourth component of complement.** *Immunol. Today* 1984, **5**:200-203.

Dodds, A.W., Xiang-Dong, R., Willis, A.C., Law, S.K.A.: **The reaction mechanism of the internal thioester in the human complement component C4.** *Nature* 1996, **379**:177-179

Oglesby, T.J., Accavitti, M.A., and Volanakis, J.E.: **Evidence for a C4b binding site on the C2b domain of C2.** *J. Immunol.* 1988, **141**:926-931.

8-25 The cell-bound C3 convertase deposits large numbers of C3b molecules on the pathogen surface.

deBruijn, M.H.L. and Fey, G.M.: **Human complement component C3: cDNA coding sequence and derived primary structure.** *Proc. Natl. Acad. Sci.* 1985, **82**:708-712.

Volanakis, J.E.: **Participation of C3 and its ligand in complement activation.** *Curr. Top. Microbiol. Immunol.* 1989, **153**: 1-21.

8-26 Bound C3b initiates the alternative pathway of complement activation to amplify the effects of the classical pathway.

Kolb, W.P., Morrow, P.R., and Tamerius, J.D.: **Ba and Bb fragments of Factor B activation: fragment production, biological activities, neoepitope expression and quantitation in clinical samples.** *Complement Inflamm.* 1989, **6**:175-204.

8-27 Some complement components bind to specific receptors on phagocytes and help to stimulate their activation.

Ahearn, J.M. and Fearon, D.T.: **Structure and function of the complement receptors of CR1 (CD35) and CR2 (CD21).** *Adv. Immunol.* 1989, **46**:183-219.

Croix, D.A., Ahearn, J.M., Rosengard, A.M., Han, S., Kelsoe, G., Ma, M., Carroll, M.C.: **Antibody response to a T-dependent antigen requires B cell expression of complement receptors.** *J. Exp. Med.* 1996, **183**:1857-1864.

Dempsey, P.W., Allison, M.E., Akkaraju, S., Goodnow, C.C., Fearon, D.T.: **C3d of complement as a molecular adjuvant: bridging innate and acquired immunity.** *Science* 1996, **271**:348-350.

8-28 Complement receptors are important in the removal of immune complexes from the circulation.

Schifferli, J.A. and Taylor, J.P.: **Physiologic and pathologic aspects of circulating immune complexes.** *Kidney Intl.* 1989, **35**:993-1003.

Schifferli, J.A., Ng, Y.C., and Peters, D.K.: **The role of complement and its receptor in the elimination of immune complexes**. *N. Engl. J. Med.* 1986, **315**:488-495.

| 8-29 | Small peptide fragments released during complement activation trigger a local response to infection. |

Frank, M.M. and Fries, L.F.: **The role of complement in inflammation and phagocytosis**. *Immunol. Today* 1991, **12**:322-326.

Gerard, C., Gerard, N.P.: **C5A anaphylatoxin and its seven transmembrane-segment receptor**. *Ann. Rev. Immunol.* 1994, **12**:775-808.

Hopken et al, **The C5a chemoattractant receptor mediates mucosal defence to infection**. *Nature* 1996, **383**:86-89.

| 8-30 | The terminal complement proteins polymerize to form pores in membranes that can kill pathogens. |

Bhakdi, S. and Tranum-Jensen, J.: **Complement lysis: a hole is a hole**. *Immunol. Today* 1991, **12**:318-320.

Esser, A.F.: **Big MAC attack: complement proteins cause leaky patches**. *Immunol. Today* 1991, **12**:316-318.

Morgan, B.P.: **Effects of the membrane attack complex of complement on nucleated cells**. *Curr. Top. Microbiol. Immunol.* 1992, **178**:115-140.

| 8-31 | Complement regulatory proteins serve to protect host cells from the effects of complement activation. |

Davies, A., Simmons, D.I., Hale, G., Harrison, R.A., Tighe, H., Lachmann, P.J., and Waldmann, H.: **CD59, an Ly-6-like protein expressed in human lymphoid cells, regulates the action of the complement membrane attack complex on homologous cells**. *J. Exp. Med.* 1989, **170**:637-654.

Meri, S., Pangburn, M.K.: **Discrimination between activators and nonactivators of the alternative pathway of complement: Regulation via a sialic acid/polyanion binding site on factor H**. *Proc. Natl. Acad. Sci.* 1990, **87**:3982-3986.

PART V

THE IMMUNE SYSTEM IN HEALTH AND DISEASE

Host Defense Against Infection

9

Throughout this book we have examined the individual mechanisms by which the adaptive immune response acts to protect the host from pathogenic infectious agents. In the remaining five chapters, we consider how the cells and molecules of the immune system work as an integrated host defense system to eliminate the infectious agent and to provide long-lasting protective immunity, how failures of immune defense and unwanted immune responses may occur, and how the immune response may be manipulated to benefit the host. In this chapter, we shall examine the role of the immune system as a whole in host defense, including those innate, non-adaptive defenses that comprise early barriers to infectious disease.

The microorganisms that are encountered daily in the life of a normal healthy individual only occasionally cause perceptible disease. Most are detected and destroyed within hours by defense mechanisms that are not antigen-specific and do not require a prolonged period of induction: these are the mechanisms of **innate immunity**. Only if an infectious organism can breach these early lines of defense will an **adaptive immune response** ensue, with the generation of antigen-specific effector cells that specifically target the pathogen, and memory cells that prevent subsequent infection with the same microorganism.

In the preceding two chapters of this book, we have discussed how an adaptive immune response is induced, and how pathogens are eliminated by the effector cells generated in such a response. Here these mechanisms will be set in the broader context of the entire array of mammalian host defenses against infection, beginning with the innate immune mechanisms that successfully prevent most infections from becoming established. This type of immunity also plays an essential part in inducing the subsequent adaptive response to those infections that overcome the first lines of defense.

The time course of the different phases of an immune response is summarized in Fig. 9.1. The innate immune mechanisms act immediately, and are followed some hours later by **early induced responses**, which can be activated by infection but do not generate lasting protective immunity. These early phases help to keep infection under control while the antigen-specific lymphocytes of the adaptive immune response are activated. Moreover, cytokines produced during these early phases play an important part in shaping the subsequent development of the adaptive immune response and can determine whether the response is predominantly T-cell mediated or humoral. Several days are required for the clonal expansion and differentiation of naive lymphocytes into effector T cells and antibody-secreting B cells that can target the pathogen for elimination. During this period, specific immunological memory is also established, ensuring a rapid re-induction of antibody and antigen-specific effector T cells on subsequent encounters with the same pathogen, thus providing long-lasting protection against re-infection. In this chapter, we shall learn how the different phases of host defense are orchestrated in space and time, and how changes in specialized cell-surface molecules guide lymphocytes to the appropriate site of action at different stages of the immune response.

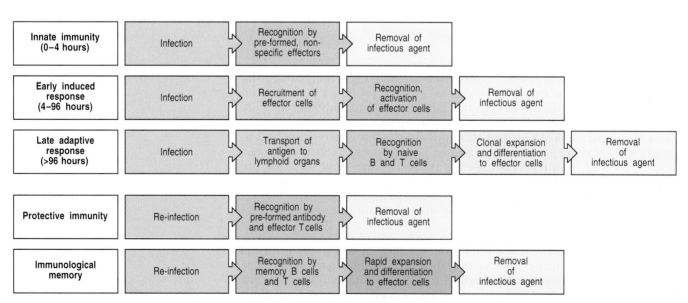

Fig. 9.1 The response to an initial infection occurs in three phases. The effector mechanisms that remove the infectious agent (eg phagocytes, NK cells, complement) are similar or identical in each phase but the recognition mechanisms differ. Adaptive immunity occurs late, because rare, antigen-specific cells must undergo clonal expansion before they can differentiate into effector cells. The response to re-infection is much more rapid; pre-formed antibodies and effector cells act immediately on the pathogen, and immunological memory speeds a renewed adaptive response.

Infection and innate immunity.

Microorganisms that cause pathology in humans and animals enter the body at different sites and produce disease by a variety of mechanisms. Such invasions are initially countered, in all vertebrates, by innate defense mechanisms that pre-exist in all individuals and act within minutes of infection. Only when the innate host defenses are bypassed, evaded, or overwhelmed is an induced or adaptive immune response required, and even then the same effector mechanisms that operate in innate immunity are ultimately harnessed to eliminate the pathogen. In this section, we shall describe briefly the infectious strategies of microorganisms, before examining the innate host defenses that, in most cases, prevent infection becoming established.

9-1 The infectious process can be divided into several distinct phases.

The process of infection can be broken down into stages, each of which can be blocked by different defense mechanisms. Before these are deployed, an infection must be established by infectious particles shed by an infected individual. The number, route, mode of transmission, and stability of an infectious agent outside the host determine its infectivity. Some pathogens, such as anthrax, are spread by spores that are highly resistant to heat and drying, while others, such as the human immunodeficiency virus, are spread only by the exchange of tissues because they are unable to survive as isolated infectious agents.

Although the body is constantly exposed to infectious agents, infectious disease is fortunately quite rare. The epithelial surfaces of the body serve as an efficient barrier to most microorganisms and those that enter are efficiently removed by innate immune mechanisms. Only when a microorganism has crossed an epithelial barrier and establishes a site of infection does infectious disease occur, and little pathology will be caused unless the agent is able to spread. Extracellular pathogens spread by direct extension of the infectious center, via the lymphatics, or via the bloodstream. Usually, spread via the bloodstream occurs only after the lymphatic system has been overwhelmed by the burden of infectious agent. Obligate intracellular pathogens must spread from cell to cell; they do so either by direct transmission from one cell to the next or by release into the extracellular fluid and re-infection of both adjacent and distant cells.

Most infectious agents show a significant degree of host specificity, causing disease only in one or a few related species. What determines host specificity for each agent is not known but the requirement for attachment to a particular cell-surface molecule is one factor. As other interactions with host cells are also commonly needed to support replication, most pathogens have a limited host range. The molecular mechanism of host specificity is an area of intense research interest known as molecular pathogenesis.

While most microorganisms are repelled by innate host defenses, an initial infection, once established, generally leads to perceptible disease followed by an effective host adaptive immune response. A cure involves the clearance of both extracellular infectious particles and intracellular residues of infection. In many infections there is little or no residual pathology after an effective primary response. In some cases, however, the infection or the response to it cause significant tissue damage.

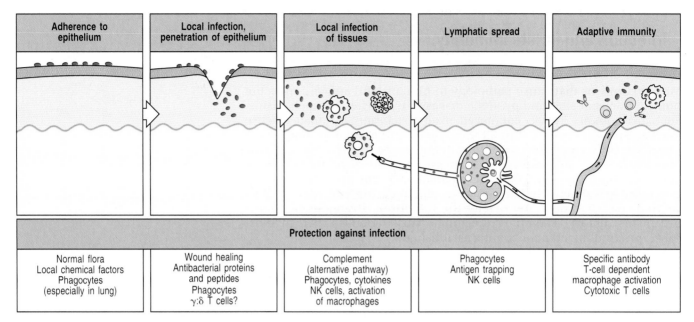

Adherence to epithelium	Local infection, penetration of epithelium	Local infection of tissues	Lymphatic spread	Adaptive immunity

Protection against infection

Normal flora Local chemical factors Phagocytes (especially in lung)	Wound healing Antibacterial proteins and peptides Phagocytes γ:δ T cells?	Complement (alternative pathway) Phagocytes, cytokines NK cells, activation of macrophages	Phagocytes Antigen trapping NK cells	Specific antibody T-cell dependent macrophage activation Cytotoxic T cells

Fig. 9.2 Infections and the responses to them can be divided into a series of stages. These are illustrated here for an infectious organism entering across an epithelium, the commonest route of entry. The infectious organism must first adhere to the epithelial cells and then cross the epithelium.

A local non-adaptive response helps contain the infection and delivers antigen to local lymph nodes, leading to adaptive immunity and clearance of the infection. The role of γ:δ T cells is uncertain, as indicated by the question mark.

In addition to clearance of the infectious agent, an effective adaptive immune response prevents re-infection. For some infectious agents, this protection is essentially absolute, while for others infection is reduced or attenuated upon re-exposure. The progress of an infection is illustrated in Fig. 9.2, which summarizes the defense mechanisms activated at each stage, each of which will be described in detail in the course of this chapter.

9-2   Infectious diseases are caused by diverse living agents that replicate in their hosts.

The agents that cause disease fall into five groups: viruses, bacteria, fungi, protozoa, and helminths (worms). Protozoa and worms are usually grouped together as parasites, and are the subject of the discipline of parasitology, whereas viruses, bacteria, and fungi are the subject of microbiology. In Fig. 9.3, the common classes of microorganisms and parasites are listed with typical examples of each. The remarkable variety of these pathogens has required potential hosts to develop two crucial features of adaptive immunity. First, the need to recognize a wide range of different pathogens has driven the development of receptors on B and T cells of equal or greater diversity. Second, the distinct habitats and life cycles of pathogens have to be countered by a range of distinct effector mechanisms. The characteristic features of each pathogen are its mode of transmission, its mechanism of replication, its pathogenesis or the means by which it causes disease, and the response it elicits. We will focus here on the immune responses to these pathogens.

Some common causes of disease in humans			
Viruses	DNA viruses	Adenoviruses	Human adenoviruses (eg types 3, 4, and 7)
		Herpesviruses	Herpes simplex, varicella zoster, Epstein-Barr virus, cytomegalovirus
		Poxviruses	Vaccinia virus
		Parvoviruses	Human parvovirus
		Papovaviruses	Papilloma virus
		Hepadnaviruses	Hepatitis B virus
	RNA viruses	Orthomyxoviruses	Influenza virus
		Paramyxoviruses	Mumps, measles, respiratory syncytial virus
		Coronaviruses	Common cold viruses
		Picornaviruses	Polio, coxsackie, hepatitis A, rhinovirus
		Reoviruses	Rotavirus, reovirus
		Togaviruses	Rubella, arthropod-borne encephalitis
		Flaviviruses	Arthropod-borne viruses, (yellow fever, dengue fever)
		Arenaviruses	Lymphocytic choriomeningitis, Lassa fever
		Rhabdoviruses	Rabies
		Retroviruses	Human T-cell leukemia virus, HIV
Bacteria	Gram +ve cocci	Staphylococci	*Staphylococcus aureus*
		Streptococci	*Streptococcus pneumoniae, S. pyogenes*
	Gram –ve cocci	Neisseriae	*Neisseria gonorrhoeae, N. meningitidis*
	Gram +ve bacilli		*Corynebacteria, Bacillus anthracis, Listeria monocytogenes*
	Gram –ve bacilli		*Salmonella, Shigella, Campylobacter, Vibrio, Yersinia, Pasteurella, Pseudomonas, Brucella, Haemophilus, Legionella, Bordetella*
	Anaerobic bacteria	Clostridia	*Clostridium tetani, C. botulinum, C. perfringens*
	Spirochetes		*Treponema pallidum, Borrelia burgdorferi, Leptospira interrogans*
	Mycobacteria		*Mycobacterium tuberculosis, M. leprae, M. avium*
	Rickettsias		*Rickettsia prowazeki*
	Chlamydias		*Chlamydia trachomatis*
	Mycoplasmas		*Mycoplasma pneumoniae*
Fungi			*Candida albicans, Cryptococcus neoformans, Aspergillus, Histoplasma capsulatum, Coccidioides immitis, Pneumocystis carinii*
Protozoa			*Entamoeba histolytica, Giardia, Leishmania, Plasmodium, Trypanosoma, Toxoplasma gondii, Cryptosporidium*
Worms	Intestinal		*Trichuris trichura, Trichinella spiralis, Enterobius vermicularis, Ascaris lumbricoides, Ancylostoma, Strongyloides*
	Tissues		*Filaria, Onchocerca volvulus, Loa loa, Dracuncula medinensis*
	Blood, liver		*Schistosoma, Clonorchis sinensis*

Fig. 9.3 A variety of microorganisms can cause disease. Pathogenic organisms are of five main types; viruses, bacteria, fungi, protozoa, and worms. Some common pathogens in each group are listed in the column on the right.

Fig. 9.4 Pathogens can be found in various compartments in the body, where they must be combated by different host defense mechanisms. Virtually all pathogens have an extracellular phase where they are vulnerable to antibody-mediated effector mechanisms. However, intracellular phases are not accessible to antibody, and these are attacked by T cells.

	Intracellular		Extracellular	
	Cytoplasmic	Vesicular	Interstitial spaces, blood, lymph	Epithelial surfaces
Site of infection	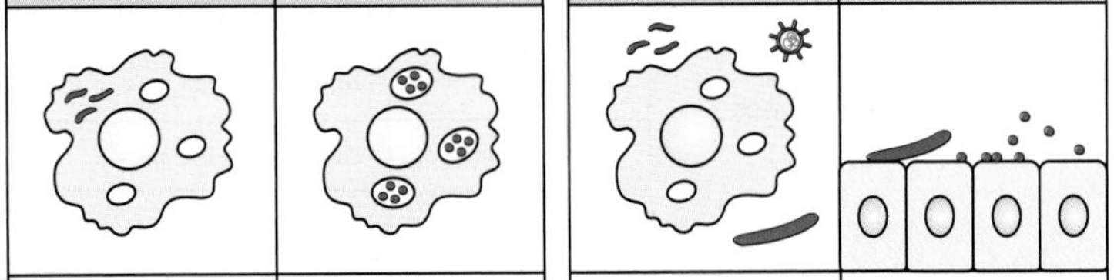			
Organisms	Viruses Chlamydia spp. Rickettsia spp. Listeria monocytogenes Protozoa	Mycobacteria Salmonella typhimurium Leishmania spp. Listeria spp. Trypanosoma spp. Legionella pneumophila Cryptococcus neoformans Histoplasma Yersinia pestis	Viruses Bacteria Protozoa Fungi Worms	Neisseria gonorrhoeae Worms Mycoplasma Streptococcus pneumoniae Vibrio cholerae Escherichia coli Candida albicans Helicobacter pylori
Protective immunity	Cytotoxic T cells NK cells T-cell dependent macrophage activation	T-cell and NK-cell dependent macrophage activation	Antibodies Complement Phagocytosis Neutralization	Antibodies, especially IgA Inflammatory cells

Infectious agents can grow in various body compartments, as shown schematically in Fig. 9.4. We have already seen that two major compartments can be defined—intracellular and extracellular. Intracellular pathogens must invade host cells in order to replicate, and must either be prevented from entering cells or detected and eliminated once they have done so. Such pathogens can be subdivided further into those that replicate freely in the cell, such as viruses and certain bacteria (species of *Chlamydia* and *Rickettsia* as well as *Listeria*), and those such as the mycobacteria, that replicate in cellular vesicles. Many microorganisms replicate in extracellular spaces, either within the body or on the surface of epithelia. Extracellular bacteria are usually susceptible to killing by phagocytes and thus have developed means to resist engulfment. The encapsulated Gram-positive cocci, for instance, grow in extracellular spaces and resist phagocytosis by means of their polysaccharide capsule; if this mechanism of resistance is overcome by opsonization, they are readily killed after ingestion by phagocytic cells.

Different infectious agents cause markedly different diseases, reflecting the diverse processes by which they damage tissues (Fig. 9.5). Many extracellular pathogens cause disease by releasing specific toxic products or toxins (see Fig. 8.19). Intracellular infectious agents frequently cause disease by damaging the cells that house them. The immune response to the infectious agent can itself be a major cause of pathology in several diseases (see Fig. 9.5). The pathology caused by a particular infectious agent also depends on the site in which it grows, so that *Streptococcus pneumoniae* in the lung causes pneumonia, whereas in the blood it causes a rapidly fatal systemic illness.

9-3   **Surface epithelia make up a natural barrier to infection.**

Our body surfaces are defended by epithelia, which provide a physical barrier between the internal milieu and the external world containing pathogens. These epithelia comprise the skin and the linings of the

	Direct mechanisms of tissue damage by pathogens			Indirect mechanisms of tissue damage by pathogens		
	Exotoxin production	Endotoxin	Direct cytopathic effect	Immune complexes	Anti-host antibody	Cell-mediated immunity
Pathogenic mechanism						
Infectious agent	*Streptococcus pyogenes* *Staphylococcus aureus* *Corynebacterium diphtheriae* *Clostridium tetani* *Vibrio cholerae*	*Escherichia coli* *Haemophilus influenzae* *Salmonella typhi* *Shigella* *Pseudomonas aeruginosa* *Yersinia pestis*	Variola Varicella-zoster Hepatitis B virus Polio virus Measles virus Influenza virus Herpes simplex virus	Hepatitis B virus Malaria *Streptococcus pyogenes* *Treponema pallidum* Most acute infections	*Streptococcus pyogenes* *Mycoplasma pneumoniae*	*Mycobacterium tuberculosis* *Mycobacterium leprae* Lymphocytic choriomeningitis virus Human immunodeficiency virus *Borrelia burgdorferi* *Schistosoma mansoni* Herpes simplex virus
Disease	Tonsilitis, scarlet fever Boils, toxic shock syndrome Food poisoning Diphtheria Tetanus Cholera	Gram-negative sepsis Meningitis, pneumonia Typhoid Bacillary dysentery Wound infection Plague	Smallpox Chickenpox, shingles Hepatitis Poliomyelitis Measles, subacute sclerosing panencephalitis Influenza Cold sores	Kidney disease Vascular deposits Glomerulonephritis Kidney damage in secondary syphilis Transient renal deposits	Rheumatic fever Hemolytic anemia	Tuberculosis Tuberculoid leprosy Aseptic meningitis AIDS Lyme arthritis Schistosomiasis Herpes stromal keratitis

Fig. 9.5 Pathogens can damage tissues in a variety of different ways. The mechanisms of damage, representative infectious agents, and the common name of the disease associated with each are shown. Exotoxins are released by microorganisms and act at the surface of host cells, for example by binding receptors. Endotoxins trigger phagocytes to release cytokines that produce local or systemic symptoms. Many pathogens directly damage cells they infect. Finally, adaptive immune responses to the pathogen can generate antigen:antibody complexes that can, in turn, activate neutrophils and macrophages, antibodies that cross-react with host tissues, or T cells that kill infected cells, all with some potential to damage the host's tissues. Neutrophils, the most abundant cells early in infection, release many proteins and small molecular mediators that both control infection and cause tissue damage.

body's tubular structures, such as the gastrointestinal, respiratory, and genitourinary tracts. Infections occur only when the pathogen can colonize or cross over these barriers. The importance of epithelia in protection against infection is obvious where the barrier is breached, as in wounds and burns, where infection is a major cause of mortality and morbidity. People with defective secretion of mucus or inhibition of ciliary movement, where bacteria can colonize the epithelial surface, frequently develop lung infections. In the absence of wounding or disruption, pathogens normally cross epithelial barriers by adhering to molecules on mucosal epithelial cells. This specific attachment allows the pathogen to infect the epithelial cell, or to damage it so that the epithelium can be crossed.

Our surface epithelia are more than mere physical barriers to infection; they also produce chemical substances that are microbicidal or inhibit microbial growth (Fig. 9.6). For instance, the acid pH of the stomach and digestive enzymes of the upper gastrointestinal tract make a substantial chemical barrier to infection. Antibacterial peptides called cryptidins are made by Paneth cells, which are resident in the base of the crypts in the small intestine beneath the epithelial stem cells. Furthermore, most epithelia are associated with a normal flora of non-pathogenic bacteria

Fig. 9.6 Surface epithelia comprise a mechanical, chemical and micro-biological barrier to infection.
Infectious agents must pass across this barrier to cause systemic infection. Normal, non-pathogenic microorganisms (the normal body flora) attach to epithelia and compete with pathogens for attachment sites and nutrients, helping to prevent infection. Antibiotic treatments that kill the normal flora can make an individual susceptible to infection with a pathogen.

Epithelial barriers to infection	
Mechanical	Epithelial cells joined by tight junctions Longitudinal flow of air or fluid across epithelium Movement of mucus by cilia
Chemical	Fatty acids (skin) Enzymes: lysozyme (saliva, sweat, tears), pepsin (gut) Low pH (stomach) Antibacterial peptides; cryptidins (intestine)
Microbiological	Normal flora compete for nutrients and attachment to epithelium and can produce antibacterial substances

that compete with pathogenic microorganisms for nutrients and for attachment sites on cells. The normal flora can also produce antimicrobial substances, such as the colicins (antibacterial proteins made by *Escherichia coli*) that prevent colonization by other bacteria. When the non-pathogenic bacteria are killed by antibiotic treatment, pathogenic microorganisms frequently replace them and cause disease.

When a pathogen crosses an epithelial barrier and begins to replicate in the tissues of the host, the host's defense mechanisms are required to remove the pathogen. The first phase of host defense depends upon the cells and molecules that mediate innate immunity.

9-4   The alternative pathway of complement activation provides a non-adaptive first line of defense against many microorganisms.

The alternative pathway of complement activation can proceed on many microbial surfaces in the absence of specific antibody (see Fig. 8.39). In this way, it triggers the same antimicrobial actions as the classical pathway without the delay of 5–7 days required for antibody production, and can be regarded as an innate humoral response.

The reaction cascade of the alternative pathway of complement activation is shown schematically in Fig. 9.7. C3 is abundant in plasma, and C3b is produced at a significant rate by spontaneous cleavage (known as 'tickover'). While much of this C3b is inactivated by hydrolysis, some attaches covalently, through its reactive thioester group, to the surfaces of host cells or to pathogens. C3b bound in this way is able to bind factor B, inducing its cleavage by the serum protease factor D, to yield the small fragment Ba, which is released, and also the active protease Bb. When this occurs on the surface of a host cell, as we learned in Chapter 8, the C3b,Bb complex is prevented from initiating further activation steps by the cell-surface proteins CR1 (complement receptor 1), DAF (delay-accelerating factor), and MCP (membrane co-factor of proteolysis), and by the plasma protein factor H. CR1 and DAF are membrane-associated molecules, while factor H has affinity for terminal sialic acids of membrane glycoproteins and thus also binds to the surfaces of host cells. All these bind to C3b, displacing Bb and thus preventing the next step in the activation pathway. In addition, factor H, CR1, and MCP render C3b susceptible to cleavage by factor I, a serine protease that circulates in active form and cleaves C3b first into iC3b and then further to C3dg, thus permanently inactivating it (see Fig. 9.7).

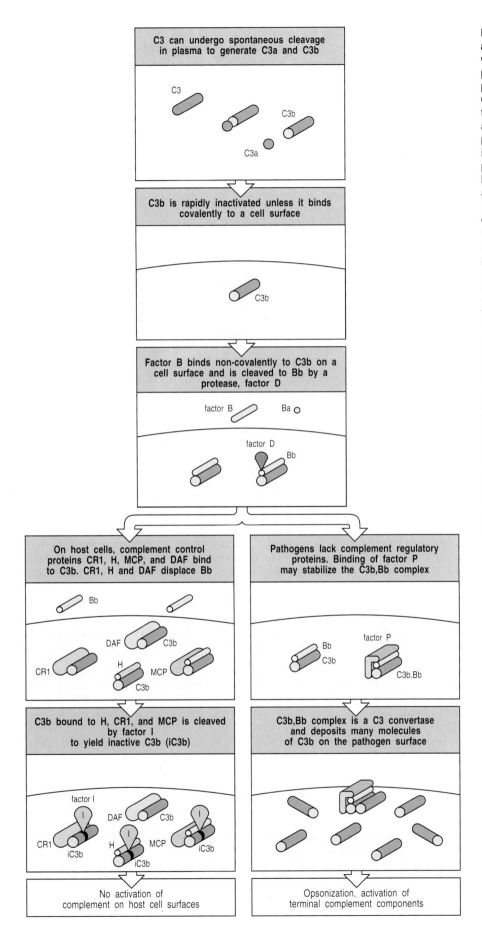

Fig. 9.7 Complement activated by the alternative pathway attacks pathogens while sparing host cells, which are protected by complement regulatory proteins. The complement component C3 is cleaved spontaneously in plasma to produce C3b (top panel), which can attach to host or pathogen (second panel) where it binds factor B. Factor B, in turn, is rapidly cleaved by a plasma protease, factor D, to Bb, which remains bound to C3b to form a C3 convertase and Ba, which is released (third panel). If C3b,Bb forms on the surface of host cells it is rapidly inactivated by complement regulatory proteins (bottom left panels). Host cells express the membrane proteins Complement Receptor 1 (CR1), Decay Accelerating Factor (DAF), and Membrane Cofactor of Proteolysis (MCP), and also favor binding of factor H from plasma; CR1, DAF, and factor H displace Bb from C3b, while CR1, MCP, and factor H catalyze the cleavage of bound C3b by factor I to produce inactive C3b (known as iC3b). Bacterial surfaces (bottom right panels) do not express complement regulatory proteins and favor binding of factor P (properdin), which stabilizes the C3b,Bb convertase activity. This convertase is the equivalent of C4b,C2b of the classical pathway (see Fig. 9.8) and initiates the cleavage of further molecules of C3 leading to opsonization by C3b and the generation of C3b$_2$Bb, the alternative pathway C5 convertase, leading to activation of the terminal complement components.

Microbial cells lack the protective proteins CR1, MCP, and DAF, and the sialic acids that allow factor H to bind preferentially to C3b on the surface of host cells. Consequently, the C3b,Bb complexes formed on the surface of a microorganism are not dissociated and function as active C3 convertases. It appears that microbial cells also favor the binding of a positive regulatory component of the alternative pathway known as **properdin**, or **factor P**, which augments activation by binding to C3b,Bb complexes and stabilizing them, preventing their dissociation by factor H and subsequent cleavage by factor I. The stabilized C3 convertase then acts in the same way as the C3 convertase of the classical pathway (see Section 8-25) and converts large numbers of free C3 molecules to C3b, which coat the adjacent surface, and C3a, which mediates local inflammation. C3b and its derivative iC3b, opsonize the pathogen for uptake by complement receptors expressed on phagocytic cells. The derivative iC3b can be further cleaved to C3dg, which also remains bound to the pathogen. C3dg is the ligand for CD21, which forms part of the B cell co-receptor complex and can engage this co-receptor to increase B-cell signaling in response to specific antigen by 100- to 1000-fold.

Some molecules of C3b bind to the existing C3b,Bb complex to form C3b2,Bb, the alternative pathway C5 convertase. This binds and cleaves C5, initiating the lytic pathway and releasing the potent inflammatory peptide C5a (see Section 8-30). Once initiated, the alternative pathway can promote its own feedback amplification, with bound C3b binding more molecules of factor B, further increasing C3 and C5 convertase activity on the pathogen surface.

Not all microbial surfaces allow activation of the alternative pathway, and it is not clear what distinguishes surfaces that allow the cascade to proceed from those that do not. Some bacterial surfaces have high levels of sialic acid residues, like the surfaces of vertebrate cells, and are therefore more resistant to attack by the alternative pathway than most bacteria which do not have surface sialic acid. These bacteria favor binding of factor H, which displaces factor B from the bound C3b and makes C3b susceptible to inactivation by factor I.

Only two events in the classical pathway of complement activation are not exactly homologous to the equivalent steps in the alternative pathway: the first is the initial cleavage that, in the classical pathway, deposits C4b on the bacterial surface; the second is the cleavage that generates C2b, the active protease of the classical pathway C3 convertase. Both of these steps are mediated in the classical pathway by activation of C1s by bound antibody; in the alternative pathway, C3 is activated spontaneously, while factor B is activated by the plasma protein factor D.

The alternative pathway of complement activation thus illustrates the general principle that most of the immune effector mechanisms that can be activated by the adaptive immune response can also be induced in a non-clonal fashion as part of the early, non-adaptive host response against infection. It is almost certain that the adaptive response evolved by adding specific recognition to the original non-adaptive system. This is illustrated particularly clearly in the complement system, because here the components are defined, and the functional homologs can be seen to be related in evolution (Fig. 9.8).

9-5 | **Phagocytes provide innate cellular immunity in tissues and initiate host-defense responses.**

Macrophages mature continuously from circulating monocytes (see Fig. 1.3) and leave the circulation to migrate into tissues throughout the body. They are found in especially large numbers in connective tissue, in

Step in pathway	Protein serving function in pathway			Relationship
	Alternative (innate)	Lectin	Classical	
Initiating serine protease	D	MBL-associated serine protease	C1s	Unknown
Covalent binding to cell surface	C3b	C4b		Homologous
C3/C5 convertase	Bb	C2b		Homologous
Control of activation	CR1 H	CR1 C4bp		Identical Homologous
Opsonization	C3b			Identical
Initiation of effector pathway	C5b			Identical
Local inflammation	C5a, C3a			Identical

Fig. 9.8 There is a close relationship between the factors of the alternative and classical pathways of complement activation. Most of the factors are either identical, or the product of genes that have duplicated and then diverged in sequence. The proteins C4 and C3 are homologous and contain the unstable thioester bond by which their large fragments, C4b and C3b, bind covalently to membranes. The proteins C2 and B are adjacent in the class III region of the MHC and arose by gene duplicaton. Factor H, CR1, and C4bp regulatory proteins share a repeat sequence common to many complement regulatory proteins. The greatest divergence between the pathways is in their initiation; the C1 complex serves to convert antibody binding into enzyme activity on a specific surface in the case of the classical pathway, mannan-binding-lectin (MBL) associates with a serine esterase to serve the same function in the lectin-mediated pathway, while this enzyme activity is provided by factor D of the alternative pathway. All other factors in the two pathways are identical.

association with the gastrointestinal tract, and along certain blood vessels in the liver (Küpffer cells), lung (both interstitial and alveolar), and spleen. The second major family of phagocytes, the neutrophils, or polymorphonuclear neutrophilic leukocytes (PMNs, or polys) are produced and lost in large numbers each day. Both these phagocytic cells play a key part in all phases of host defense. In addition to engulfing opsonized particles coated with antibodies and/or complement, they can recognize and ingest many pathogens directly. Indeed, the same complement receptors by which they engulf opsonized particles recognize various microbial constituents. For example, the leukocyte integrins CD11b/CD18, also known as CR3 or Mac-1, and CD11c/CD18 or CR4, are able to recognize several microbial substances, including bacterial lipopolysaccharide (LPS), the lipophosphoglycan of *Leishmania*, the filamentous hemagglutinin of *Bordetella*, and structures on yeasts such as *Candida* and *Histoplasma*. Tissue macrophages and neutrophils also have on their surface other receptors able to recognize components common to many pathogens. These receptors include the macrophage mannose receptor, which is found on macrophages but not on monocytes or neutrophils, the scavenger receptor, which binds many sialic acid ligands, and CD14, a molecule that binds LPS (Fig. 9.9). Neutrophils have granules which contain enzymes, proteins, and peptides which can mediate a host-anti-bacterial response when they are released upon activation.

When pathogens cross an epithelial barrier, they are thus immediately recognized by phagocytes in the subepithelial connective tissues, with three important consequences. The first is the trapping, engulfment,

Fig. 9.9 Phagocytes bear several different receptors that recognize microbial components and induce phagocytosis and the release of cytokines. The figure illustrates this for two such receptors, CD14 and CD11c/CD18 (CR4), both of which are specific for bacterial lipopolysaccharide (LPS).

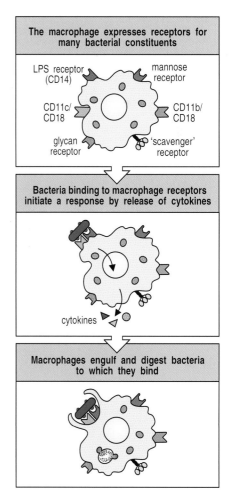

The macrophage expresses receptors for many bacterial constituents

LPS receptor (CD14) · mannose receptor · CD11c/CD18 · CD11b/CD18 · glycan receptor · 'scavenger' receptor

Bacteria binding to macrophage receptors initiate a response by release of cytokines

cytokines

Macrophages engulf and digest bacteria to which they bind

and destruction of the pathogen by tissue macrophages and migrating neutrophils, thereby providing an immediate innate cellular immune response. This process may be sufficient to prevent an infection from becoming established, even after a microbe has crossed an epithelial barrier. Indeed, the great cellular immunologist Elie Metchnikoff believed that the innate response of macrophages and neutrophils encompassed all host defense. For a microbe to become pathogenic, it must devise strategies to avoid engulfment by phagocytes, or, like the mycobacteria, devise ways to grow inside the phagosome. The strategy employed by many extracellular bacteria is to coat themselves with a thick polysaccharide capsule that is not recognized by any phagocyte receptor. Even without such devices, if sufficient bacteria enter the body to simply overwhelm this innate system of host defense, they can also establish a focus of infection.

The second important effect of the interaction of phagocytes with pathogens is the secretion of cytokines by the phagocyte. It is thought that the pathogen induces cytokine secretion by binding to the same receptors used for engulfment. Cytokines are an important component of the next phase of host defense, which comprises a series of induced but non-adaptive responses, as discussed in the next part of this chapter.

Finally, as we learned in Chapter 7, receptors on macrophages (but not neutrophils) play an important role in antigen uptake and processing, and signals transmitted by these receptors are likely to be responsible for inducing the expression of co-stimulatory molecules that allow the macrophage to function as a professional antigen-presenting cell. Thus, macrophages are important in the induction of the adaptive immune response, and their released cytokines play an additional role in determining the form of the adaptive immune response, as we shall see in the third part of this chapter.

Summary.

The mammalian body is susceptible to infection by many pathogens, which must first make contact with the host and then establish a focus of infection in order to cause disease. These pathogens differ greatly in their lifestyles and means of pathogenesis, which requires an equally diverse set of defensive responses from the host immune system. The first phase of host defense is called innate immunity, and comprises those mechanisms that are present and ready to attack an invader at any time. The epithelial surfaces of the body keep pathogens out as a first line of defense, and many viruses and bacteria can enter tissues only through specialized cell-surface interactions. Bacteria that overcome this barrier are faced with two immediate lines of defense. First, they are subject to humoral attack by the alternative pathway of complement activation, which is spontaneously active in plasma and can opsonize or destroy bacteria while sparing host cells, which are protected by complement regulatory proteins. Second, they may be recognized directly and engulfed by phagocytic macrophages and neutrophils with receptors for common bacterial components.

Innate immunity involves the direct engagement of an effector mechanism by the pathogen, acts immediately on contact with it, and is unaltered in its ability to resist a subsequent challenge. This distinguishes innate immunity from the induced responses we shall consider next and from the adaptive immune response that provides long-lasting protection against re-infection.

Non-adaptive host responses to infection.

The activation of complement by the alternative pathway and the engulfment of microorganisms by phagocytes occur in the early hours of local infection. If the microorganism evades or overwhelms these innate defenses, the infection may still be contained by a second wave of responses involving the activation of a variety of humoral and cell-mediated effector mechanisms that are strikingly similar to those discussed in Chapters 7 and 8. These are the early induced responses. Unlike the adaptive response, these responses to pathogens involve recognition mechanisms that are based on relatively invariant receptors, and they do not lead to the lasting protective immunity against the inducing pathogen that is the hallmark of adaptive immunity. Instead, as we shall see, the same response is usually made to all pathogens of a given type.

The early induced but non-adaptive responses are important for two main reasons. First, they can repel a pathogen or, more often, hold it in check until an adaptive immune response can be mounted. The early responses occur rapidly, because they do not require clonal expansion, whereas adaptive responses have a latent period of clonal expansion before the proliferating lymphocytes mature into effector cells capable of eliminating an infection. Second, these early responses influence the adaptive response in several ways, as we shall see when we consider this later phase of host defense in the next part of this chapter.

| 9-6 | **The innate immune response produces inflammatory mediators that recruit new phagocytic cells to local sites of infection.** |

One important function of the innate immune response is to recruit more phagocytic cells and effector molecules to the site of the infection through the release of a battery of cytokines and other inflammatory mediators that have profound effects on subsequent events. The cytokines secreted by phagocytes in response to infection comprise a structurally diverse group of molecules and include interleukin-1 (IL-1), interleukin-6 (IL-6), interleukin-8 (IL-8), interleukin-12 (IL-12), and tumor necrosis factor-α (TNF-α). All have important local and systemic effects, which are summarized in Fig. 9.10. Phagocytes also release other proteins with potent local effects, such as the enzymes plasminogen activator and phospholipase.

The other mediators released by phagocytes in response to infectious agents comprise a variety of molecules, including prostaglandins, oxygen radicals, peroxides, nitric oxide (NO), leukotrienes, particularly leukotriene B4 (LTB4), and platelet-activating factor (PAF) (see Section 8-18 for the effects of prostaglandins, leukotrienes, and other lipid mediators of inflammation). In addition to these products of phagocytes, the activation of complement by infectious agents contributes the inflammatory mediators C5a (the most potent), C3a, and to a lesser extent, C4a. As well as being an inflammatory mediator in its own right, C5a is also able to activate mast cells, causing them to release their granule contents, which include histamine, serotonin (in mice), and LTB4. These contribute to the changes in endothelial cells that occur in sites of infection.

We have already discussed the activation of mast cells and the actions of the inflammatory mediators they release in Sections 8-20 and 8-21; however, when an individual first encounters a new pathogen there is

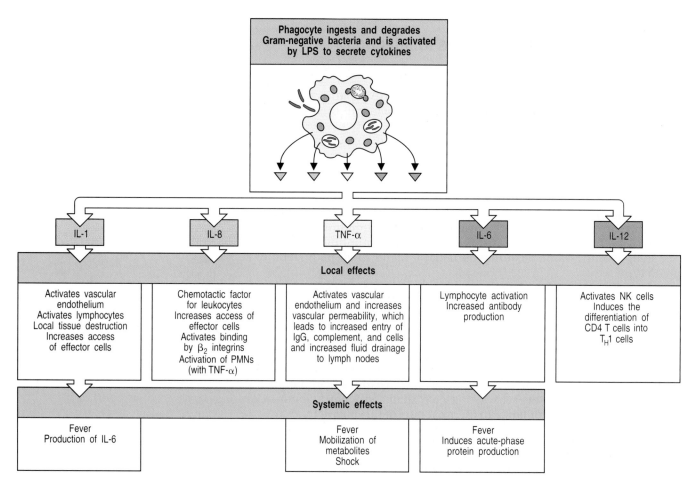

Fig. 9.10 Important cytokines secreted by macrophages in response to bacterial products include IL-1, IL-6, IL-8, IL-12 and TNF-α. In particular, TNF-α is an inducer of a local inflammatory response that helps to contain infections (see Fig. 9.12). It also has systemic effects, many of which are harmful. IL-1, IL-6 and TNF-α play a critical role in inducing the acute-phase response in the liver (see Fig. 9.15) and induce fever, which favors effective host defense in several ways. IL-8 is particularly important in directing neutrophil migration to sites of infection. IL-12 activates NK cells and favors the differentiation of T_H1 cells.

unlikely to be any IgE of an appropriate specificity bound to the mast cells, so this route of activation is only likely to occur on re-infection. We will return to the role of mast cells in inflammatory responses in Chapter 11, when we discuss allergic responses mediated by IgE.

The combined local effects of these mediators results in an **inflammatory response**, which is usually one of the immediate local reactions to infection. Inflammatory responses, which are operationally characterized by pain, redness, heat, and swelling at the site of an infection, reflect two types of changes in the local blood vessels. The first of these is an increase in vascular diameter, leading to increased local blood flow—hence the heat and redness—and a reduction in the velocity of blood flow, especially along the surfaces of local blood vessels.

Under normal conditions, leukocytes are restricted to the center of blood vessels, where the flow is fastest. In inflammatory sites, where the vessels are dilated, the slower blood flow allows the leukocytes to move out of the center of the blood vessel and interact with the vascular endothelium. In addition to these changes, there is an increase in vascular permeability, leading to the local accumulation of fluid—hence the swelling and pain—as well as the accumulation of immunoglobulins, complement, and other blood proteins in the tissue.

The second effect of these mediators on endothelium is to induce the expression of adhesion molecules, which bind to the surface of circulating monocytes and neutrophils and greatly enhance the rate at which these phagocytic cells migrate across local small blood vessel walls into the tissues. Monocytes migrate continuously into the tissues where they differentiate into macrophages. During an inflammatory response, the induction of adhesion molecules on the endothelial cells of local blood vessels, as well as induced changes in the adhesion molecules expressed on the leukocytes, recruit large numbers of circulating leukocytes, initially neutrophils and later monocytes, into the site of an infection.

9-7 | **The migration of leukocytes out of blood vessels depends on adhesive interactions activated by the local release of inflammatory mediators.**

The migration of leukocytes out of blood vessels, a process known as **extravasation**, is thought to occur in four steps. We shall describe this process as it is known to occur for monocytes and neutrophils (Fig. 9.11). Similar processes are thought to account for the homing of naive T lymphocytes to peripheral lymphoid organs and the delivery of effector T cells to sites of infection, as we shall see later.

The first step in this process is mediated by selectins (see Fig. 7.5). The adhesive molecule P-selectin, which is carried inside endothelial cells in granules known as **Weibel-Palade bodies**, appears on endothelial cell surfaces within a few minutes of exposure to LTB4, C5a, or histamine. A second selectin, E-selectin, appears a few hours after exposure to lipopolysaccharide or TNF-α. These selectins recognize carbohydrate epitopes, in this case the sialyl-Lewis^x moiety of certain leukocyte glycoproteins. The interaction of P-selectin and E-selectin with these surface glycoproteins allows monocytes and neutrophils to adhere reversibly to the vessel wall, so that circulating leukocytes can be seen to 'roll' along endothelium that has been treated with inflammatory cytokines (see Fig. 9.11, top panel). This adhesive interaction permits the stronger interactions of the second step in leukocyte migration.

The second step depends upon interactions between the leukocyte integrins known as LFA-1 (CD11a:CD18) and CR3 (CD11b:CD18—also called Mac-1) with molecules on endothelium such as the immunoglobulin-related adhesion molecule ICAM-1, which is also induced on endothelial cells by TNF-α (see Fig. 9.11, bottom panel). LFA-1 and CR3 normally adhere only weakly, but IL-8 or other chemoattractants trigger a conformational change in LFA-1 and CR3 on the rolling leukocyte, which greatly increases its adhesive capacity. In consequence, the leukocyte attaches firmly to the endothelium and the rolling is arrested.

In the third step, the leukocyte extravasates, or crosses the endothelial wall. This step also involves the leukocyte integrins LFA-1 and Mac-1, as well as a further adhesive interaction. This involves an immunoglobulin-related molecule called PECAM or CD31, which is expressed both on the leukocyte and at the intercellular junctions of endothelial cells. These interactions enable the phagocyte to squeeze between the endothelial cells. It then penetrates the basement membrane (an extracellular matrix structure) with the aid of proteolytic enzymes that break down the proteins of the basement membrane. The movement through the vessel wall is known as **diapedesis**, and allows phagocytes to enter the site of infection. The fourth and final step in extravasation is the migration of the leukocytes through the tissues under the influence of chemoattractant cytokines (chemokines), discussed in more detail later in this chapter.

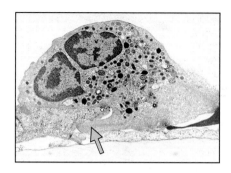

Fig. 9.11 Phagocytic leukocytes are directed to sites of infection through interactions between adhesion molecules induced by cytokines. The first step (top panel) involves reversible binding of leukocytes to vascular endothelium through interactions between selectins induced on the endothelium and their carbohydrate ligands on the leukocyte, shown here for E-selectin and its ligand the sialyl-Lewis^x moiety (s-Le^x). This interaction cannot anchor the cells against the shearing force of the flow of blood and instead they roll along the endothelium, continually making and breaking contact. The binding does, however, allow stronger interactions, which occur as a result of the induction of ICAM-1 on the endothelium and the activation of its receptors LFA-1 and Mac-1 (not shown) on the leukocyte. Tight binding between these molecules arrests the rolling and allows the leukocyte to squeeze between the endothelial cells forming the wall of the blood vessel (extravasate). The leukocyte integrins LFA-1 and Mac-1 are required for extravasation, and for migration toward chemoattractants. Adhesion between molecules of CD31, expressed on both the leukocyte and the junction of the endothelial cells, is also thought to contribute to diapedesis. The leukocyte also needs to traverse the basement membrane. Finally, the leukocyte migrates along a concentration gradient of chemokines (here shown as IL-8) secreted by cells at the site of infection. The electron micrograph, above left, shows a neutrophil that has just started to migrate between two endothelial cells but has not yet broken through the basement membrane (bottom of photograph). Note the pseudopod (arrow) that the neutrophil has inserted between adjacent endothelial cells. The dark mass at the bottom right is an erythrocyte that has become trapped underneath the neutrophil. Photograph (x 5500) courtesy of I Bird and J Spragg.

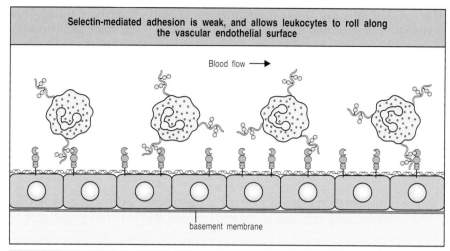

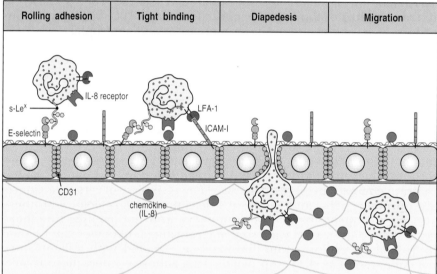

9-8 TNF-α induces blood vessel occlusion and plays an important role in containing local infection but can be fatal when released systemically.

The molecular changes induced by the inflammatory mediators at the endothelial cell surface also induce expression of molecules on endothelial cells that trigger blood clotting in the local small vessels, occluding them and cutting off blood flow. This may be important in preventing the pathogen from entering the bloodstream and spreading via the blood to organs all over the body. Instead, the fluid that has leaked into the tissue from the plasma early on carries the pathogen, either directly or enclosed in phagocytic cells, via the lymph to the regional lymph nodes, where an adaptive immune response can be initiated. The importance of TNF-α in this process is illustrated by experiments in which rabbits are infected locally with a bacterium. Normally, the infection will be contained at the site of the inoculation; if, however, an injection of anti-TNF-α antibody is also given, the infection spreads via the blood to other organs.

Once an infection spreads to the bloodstream, however, the same mechanisms whereby TNF-α so effectively contains local infection instead become catastrophic (Fig. 9.12). This condition, known as **sepsis**, is accompanied by the release of TNF-α by macrophages in the liver,

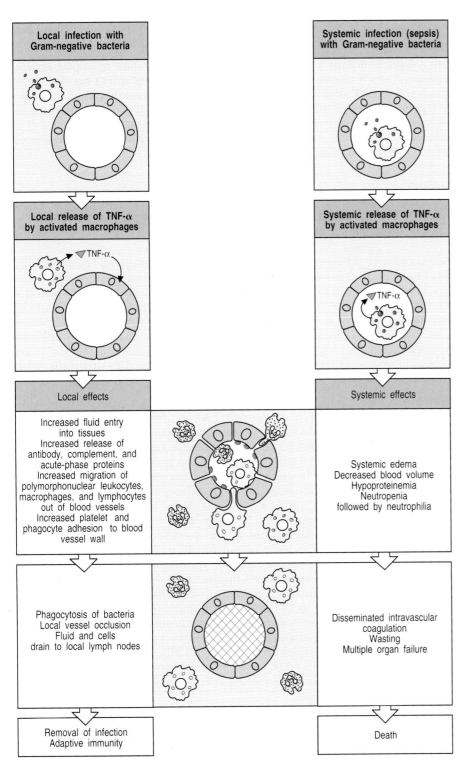

Fig. 9.12 The release of TNF-α by macrophages induces local protective effects, but TNF-α can have damaging effects when released systemically. The panels on the left show the causes and consequences of local release of TNF-α. The panels on the right, however, show the causes and consequences of systemic release. The central panels illustrate the common effects of TNF-α, which acts on blood vessels, especially venules, to increase blood flow, increase vascular permeability to fluid, proteins, and cells, and to increase endothelial adhesiveness for white blood cells and platelets. Local release thus allows an influx into the infected tissue of fluid, cells, and proteins that participate in host defense. The small vessels later clot, preventing spread of the infection to the blood, and the fluid drains to regional lymph nodes where the adaptive immune response is initiated. When there is a systemic infection, or sepsis, with bacteria that elicit TNF-α production, then TNF-α acts in similar ways on all small blood vessels. The result is shock, disseminated intravascular coagulation with depletion of clotting factors and consequent bleeding, multiple organ failure, and death.

spleen, and other sites. The systemic release of TNF-α causes vasodilation and loss of plasma volume owing to increased vascular permeability, leading to shock. In **septic shock**, disseminated intravascular coagulation is also triggered by TNF-α, leading to the generation of blood clots in the small vessels and the massive consumption of clotting proteins. The patient's ability to clot blood appropriately is lost. This condition frequently leads to failure of vital organs such as the kidneys, liver, heart, and lungs, which are quickly compromised by failure of normal perfusion; consequently, septic shock has a high mortality rate.

Mice with a mutant TNF-α receptor gene are resistant to septic shock; however, such mice are also unable to control local infection. Although the features of TNF-α that make it so valuable in containing local infection are precisely those that allow it to play a central role in the pathogenesis of septic shock, it is clear from the evolutionary conservation of TNF-α that its benefits in the former arena outweigh the devastating consequences of its systemic release.

9-9	**Small proteins called chemokines recruit new phagocytic cells to local sites of infection.**

Some of the cytokines released in response to infection belong to a family of closely related proteins called **chemokines**, small polypeptides that are synthesized not only by phagocytes but also by endothelial cells, the keratinocytes of the skin, and the fibroblasts and smooth muscle cells of connective tissue. IL-8, whose contribution to extravasation we have just discussed, belongs to this subset of cytokines. All the chemokines are related in amino acid sequence and function mainly as chemoattractants for phagocytic cells, recruiting monocytes and neutrophils from the blood to sites of infection.

Members of the chemokine family fall into three broad groups: CC chemokines with two adjacent cysteines; CXC chemokines, in which the same two cysteine residues are separated by another amino acid; and C chemokines, where only one cysteine residue is present at the same site as in other chemokines. The three groups of chemokines act on different cell types: in general, the CXC chemokines promote migration of neutrophils; while the CC chemokines promote the migration of monocytes; the C chemokines that have been identified to date have individual specialized functions. IL-8 is an example of a CXC chemokine; a representative CC chemokine is the so-called human macrophage chemoattractant and activating factor (MCAF or MCP-1). IL-8 and MCAF have similar, although complementary, functions. IL-8 induces neutrophils to leave the bloodstream and migrate into the surrounding tissues. MCAF, on the other hand, acts on monocytes, inducing their migration from the bloodstream to become tissue macrophages. Other chemokines such as RANTES may promote the infiltration into tissues of other cell types including effector T cells (see Section 9-20), with individual chemokines acting on different subsets of cells. The known C chemokines are more specialized. Lymphotactin attracts T-cell precursors to the thymus, while eotaxin is a product of T_H2 cells and is a chemoattractant for eosinophils (Fig. 9.13).

The role of chemokines such as IL-8 and MCAF in cell recruitment is two-fold: firstly to convert the initial rolling interaction of the leukocyte with endothelial cells into stable binding; and secondly to direct its migration along a gradient of the chemokine that increases in concentration towards the site of infection. This is achieved by the binding of the small, soluble chemokines to proteoglycan molecules, both in the extracellular matrix and on endothelial cell surfaces, thus displaying the chemokines on a solid substrate along which the leukocytes can migrate. Once the leukocytes have crossed the endothelium and the basement membrane to enter the tissues, their migration to the focus of infection is directed by the gradient of matrix-associated chemokine molecules.

Chemokines can be produced by a wide variety of cell types in response to bacterial products, viruses, and agents that cause physical damage,

Chemokine	Subclass	Produced by	Effects on		
			T cells	Monocytes	Neutrophils
IL-8	CXC	Monocytes Macrophages Fibroblasts Keratinocytes	Chemoattractant for naive T cells		Chemoattractant Activation
PBP/β-TG/ NAP-2	CXC	Platelets			Chemoattractant Induction of degranulation
MIP-1β	CC	Monocytes Macrophages Neutrophils Endothelium	Chemoattractant for CD8 T cells		
MCP-1 or MCAF	CC	Monocytes Macrophages Fibroblasts Keratinocytes	Chemoattractant for memory T cells	Chemoattractant Activation	
RANTES	CC	T cells	Chemoattractant for memory CD4 T cells	Chemoattractant	
Lymphotactin	C	Thymic stroma Some T cells	Chemoattractant for pre-T cells to thymus		
Eotaxin	C	T$_H$2 cells			Eosinophil chemoattractant Eosinophil activation

Fig. 9.13 Properties of selected chemokines. Chemokines fall into three related but distinct groups: the CC chemokines having two adjacent cysteine residues, which in humans are all encoded in one region of chromosome 4; the CXC chemokines, which have a residue between the same two cysteines, and which are found in a cluster on chromosome 17; and the C chemokines that have only one cysteine at this location. The table lists the actions of some chemokines in each group.

such as silica or the urate crystals that occur in gout. Thus, infection or physical damage to tissues sets in motion the recruitment of phagocytic cells to the site of damage. Both IL-8 and MCAF also activate their respective target cells, so that not only are neutrophils and macrophages brought to potential sites of infection but, in the process, they are armed to deal with any pathogens they may encounter. In particular, neutrophils exposed to IL-8 and TNF-α are activated to mediate a respiratory burst that generates oxygen radicals and nitric oxide, and to release their stored granule contents, thus contributing both to host defense and to local tissue destruction seen in local sites of infection with pyogenic (pus-forming) bacteria. Just as all the chemokines have similar structures, all their receptors are similar in structure (see Fig. 7.33); all are integral membrane proteins containing seven membrane-spanning helices. This structure is characteristic of receptors such as rhodopsin and the muscarinic acetylcholine receptor, which are coupled to guanine nucleotide binding proteins (G proteins), and the chemokines also activate G proteins.

Thus, tissue phagocytes initiate host responses in tissues, and their numbers are soon augmented through the action of chemokines, which recruit large numbers of circulating phagocytic cells to sites of infection and tissue damage. Why there are so many chemokines, and the exact role of each one in host defense and in pathological responses, is not yet known.

9-10   **Neutrophils predominate in the early cellular infiltrate into inflammatory sites.**

Neutrophils are abundant in the blood but are absent from normal tissues. They are short-lived, surviving only a few hours after leaving the bone marrow. The innate immune response produces a variety of factors that are chemotactic for neutrophils and they rapidly emigrate from the blood to enter sites of infection, where they are the earliest phagocytic cells to be recruited. Once in an inflammatory site, the neutrophils are able to eliminate many pathogens by phagocytosis.

The role of neutrophils in the phagocytosis of antibody-coated pathogens was discussed in Chapter 8, and where the individual has had a previous encounter with the pathogen this is likely to be the dominant mechanism by which microorganisms are removed. However, neutrophils are able to phagocytose bacteria even in the absence of specific antibodies and can thus provide a protective response in the first encounter with a pathogen. Bacterial cell wall components can be bound directly by neutrophils, or indirectly in the case of LPS, which is first bound by a serum protein, lipopolysaccharide-binding protein (LBP) which catalyzes the binding of LPS by CD14 on the surface of the neutrophil. Neutrophils can also phagocytose microorganisms coated with the complement components C3b and its inactive derivative iC3b, which are deposited on the surface of the pathogen by the alternative pathway of complement activation (see Sections 8-26 and 9-4).

Neutrophils produce several bacteriostatic and toxic products such that phagocytosed pathogens are killed rapidly(see Section 8-18). The combination of toxic oxygen metabolites, nitric oxide, proteases, phospholipases, and antibacterial proteins is able to eliminate Gram-positive and Gram-negative bacteria, fungi, and even some enveloped viruses. The importance of neutrophils in host defense is best illustrated by considering inherited defects in neutrophil maturation or antibacterial functions; patients with such deficiencies suffer recurrent infections, often of bacteria and fungi that form part of the normal flora. In patients with no neutrophils such infections frequently escape from the local site to produce a life-threatening septicemia. Neutrophils themselves are short-lived and the pus formed at sites of inflammation contains many dead and dying neutrophils. Any microorganisms that have been phagocytosed but not killed are released at this point and can be re-phagocytosed by other neutrophils or by macrophages that accumulate later in the inflammatory response. Even this sequestration of microorganisms can be important in host defense; in individuals whose neutrophils are unable to kill phagocytosed organisms, in contrast to those with no neutrophils at all, infections only rarely spread beyond the local inflammatory site.

9-11   Cytokines released by phagocytes also activate the acute phase response.

As well as their important local effects, the cytokines produced by macrophages and neutrophils have long-range effects that contribute to host defense. One of these is the elevation of body temperature, which is caused by TNF-α, IL-1, IL-6, and other cytokines. These are termed 'endogenous pyrogens' because they cause fever and derive from an endogenous source rather than from bacterial components. Fever is generally beneficial to host defense; most pathogens grow better at lower temperatures and adaptive immune responses are more intense at raised temperatures. Host cells are also protected from deleterious effects of TNF-α at raised temperatures.

The effects of TNF-α, IL-1, and IL-6 are summarized in Fig. 9.14. One of the most important of these is the initiation of a response known as the

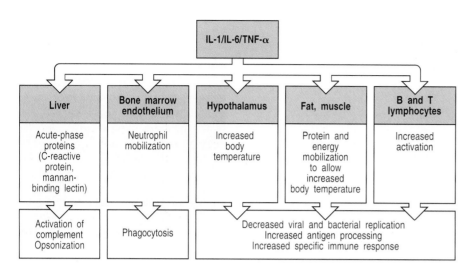

Fig. 9.14 The cytokines TNF-α, IL-1, and IL-6 have a wide spectrum of biological activities that help coordinate the body's responses to infection. IL-1, IL-6, and TNF-α activate hepatocytes to synthesize acute-phase proteins, and bone-marrow endothelium to release neutrophils. The acute-phase proteins act as opsonins, while the disposal of opsonized pathogens is augmented by enhanced recruitment of neutrophils from the bone marrow. IL-1, IL-6, and TNF-α are also endogenous pyrogens, raising body temperature, which is believed to help eliminate infections. A major effect of these cytokines is to act on the hypothalamus, altering the body's temperature regulation, and on muscle and fat cells, altering energy mobilization to increase the body temperature. At elevated temperatures, bacterial and viral replication are decreased, while processing of antigen is enhanced. Finally, they help activate B and T cells, which, together with the enhanced processing of antigen, increase the adaptive immune response.

acute-phase response (Fig. 9.15). This involves a shift in the proteins secreted by the liver into the blood plasma and results from the action of IL-1, IL-6, and TNF-α on hepatocytes. In the acute-phase response, levels of some plasma proteins go down, while levels of others increase markedly. The proteins whose synthesis is induced by TNF-α, IL-1, and IL-6 are called acute-phase proteins. Of the acute-phase proteins, two are of particular interest because they mimic the action of antibodies.

One of these proteins, **C-reactive protein**, is a member of the **pentraxin** protein family, so called because they are formed from five identical subunits. C-reactive protein binds to the phosphorylcholine portion of certain bacterial and fungal cell wall lipopolysaccharides. Phosphorylcholine is also found in mammalian cell membrane phospholipids but in a form that cannot react with C-reactive protein. When C-reactive protein binds to a bacterium, it is not only able to opsonize it but can also activate the complement cascade by binding to C1q, the first component of the classical pathway of complement activation. The interaction with C1q involves the collagen-like parts of C1q, rather than the globular heads contacted by antibody, but the same cascade of reactions is initiated.

The second acute-phase protein of interest is **mannan-binding lectin** (**MBL**). This is found in normal serum at low levels but is also produced in increased amounts during the acute-phase response. It is a calcium-dependent sugar-binding protein, or lectin, a member of a structurally related family of proteins known as the **collectins**. It binds to mannose residues, which are accessible on many bacteria but are covered by other sugar groups in the carbohydrates on vertebrate cells. Mannan-binding lectin also acts as an opsonin for monocytes, which, unlike tissue macrophages, do not express the macrophage mannose receptor. The structure of mannan-binding lectin resembles that of the C1q component of complement, although the two proteins do not share sequence homology. When it binds to bacteria, mannan-binding lectin can, like C1q, activate a proteolytic enzyme complex that cleaves C4 and C2, to initiate complement activation by the lectin pathway (see Fig. 9.8). The collectins also include the pulmonary surfactant proteins A and D (SP-A and SP-D), which are probably important in binding and opsonizing pulmonary pathogens such as *Pneumocystis carinii*.

Thus, within a day or two, the acute-phase response provides the host with two proteins with the functional properties of antibodies and which can bind a broad range of bacteria. However, unlike antibodies, they have no structural diversity, and are made in response to any

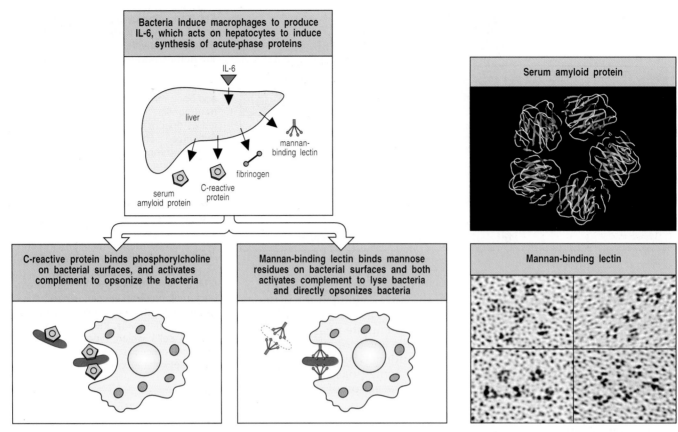

Fig. 9.15 The acute-phase response produces molecules that bind bacteria but not host cells. Acute-phase proteins are produced by liver cells in response to cytokines released by phagocytes in the presence of bacteria. They include serum amyloid protein (SAP) (in mice but not humans), C-reactive protein (CRP), fibrinogen and mannan-binding lectin (MBL). SAP and CRP are homologous in structure; both are pentraxins, forming five-membered disks, as shown for SAP (upper photograph). CRP binds phosphorylcholine on bacterial surfaces but does not recognize it in the form in which it is found in host-cell membranes, and can both act as an opsonin in its own right and activate the classical complement pathway by binding C1q to augment opsonization. MBL is a member of the collectin family, which includes C1q, which it resembles in its structure (see lower photograph and Fig. 8.33). MBL binds mannose residues on bacterial cell surfaces, and like CRP, can act both as an opsonin in its own right and activate complement. MBL activates the lectin complement pathway by binding and activating a serine esterase resembling C1rs, that in turn activates C4 and C2. Thus, CRP and MBL can lead to bacterial clearance in the same way as an IgM antibody. Photographs courtesy of J Emsley (SAP) and K Reid (MBL).

stimulus that triggers TNF-α, IL-1, and IL-6 release, so their synthesis is not specifically induced and targeted.

A final distant effect of the cytokines produced by phagocytes is to induce a leukocytosis, an increase in circulating neutrophils. The leukocytes come from two sources: the bone marrow, from which mature leukocytes are released in increased numbers; and sites in blood vessels where the leukocytes are attached loosely to endothelial cells. All these effects of cytokines produced in response to infection contribute to the control of infection while the adaptive immune response is being developed.

9-12 Interferons inhibit viral replication and activate certain host-defense responses.

Infection of cells with viruses induces the production of proteins known as **interferons** because they were found to interfere with viral replication in previously uninfected tissue culture cells. They are believed to play a similar role *in vivo*, blocking the spread of viruses to uninfected cells. These antiviral interferons, called **interferon-α (IFN-α)** and interferon-β (**IFN-β**), are quite distinct from interferon-γ (IFN-γ), which is produced by activated NK cells and in larger amounts by effector T cells and thus appears mainly after the induction of the adaptive immune response. IFN-α, actually a family of several closely related proteins, and IFN-β, the product of a single gene, are synthesized by many cell types after viral infection. Double-stranded RNA is not found in mammalian cells but forms the genome of some viruses and may be made as part of the infectious cycle of all viruses. It is a potent inducer of interferon synthesis and may be the common element in interferon induction. These proteins make several contributions to host defense against viral infection (Fig. 9.16).

An obvious and important effect of interferons is the induction of a state of resistance to viral replication in all cells. IFN-α and IFN-β bind to a common cellular receptor on cells. The interferon receptor, like other cytokine receptors (see Chapter 7), is coupled to a Janus-family tyrosine kinase, which in turn phosphorylates signal-transducing activators of transcription known as STATs. The binding of phosphorylated STATs to the promoters of several genes induces the synthesis of host-cell proteins that contribute to the inhibition of viral replication. One of these is the enzyme oligo-adenylate synthetase, which polymerizes ATP into a series of 2′-5′ linked oligomers (nucleotides in nucleic acids are normally linked 3′-5′). These activate an endoribonuclease that then degrades viral RNA. A second protein activated by IFN-α and IFN-β is a serine/threonine kinase called P1 kinase. This enzyme phosphorylates the eukaryotic protein synthesis initiation factor eIF-2, thereby inhibiting translation and thus contributing to the inhibition of viral replication. The importance of interferon-induced inhibition of viral replication can be seen in mice that lack the gene for an interferon-inducible protein called Mx, which is required for cellular resistance to influenza virus replication. These animals are highly susceptible to infection with the influenza virus, while genetically normal mice are resistant to influenza virus infection.

The second effect of interferons in host defense is to increase expression of MHC class I molecules, TAP transporter proteins, and the Lmp2 and Lmp7 components of the proteasome. This enhances the ability of host cells to present viral peptides to CD8 T cells should infection occur (see Section 4-8). At the same time, this increase in MHC class I expression protects uninfected host cells against attack by natural killer cells (NK cells). Natural killer cells are strongly activated by IFN-α and IFN-β, and make several important contributions to early host responses to viral infections, as we shall see next.

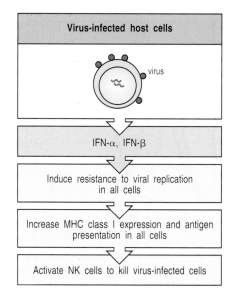

Virus-infected host cells

virus

IFN-α, IFN-β

Induce resistance to viral replication in all cells

Increase MHC class I expression and antigen presentation in all cells

Activate NK cells to kill virus-infected cells

Fig. 9.16 Interferons are antiviral proteins produced by cells in response to viral infection. The α- and β- interferons have three major functions. First, they induce resistance to viral replication by activating cellular genes that destroy mRNA and inhibit the translation of viral and some host proteins. Second, they induce MHC class I expression in most uninfected cells in the body, thus enhancing the resistance to NK cells, and increasing the susceptibility of cells newly-infected by virus to killing by CD8 cytotoxic T cells. Third, they activate natural killer (NK) cells, which then kill virus-infected cells selectively (see Figs 9.17 and 9.18).

9-13   **Natural killer cells serve as an early defense against certain intracellular infections.**

Natural killer, or NK cells, which we introduced in Chapter 8 as the effectors in antibody-dependent cell-mediated cytotoxicity, are identified by their ability to kill certain lymphoid tumor cell lines *in vitro* without the need for prior immunization or activation. However, their known function in host defense is in the early phases of infection with several intracellular pathogens, particularly herpes virus and *Listeria monocytogenes*, and we shall consider them here from that point of view.

Although NK cells that can kill sensitive targets can be isolated from uninfected individuals, this activity is increased by between 20- and 100-fold when NK cells are exposed to IFN-α and IFN-β or to the NK-cell activating factor IL-12, which is one of the cytokines produced early in many infections (Fig. 9.17). IL-12, in synergy with TNF-α, can also elicit

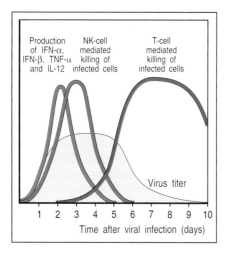

Fig. 9.17 Natural killer cells (NK cells) are an early component of the host response to virus infection. Interferons α and β and the cytokines TNF-α and IL-12 appear first, followed by a wave of NK cells, which together control virus replication but do not eliminate the virus. Virus elimination is accomplished when specific CD8 T cells are produced. Without NK cells, levels of certain viruses are much higher in the early days of the infection.

production of large amounts of IFN-γ by NK cells, and this secreted IFN-γ is crucial in controlling some infections before T cells have been activated to produce this cytokine. One example is the response to the intracellular bacterium *Listeria monocytogenes*. Mice that lack T and B lymphocytes are initially quite resistant to this pathogen; however, depletion of NK cells or mutations in the genes encoding TNF-α or IFN-γ or their receptors renders them highly susceptible, so that they die a few days after infection, before adaptive immunity can be induced.

If NK cells are to mediate host defense against infection with viruses and other pathogens, they must have some mechanism for distinguishing infected from uninfected cells. Exactly how this is achieved is not yet worked out; the observation, however, that NK cells selectively kill target cells bearing low levels of MHC class I molecules suggests one possible mechanism (Fig. 9.18). Another is that they recognize changes in cell surface glycoproteins induced by viral or bacterial infection.

Fig. 9.18 Possible mechanisms whereby NK cells distinguish infected from non-infected cells. A proposed mechanism of NK cell recognition is shown. NK cells have lectin-like receptors, called NKR-P1, that recognize carbohydrate on self cells. This recognition event signals NK cells to kill. However, another set of receptors, called Ly49 in the mouse and killer inhibitory receptors (KIR) in the human, recognize MHC class I molecules and inhibit killing by NK cells in a dominant way. This inhibitory signal is lost when host cells do not express MHC class I and perhaps also in cells infected with virus, which may inhibit MHC class I expression or alter its conformation. Normal cells respond to interferons α and β by increasing levels of MHC class I expression, making them resistant to activated NK killing. Infected cells may fail to increase MHC class I expression, making them targets for activated NK cells. Ly49 and KIR are encoded in different families of genes, the C-type lectins for Ly49 and the immunoglobulin gene super-family for the KIRs. The KIRs are made in two forms, p58 and p70, which differ by the presence of one immuno-globulin domain.

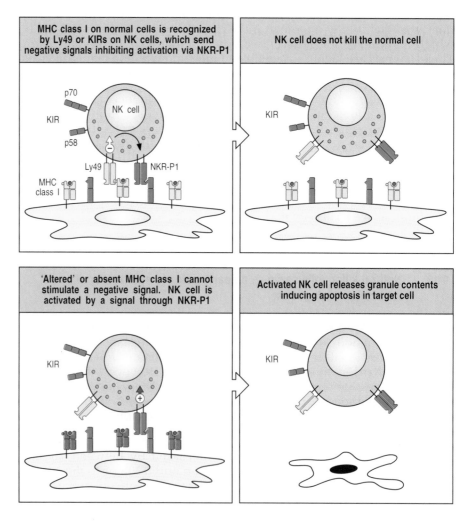

NK cells have two types of surface receptor. One, which triggers killing by NK cells, is known as NKR-P1. This receptor has the characteristics of a calcium-binding or C-type lectin, like the macrophage mannose receptor, and recognizes a wide variety of carbohydrate ligands that are thought to be found on many cells. The activation of NK cells to kill normal cells through this receptor is prevented by a second receptor. In mice, this inhibitory receptor is a C-type lectin, which recognizes self (and some non-self) MHC class I molecules. The mouse inhibitory receptors are encoded by a multigene family called Ly49 whose members recognize different H-2D alleles. In humans, there are also inhibitory receptors, which recognize distinct HLA-B and HLA-C alleles. However, the inhibitory receptors on human NK cells are structurally different from those of the mouse, being members of the immunoglobulin gene superfamily; they are usually called p58 and p70, or killer inhibitory receptors (KIRs).

Why two such distinct classes of molecule should serve equivalent functions in two species that share so many homologous genes is a major mystery. Either we will discover that human NK cells have molecules belonging to the Ly49 family, and that mouse NK cells have receptors equivalent to p58 and p70, or we will have to re-evaluate the hypothesis that NK cells are primitive or primordial killer cells.

Since the binding of the inhibitory receptors to MHC class I molecules inhibits NK activity, normal syngeneic cells are not susceptible to cytotoxic attack by NK cells. Both NKR-P1 and Ly49 are encoded by members of a small family of related genes that are differentially expressed on different subsets of NK cells and thus allow some variability in the structures that can be recognized by NK cells. Other NK receptors, specific for the products of other MHC class I loci, are being defined at a rapid rate.

Virus-infected cells, therefore, may be made susceptible to killing by NK cells by a variety of mechanisms. First, some viruses inhibit all host-protein synthesis, so the augmented synthesis of MHC class I proteins induced by interferon would be blocked selectively in infected cells, and NK cells would no longer be inhibited through their MHC-specific receptors. Second, some viruses can selectively prevent export of MHC class I molecules, which might allow the infected cell to evade recognition by CD8 T cells but would make it sensitive to NK cell killing. There is also evidence that introduction of new peptides into self MHC class I is detectable by NK cells. Whether these peptides are recognized directly, or whether they alter MHC conformation is not known. Finally, virus infection alters the glycosylation of cellular proteins, perhaps allowing dominant recognition by NKR-P1 or removing the normal ligand for Ly49 and other inhibitory NK receptors. Either of these mechanisms could allow infected cells to be detected even when the level of MHC class I expression is not altered by infection.

Clearly, much remains to be learned about this innate mechanism of cytotoxic attack and its physiological significance. At present, the only clue to the function of NK cells in humans comes from a rare patient deficient in NK cells who proved highly susceptible to early phases of herpes virus infection. The ability of NK cells to operate early in host defense by mechanisms that involve recognition of self MHC molecules, suggests they may represent the modern remnants of the evolutionary forebears of T cells. Two other 'primitive' lymphocyte types, γ:δ T cells and B-1 (or CD5) B cells, may also participate in the pre-adaptive immune response: of these, the γ:δ T cells, which we discuss first, are the more enigmatic.

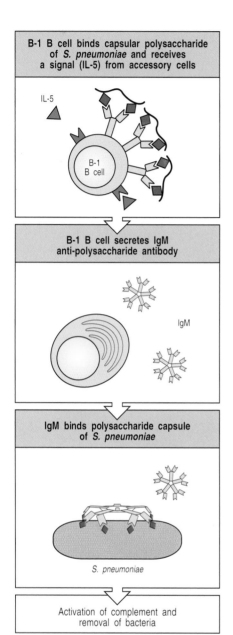

Fig. 9.19 B-1 B cells may be important in the response to carbohydrate antigens such as bacterial polysaccharides. These TI-2 responses may require IL-5 provided by T cells but this help is not antigen-specific and its mechanism is not clear. These responses are rapid, with antibody appearing in 48 hours, presumably because there is a high precursor frequency so that little clonal expansion is required. In the absence of antigen-specific T-cell help, only IgM is produced and, in mice, these responses therefore work mainly through the activation of complement.

9-14 | **T cells bearing γ:δ T-cell receptors are found in most epithelia and may contribute to host defense at the body surface.**

One of the most striking features of γ:δ T cells, whose discovery was accidental and whose function remains obscure, is the relative lack of diversity in their receptors (see Section 4-31). This is particularly striking in the γ:δ T cells found in surface epithelia, whose receptors are essentially homogeneous in any one epithelium. Moreover, although gut intra-epithelial lymphocytes appear to have diverse receptor sequences, they show the same pattern of responsiveness to different cell lines, and thus appear functionally, if not absolutely, homogeneous. What might cells with such invariant receptors be able to recognize, and why are these homogeneous lymphocytes found at the body surfaces? A possible explanation is that epithelial γ:δ T cells, although expressing receptors encoded in rearranging genes, are really part of a non-adaptive, early acting line of host defense. It has been proposed that because epithelial γ:δ T cells express but a single receptor within any epithelium, and also because they do not recirculate, they must recognize alterations on the surfaces of epithelial cells infected with any agent, rather than specific features of the pathogen. For instance, infected cells could make stress or heat-shock proteins in response to infection, and indeed, many γ:δ T cells do respond to such ligands. Equally, they may recognize the aberrant expression of MHC class IB genes that occurs when epithelial cells are infected. Recently, it has been shown that IL-1 and IL-12, released by phagocytes upon infection, can activate γ:δ T cells for production of IFN-γ. This IFN-γ contributes to macrophage activation. However, the true function of epithelial γ:δ T cells remains to be established definitively.

9-15 | **B-1 B cells form a separate population of B cells, producing antibodies to common bacterial polysaccharides.**

The production of antibody by conventional B cells plays a major part in the adaptive immune response. However, there is a separate lineage of B cells marked by the cell-surface protein CD5 that have properties quite distinct from those of conventional B cells (see Section 5-14). These so-called CD5 B cells, or B-1 B cells, are in many ways analogous to epithelial γ:δ T cells: they arise early in ontogeny, they use a distinctive and limited set of V genes to make their receptors, they are self-renewing in the periphery, and they are the predominant lymphocyte in a distinctive microenvironment, the peritoneal cavity.

B-1 B cells appear to make antibody responses mainly to polysaccharide antigens of the TI-2 type. These T-cell independent responses do not induce significant class switching or somatic hypermutation of immunoglobulin variable regions; as a consequence, the predominant antibody isotype produced is IgM (Fig. 9.19). Although these responses can be augmented by T cells, with IL-5 playing an important part (see Section 8-10), this interaction is not antigen specific and does not generate immunological memory: repeated exposures to the same TI-2 antigen elicit similar responses each time. Moreover, these responses appear within 48 hours of exposure to antigen, which is too soon for the generation of antigen-specific T cells. Thus, these responses, although generated by lymphocytes with rearranging receptors, resemble innate rather than adaptive immune responses.

As with γ:δ T cells, the precise role of B-1 B cells in host defense is uncertain. Mice that are deficient in B-1 B cells are more susceptible to infection with *Streptococcus pneumoniae*; this is because they fail to produce an antibody to phosphatidylcholine that effectively protects against this organism. A significant fraction of the B-1 B cells can make antibodies of this specificity, and since no antigen-specific T-cell help is required, a potent response can be produced early in infection with this pathogen. Whether human B-1 B cells play the same role is uncertain. In terms of evolution, it is interesting to note that γ:δ T cells appear to defend the body surfaces, while B-1 B cells defend the body cavity. Both cell types are relatively limited in their range of specificities and in the efficiency of their responses. It is possible that these two cell types represent a transitional phase in the evolution of the adaptive immune response, guarding the two main compartments of primitive organisms—the epithelial surfaces and the body cavity. Whether they are still critical to host defense, or whether they represent an evolutionary relic, is not yet clear. Nevertheless, as each cell type is prominent in certain sites in the body and contributes to certain responses, they must be incorporated into our thinking about host defense.

Summary.

The early induced but non-adaptive responses to infection involve a wide variety of effector mechanisms directed at distinct classes of pathogen. These responses are triggered by receptors that are either non-clonal or of very limited diversity, and are distinguished from adaptive immunity by their failure to provide lasting immunity or immunological memory. Some are induced by cytokines released by phagocytes in response to microbial infection, and these have three major effects. First, they induce the production of acute-phase proteins by the liver, which can bind to bacterial surface molecules and activate complement or phagocytes. Second, they can elevate body temperature, which is thought to be deleterious to the microorganism but to enhance the immune response. Third, they induce inflammation, in which the surface properties and permeability of blood vessels are changed, recruiting phagocytes, immune cells, and molecules to the site of infection. Interferons are produced by cells infected with viruses, and these slow viral replication and enhance the presentation of viral peptides to cytotoxic T cells, as well as activating natural killer cells (NK cells), which can distinguish infected from uninfected host cells. NK cells, B-1 B cells, and γ:δ T cells are lymphocytes with receptors of limited diversity that seem to provide early protection from a limited range of pathogens but do not generate lasting immunity. All these mechanisms play an important role, both on their own in holding infection in check during its early phases while the adaptive immune response is being developed, and also in their impact on the adaptive immune response that develops subsequently.

Adaptive immunity to infection.

It is not known how many infections are dealt with solely by non-adaptive mechanisms of host defense; this is because they are eliminated early and such infections produce little in the way of symptoms or pathology. Moreover, deficiencies in non-adaptive defenses are rare, so it has seldom been possible to study their consequences. Adaptive immunity is triggered when an infection eludes the innate defense mechanisms and

Fig. 9.20   The course of a typical acute infection. 1. The level of infectious agent increases with pathogen replication. 2. When the pathogen level exceeds the threshold dose of antigen required for an adaptive response, the response is initiated; the pathogen continues to grow, retarded only by the innate and early, non-adaptive responses. 3. After 4–5 days, effector cells and molecules of the adaptive response start to clear the infection. 4. When the infection is cleared, and the dose of antigen falls below the response threshold, the response ceases but antibody, residual effector cells, and also immunological memory provide lasting protection against re-infection.

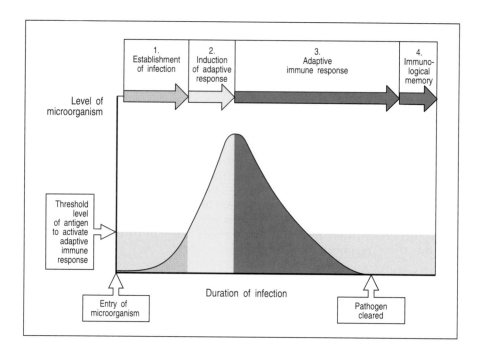

generates a threshold dose of antigen (Fig. 9.20). This antigen then initiates an adaptive immune response, which becomes effective only after several days, the time required for antigen-specific T and B cells to proliferate and differentiate into effector cells. Meanwhile, the pathogen continues to grow in the host, held in check mainly by innate and non-adaptive mechanisms (Fig. 9.21). In the earlier chapters of this book we discussed the cells and molecules that mediate the adaptive immune response, and the interactions between cells that stimulate individual steps in its development. We are now ready to see how each cell type is recruited in turn in the course of a primary immune response to a pathogen, and how the effector cells and molecules that are generated in response to antigen are dispersed to their sites of action, leading to clearance of the infection and the establishment of a state of protective immunity.

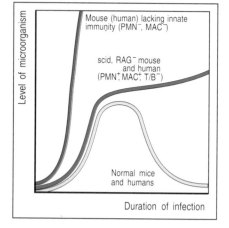

Fig. 9.21   The time course of infections in various types of immunodeficient mice and humans. The red curve shows the growth of microorganisms in the absence of innate immunity. The green curve shows mice and humans that have innate immunity but lack adaptive immunity. The yellow curve shows the normal course of an infection in immunocompetent mice or humans.

9-16   T-cell activation is initiated when recirculating T cells encounter specific antigen in draining lymphoid tissues.

The first step in any adaptive immune response leading to protective immunity is the activation of T cells in the draining lymphoid organs. The importance of the peripheral lymphoid organs was first shown by ingenious experiments in which a skin flap was isolated from the body wall so that it had a blood circulation but no lymphatic drainage. Antigen placed in this site did not elicit a T-cell response, showing that T cells do not become sensitized in peripheral tissues. We now know that T lymphocytes generally become sensitized in lymphoid organs: antigens in tissues are trapped in draining lymph nodes through which T cells circulate, while antigens introduced directly into the bloodstream, or that reach the bloodstream from an infected lymph node, are picked up by antigen-presenting cells in the spleen, and lymphoid cell sensitization then occurs in the splenic white pulp (see Fig. 1.8). The trapping of antigen by antigen-presenting cells that migrate to these lymphoid tissues and the continuous recirculation of T cells through the tissues ensures that rare antigen-specific T cells will encounter their specific antigen on a professional antigen-presenting cell.

The recirculation of naive T cells through the lymphoid organs is orchestrated by adhesive interactions between lymphocytes and endothelial cells. Naive T cells enter the lymphoid organs in essentially the same way to that described earlier for the entry of phagocytes into sites of infection (see Fig. 9.11), except that in this case the selectin is expressed on the T cell rather than the endothelium. L-selectin on naive T cells binds to sulfated carbohydrates on the vascular addressins GlyCAM-1 and CD34. CD34 is expressed on endothelial cells in many tissues but is properly glycosylated for L-selectin binding only on the high endothelial venule cells of lymph nodes. L-selectin binding promotes a rolling interaction like that mediated by P- and E-selectin when they bind to the surface of phagocytes. This interaction is critical to the selectivity of naive lymphocyte homing. Although this interaction is too weak to promote extravasation, it is essential for the initiation of the stronger interactions that then follow between the T cell and the high endothelium, which are mediated by molecules with a relatively broad tissue distribution.

Stimulation by locally bound chemokines activates the adhesion molecule LFA-1 on the T cell, increasing its affinity for ICAM-2, which is expressed constitutively on all endothelial cells, and ICAM-1, which, in the absence of inflammation, is expressed only on the high endothelial venule cells of peripheral lymphoid tissues. The binding of LFA-1 to its ligands ICAM-1 and ICAM-2 plays a major role in T-cell adhesion to and migration through the wall of the blood vessel into the lymph node (Fig. 9.22).

The high endothelial venules are located in the T-cell rich zone of the lymph nodes. This area is also inhabited by dendritic cells, which have recently migrated from the periphery and developed co-stimulatory capacity. The migrating T cells scan the surface of these professional antigen-presenting cells for specific peptide:MHC complexes. If they do not recognize antigen presented by these cells, they eventually leave the node via an efferent lymphatic vessel, which returns them to the blood so that they can recirculate through other lymph nodes. Rarely, a naive T cell recognizes its specific peptide:MHC complex on the surface

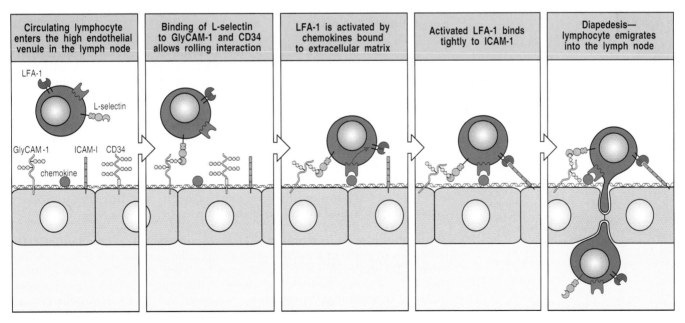

| Circulating lymphocyte enters the high endothelial venule in the lymph node | Binding of L-selectin to GlyCAM-1 and CD34 allows rolling interaction | LFA-1 is activated by chemokines bound to extracellular matrix | Activated LFA-1 binds tightly to ICAM-1 | Diapedesis— lymphocyte emigrates into the lymph node |

Fig. 9.22　Lymphocytes in the blood enter lymphoid tissue by crossing high endothelial venules. The first step in lymphocyte entry is the binding of L-selectin on the lymphocyte to sulfated carbohydrates of GlyCAM-1 and CD34 on the high endothelial venule cell. Local chemokines activate LFA-1 on the lymphocyte and cause it to bind tightly to ICAM-1 on the endothelial cell, allowing transendothelial migration.

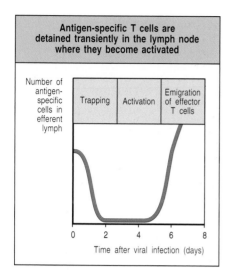

Antigen-specific T cells are detained transiently in the lymph node where they become activated

Fig. 9.23 Naive T cells migrate from blood through lymphoid tissue continually. In the cortex of the lymph node, T cells encounter many antigen-presenting cells. T cells that do not recognize their specific antigen in the lymph node cortex leave via the efferent lymphatics and re-enter the blood. T cells that do recognize their specific antigen bind in a stable manner to the antigen-presenting cell and are activated through their T-cell receptor, resulting in the production of armed effector T cells. Lymphocyte recirculation is so active that all specific T cells can be trapped by antigen in one node within 2 days. By 5 days after antigen arrives, activated effector T cells are leaving the lymph node in large numbers via the afferent lymphatics.

of a professional antigen-presenting cell, which signals the activation of LFA-1, causing the T cell to adhere strongly to the antigen-presenting cell and cease migrating. Binding to the peptide:MHC complex also activates the cell to proliferate and differentiate, resulting in the production of armed, antigen-specific effector T cells (see Fig. 7.2). The number of T cells that interact with each antigen-presenting cell in lymph nodes is very high, as can be seen by the rapid trapping of antigen-specific T cells in a single lymph node containing antigen: all antigen-specific T cells can be trapped in a lymph node within 48 hours of antigen deposition there (Fig. 9.23).

9-17 | Cytokines made in the early phases of an infection influence the functional differentiation of CD4 T cells.

It is during the initial response of naive CD4 T cells to antigen in the peripheral lymphoid tissues that the differentiation of these cells into the two major classes of CD4 effector T cells occurs. This step, at which a naive CD4 T cell becomes either an armed T_H1 cell or an armed T_H2 cell, has a critical impact on the outcome of an adaptive immune response, determining whether it will be dominated by macrophage activation or by antibody production. This is one of the most important events in the induction of adaptive immune responses.

The mechanism controlling this step in CD4 T-cell differentiation is not fully defined; however, it is clear that it can be influenced profoundly by cytokines present during the initial proliferative phase of T-cell activation. Experiments *in vitro* have shown that CD4 T cells initially stimulated in the presence of IL-12 and IFN-γ tend to develop into T_H1 cells, in part because IFN-γ inhibits the proliferation of T_H2 cells. As IL-12 and IFN-γ are produced by macrophages and NK cells in the early phases of responses to viruses and some intracellular bacteria, such as *Listeria* spp., T-cell responses in viral and *Listeria* infections tend to be dominated by T_H1 cells. By contrast, CD4 T cells activated in the presence of IL-4 and especially IL-6 tend to differentiate into T_H2 cells, as IL-4 and IL-6 promote differentiation of T_H2 cells, while IL-4 and IL-10 inhibit the generation of T_H1 cells.

One possible source of the IL-4 needed to generate T_H2 cells is a specialized subset of CD4 T cells that express the NK1.1 marker normally associated with NK cells. These T cells have a nearly invariant T-cell receptor; in fact, essentially the same receptor appears to be used in the NK1.1$^+$ cells of mice and their counterparts in humans. Unlike other CD4 T cells, the development of the **NK1.1 CD4 T cells** does not depend on the expression of MHC class II molecules. Instead, these T cells recognize an MHC class IB molecule, CD1, which is not encoded within the MHC. In mice there are two CD1 genes (CD1.1 and CD1.2), while in humans there are five (CD1a–e) of which only CD1d is homologous to the murine CD1.1 and CD1.2. CD1 molecules are expressed by thymocytes, antigen-presenting cells, and intestinal epithelium.

Although the exact function of CD1 molecules is not well defined, CD1b is known to present a bacterial lipid, mycolic acid, to α:β T cells, while other CD1 molecules are recognized by γ:δ T cells. The activation of NK1.1 CD4 T cells is thought to depend on the expression of CD1 molecules induced in response to infection; whether the NK1.1 CD4 cells recognize a specific antigen presented by these CD1 molecules is not known. Upon activation, these NK1.1 CD4 cells secrete very large amounts of IL-4 and can therefore enhance the development of T_H2 cells (Fig. 9.24), which promotes the production of IgG1 (mouse) and IgE (mouse, human) in subsequent humoral immune responses.

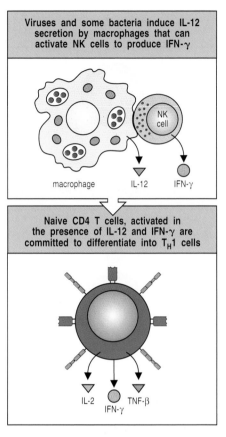

| Viruses and some bacteria induce IL-12 secretion by macrophages that can activate NK cells to produce IFN-γ |
| Naive CD4 T cells, activated in the presence of IL-12 and IFN-γ are committed to differentiate into T$_H$1 cells |

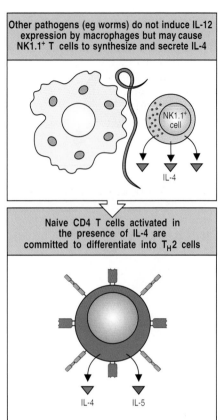

| Other pathogens (eg worms) do not induce IL-12 expression by macrophages but may cause NK1.1$^+$ T cells to synthesize and secrete IL-4 |
| Naive CD4 T cells activated in the presence of IL-4 are committed to differentiate into T$_H$2 cells |

Fig. 9.24 The differentiation of naive CD4 T cells into armed effector cell types is influenced by cytokines elicited by the pathogen. Many pathogens, especially intracellular bacteria and viruses, activate macrophages and NK cells to produce IL-12 and IFN-γ, which act on proliferating CD4 T cells causing them to differentiate into T$_H$1 cells. IL-4 can inhibit these responses. IL-4, produced by an NK1.1$^+$, CD4$^+$ T cell in response to parasitic worms or other pathogens, acts on proliferating CD4 T cells to cause them to become T$_H$2 cells. The mechanism by which these cytokines induce the selective differentiation of CD4 T cells is not known. They could act either when the CD4 T cell is first activated by an antigen-presenting cell (bottom panels) or during the proliferative phase that ensues.

The differential capacity of pathogens to interact with macrophages, NK cells, and NK1.1 CD4 T cells may therefore influence the overall balance of cytokines present early in the immune response and thus determine whether T$_H$1 or T$_H$2 cells develop preferentially to bias the adaptive immune response towards a cellular or a humoral response. This may in turn determine whether the pathogen is eliminated or survives within the host, and some pathogens may have evolved to interact with the innate immune system so as to generate responses that are beneficial to them, rather than to the host.

9-18   **Distinct subsets of T cells can regulate the growth and effector functions of other T-cell subsets.**

The two subsets of CD4 T cells, T$_H$1 cells and T$_H$2 cells, have very different functions: T$_H$2 cells are the most effective activators of B cells, especially in primary responses, while T$_H$1 cells are crucial for activating macrophages. It is also clear that the two CD4 T-cell subsets can regulate each other; once one subset becomes dominant, it is often hard to shift the response to the other type. One reason for this is that cytokines from one type of CD4 T cell inhibit the activation of the other. Thus, IL-10, a product of T$_H$2 cells, can inhibit the development of T$_H$1 cells by acting on the antigen-presenting cell, while interferon-γ, a product of T$_H$1 cells, can prevent the activation of T$_H$2 cells (Fig. 9.25). If a particular CD4 T-cell subset is activated first or preferentially in a response, it can suppress the development of the other subset. The overall effect is that certain responses are dominated by either humoral (T$_H$2) or cell-mediated (T$_H$1) immunity.

This interplay of cytokines plays an important role in human disease, but it has been explored at present mainly in certain mouse models, where such polarized responses are easier to study. For example, when

Fig. 9.25 The two subsets of CD4 T cell each produce cytokines that can negatively regulate the other subset. T$_H$2 cells make IL-10, which acts on macrophages to inhibit T$_H$1 activation, perhaps by blocking macrophage IL-12 synthesis and TGF-β, which acts directly in T$_H$1 cells (left panels). T$_H$1 cells make IFN-γ, which blocks the growth of T$_H$2 cells (right panels). These effects allow either subset to dominate a response by suppressing outgrowth of cells of the other subset.

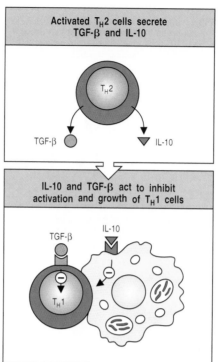

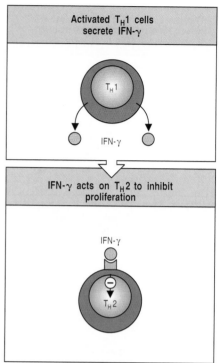

CD4 T cells in BALB/c mice are stimulated with the protozoan parasite *Leishmania*, their CD4 T cells fail to differentiate into T$_H$1 effector cells; instead, they preferentially make T$_H$2 cells in response to this pathogen. These T$_H$2 cells are unable to activate macrophages to inhibit leishmanial growth, resulting in susceptibility to disease. By contrast, C57BL/6 mice respond by producing T$_H$1 cells that protect the host by activating infected macrophages to kill the *Leishmania*. The activation of T$_H$2 cells in BALB/c mice can be reversed if IL-4 is blocked in the first days of infection by injecting anti-IL-4 antibody. This treatment is ineffective after a week or so.

A second aspect of this balancing is that one type of effector CD4 T cell can directly inhibit the effector functions of the other type. Thus, armed T$_H$1 cells can block B-cell activation by armed T$_H$2 cells, at least in some systems. This occurs mainly through killing of activated B cells by armed T$_H$1 cells; these express the Fas ligand, which induces apoptosis by binding to Fas on activated B cells (Fig. 9.26). Likewise, there is evidence that armed T$_H$2 cells may prevent expression of armed T$_H$1 cell function by secreting the cytokine IL-10.

Fig. 9.26 T$_H$1 cells can suppress the activation of B cells by T$_H$2 cells. T$_H$2 cells activate B cells to produce antibody. When both T$_H$2 cells and T$_H$1 cells recognizing peptides from the same antigen are added to antigen-specific B cells, suppression can dominate so that no antibody production is seen. Most T$_H$1 cells can kill B cells, perhaps explaining their suppressive effects.

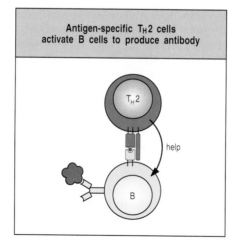

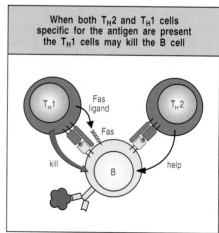

Since cytokines appear to regulate the balance between T$_H$1 and T$_H$2 cells, one might expect that it would be possible to shift this balance by administering appropriate cytokines. IL-2 and IFN-γ have been used to stimulate cell-mediated immunity in diseases such as lepromatous leprosy and can cause both a local resolution of the lesion and a systemic change in T-cell responses, as we shall see in Chapter 10. IL-12, which we have seen is a potent inducer of T$_H$1 cells, may be an even more attractive potential therapy.

CD8 T cells are also able to regulate the immune response by producing cytokines. It has become clear recently that CD8 T cells can, in addition to their familiar cytolytic function, also respond to antigen by secreting cytokines typical of either T$_H$1 or T$_H$2 cells. Such CD8 T cells appear to be responsible for the development of leprosy in its lepromatous rather than its tuberculoid form, which we discuss in detail in Chapter 10 (see Fig. 10.6). Patients with the less destructive tuberculoid leprosy make only T$_H$1 cells, which can activate macrophages to rid the body of leprosy bacilli. Patients with lepromatous leprosy have CD8 T cells that suppress the T$_H$1 response by making IL-10 and TGF-β. Thus, the suppression by CD8 T cells that has been observed in various situations may be explained by their expression of different sets of cytokines.

9-19 The nature and amount of antigenic peptide can also affect the differentiation of CD4 T cells.

Another factor that influences the differentiation of CD4 T cells into distinct effector subsets is the amount and exact sequence of the antigenic peptide that initiates the response. Large amounts of peptides that achieve a high density on the surface of antigen-presenting cells tend to stimulate T$_H$1 cell responses, while low-density presentation tends to elicit T$_H$2 cell responses. Moreover, peptides that interact strongly with the T-cell receptor tend to stimulate T$_H$1-like responses, while peptides that bind weakly tend to stimulate T$_H$2-like responses (Fig. 9.27).

This difference may be very important in several circumstances. For instance, allergy is caused by the production of IgE antibody, which as we learned in Chapter 8, requires high levels of IL-4 but does not occur in the presence of IFN-γ, a potent inhibitor of IL-4-driven class switching to IgE. We shall see in Chapter 11 that antigens that elicit IgE-mediated allergy are generally delivered in minute doses, and that they elicit T$_H$2 cells that make IL-4 and no IFN-γ. It is also relevant that allergens do not elicit any of the known innate immune responses, which produce cytokines that tend to bias CD4 T-cell differentiation toward T$_H$1 cells.

Most protein antigens that elicit CD4 T-cell responses stimulate the production of both T$_H$1 and T$_H$2 cells. This reflects the presence in most proteins of several different peptide sequences that can bind to MHC class II molecules and be presented to T cells. Some of these peptides are likely to bind to MHC class II molecules with high affinity, and consequently may be present at high density on the antigen-presenting cell,

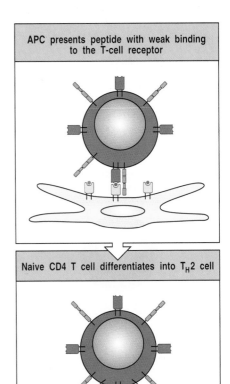

APC presents peptide with weak binding to the T-cell receptor

Naive CD4 T cell differentiates into T$_H$2 cell

IL-4   IL-5

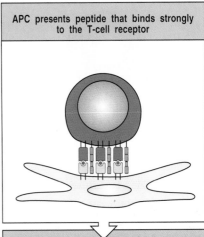

APC presents peptide that binds strongly to the T-cell receptor

Naive CD4 T cell differentiates into T$_H$1 cell

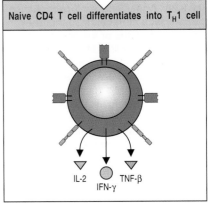

IL-2   IFN-γ   TNF-β

Fig. 9.27 The nature and amount of ligand presented to a CD4 T cell during primary stimulation can determine its functional phenotype. CD4 T cells presented with low levels of a ligand that binds the T-cell receptor poorly, differentiate preferentially into T$_H$2 cells making IL-4 and IL-5. Such T cells are active in stimulating naive B cells to differentiate into plasma cells and make antibody. T cells presented with a high density of a ligand that binds the T-cell receptor strongly differentiate into T$_H$1 cells that secrete IL-2, TNF-β and IFN-γ, and are effective in activating macrophages.

while others may bind with low affinity and be present only at low density. Naive T cells specific for peptide antigens that have high affinity for MHC molecules are likely therefore to encounter a high density of their ligand, while others may only encounter a low density, and these differences in ligand density may affect the subsequent response of the T cell. Indeed, it can be demonstrated experimentally that some peptides in a protein tend to elicit T_H2 cells, while others tend to elicit T_H1 cells.

The difference in ligand density or T-cell receptor avidity required to elicit and activate T_H1 and T_H2 cells may be an adaptation to differences in the behavior of the infectious agents against which the two types of CD4 T cell are directed. T_H2 cells are required for effective immunity to extracellular forms of pathogens; they must mount a rapid response to combat these rapidly proliferating microorganisms. Since these pathogens do not multiply inside the antigen-presenting cells that take them up, their antigens will tend to be presented at a relatively low density. Thus, it is advantageous for T_H2 cells to be produced in response to low levels of foreign peptide presented by a macrophage. In contrast, T_H1 cells are required primarily to combat intracellular pathogens that initially infect single cells, proliferate more slowly, and cause little damage early in the course of an infection. Thus, the responses that produce T_H1 cells can afford a higher threshold of antigen density for activation, and this is readily achieved through the growth of many bacteria or viruses within a single infected cell, providing a large endogenous source of antigenic peptides for shipment to the cell surface by MHC class II molecules.

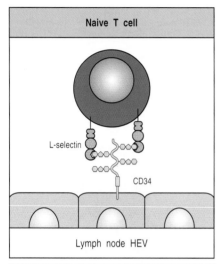

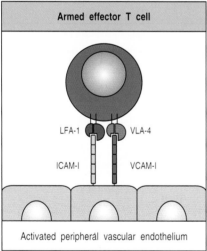

Fig. 9.28 Armed effector T cells change their surface molecules so that they can home to sites of infection via the blood. Naive T cells home to lymph nodes through L-selectin binding to sulfated carbohydrates displayed by CD34 and GlyCAM-1 (upper panel). If they encounter antigen and differentiate into effector cells, many lose expression of L-selectin, leave the lymph node about 4–5 days later, and now express VLA-4 and increased levels of LFA-1, which bind to VCAM-1 and ICAM-1 respectively on peripheral vascular endothelium at sites of inflammation (lower panel).

| 9-20 | **Armed effector T cells are guided to sites of infection by newly expressed surface molecules.** |

The full activation of naive T cells takes 4–5 days and is accompanied by changes in cell-surface adhesion molecules that direct the newly differentiated armed effector T cells to the site of infection in the peripheral tissues. Thus, most armed effector T cells lose expression of the L-selectin molecule that mediates homing to the lymph nodes, while the expression of other adhesion molecules is increased (Fig. 9.28). One important change is a marked increase in the expression of the α_4 integrin VLA-4 (see Section 7-2), which binds to vascular cell adhesion molecule-1 (VCAM-1); cytokines induce expression of VCAM-1 on endothelial cells at sites of infection in peripheral tissues.

Differential expression of adhesion molecules may also direct different subsets of armed effector T cells to specific sites. Some, for example, migrate to Peyer's patches, where they are thought to contribute to mucosal immunity. Homing to Peyer's patches and to the lamina propria of the gut involves the binding of both L-selectin and the $\alpha_4\beta_7$ integrin expressed on the T cell to separate sites on MAdCAM-1. T cells that home to the epithelium of the gut express a novel integrin, called $\alpha_e\beta_7$, and bind to E-cadherin expressed on epithelial cells. Cells that home to the skin, by contrast, express the **cutaneous lymphocyte antigen (CLA)** and may bind E-selectin.

Not all infections trigger innate immune responses that activate local endothelial cells, and it is not so clear how T cells are guided to the sites of infection in these cases. Armed effector T cells appear to enter all tissues in very small numbers, perhaps via adhesive interactions such as the binding of LFA-1 to ICAM-2, which is constitutively expressed on all endothelial cells. If these T cells recognize specific antigen in the tissue they enter, they produce cytokines, such as TNF-α, which activates endothelial cells to express E-selectin, VCAM-1, and ICAM-1, and chemokines such as RANTES (see Fig. 9.13), which can then act on effector T cells to activate their adhesion molecules. The increased levels of VCAM-1 and ICAM-1 on endothelial cells bind VLA-4 and LFA-1, respectively, on armed effector T cells, recruiting more of these cells into tissues that contain antigen. At the same time, monocytes and polymorphonuclear leukocytes are recruited to these sites by adhesion to E-selectin. The TNF-α and IFN-γ released by the activated T cells also act synergistically to change the shape of endothelial cells, allowing increased blood flow, increased vascular permeability, and increased emigration of leukocytes, fluid, and protein into a site of infection.

Thus, one or a few specific effector T cells encountering antigen in a tissue can initiate a potent local inflammatory response that recruits both more specific effector cells and many accessory cells to that site. Most of the armed effector T cells that migrate at random into tissues will of course not encounter specific antigen, and these cells either enter afferent lymph and return to the bloodstream, or undergo apoptotic death in the tissues. Many of the T cells in afferent lymph draining peripheral tissues are memory or effector T cells that express CD45R0 and lack L-selectin. They appear to be committed to migration through potential sites of infection.

9-21 | Antibody responses develop in lymphoid tissues under the direction of armed T$_H$2 cells.

Migration into the periphery is clearly important for the effector actions of CD8 cytotoxic T cells, and for T$_H$1 cells, which need to activate macrophages at the site of an infection. The most important functions of T$_H$2 cells, however, depend upon their interactions with B cells, and these interactions occur in the lymphoid tissues. B cells specific for protein antigens cannot be activated to proliferate, form germinal centers, or differentiate into plasma cells until they encounter a T$_H$2 cell that is specific for one of the peptides derived from that antigen or antigenic complex. It follows, therefore, that humoral immune responses to protein antigens cannot occur until after antigen-specific T$_H$2 cells have been generated.

One of the most interesting questions in immunology is how two antigen-specific lymphocytes, the naive antigen-binding B cell and the armed helper T cell, find one another to initiate a T-cell dependent antibody response. As we learned in Chapter 8, the likely answer lies in the migratory path of B cells through the lymphoid tissues and the presence of armed helper T cells on that path (Fig. 9.29).

B cells migrate through peripheral lymphoid organs in much the same way as T cells (see Fig. 9.29, first panel), and it is thought that the trapping and activation of naive CD4 T cells in the T-cell areas of lymphoid tissues provides a concentration of antigen-specific helper T cells capable of activating those rare B cells that are specific for the same antigen. Antigen-specific B cells are also enriched in these same areas by binding their cognate antigen; such cells are observed to accumulate in T-cell areas of the spleen and lymph nodes when exposed to their specific antigen. If the B cells receive specific signals from armed T$_H$2 cells, they proliferate in the T-cell areas of lymphoid tissues (see Fig. 9.29, second panel). In the absence of T-cell signals, these antigen-specific B cells die in less than 24 hours.

About 5 days after primary immunization, primary foci of proliferating B cells appear in the T-cell areas, correlating with the time needed for helper T cells to differentiate. Some of the B cells activated in the primary focus may migrate to the medullary cords of the lymph node or to those parts of the red pulp that are next to the T-cell zones of the spleen

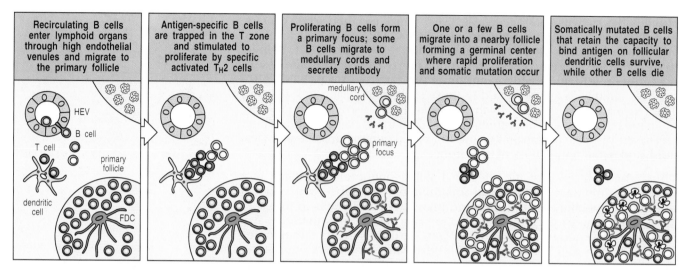

| Recirculating B cells enter lymphoid organs through high endothelial venules and migrate to the primary follicle | Antigen-specific B cells are trapped in the T zone and stimulated to proliferate by specific activated T$_H$2 cells | Proliferating B cells form a primary focus; some B cells migrate to medullary cords and secrete antibody | One or a few B cells migrate into a nearby follicle forming a germinal center where rapid proliferation and somatic mutation occur | Somatically mutated B cells that retain the capacity to bind antigen on follicular dendritic cells survive, while other B cells die |

Fig. 9.29   The specialized regions of lymphoid tissue provide an environment where antigen-specific B cells can interact with armed helper T cells specific for the same antigen. The initial encounter of antigen-specific B cells with the appropriate helper T cells occurs in the T-cell areas in lymphoid tissue and stimulates proliferation of B cells in contact with the helper T cells, resulting in some isotype switching. Some activated B-cell blasts then migrate to medullary cords, where they divide, differentiate into plasma cells, and secrete antibody for a few days. Other cells migrate into primary lymphoid follicles where they proliferate rapidly to form a germinal center under the influence of helper T cells and antigen trapped on follicular dendritic cells. The germinal center is the site of somatic hypermutation and selection of high-affinity B cells on the follicular dendritic cell network. In the primary response, antigen trapping occurs only after initial production of antibody by B cells in the primary focus and the medullary cords. HEV, high endothelial venule; FDC, follicular dendritic cell.

and secrete specific antibody for a few days (see Fig. 9.29, third panel). Others migrate to the follicle (see Fig. 9.29, fourth panel), where they proliferate further, forming a germinal center in which they undergo somatic hypermutation (see Chapter 8). The antibodies secreted by B cells differentiating early in the response not only provide early protection; they may also be important in trapping antigen, in the form of antigen:antibody complexes, on the surface of the local follicular dendritic cells. This contributes to the selection of B cells by antigen that underlies the affinity maturation observed during an antibody response. The antigen is held by a non-phagocytic Fc receptor on the follicular dendritic cells in the form of antigen:antibody complexes. Antigen can be retained in lymphoid follicles in this form for very long periods.

The proliferation, somatic hypermutation, and selection that occur in the germinal centers during a primary antibody response have been described in Chapter 8. The adhesion molecules that govern the migratory behavior of B cells are likely to be very important to this process but, as yet, little is known of their nature or of the ligands to which they bind.

9-22   Antibody responses are sustained in medullary cords and bone marrow.

Antibody-secreting cells are generated either as the result of B cells proliferating in primary foci or after migration to follicles. The proliferative response is started by B cells that have taken up antigen interacting in the T-cell zone with T$_H$2 cells specific for the same antigen. The B cells activated in primary foci then migrate either to adjacent follicles or to local extrafollicular sites of proliferation. The extrafollicular sites in lymph nodes are the medullary cords and in the spleen are those parts of the red pulp directly adjoining the T-cell zone. B cells grow exponentially in these sites for 2–3 days and undergo six or seven cell divisions before the progeny come out of the cell cycle and form antibody-pro-

Fig. 9.30 Plasma cells are dispersed in medullary cords and bone marrow. In these sites they secrete antibody at high rates directly into the blood for distribution to the rest of the body. In the upper micrograph, plasma cells in lymph node medullary cords are stained green (with fluorescein anti-IgM) if they are secreting IgM and red (with rhodamine anti-IgG) if they are secreting IgG. These plasma cells are short-lived (2–4 days).

In the lower micrograph, longer-lived plasma cells (3–6 weeks) in the bone marrow are revealed with light-chain specific antibodies (fluorescein anti-λ and rhodamine anti-κ stain). Plasma cells secreting immunoglobulins containing λ light chains are stained green while those secreting immunoglobulins containing κ chains are stained red. Photographs courtesy of P Brandtzaeg.

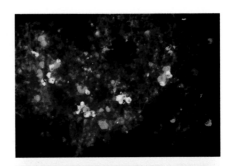

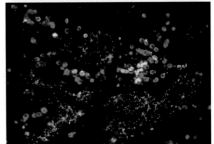

ducing plasma cells *in situ*. Most of these plasma cells have a life-span of 2–3 days, after which they undergo apoptosis. About 10% of plasma cells in these extrafollicular sites live longer; their origin and ultimate fate is unknown. B cells that migrate to the primary follicles to form germinal centers have been discussed in Chapter 8 (see Sections 8-6 to 8-8). Some B cells leave germinal centers as **plasmablasts** (pre-plasma cells). These migrate to distant sites of antibody production where they differentiate into plasma cells that have a life span of about 1 month. Plasmablasts originating in the follicles of Peyer's patches and mesenteric lymph nodes migrate via lymph and blood to the lamina propria of the gut and other epithelial surfaces. Those originating in peripheral lymph node or splenic follicles migrate to the bone marrow (Fig. 9.30, lower panel). In responses to non-replicating antigens, germinal centers are only present for 3–4 weeks after the supply of extrafollicular antigen is exhausted. Small numbers of B cells, however, continue to proliferate in the follicles for months, and are likely the precursors of antigen-specific plasma cells in the mucosa and bone marrow throughout the subsequent months and years.

9-23   The effector mechanisms used to clear an infection depend on the infectious agent.

A primary adaptive immune response to an infection serves to clear the primary infection from the body and to provide protection against re-infection with the same pathogen in most cases. However, some pathogens persist for life, such as *Leishmania*, toxoplasma, and herpes viruses. Fig. 9.31 summarizes the different types of infection and the ways in which they can be eliminated effectively by an initial adaptive immune response.

Immunity to re-infection is called **protective immunity**, and inducing protective immunity is the goal of vaccine development. Protective immunity consists of two components, immune reactants generated in the initial infection or by vaccination, and long-lived immunological memory (Fig. 9.32), which we shall consider in the last part of this chapter. Protective immunity may require the presence of pre-formed reactants, such as antibody molecules or armed effector T cells. For instance, effective protection against polio virus requires pre-existing antibody, because the virus will rapidly infect motor neurons and lead to their destruction unless it is neutralized by antibody as soon as it enters the body. Specific IgA on epithelial surfaces may also neutralize the virus before it enters the body. Thus, protective immunity may involve effector mechanisms (IgA in this case) that do not operate in the elimination of the primary infection (see Fig. 9.31). Pre-formed reactants may also allow the immune system to respond more rapidly and efficiently to a second exposure to a pathogen. Thus, when antibody is present, opsonization and phagocytosis of pathogens will be more efficient. If specific IgE is present, then pathogens will also be able to activate mast cells, rapidly initiating an inflammatory response through the release of histamine and leukotrienes.

	Infectious agent	Disease	Humoral immunity				Cell-mediated Immunity	
			IgM	IgG	IgE	IgA	CD4 T cells (macrophages)	CD8 killer T cells
Viruses	Variola	Smallpox						
	Varicella zoster	Chickenpox						
	Epstein-Barr virus	Mononucleosis						
	Influenza virus	Influenza						
	Mumps virus	Mumps						
	Measles virus	Measles						
	Polio virus	Poliomyelitis						
	Human immunodeficiency virus	AIDS						
Bacteria	*Staphylococcus aureus*	Boils						
	Streptococcus pyogenes	Tonsilitis						
	Streptococcus pneumoniae	Pneumonia						
	Neisseria gonorrhoeae	Gonorrhea						
	Neisseria meningitidis	Meningitis						
	Corynebacterium diphtheriae	Diphtheria						
	Clostridium tetani	Tetanus						
	Treponema pallidum	Syphilis			Transient			
	Borrelia burgdorferi	Lyme disease			Transient			
	Salmonella typhi	Typhoid						
	Vibrio cholerae	Cholera						
	Legionella pneumophilia	Legionnaire's disease						
	Rickettsia prowazeki	Typhus						
	Chlamydia trachomatis	Trachoma						
	Mycobacteria	Tuberculosis, leprosy						
Fungi	*Candida albicans*	Candidiasis						
Protozoa	*Plasmodium* spp.	Malaria						
	Toxoplasma gondii	Toxoplasmosis						
	Trypanosoma spp.	Trypanosomiasis						
	Leishmania spp.	Leishmaniasis						
Worms	Schistosome	Schistosomiasis						

Fig. 9.31 Different effector mechanisms are used to clear primary infections with different pathogens and to protect against subsequent re-infection. The pathogens are listed in order of increasing complexity, and the defense mechanisms used to clear a primary infection are identified by the red shading of the boxes where these are known. Yellow shading indicates a role in protective immunity. Paler shades indicate less well-established mechanisms. Much has to be learned about such host–pathogen interactions. It is clear that classes of pathogens elicit similar protective immune responses, reflecting similarities in their lifestyles.

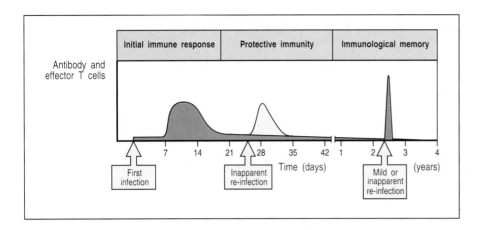

Fig. 9.32 Protective immunity consists of pre-formed immune reactants and immunological memory. Antibody levels and effector T-cell activity gradually decline after an infection is cleared. An early re-infection is rapidly cleared by these immune reactants, with few symptoms but levels of immune reactants increase. Re-infection at later times leads to rapid increases in antibody and effector T cells owing to immunological memory, and infection may be mild or even inapparent.

Summary.

The adaptive immune response is required for effective protection of the host against pathogenic microorganisms. Adaptive immunity occurs when pathogens have overwhelmed or evaded non-adaptive mechanisms of host defense and established a focus of infection. The antigens of the pathogen are transported to local lymphoid organs by migrating antigen-presenting cells, or trapped there by resident cells. This antigen is processed and presented to antigen-specific naive T cells that continuously recirculate through the lymphoid organs. T-cell priming and the differentiation of armed effector T cells occurs here, and the armed effector T cells either leave the lymphoid organ to effect cell-mediated immunity in sites of infection in the tissues, or remain in the lymphoid organ to participate in humoral immunity by activating antigen-binding B cells. Which response occurs is determined by the differentiation of CD4 T cells into T_H1 or T_H2 cells, which is in turn determined by the cytokines produced in the early non-adaptive phase. CD4 T-cell differentiation is also affected by ill-defined characteristics of the activating antigen and by its overall abundance. Ideally, the adaptive immune response eliminates the infectious agent and provides the host with a state of protective immunity against re-infection with the same pathogen.

Immunological memory.

One of the most important consequences of an adaptive immune response is the establishment of a state of immunological memory. Immunological memory is the ability of the immune system to respond more rapidly and effectively to pathogens that have been encountered previously, and reflects the pre-existence of a clonally expanded population of antigen-specific lymphocytes. Memory responses, which are called secondary, tertiary, and so on, depending on the number of exposures to antigen, also differ qualitatively from primary responses.

This is particularly clear in the case of the antibody response, where the characteristics of antibodies produced in secondary and subsequent responses are distinct from those produced in the primary response to the same antigen. How immunological memory is maintained, however, is still poorly understood. The principal focus of this section will therefore be the altered character of memory responses, although we shall also outline the mechanisms that have been suggested to explain the persistence of immunological memory after exposure to antigen.

9-24   Immunological memory is long-lived following infection.

Most children in the United States are now vaccinated against measles virus; before vaccination was widespread, most were naturally exposed to this virus and suffered from an acute, unpleasant, and potentially dangerous viral illness. Whether through vaccination or through infection, children exposed to the virus acquire long-term protection from measles. The same is true of many other acute infectious diseases: this state of protection is the consequence of immunological memory.

The basis for immunological memory has been hard to explore experimentally; although the phenomenon was first recorded by the ancient Greeks and has been exploited routinely in vaccination programs for 200 years, it is still not clearly established whether memory reflects a long-lived population of specialized memory cells or depends upon the persistence of undetectable levels of antigen that continuously re-stimulate antigen-specific lymphocytes. It can be demonstrated, however, that only individuals who were themselves previously exposed to a given infectious agent are immune, and that memory is not dependent on repeated exposure to infection as a result of contacts with other infected individuals. This was established by observations on remote island populations, where a virus such as measles can cause an epidemic, infecting all people living on the island at that time, after which the virus disappears for many years. On re-introduction from outside the island, the virus does not affect the original population but causes disease in those people born since the initial epidemic. This means that immunological memory cannot be caused by repeated exposure to infectious virus and leaves two alternative explanations.

The first is that memory is sustained by long-lived lymphocytes induced by the original exposure that persist in a resting state until a second encounter with the pathogen. The second is that the lymphocytes activated by the original exposure to antigen are re-stimulated repetitively, even in the absence of further encounters with infectious antigen. This could occur by the persistence in each individual of small amounts of the pathogen sufficient to restimulate the activated cells but not to spread the infection to others, by the existence of other, cross-reactive, antigens that would not be able to activate naive cells but which could stimulate previously activated cells, or by cytokine-mediated stimulation of bystander memory but not naive cells, in the course of an antigen-specific immune response.

The experimental measurement of immunological memory has been carried out in various ways. Adoptive transfer assays of lymphocytes from animals immunized with simple, non-living antigens have been favored for such studies, as the antigen cannot proliferate. When an animal is immunized with a protein antigen, helper T cells appear abruptly after 5 days or so, while antigen-specific B cells appear some days later, because B-cell activation cannot begin until armed helper T cells are available and B cells must then enter a phase of proliferation and selection in lymphoid tissue. By 1 month after immunization, both memory B cells and memory helper T cells can be detected at what will be their maximal levels. These levels are then maintained with little alteration for the lifetime of the animal. In these experiments, the existence of memory cells is measured purely in terms of the transfer of specific responsiveness from an immunized or 'primed' animal to an irradiated, immuno-incompetent host (see Sections 2-29 and 2-32). In succeeding sections, we shall look in more detail at the changes that occur in lymphocytes after antigen priming and discuss the mechanisms that may account for these changes.

9-25   Both clonal expansion and clonal differentiation contribute to immunological memory in B cells.

Immunological memory in B cells can be examined by isolating B cells from immunized mice and restimulating them with antigen in the presence of armed helper T cells specific for the same antigen. In this way, it is possible to show that antigen-specific memory B cells differ both quantitatively and qualitatively from naive B cells. B cells that can respond to antigen increase in frequency after priming by about 10- to 100-fold (Fig. 9.33) and produce antibody of higher average affinity than unprimed B lymphocytes; the affinity of that antibody continues to increase during the ongoing secondary and subsequent antibody responses (Fig. 9.34). The secondary antibody response is characterized in its first few days by production of small amounts of IgM antibody and large amounts of IgG antibody, with some IgA and IgE. These antibodies are produced by memory B cells that have already switched from IgM to these more mature isotypes and express IgG, IgA, or IgE on their surface, as well as a somewhat higher level of MHC class II molecules than is characteristic of naive B cells. Increased affinity for antigen and increased levels of MHC class II expression facilitate antigen uptake and presentation, and allow memory B cells to initiate their critical interactions with armed helper T cells at lower doses of antigen. Recent evidence from mice injected with antibody against nerve growth factor show a profound loss of the capacity to make IgG antibody in a secondary response. These results suggest a role for this hormone in sustaining B cell memory.

The distinction between primary and secondary antibody responses is most clearly seen in those cases where the primary response is dominated by antibodies that are closely related and show few if any somatic hypermutations. This occurs in inbred mouse strains in response to certain haptens that may by chance activate a pre-existing set of naive B cells poised to respond to such antigens. Such antibodies are encoded by the same V_H and V_L genes in all animals of the strain, suggesting that these variable regions may have been selected during evolution for recognition of determinants on pathogens that happen to cross-react with some haptens. As a result of the uniformity of these primary responses, changes in the antibody molecules produced in secondary responses to the same antigens are easy to observe. These differences include not only numerous somatic mutations in antibodies containing the dominant variable regions but also the addition of antibodies containing V_H and V_L gene segments not detected in the primary response. These are thought to derive from B cells that were activated at low frequency during the primary response (and thus were not detected) and which differentiated into memory B cells.

Fig. 9.33 The generation of secondary antibody responses from memory B cells is distinct from the generation of the primary antibody response. The primary response usually consists of antibody molecules from a relatively large number of different precursors of relatively low affinity with few somatic mutations, while the secondary response comes from far fewer, high-affinity precursors whose receptors show extensive somatic mutation and which have undergone significant clonal expansion. Thus, there is usually only a 10- to 100-fold increase in the frequency of activatable B cells after priming; however, the quality of the antibody response is altered radically, such that these precursors induce a far more intense and effective response.

	Source of B cells	
	Unimmunized donor Primary response	Immunized donor Secondary response
Frequency of specific B cells	$1:10^4 - 1:10^5$	$1:10^3$
Isotype of antibody produced	IgM > IgG	IgG, IgA
Affinity of antibody	Low	High
Somatic hypermutation	Low	High

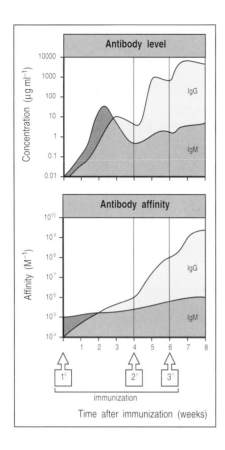

Fig. 9.34 The affinity as well as the amount of antibody increases with repeated immunization. (Note that these graphs are on a logarithmic scale). The upper panel shows the increase in the level of antibody with time after primary followed by secondary and tertiary immunization; the lower panel shows the increase in the affinity of the antibodies. The increase in affinity (affinity maturation) is seen largely in IgG antibody (as well as IgA and IgE, which are not shown), coming from mature B cells that have undergone isotype switching and somatic hypermutation to yield higher-affinity antibodies. Although some affinity maturation occurs in the primary antibody response, most arises in later responses to repeated antigen injections.

9-26   **Repeated immunizations lead to increasing affinity of antibody owing to somatic hypermutation and selection by antigen in germinal centers.**

As we saw in Section 9-21 and Figure 9.29, in a primary antibody response naive B cells stimulated by armed T_H2 cells form a primary extrafollicular focus in lymphoid tissues, where some differentiate and secrete antibody that helps to localize antigen on the surface of follicular dendritic cells (Fig. 9.35). Some B cells that have not yet undergone terminal differentiation migrate into the follicle and become germinal center B cells. Stimulated by the antigen-bearing follicular dendritic cells, these B cells enter a second proliferative phase, during which the DNA encoding their immunoglobulin variable domains undergoes somatic hypermutation before the B cells differentiate into antibody-secreting plasma cells (see Section 8-6).

The antibodies produced by plasma cells in the primary response play an important part in driving the secondary response. In secondary and subsequent immune responses, any persisting antibodies produced by the B cells that differentiated in the primary response are immediately available to bind to the newly introduced antigen. Some of these antibodies divert antigen to phagocytes for degradation and disposal; however, some seem to be trapped by special antigen-transporting cells in the marginal zones of the spleen and the marginal sinus of lymph nodes. These cells bind antigen:antibody complexes and, instead of ingesting

Fig. 9.35 B cells recognize antigen as immune complexes bound to the surface of follicular dendritic cells. Radiolabeled antigen localizes to, and persists in, lymphoid follicles of draining lymph nodes (see light micrograph and schematic representation, showing a germinal center in a lymph node). Radio-labeled antigen has been injected 3 days previously and its localization in the germinal center is shown by the intense dark staining. The antigen is in the form of antigen:antibody:complement complexes bound to Fc and complement receptors on the surface of the follicular dendritic cell (FDC). These complexes are not internalized, as depicted schematically for antigen:antibody complexes bound to the Fc receptor in the right panel and insert. Antigen can persist in this form for long periods. Photograph courtesy of J Tew.

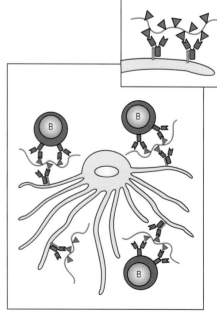

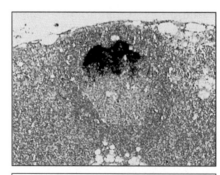

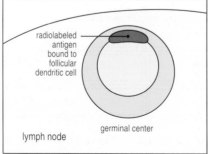

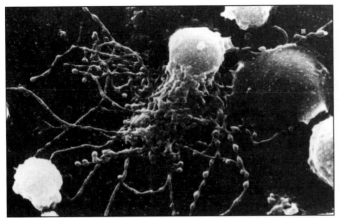
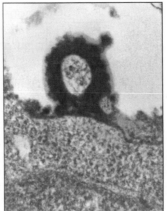
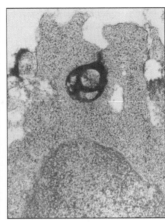

Fig. 9.36 Immune complexes bound to follicular dendritic cells form iccosomes, which are released and can be taken up by B cells in the germinal center. Follicular dendritic cells have a prominent cell body and many dendritic processes. Immune complexes, bound to Fc receptors on the follicular dendritic cell surface, become clustered, forming prominent 'beads' along the dendrites (left panel). An intermediate form of FDC is shown with both straight filiform dendrites and those that are becoming beaded. These beads are shed from the cell as iccosomes (immune complex coated bodies) and can bind (center panel) and be taken up by B cells in the germinal center (right panel). In the center and right panels, the iccosome has been formed with immune complexes containing horseradish peroxidase, which is electron-dense and thus appears dark in the transmission electron micrographs. Photographs courtesy of A K Szakal.

them, transport them to the lymphoid follicles, where the complexes are subsequently found on the surface of follicular dendritic cells. It is possible that the antigen-transporting cells in the spleen are B cells. In the lymph nodes, the transporter cells are resistant to ionizing radiation and their nature is obscure.

The follicular dendritic cells package the antigen into bundles of membrane coated with antigen:antibody complexes that bud off the follicular dendritic cell surface; these structures are called **iccosomes** (Fig. 9.36). It is believed that B cells whose receptors bind the antigen with sufficient avidity to compete with the existing antibody take up these iccosomes, process the antigen into peptide fragments, and present them to armed helper T cells surrounding and infiltrating the germinal centers (see Section 8-8). Contact between B cells presenting antigen fragments and armed helper T cells specific for the same peptides leads to an exchange of activating signals and rapid proliferation of both activated antigen-specific B cells and helper T cells. This process depends on bi-directional signaling through CD40L on the activated T cell, and CD40 on the B cell, and on the induction of other co-stimulatory molecules. In this way, the affinity of the antibody produced rises progressively, as only B cells with high-affinity antigen receptors can bind antigen efficiently and be driven to proliferate by antigen-specific helper T cells (Fig. 9.37).

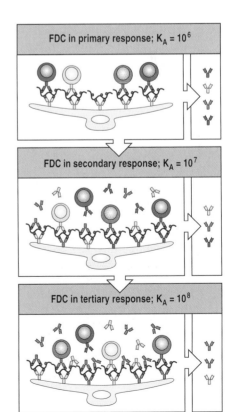

Fig. 9.37 The mechanism of affinity maturation in an antibody response. High concentrations of antigen in the presence of small amounts of antibody can interact with B cells of a wide variety of affinities, most of which will bind antigen with low affinity. In a primary response, those B cells with receptors of the highest affinity (K_A) are most efficient at extracting antigen from follicular dendritic cells (FDCs) in germinal centers, and these are then selected to survive by interaction with helper T cells, even if the high-affinity B cells are actually quite infrequent. On re-introduction of antigen, antibody produced in the primary response competes with B-cell receptors for binding, and in the secondary response, only B cells with receptors of high enough affinity to compete with existing antibodies can bind antigen and contribute to the response. In the tertiary response, the same mechanism selects for B-cell receptors with still higher affinity.

9-27   **Memory T cells are increased in frequency and have distinct activation requirements and cell-surface proteins that distinguish them from armed effector T cells.**

Since the T-cell receptor does not undergo isotype switching or affinity maturation, memory T cells have been more difficult to characterize than memory B cells. The number of T cells reactive to an antigen increases markedly after immunization, persisting at a level significantly (10- to 100-fold) above the initial frequency for the rest of the animal's or person's life. These cells carry cell-surface proteins more characteristic of armed effector cells than of naive T cells. However, it is not easy to establish whether these cells really are long-lived armed effector T cells, or whether they are cells with distinct properties that should be specifically designated memory T cells. This issue does not arise with B cells because effector B cells, as we saw in Chapter 8, are terminally differentiated plasma cells, which die between 3 days and 6 weeks after antigen exposure.

A major problem in experiments aimed at establishing the existence of memory T cells is that most assays for T-cell effector function take several days, during which the putative memory T cells are re-induced to armed effector cell status, so that the assays do not distinguish pre-existing effector cells from memory T cells. This problem does not apply in the case of cytotoxic T cells, however, which can program a target cell for lysis in 5 minutes. Experiments with memory CD8 T cells from primed animals show that exposure to antigen in a form that cannot activate naive CD8 T cells readily generates armed effector CD8 T cells, but only after 1–2 days of culture. Such studies can be carried out in the presence of mitotic inhibitors, proving that cell division is not required. Thus, it is clear that in the case of CD8 T cells, long-term protective immunity need not be mediated by long-lived effector T cells (which, in the above experiment, would be activated immediately), and that a distinct population of memory CD8 T cells can be defined.

The issue is more difficult to address for CD4 T-cell responses, and the identification of memory CD4 T cells rests largely on the existence of a population of cells with the surface characteristics of activated armed effector T cells (Fig. 9.38) but distinct from them in that they require additional restimulation before acting on target cells. Changes in three cell-surface proteins—L-selectin, CD44, and CD45—are particularly significant after exposure to antigen. L-selectin is lost on most memory T cells, while CD44 levels increase on all memory T cells after priming, and the isoform of CD45 changes because of alternative splicing of exons that encode the extracellular domain of CD45 (Fig. 9.39), leading to isoforms that bind to the T-cell receptor and facilitate antigen recognition. These changes are characteristic of cells that have been activated to become armed effector T cells, yet some of the cells on which these changes have occurred have many characteristics of resting CD4 T cells, suggesting that they represent memory CD4 T cells. Only after re-exposure to antigen on a professional antigen-presenting cell do they achieve armed effector T-cell status, and acquire all the characteristics of armed T_H2 or T_H1 cells, secreting IL-4 and IL-5, or IFN-γ and TNF-β, respectively.

It thus seems reasonable to designate these cells as memory CD4 T cells. These observations together suggest that naive CD4 T cells can differentiate into armed effector T cells or into memory T cells; whether armed effector T cells can persist *in vivo*, and whether they can differentiate into memory T cells, is not yet clear.

Molecule	Other names	Relative expression on cells of indicated subset		Comments
		Naive	Memory	
LFA-3	CD58	1	>8	Ligand for CD2, involved in adhesion and signaling
CD2	T11	1	3	Mediates T-cell adhesion and activation
LFA-1	CD11a/CD18	1	3	Mediates leukocyte adhesion and signaling
α₄ integrin	VLA4	1	4	Involved in T-cell homing to tissues
CD44	Ly24 Pgp-1	1	2	Lymphocyte homing to tissues
CD45RO		1	30	Lowest molecular weight isoform of CD45
CD45RA		10	1	High molecular weight isoform of CD45
L-selectin		High	Most high, some low	Lymph node homing receptor
CD3		1.0	1.0	Part of antigen-specific receptor complex

Fig. 9.38 Many cell-surface molecules alter their expression on memory T cells. This is seen most clearly with CD45, where there is a change in the isoforms expressed (see Fig. 9.39). Many of these changes are also seen on cells that have been activated to become armed effector T cells. The changes increase the adhesion of the T cell to antigen-presenting cells and to endothelial cells. They also increase the sensitivity of the memory T cell to antigen stimulation.

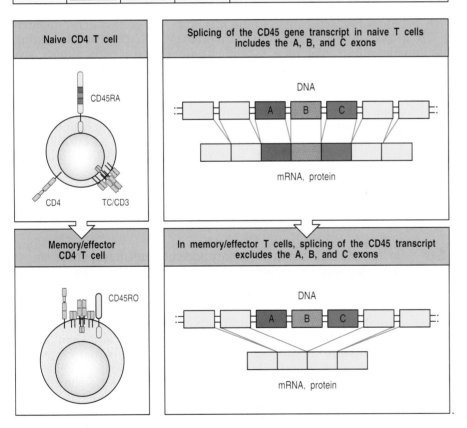

Naive CD4 T cell

CD45RA

CD4 TC/CD3

Memory/effector CD4 T cell

CD45RO

Splicing of the CD45 gene transcript in naive T cells includes the A, B, and C exons

DNA

A B C

mRNA, protein

In memory/effector T cells, splicing of the CD45 transcript excludes the A, B, and C exons

DNA

A B C

mRNA, protein

Fig. 9.39 Memory CD4 T cells express altered CD45 isoforms that regulate the interaction of the T-cell receptor with its co-receptors. CD45 is a transmembrane tyrosine phosphatase with three variable exons (A,B, and C) that encode part of its external domain. In naive T cells, high molecular weight isoforms (CD45RA) are found that do not associate with either the T-cell receptor or co-receptors. In memory T cells, the variable exons are removed by alternative splicing of CD45 RNA, and this isoform, known as CD45RO, associates with both the T-cell receptor and the co-receptor. This assembled receptor appears to transduce signals more effectively than the receptor on naive T cells.

9-28 Retained antigen may play a role in immunological memory.

A successful adaptive immune response clears antigen from the body, halting further activation of naive lymphocytes. Antibody levels gradually decline, and effector T cells can no longer be detected. Residual

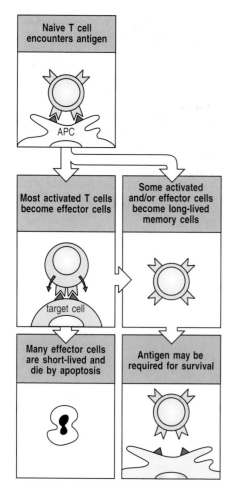

Fig. 9.40 Encounter with antigen generates effector T cells and long-lived memory T cells. Most of the effector T cells that are derived from antigen-stimulated naive T cells are relatively short lived, dying either from antigen overload or the absence of antigenic stimulus. Some may become long-lived memory T cells, which may also differentiate directly from armed effector T cells; antigenic stimulation may be required for these cells to persist. APC, antigen presenting cell.

antigen is difficult to detect, either in the form of surviving infectious agents or as antigens derived from them. Nevertheless, some antigen is probably retained for long periods as immune complexes bound to follicular dendritic cells in lymphoid follicles (see Fig. 9.35). Some intact virions may persist in this site as well, and a few infected cells may escape immune elimination. It has been proposed that this residual antigen is crucial for sustaining the cells that mediate immunological memory.

The long-lived cells that mediate immunological memory may be derived from activated naive T cells that differentiate directly into memory T cells, or they may first differentiate into effector T cells, which then either become long-lived memory T cells or are short-lived and undergo apoptosis (Fig. 9.40). Antigen plays a critical role in determining the fate of the activated T cells, in a fashion reminiscent of positive selection in the thymus (see Chapter 6). Thus, high doses of antigen can trigger apoptosis of the effector T cells, in much the same way as happens in clonal deletion; however, the absence of antigen can also lead to their apoptosis, just as developing T cells die if they are not positively selected. Memory T cells persist either because antigen has programmed them for a longer life-span or because a low level of residual antigen preserves them by repetitive sub threshold signaling.

Attempts to clarify the role of antigen in the persistence of immunological memory are fraught with difficulty. Transferring primed lymphocytes to irradiated recipient mice does not produce clear evidence of long-term immunological memory, while administering antigen along with the cells prolongs responsiveness to the priming antigen. However, the antigen treatment also increases the number of specific cells by stimulating their proliferation, making it difficult to determine whether there are simply more precursors in the mice that received antigen, or whether the life-span of individual cells is also increased. Although it is hard to determine whether antigen is absolutely required for the persistence of immunological memory, persistent antigen can clearly help to maintain a population of lymphocytes able to respond rapidly to the priming antigen. Thus, antigen retention in specialized sites, such as on follicular dendritic cells (see Section 9-21), where antigen persists for months or years, may be very important in immunological memory.

9-29   In immune individuals, secondary and subsequent responses are mediated solely by memory lymphocytes and not by naive lymphocytes.

In the normal course of an infection, a pathogen first proliferates to a level sufficient to elicit an adaptive immune response and then stimulates the production of antibodies and effector T cells that eliminate the pathogen from the body. Most of the armed effector T cells subsequently die and antibody levels gradually decline after the pathogen is eliminated, because the antigens that elicited the response are no longer present at the level needed to sustain it; we can think of this as feedback inhibition of the response. However, memory T and B cells remain and maintain a heightened ability to mount a response to a recurrence of the infection.

The antibody and effector T cells remaining in an individual that has already been immunized also prevent the activation of naive B and T cells by the same antigen. Such a response would be wasteful given the presence of memory cells that can respond much more quickly. The

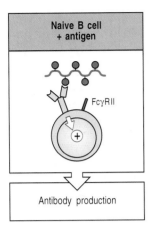 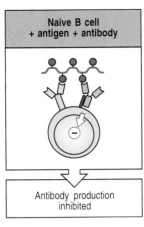 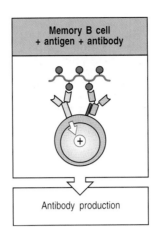

Fig. 9.41 Antibody can suppress naive B-cell activation by crosslinking the specific antigen receptor on B cells to the B-cell specific Fcγ receptor IIb (FcγRIIb). Antigen binding to the B-cell antigen receptor delivers an activating signal (left panel), while simultaneous signaling via the antigen receptor and FcγRIIb delivers a negative signal to naive B cells (center panel). Such crosslinking does not appear to affect memory B cells (right panel). This mechanism may play a role in suppressing naive B-cell responses in already primed individuals.

suppression of naive lymphocyte activation can be shown by passively transferring antibody or effector T cells to naive recipients; when the recipient is then immunized, naive lymphocytes do not respond to the original antigen while responses to other antigens are unaffected. This has been put to practical use to prevent the response of Rh⁻ mothers to their Rh⁺ children (see Section 2-9); if anti-Rh antibody is given to the mother before she reacts to her child's red blood cells, her response will be inhibited. The mechanism of this suppression is known to involve the crosslinking of the antigen receptor on B cells to the isoform of FcγRII on the B-cell surface (FcγRIIb), which inhibits the activation of naive B cells (Fig. 9.41). FcγRIIb is expressed only by B cells and has an insertion in its intracellular domain that inhibits phagocytosis; this inactivates signaling via the B-cell antigen receptor when both structures are bound by the same ligand. For some reason, memory B-cell responses are not inhibited by antibody to the antigen, so the Rh⁻ mothers at risk must be identified and treated before a response has occurred. The fact that memory B cells can be activated to produce antibody even when exposed to pre-existing antibody allows secondary antibody responses to occur in individuals who are already immune.

Adoptive transfer of immune T cells to naive syngeneic mice also prevents the activation of naive T cells by antigen. This has been shown most clearly for cytotoxic T cells. It is possible that these memory CD8 T cells are activated to regain cytotoxic activity sufficiently rapidly that they can kill the antigen-presenting cells that are required to activate naive CD8 T cells, thereby inhibiting their activation.

These mechanisms may also explain the phenomenon known as **original antigenic sin**. This term was coined to describe the tendency of people to make antibodies only to epitopes expressed on the first influenza virus variant to which they were exposed, even in subsequent infections with variants that bear additional, highly immunogenic epitopes (Fig. 9.42). Antibodies to the original virus will tend to suppress responses of naive B cells specific for the new epitopes by crosslinking their antigen receptors to FcγRIIb. This may benefit the host by using only those B cells that can respond most rapidly and effectively to the virus. This pattern is broken only if the person is exposed to an influenza virus that lacks all epitopes seen in the original infection, since now no pre-existing antibodies bind the virus and naive B cells are able to respond.

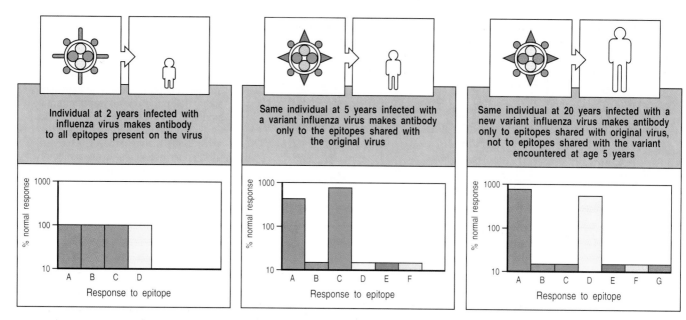

Fig. 9.42 Individuals who have already been infected with one variant of influenza virus make antibodies only to epitopes that were present on the initial virus variant when infected with a second variant. A child infected for the first time with an influenza virus makes a response to all epitopes (left panel). At age 5 years, the same child exposed to a variant virus responds preferentially to those epitopes shared with the original virus, and makes a less than normal response to new epitopes on the virus (middle panel). Even at age 20 years, this commitment to respond to epitopes shared with the original virus, and the subnormal response to new epitopes, is retained (right panel). This phenomenon is called 'original antigenic sin'.

Summary.

Protective immunity against re-infection is one of the most important consequences of adaptive immunity operating through clonal selection of lymphocytes. Protective immunity depends not only on pre-formed antibody and armed effector T cells, but also on immunological memory, an increased responsiveness to previously encountered pathogens that is long-lived, and upon the establishment of a new population of memory lymphocytes. The capacity of these cells to respond rapidly to antigen can be transferred to naive recipients with primed B and T cells. The precise changes that distinguish naive, effector, and memory lymphocytes are not well characterized, and in the case of T cells, the relative contributions of clonal expansion and differentiation to the memory phenotype are not yet clear. Memory B cells, however, can be distinguished by changes in their immunoglobulin genes because of isotype switching and somatic hypermutation, and secondary and subsequent immune responses are characterized by antibodies of increasing affinity for antigen. It seems likely that residual antigen or infection is important in sustaining memory lymphocytes, although it may not be essential.

Summary to Chapter 9.

Vertebrates resist infection by pathogenic microorganisms in several ways. First, innate defenses against infection exclude infectious agents or kill them on first contact. For those pathogens that establish an infection, several early, non-adaptive responses are crucial to control infections and hold them in check until an adaptive immune response can be generated. Adaptive immunity takes several days to develop, as T and B lymphocytes must encounter their specific antigen, proliferate, and differentiate into effector cells. T-cell dependent B-cell responses cannot be initiated until antigen-specific T cells have had a chance to proliferate and differentiate. The same final effector mechanisms are used in all three phases of immunity, only the recognition mechanism changes (Fig. 9.43). Once an adaptive immune response has occurred, the infection is usually controlled and the pathogen contained or eliminated, and a state of protective immunity ensues. This state consists of the presence of effector cells and molecules produced in the initial response, and immunological memory. Immunological memory is manifest as a heightened ability to respond to pathogens that have been encountered previously and successfully eliminated. It is a property of memory T and B lymphocytes, which can transfer memory to naive recipients. However, the precise mechanism of immunological memory, which is a crucial feature of adaptive immunity, remains obscure. The artificial induction of protective immunity including immunological memory by vaccines is the most outstanding accomplishment of immunology in the field of medicine. Understanding how this is accomplished still lags behind its practical success.

Phases of the immune response		
Immediate (0–4 hours)	**Early (4–96 hours)**	**Late (after 96 hours)**
Non-specific Innate No memory No specific T cells	Non-specific + specific Inducible No memory No specific T cells	Specific Inducible Memory Specific T cells

	Immediate (0–4 hours)	Early (4–96 hours)	Late (after 96 hours)
Barrier functions	Skin, epithelia	Local inflammation (C5a) Local TNF-α	IgA antibody in luminal spaces IgE antibody on mast cells
Response to extracellular pathogens	Phagocytes Alternative complement pathway	Mannan-binding lectin C-reactive protein T-cell independent B-cell antibody plus complement	IgG antibody and Fc receptor-bearing cells IgG, IgM antibody + classical complement pathway
Response to intracellular bacteria	Macrophages	Activated NK-dependent macrophage activation IL-1, IL-6, TNF-α, IL-12	T-cell activation of macrophages by IFN-γ
Response to virus-infected cells	Natural killer (NK) cells	Interferon-α and -β IL-12-activated NK cells	Cytotoxic T cells IFN-γ

Fig. 9.43 The components of the three phases of the immune response involved in defense against different classes of microorganisms. There are striking similarities in the effector mechanisms at each phase of the response; the main change is in the recognition structures used.

General references.

Fearon, D.T., and Locksley, R.M.: **The instinctive role of innate immunity in the acquired immune response**. *Science* 1996, **272**:50-53.

Gallin, J.I., Goldstein, I.M., and Snyderman, R. (eds): *Inflammation—Basic Principles and Clinical Correlates*, 2nd edn. New York, Raven Press, 1992.

Gorbach, S.L., Bartlett, J.G., and Blacklow, N.R. (eds): In: *Infectious Diseases*, 1st edn. Philadelphia, W.B. Saunders, 1992.

Picker, L.J. and Butcher, E.C.: **Physiological and molecular mechanisms of lymphocyte homing**. *Ann. Rev. Immunol.* 1993, **10**:561-591.

Salyers, A.A., and Whitt, D.D.: **Bacterial pathogenesis, A molecular approach**. ASM Press, Washington, DC, 1994.

Section references.

9-1 & 9-2 The infectious process can be divided into several distinct phases.

Infectious diseases are caused by diverse living agents that replicate in their hosts.

Gibbons, R.J.: **How microorganisms cause disease**. In: Gorbach, S.L., Bartlett, J.G., and Blacklow, N.R. (eds): *Infectious Diseases*, 1st edn. 1992, 7-106.

9-3 Surface epithelia make up a natural barrier to infection.

Boman, H.G.: **Peptide antibiotics: holy or heretic grails of innate immunity?** *Scand. J. Immunol*.1996, **43**:475-482.

Isberg, R.R.: **Discrimination between intracellular uptake and surface adhesion of bacterial pathogens.** *Science* 1991, **252**:934-938.

Lehrer, R.I., Lichtenstein, A.K., Ganz, T.: **Defensins: antimicrobial and cytotoxic peptides of mammalian cells.** *Ann. Rev. Immunol.* 1993, **11**:105-128.

| 9-4 | The alternative pathway of complement activation provides a non-adaptive first line of defense against many microorganisms. |

Liszewski, M.K., Post, T.W., and Atkinson, J.P.: **Membrane co-factor protein (MCP or CD46): newest member of the regulators of complement activation gene cluster.** *Ann. Rev. Immunol.* 1993, **9**:431-455.

Pangburn, M.K.: **The alternative pathway.** In: Ross, G.D. (ed.): *Immunobiology of the Complement System.* Orlando, Academic Press, 1986, pp. 45-62.

| 9-5 | Phagocytes provide innate cellular immunity in tissues and initiate host-defense responses. |

Ezekowitz, R.A.B., Williams, D.J., Koziel, H., Armstrong, M.Y.K., Warner, A., Richards, F.F., and Rose, R.M.: **Uptake of *Pneumocystis carinii* mediated by the macrophage mannose receptor.** *Nature* 1991, **351**:155-158.

Hauschildt, S., Kleine, B.: **Bacterial stimulators of macrophages.** *Intl. Rev. Cytology.* 1995, **161**:263

Ulevitch, R.J., and Tobias, P.S.: **Receptor-dependent mechanism of cell stimulation by bacterial endotoxin.** *Ann. Rev. Immunol.* 1995, **13**:437-457.

| 9-6 | The innate immune response produces inflammatory mediators that recruit new phagocytic cells to local sites of infection. |

Bevilacqua, M.P.: **Endothelial leukocyte adhesion molecules.** *Ann. Rev. Immunol.* 1993, **11**:767-804.

Downey, G.P.: **Mechanisms of leukocyte motility and chemotaxis.** *Curr. Opin. Immunol.* 1994, **6**:113–124.

Springer, T.A.: **Traffic signals for lymphocyte recirculation and leukocyte emigration: the multi-step paradigm.** *Cell* 1994, **76**:301-304.

| 9-7 | The migration of leukocytes out of blood vessels depends on adhesive interactions activated by the local release of inflammatory mediators. |

Ebnet, K., Kaldjian, E.P., Anderson, A.O., Shaw, S.: **Orchestrated information transfer underlying leukocyte endothelial interactions.** *Ann. Rev. Immunol,* 1996, **14**:155-177.

| 9-8 | TNF-α induces blood vessel occlusion and plays an important role in containing local infection but can be fatal when released systemically |

Pfieffer, K., Matsuyama, T., Kundig, T.M., Wakeham, A., Kishihara, K., Shahinian, A., Wiegmann, K., Ohashi, P.S., Kromke, M., and Mak, T.W.: **Mice deficient for the 55kd tumor necrosis factor receptor are resistant to endotoxic shock, yet succumb to *L. monocytogenes* infection.** *Cell* 1993, **73**:457-467.

| 9-9 | Small proteins called chemokines recruit new phagocytic cells to local sites of infection. |

Gerard, C., and Gerard, N.P: **The pro-inflammatory seven transmembrane spanning receptors of the leukocyte.** *Curr. Opin. Immunol.* 1994, **6**:140.

Miller, M.D. and Krangel, M.S.: **Biology and biochemistry of the chemokines: a family of chemotactic and inflammatory cytokines.** *CRC Crit. Rev. Immunol.* 1992, **12**:30.

Murphy, P.M.: **The molecular biology of leukocyte chemoattractant receptors.** *Ann. Rev. Immunol.* 1994 **12**:593-633.

| 9-10 | Neutrophils predominate in the early cellular infiltrate into inflammatory sites. |

Rosales, C., and Brown, E.J.: **Neutrophil receptors and modulation of the immune response.** In: Abramson, J.S., and Wheeler, J.G. (eds): *The Natural Immune System,* New York, IRL Press, 1993, pp. 24-62.

| 9-11 | Cytokines released by phagocytes also activate the acute phase response. |

Emsley, J., White, H.E., O'Hara, B.P., Oliva, G., Srinivasan, N., Tickle. I.J., Blundell, T.L., Pepys, M.B., and Wood, S.P.: **Structure of pentameric human serum amyloid P component.** *Nature* 1994, **367**:338.

Sastry, K. and Ezekowitz, R.A.: **Collectins: pattern-recognition molecules involved in first-line host defense.** *Curr. Opin. Immunol.* 1993, **5**:59-66.

Weiss, W.I., Drickamer, K., Hendrickson, W.A.: **Structure of a C-type mannose-binding protein complexed with an oligosaccharide.** *Nature* 1992, **360**:127-134.

| 9-12 | Interferons inhibit viral replication and activate certain host-defense responses. |

Biron, C.A.: **Cytokines in the generation of immune responses to, and resolution of, virus infection.** *Curr. Opin. Immunol.* 1994, **6**:530-538.

Sen, G.C., and Lengyel, P.: **The interferon system. A bird's eye view of its biochemistry.** *J. Biol. Chem.* 1992, **267**:5017-5020.

| 9-13 | Natural killer cells serve as an early defense against certain intracellular infections. |

Gumperez, J.E., Parham, P.: **The enigma of the natural killer cell.** *Nature* 1995, **378**:245-298.

Karlhofer, F.M., Ribaudo, R.K., and Yokoyama, W.M.: **MHC class I alloantigen specificity of Ly-49$^+$ IL-2 activated natural killer cells.** *Nature.* 1992, **358**:66-70.

Moretta, A., Bottino, C., Vitale, M., Pende, D., Biassoni, R., Mingari, M.C., Moretta, L.: **Receptors for HLA class-1 molecules in human natural killer cells.** *Ann. Rev. Immunol.* 1996, **14**:619-648.

| 9-14 | T cells bearing $\gamma{:}\delta$ T-cell receptors are found in most epithelia and may contribute to host defense at the body surface. |

Davis, M.M., and Chien, Y-H.: **Issues concerning the nature of antigen recognition by $\alpha\beta$ and $\gamma\delta$ T cell receptors.** *Immunol. Today.* 1995, **16**:316-318.

Haas, W., Pereira, P., and Tonegawa, S.: **$\gamma{:}\delta$ cells.** *Ann. Rev. Immunol.* 1993, **11**:637-685.

Raulet, D.H.: **The structure, function, and molecular genetics of the $\gamma{:}\delta$ T-cell receptor.** *Ann. Rev. Immunol.* 1993, **7**:175-207.

| 9-15 | B-1 B cells form a separate population of B cells, producing antibodies to common bacterial polysaccharides. |

Kantor, A.B. and Herzenberg, L.A.: **Origin of murine B-cell lineages.** *Ann. Rev. Immunol.* 1993, **11**:501-538.

9-16 T-cell activation is initiated when recirculating T cells encounter specific antigen in draining lymphoid tissues.

Finger, E.B., Purl, K.D., Alon, R., Lawrence, M.B., von Andrian, U.H., Springer, T.A.: **Adhesion through L-selectin requires a threshold hydrodynamic shear.** *Nature* 1996, **379**:266-269.

Roake, J.A., Rao, A.S., Morris, P.J., Larson, C.P., Hankins, D.F., Austyn, J.M.: **Dendritic cell loss from nonlymphoid tissues after systemic administration of lipopolysaccharide, tumor necrosis factor, and interleukin-1.** *J. Exp. Med.* 1995, **181**:2237-2247.

Tanaka, Y., Adams, D.H., Hubscher, S., Hirano, H., Siebenlist, U., and Shaw, S.: **T cell adhesion induced by proteoglycan-immobilized cytokine MIP-1β.** *Nature* 1993, **361**:79-82.

9-17 Cytokines made in the early phases of an infection influence the functional differentiation of CD4 T cells.

Bendelac, A., Lantz, O., Quimby, M.E., Yewdell, J.W., Bennick, J.R., and Brutkiewicz, R.R.: **CD1 recognition by mouse NK1.1+ T lymphocytes.** *Science* 1995, **268**:863-865.

Hsieh, C.-S., Macatonia, S.E., Tripp, C.S., Wolf, S.F., O'Garra, A., and Murphy, K.M.: **Development of TH1 CD4+ T cells through IL-12 produced by** *Listeria*-**induced macrophages.** *Science* 1993, **260**:547-549.

Paul, W.E., Seder, R.A.: **Lymphocyte responses and cytokines.** *Cell* 1994, **76**:241-251.

Scott, P.: **Selective differentiation of CD4+ T-helper cell subsets.** *Curr. Opin. Immunol.* 1993, **5**:391-397.

Sher, A. and Coffman, R.L.: **Regulation of immunity to parasites by T cells and T cell-derived cytokines.** *Ann. Rev. Immunol.* 1992, **10**:385-409.

Yoshimoto, T., Bendelac, A., Watson, C., Hu-Li, J., Paul, W.E.: **Role of NK1.1+ T cells in a TH2 response and in immunoglobulin E production.** *Science* 1995, **270**:1845-1848.

9-18 Distinct subsets of T cells can regulate the growth and effector functions of other T cell subsets.

Croft, M., Carter, L., Swain, S.L., Dutton, R.W.: **Generation of polarized antigen-specific CD8 effector populations: reciprocal action of interleukin-4 and IL-12 in promoting type 2 versus type 1 cytokine profiles.** *J. Exp. Med.* 180:1715-1728.

Seder. R.A., and Paul, W.E.: **Acquistion of lymphokine producing phenotype by CD4+ T cells.** *Ann. Rev. Immunol.* 1994, **12**:635-673.

9-19 The nature and amount of antigenic peptide can also affect the differentiation of CD4 T cells.

Constant, S., Pfeiffer, C., Woodard, A., Pasqualini, T., and Bottomly, K.: **Extent of T cell receptor ligation can determine the functional differentiation of naive CD4 T cells.** *J. Exp. Med.* 1995, **182**:1591-1596.

Pfeiffer, C., Stein, J., Southwood, S., Ketelaar, H., Sette, A., and Bottomly, K.: **Altered peptide ligands can control CD4 T lymphocyte differentiation** *in vivo.* *J.Exp. Med.* 1995, **181**:1569-1574.

Wang, L-F., Lin J-Y., Hsieh, K-H., Lin, R-H.: **Epicutaneous exposure of protein antigen induces a predominant TH2-like response with high IgE production in mice.** *J. Immunol.* 1996, **156**:4079-4082.

9-20 Armed effector T cells are guided to sites of infection by newly expressed surface molecules.

Baron, J.L., Madri, J.A., Ruddle, N.H., Hashim, G., and Janeway, C.A. Jr: **Surface expression of α4 integrin by CD4 T cells is required for their entry into brain parenchyma.** *J. Exp. Med.* 1993, **177**:57-68.

MacKay, C.R., Marston, W., and Dudler, L.: **Altered patterns of T-cell migration through lymph nodes and skin following antigen challenge.** *Eur. J. Immunol.* 1992, **22**:2205-2210.

9-21 Antibody responses develop in lymphoid tissues under the direction of armed TH2 cells.

Jacob, J. and Kelsoe, G.: *In situ* **studies of the primary immune response to (4-hydroxy-3-nitrophenyl)acetyl II. A common clonal origin for periarteriolar lymphoid sheath-associated foci and germinal centers.** *J. Exp. Med.* 1992, **176**:679-687.

Kelsoe, G.: **Life and death in germinal centres (Redux).** *Immunity* 1996, **4**:107-111.

Liu, Y.J., Johnson, G.D., Gordon, J., and MacLennan, I.C.M.: **Germinal centres in T cell-dependent antibody responses.** *Immunol. Today* 1992, **13**:17-21.

MacLennan, I.C.M.: **Germinal centres.** *Ann. Rev. Immunol.* 1994, **12**:117-139.

9-22 Antibody responses are sustained in medullary cords and bone marrow.

Benner, R., Hijmans, W., and Haaijman, J.J.: **The bone marrow: the major source of serum immunoglobulins, but still a neglected site of antibody formation.** *Clin. Exp. Immunol.* 1981, **46**:1-8.

MacLennan, I.C.M. and Gray, D.: **Antigen-driven selection of virgin and memory B cells.** *Immunol. Rev.* 1986, **91**:61.

9-23 The effector mechanisms used to clear an infection depend on the infectious agent.

Mims, C.A.: *The pathogenesis of infectious disease.* 3rd edn. London. Academic Press, 1987.

9-24 Immunological memory is long-lived following infection.

Black, F.L. and Rosen, L.: **Patterns of measles antibodies in residents of Tahiti and their stability in the absence of re-exposure.** *J. Immunol.* 1962, **88**:725-731.

Sprent, J.: **T and B memory cells.** *Cell* 1994, **76**:315-322.

Zinkernagel, R.M., Bachmann, M.F., Kündig, T.M., Oehen, S., Pirchet, H., Hengartner, H.: **On immunological memory.** *Ann. Rev. Immunol.* 1996, **14**:333-367.

9-25 Both clonal expansion and clonal differentiation contribute to immunological memory in B cells.

Lane, P.: **Development of B-cell memory and effector function.** *Curr. Opin. Immunol.* 1996, **8**:331-335.

Linton, P.J., Lai, L., Lo, D., Thorbecke, G.R., and Klinman, N.R.: **Among naive precursor cell subpopulations only progenitors of memory B cells originate germinal centers.** *Eur. J. Immunol.* 1992, **22**:1293-1297.

Shittek, B. and Rajewsky, K.: **Natural occurrence and origin of somatically mutated memory in mice.** *J. Exper. Med.* 1992, **176**:427.

Torcia, M., Bracci-Laudiero, L., Lucibello, M., Nencioni, L., Labardi, D., Rubartelli, A., Cozzolino, F., Aloe, L., and Garaci, E.: **Nerve growth factor is an autocrine survival factor for memory B lymphocytes.** *Cell* 1996, **85**:345-356.

9-26 Repeated immunizations lead to increasing affinity of antibody owing to somatic hypermutation and selection by antigen in germinal centers.

Szakal, A.K. Gieringer, R.L., Kosco, M.H., Tew, J.G.: **Isolated follicular dendritic cells: cytochemical antigen localization, Nomarski, SEM and TEM morphology.** *J. Immunol.* 1985. **134**:1349-1359.

Szakal, A.K., Kosco, M.H., Tew, J.G.: **Microanatomy of lymphoid tissue during humoral immune responses: structure function relationships**. *Ann. Rev. Immunol.* 1989. **7**:91-109.

9-27 Memory T cells are increased in frequency and have distinct activation requirements and cell-surface proteins that distinguish them from armed effector T cells.

Beverley, P.: **Immunological memory in T cells**. *Curr. Opin. Immunol.* 1991, **3**:355-360.

MacKay, C.R.: **Immunological memory**. *Adv. Immunol.* 1993, **53**:217-265.

Michie, C.A., McLean, A., Alcock, C., Beverly, P.C.L.: **Lifespan of human lymphocyte subsets defined by CD45 isoforms**. *Nature* 1992, **360**:264-265.

Novak. T.J., Farber, D., Leitenberg, D., Hong, S., Johnson, P., and Bottomly, K.: **Isoforms of the transmembrane tyrosine phosphatase CD45 differentially affect T-cell recognition**. *Immunity* 1994,**1**:81-92.

9-28 Retained antigen may play a role in immunological memory.

Gray, D.: **The dynamics of immunological memory**. *Semin. Immunol.* 1992, **4**:29-34.

Sprent, J.: **Lifespan of naive, memory and effector lymphocytes**. *Curr. Opin. Immunol.* 1993, **5**:433-438.

9-29 In immune individuals, secondary and subsequent responses are mediated solely by memory lymphocytes and not by naive lymphocytes.

Fazekas de St Groth, B., and Webster, R.G.: **Disquisitions on original antigenic sin. I. Evidence in man**. *J. Exp. Med.* 1966, **140**:2893-2898.

Fridman, W.H.: **Regulation of B cell activation and antigen presentation by Fc receptors**. *Curr. Opin. Immunol.* 1993, **5**:355-360.

Pollack, W. *et al.*: **Results of clinical trials of RhoGAm in women**. *Transfusion* 1968, **8**:151.

Failures of Host Defense Mechanisms

10

In the normal course of an infection, disease is followed by an adaptive immune response that clears the infection and establishes a state of protective immunity. This does not always happen, however, and in this chapter we will examine three circumstances in which there are failures of host defense against infection: avoidance or subversion of a normal immune response by the pathogen; inherited failures of defense because of gene defects; and the acquired immune deficiency syndrome (AIDS), a generalized susceptibility to infection which is itself due to the failure of the host to control and eliminate the human immunodeficiency virus (HIV).

The propagation of a pathogen depends upon its ability to replicate in a host and to spread to new hosts. Common pathogens must therefore grow without activating too vigorous an immune response, and conversely, must not kill the host too quickly. The most successful pathogens persist either because they do not elicit an immune response, or by evading the response once it has occurred. Over millions of years of co-evolution with their hosts, pathogens have developed various strategies for avoiding destruction by the immune system, and we have encountered some of them in earlier chapters. In the first part of this chapter, we shall examine these in more detail, and discuss some that have not yet been mentioned.

In the second part of the chapter, we turn to the **immunodeficiency diseases**, in which host defense fails. In most of these diseases, a defective gene eliminates one or more components of the immune system, leading to heightened susceptibility to infection with specific classes of pathogen. Immunodeficiency diseases caused by defects in T- or B-lymphocyte development, phagocyte function, and components of the complement system have all been described. Finally, we shall consider how the persistent infection of immune system cells by the human immunodeficiency virus, HIV, leads to the acquired immune deficiency syndrome, AIDS.

The analysis of all these diseases has already made an important contribution to our understanding of host defense mechanisms and in the longer term may help to provide new methods for controlling or preventing infectious diseases, including AIDS.

Pathogens have evolved various means of evading or subverting normal host defenses.

Just as vertebrates have developed many different defenses against pathogens, so pathogens have evolved elaborate strategies to evade these defenses. Many pathogens use one or more of these strategies to evade the immune system and we shall see that HIV may succeed in defeating the immune response by using several of them in combination.

10-1	Antigenic variation can allow pathogens to escape from immunity.

One way in which an infectious agent can evade immune surveillance is by altering its antigens; this is particularly important for extracellular pathogens, against which the principal defense is production of antibody to their surface structures. There are three ways in which **antigenic variation** can occur. First, many infectious agents exist in a wide variety of antigenic types. There are, for example, 84 known types of *Streptococcus pneumoniae*, an important cause of bacterial pneumonia. Each type differs from the others in the structure of its polysaccharide capsule. The different types are distinguished by serological tests and so are often known as serotypes. Infection with one serotype of such an organism can lead to type-specific immunity, which protects against re-infection with that type but not with a different serotype. Thus, from the point of view of the immune system, each serotype of *S. pneumoniae* represents a distinct organism. The result is that essentially the same pathogen can cause disease many times in the same individual (Fig. 10.1).

Fig. 10.1 Host defense against *Streptococcus pneumoniae* is type specific. The different strains of *S. pneumoniae* have antigenically distinct capsular polysaccharides. The capsule prevents effective phagocytosis until the bacterium is opsonized by specific antibody and complement, allowing phagocytes to destroy it. Antibody to one type of *S. pneumoniae* does not cross-react with the other types, so an individual immune to one type has no protective immunity to a subsequent infection with a different type. An individual must generate a new immune response each time he or she is infected with a different type of *S. pneumoniae*.

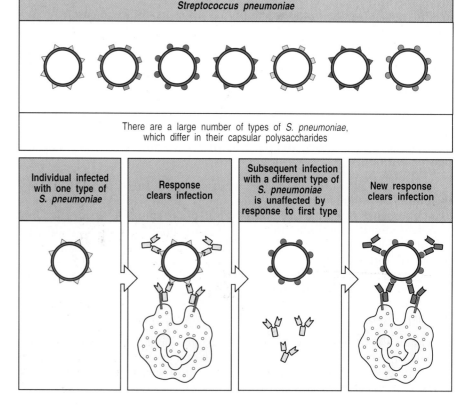

A second, more dynamic mechanism of antigenic variation is seen in the influenza virus. At any one time, a single virus type is responsible for most infections throughout the world. The human population gradually develops protective immunity to this virus type, chiefly by directing neutralizing antibody against the major surface protein of the influenza virus, the hemagglutinin. Since the virus is rapidly cleared from individual hosts, its survival depends on having a large pool of unprotected individuals among whom it spreads very readily. The virus might therefore be in danger of running out of potential hosts if it had not evolved two distinct ways of changing its antigenic type (Fig. 10.2).

The first of these, **antigenic drift**, is caused by point mutations in the genes encoding hemagglutinin and a second surface protein, neuraminidase. Every 2–3 years, a variant arises with mutations that allow the virus to evade neutralization by antibodies in the population; other mutations affect epitopes that are recognized by T cells, and in particular CD8 T cells, so that cells infected with the mutant virus also escape destruction. Individuals who were previously infected with, and hence immune to, the old variant are thus susceptible to the new variant. This causes an epidemic that is relatively mild because there is still some cross-reaction with antibodies and T cells produced against the previous variant of the virus, and therefore most of the population have some level of immunity (see Section 9-27).

Major influenza pandemics resulting in widespread and often fatal disease occur as the result of the second process, which is termed **antigenic shift**. This happens when there is reassortment of the segmented RNA genome of the influenza virus and related viruses in an animal host, leading to major changes in the hemagglutinin protein on the viral surface. The resulting virus is recognized poorly, if at all, by antibodies and T cells directed at the previous variant, so that most people are highly susceptible to the new virus, and severe infection results.

The third mechanism of antigenic variation involves programmed rearrangements in the DNA of the pathogen. The most striking example occurs in African trypanosomes, where changes in the major surface antigen occur repeatedly within a single infected host. Trypanosomes are insect-borne protozoa that replicate in the extracellular tissue spaces of the body and cause sleeping sickness in humans. The trypanosome is coated with a single type of glycoprotein, the variant-specific

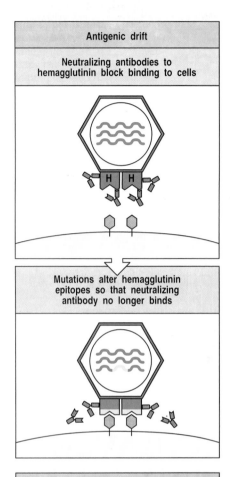

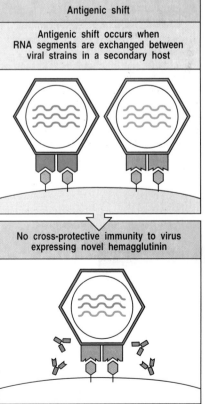

Fig. 10.2 Two types of variation allow repetitive infection with type A influenza virus. Neutralizing antibody that mediates protective immunity is directed at the surface protein hemagglutinin (H), which mediates viral binding to and entry into cells. Antigenic drift (upper two panels) involves the emergence of point mutants that alter the binding sites of protective antibodies on the hemagglutinin. When this happens, the new virus can grow in a host that is immune to the previous strain of virus. However, as T cells and some antibodies can still recognize epitopes that have not been altered, the new variants cause only mild disease in previously infected individuals. Antigenic shift (lower two panels) is a rare event involving reassortment of the segmented RNA viral genome between two influenza viruses, probably in avian hosts. These antigen-shifted viruses have large changes in their hemagglutinin molecule and therefore T cells and antibodies produced in earlier infections are not protective. For this reason, these shifted strains cause severe infection that spreads widely, causing the influenza pandemics that occur every 10–50 years. (There are eight RNA segments in each viral genome but for simplicity only three are shown.)

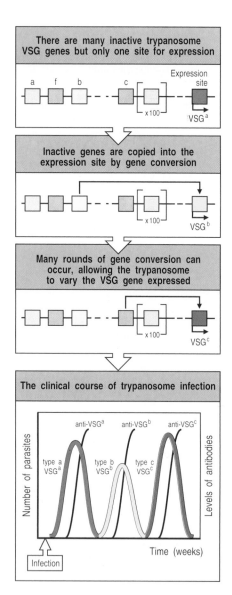

Fig. 10.3 Antigenic variation in trypanosomes allows them to escape immune surveillance. The surface of a trypanosome is covered with a variant-specific glycoprotein (VSG). Each trypanosome has about 1000 genes encoding different VSGs but only the gene in a specific telomeric expression site is active. Although several genetic mechanisms have been observed for changing the VSG gene expressed, the usual mechanism is gene duplication. Here an inactive gene, which is not at the telomere, is copied and transposed into the telomeric expression site, becoming active. When an individual is first infected, antibodies are raised against the VSG initially expressed by the trypanosome population. A small number of trypanosomes spontaneously switch their VSG gene to a new type, and while the host antibody eliminates the initial variant, the new variant is unaffected. As the new variant grows, the whole sequence of events is repeated.

glycoprotein (VSG), which elicits a potent protective antibody response that rapidly clears most of the parasites. The trypanosome genome, however, contains about 1000 VSG genes, each with distinct antigenic properties. To escape surveillance by a system capable of generating many distinct antibodies by gene rearrangment, the trypanosome has developed its own system of gene rearrangement that causes a change in the pattern of expression of VSG genes. A few trypanosomes with such changed surface glycoproteins escape the antibodies, and these soon grow and cause a recurrence of disease (Fig. 10.3). Antibodies are then made to the new VSG, and the whole cycle repeats. This chronic cycle of antigen clearance leads to immune complex damage and inflammation, and eventually to neurological damage, finally resulting in coma. This gives the disease, sleeping sickness, its name. These cycles of evasive action make trypanosome infections very difficult for the immune system to defeat and they are a major health problem in Africa. Malaria is another major disease caused by a protozoan parasite that varies its antigens in order to evade elimination by the immune system.

Antigenic variation also occurs in bacteria; DNA rearrangements help to account for the success of two important bacterial pathogens—*Salmonella typhimurium*, a common cause of salmonella food poisoning, and *Neisseria gonorrhoeae*, which causes gonorrhea, a major sexually transmitted disease and an increasing public health problem in the USA. *S. typhimurium* regularly alternates its surface flagellin protein by inverting a segment of its DNA containing the promoter for one flagellin gene. This turns off expression of the gene and allows expression of the second gene, which encodes an antigenically distinct protein. *N. gonorrhoeae* has several variable antigens, the most dramatic of which is the pilin protein, which, like the variable surface glycoproteins of the African trypanosome, is encoded by several variant genes only one of which is active at any given time. Silent versions of the gene from time to time replace the active version downstream of the pilin promoter. All of these mechanisms help the pathogen to evade an otherwise specific and effective immune response.

10-2   Some viruses persist *in vivo* by ceasing to replicate until immunity wanes.

Viruses usually betray their presence to the immune system once they have entered cells by directing the synthesis of viral proteins, fragments of which are displayed on the surface MHC molecules of the infected cell, where they are detected by T lymphocytes. To replicate, a virus must make viral proteins, and rapidly replicating viruses which produce acute viral illnesses, are therefore readily detected by T cells, which normally control them. Some viruses, however, can enter a state known as **latency** in which the virus is not transcriptionally active. In the latent state, the virus does not cause disease but, because there are no viral peptides to flag its presence, it cannot be eliminated. Such latent infections can later be reactivated and this results in recurrent illness.

Herpes viruses often enter latency. Herpes simplex virus, the cause of cold sores, infects epithelia and spreads to sensory neurons serving the area of infection. After an effective immune response controls the epithelial infection, the virus persists in a latent state in the sensory neurons. Factors such as sunlight, bacterial infection, or hormonal changes reactivate the virus, which then travels down the axons of the sensory neuron and re-infects the epithelial tissues (Fig. 10.4). At this point, the immune response again becomes active and controls the local infection by killing the epithelial cells, producing a new sore. This cycle can be repeated many times. There are two reasons why the sensory neuron remains infected: first, the virus is quiescent in the nerve and therefore few viral proteins are produced, generating few virus-derived peptides to present on MHC class I; and second, neurons carry very low levels of MHC class I molecules, which makes it harder for CD8 T cells to recognize infected cells and attack them. This low level of MHC class I expression may be beneficial, as it reduces the risk that neurons, which cannot regenerate, will be attacked inappropriately by CD8 T cells. It also makes neurons unusually vulnerable to persistent infections. Similarly, herpes zoster (or varicella zoster), which causes chickenpox, remains latent in one or a few dorsal root ganglia after the acute illness is over.

Stress or immunosuppression can reactivate the virus, which spreads down the nerve and infects the skin. This re-infection causes the reappearance of the classic rash of varicella in the area of skin served by the infected dorsal root, a disease commonly called shingles. Herpes simplex reactivation is frequent but herpes zoster usually reactivates only once in a lifetime in an immunocompetent host.

The Epstein-Barr virus (EBV), yet another herpes virus, causes infectious mononucleosis (glandular fever), an acute infection of B lymphocytes. EBV infects B cells by binding to CR2 (CD21), a component of the B cell CD19 co-receptor complex. The infection causes most of the infected cells to proliferate and produce virus, leading in turn to the proliferation of antigen-specific T cells and the excess of mononuclear white cells in the blood that gives the disease its name. The infection is controlled eventually by specific CD8 T cells, which kill the infected proliferating B cells. A fraction of B lymphocytes become latently infected, however, and EBV remains quiescent in these cells. These cells express a viral protein, EBNA-1, which is needed to maintain the viral genome, but EBNA-1 interacts with the proteasome (see Chapter 4) to prevent its own degradation into peptides that would elicit a T-cell response.

Latently infected B cells can be detected by taking B cells from individuals who have apparently cleared their EBV infection and placing them in tissue culture: in the absence of T cells, the latently infected cells that have retained the EBV genome transform into continuously growing cell lines. *In vivo*, EBV-infected B cells sometimes undergo malignant transformation, giving rise to a B-cell lymphoma called Burkitt's lymphoma (see Section 5-17). This is a rare event and it seems likely that a crucial part of this process is a failure of T-cell surveillance. Further evidence in support of this hypothesis comes from the observations of the increased risk of development of EBV-associated B-cell lymphomas in patients with acquired and inherited immunodeficiencies of T-cell function

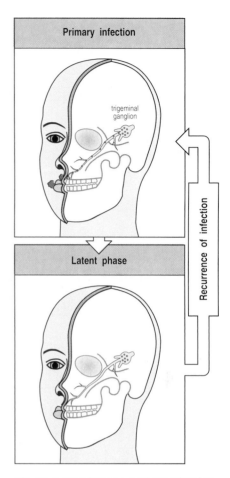

Fig. 10.4 Persistence and reactivation of herpes simplex virus infection. The initial infection in the skin is cleared by an effective immune response but residual infection persists in sensory neurons such as those of the trigeminal ganglion, whose axons innervate the lips. When the virus is reactivated, usually by some environmental stress and/or alteration in immune status, the skin in the area served by the nerve is re-infected from virus in the ganglion and a new cold sore results. This process can be repeated many times.

(see Sections 10-6 and 10-23). Recent evidence suggests that EBV may also infect dendritic cells and transform them into the malignant cell in Hodgkin's disease (see Section 6-20).

| 10-3 | **Some pathogens resist destruction by host defense mechanisms or exploit them for their own purposes.** |

Some pathogens induce a normal immune response but have evolved specialized mechanisms for resisting its effects. For instance, some bacteria that are engulfed in the normal way by macrophages have evolved ways of avoiding destruction by these phagocytes; indeed they use macrophages as their primary host. *Mycobacterium tuberculosis*, for example, is taken up by macrophages but prevents the fusion of the phagosome with the lysosome, protecting itself from the bactericidal actions of the lysosomal contents. Other microorganisms, such as *Listeria monocytogenes*, escape from the phagosome into the cytoplasm of the macrophage, where they can multiply readily, and then spread to adjacent cells in tissues without emerging from the cell into the extracellular medium. Hence they resist antibody-mediated killing. However, cells infected with *L. monocytogenes* are susceptible to killing by cytotoxic T cells.

The protozoan parasite *Toxoplasma gondii* can apparently generate its own vesicle, which isolates it from the rest of the cell because it does not fuse with any cellular vesicle. This may actually enable *T. gondii* to avoid making peptides derived from its proteins accessible for loading onto MHC molecules, and thereby to remain invisible to the immune system.

Two prominent spirochetal infections, **Lyme disease** and syphilis, avoid elimination by antibodies through less well understood mechanisms, and establish a persistent and extremely damaging infection in tissues. Lyme disease is caused by the spirochete *Borrelia burgdorferi*, while syphilis is caused by *Treponema pallidum*. Syphilis is the more widespread and much the better understood of the two diseases, and the bacterium is believed to avoid recognition by antibodies by coating its surface with host molecules until it has invaded the tissues, where it is less easily reached by antibodies.

Finally, many viruses have evolved mechanisms to subvert various arms of the immune system. These range from capturing cellular genes for cytokines or cytokine receptors, to synthesizing complement regulatory molecules or inhibiting MHC class I synthesis or assembly. This area is one of the most rapidly expanding areas in the field of host–pathogen relationships. Examples of how members of the herpes and poxvirus families subvert host responses are shown in Fig. 10.5.

| 10-4 | **Immunosuppression or inappropriate immune responses can contribute to persistent disease.** |

Many pathogens suppress immune responses in general. For example, staphylococcal bacteria produce toxins, such as the **staphylococcal enterotoxins** and **toxic shock syndrome toxin-1**, that act as **superantigens**. Superantigens are proteins that bind the antigen receptor of very large numbers of T cells (see Section 4-26), stimulating them to produce cytokines that cause significant suppression of all immune responses. The details of this suppression are not understood.

Viral strategy	Specific mechanism	Result	Virus examples
Inhibition of humoral immunity	Virally encoded Fc receptor	Blocks effector functions of antibodies bound to infected cells	Herpes simplex Cytomegalovirus
	Virally encoded complement receptor	Blocks complement-mediated effector pathways	Herpes simplex
	Virally encoded complement control protein	Inhibits complement activation of infected cell	Vaccinia
Inhibition of inflammatory response	Virally encoded cytokine homolog, eg β-chemokine receptor	Sensitizes infected cells to effects of β-chemokine; advantage to virus unknown	Cytomegalovirus
	Virally encoded soluble cytokine receptor, eg IL-1 receptor homolog TNF receptor homolog γ-interferon receptor homolog	Blocks effects of cytokines by inhibiting their interaction with host receptors	Vaccinia Rabbit myxoma virus
	Viral inhibition of adhesion molecule expression, eg LFA-3 ICAM-1	Blocks adhesion of lymphocytes to infected cells	Epstein-Barr virus
Blocking of antigen processing and presentation	Inhibition of MHC-class I expression	Impairs recognition of infected cells by cytotoxic T cells	Herpes simplex Cytomegalovirus
	Inhibition of peptide transport by TAP	Blocks peptide association with MHC class I	Herpes simplex
Immunosuppression of host	Virally encoded cytokine homolog of IL-10	Inhibits T_H1 lymphocytes Reduces γ-interferon production	Epstein-Barr virus

Fig. 10.5 Mechanisms of subversion of the host immune system by viruses of the herpes and pox families.

The stimulated T cells proliferate and then rapidly undergo apoptosis, leaving a generalized suppression together with peripheral deletion of many T cells.

Many other pathogens cause mild or transient immunosuppression during acute infection. These forms of suppressed immunity are poorly understood but important, as they often make the host susceptible to secondary infections by common environmental organisms. A crucially important example of immune suppression follows trauma, burns, or even major surgery. The burned patient has a clearly diminished capability to respond to infection, and generalized infection is a common cause of death in these patients. The reasons for this are not fully understood.

The most extreme case of immune suppression caused by a pathogen is infection with HIV. The ultimate cause of death in AIDS is usually infection with an **opportunistic pathogen**, a term used to describe a micro-organism that is present in the environment but does not usually cause disease because it is well controlled by the normal immune response. HIV infection leads to gradual loss of immune competence, allowing infection with organisms that are not normally pathogenic.

Leprosy, which we discussed in Section 7-12, is a more complex case, in which the causal bacterium, *Mycobacterium leprae*, may suppress either cell-mediated immunity or humoral immunity, leading to two major forms of the disease: lepromatous and tuberculoid leprosy. In **lepromatous leprosy**, cell-mediated immunity is profoundly depressed, *M. leprae* are present in great profusion, and immune responses to many antigens are suppressed. This leads to a phenotypic state in such patients called **anergy**, here meaning the absence of delayed-type hypersensitivity to a wide range of antigens unrelated to *M. leprae*. In **tuberculoid leprosy**, by contrast, there is potent cell-mediated immunity with macrophage activation, which controls but does not eradicate infection. Few viable microorganisms are found in tissues, the patients usually survive, and most of the symptoms and pathology are caused by the inflammatory response to these persistent microorganisms. The difference between the two forms of disease may lie in a difference in the ratio of T_H1 to T_H2 cells (Fig. 10.6), and this is thought to be caused by cytokines produced by CD8 T cells, as we learned in Chapter 9 (see Section 9-18).

| 10-5 | **Immune responses can contribute directly to pathogenesis.** |

Tuberculoid leprosy is just one example of an infection in which the pathology is caused largely by the immune response. This is true to some degree in most infections. For example, the fever that accompanies a bacterial infection is caused by the release of cytokines by macrophages. A particularly relevant example is the wheezy broncheolitis caused by **respiratory syncytial virus** (**RSV**). Broncheolitis caused by RSV is the major cause of admission of young children to hospital in the Western world, with as many as 90 000 admissions and 4500 deaths per annum in the USA alone. The first indication that the immune response to the virus may play a role in the pathogenesis of disease came from the observation that young infants vaccinated with an alum-precipitated killed virus preparation suffered a worse disease than unvaccinated children. This occurred because the vaccine failed to induce neutralizing antibodies but succeeded in producing T_H2 cells. Upon infection, the T_H2 cells released IL-3, IL-4, and IL-5, which induced bronchospasm, increased mucus secretion, and tissue eosinophilia. Mice can be infected with RSV and develop a disease similar to that seen in humans.

Another example of a pathogenic immune response is the response to the eggs of the schistosome. Schistosomes are parasitic worms that lay eggs in the hepatic portal vein. Some of the eggs reach the intestine and are shed in the feces, spreading the infection; others lodge in the portal circulation of the liver, where they elicit a potent immune response leading to chronic inflammation, hepatic fibrosis, and eventually to liver failure. This process reflects the excessive activation of T_H2 cells, and can be modulated by T_H1 cells, interferon-γ (IFN-γ), or CD8 T cells, which may act by producing IFN-γ.

In the case of the **mouse mammary tumor virus** (**MMTV**), which causes mammary tumors in mice, the immune response is required for the infective cycle of the pathogen. MMTV is transferred from the mother's mammary gland to her pups in milk. The virus then enters the B lymphocytes of the new host, where it must replicate in order to be transported to the mammary epithelium to continue its life cycle. As it is a retrovirus, however, MMTV can only replicate in dividing cells. The virus ensures that infected B cells will proliferate by causing them to express on their surface a superantigen encoded within the MMTV genome. This superantigen enables the B cells to bypass the requirement for specific antigen and stimulate large numbers of CD4 T cells with the appropriate T-cell receptor $V\beta$ domain (see Section 4-26), causing

Pathogens have evolved various means of evading or subverting normal host defenses.

10:9

Infection with *Mycobacterium leprae* can result in different clinical forms of leprosy

There are two polar forms, tuberculoid and lepromatous leprosy, but several intermediate forms also exist

Tuberculoid leprosy	Lepromatous leprosy

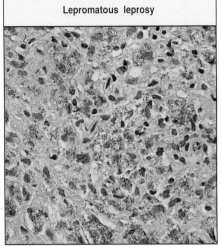

Organisms present at low to undetectable levels	Organisms show florid growth in macrophages
Low infectivity	High infectivity
Granulomas and local inflammation. Peripheral nerve damage	Disseminated infection. Bone, cartilage, and diffuse nerve damage
Normal serum immunoglobulin levels	Hypergammaglobulinemia
Normal T-cell responsiveness. Specific response to *M. leprae* antigens	Low or absent T-cell responsiveness. No response to *M. leprae* antigens

Cytokine patterns in leprosy lesions

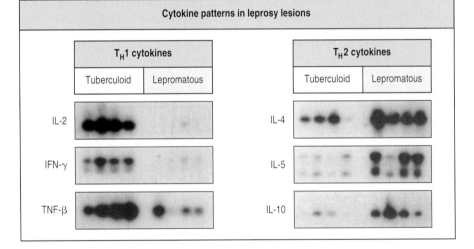

T$_H$1 cytokines		T$_H$2 cytokines	
Tuberculoid	Lepromatous	Tuberculoid	Lepromatous
IL-2		IL-4	
IFN-γ		IL-5	
TNF-β		IL-10	

Fig. 10.6 T-cell and macrophage responses to *Mycobacterium leprae* are sharply different in the two polar forms of leprosy. Infection with *M. leprae*, which stain red in the photographs, can lead to two very different forms of disease. In tuberculoid leprosy (left), growth of the organism is well controlled by T$_H$1-like cells that activate infected macrophages. The tuberculoid lesion contains granulomas and is inflamed but the inflammation is local and causes only local effects, such as peripheral nerve damage. In lepromatous leprosy (right), infection is widely disseminated and the bacilli grow uncontrolled in macrophages; in the late stages of disease there is major damage to connective tissues and to the peripheral nervous system. There are several intermediate stages between these two polar forms. The cytokine patterns in the two polar forms of the disease are sharply different, as shown by analysis of mRNA isolated from lesions of three patients with lepromatous leprosy and three patients with tuberculoid leprosy (Northern blots, lower panel). Cytokines typically produced by T$_H$2 cells (IL-4, IL-5, and IL-10) dominate in the lepromatous form, while cytokines produced by T$_H$1 cells (IL-2, IFN-γ, and TNF-β) dominate in the tuberculoid form. It appears therefore that T$_H$1-like cells predominate in tuberculoid leprosy, and T$_H$2-like cells in lepromatous leprosy. IFN-γ would be expected to activate macrophages, enhancing killing of *M. leprae*, whereas IL-4 can actually inhibit the induction of bactericidal activity in macrophages. High levels of IL-4 would also explain the hypergammaglobulinemia observed in lepromatous leprosy. The determining factors in the initial induction of T$_H$1- or T$_H$2-like cells are not known, and the mechanism for the anergy or generalized loss of effective cell-mediated immunity in lepromatous leprosy is also not understood. Photographs courtesy of G Kaplan; cytokine patterns courtesy of R L Modlin.

them to produce cytokines and express CD40 ligand, which in turn stimulates the B cells to divide (Fig. 10.7). The mouse host can protect itself against the virus by deleting the particular subset of T cells carrying the V$_β$ domain recognized by the viral superantigen.

There are several different strains of MMTV whose superantigens bind to different V$_β$ domains. As we learned in Section 6-17, most mouse strains have MMTV genomes stably integrated into their DNA. These

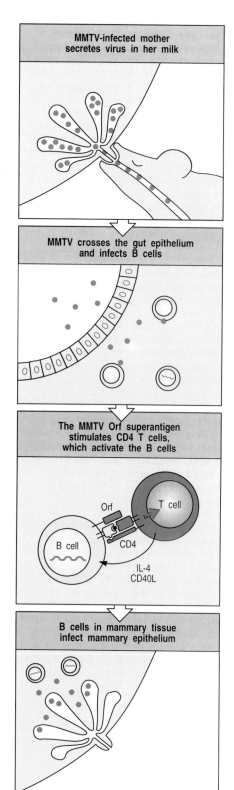

MMTV-infected mother secretes virus in her milk

MMTV crosses the gut epithelium and infects B cells

The MMTV Orf superantigen stimulates CD4 T cells, which activate the B cells

Orf

T cell

B cell

CD4

IL-4
CD40L

B cells in mammary tissue infect mammary epithelium

Fig. 10.7 Activation of T cells by the MMTV superantigen is crucial for the virus life cycle. MMTV is transferred from mother to pup in milk, and crosses the gut epithelium to reach the lymphoid tissue of its new host and infect B lymphocytes. The superantigen encoded by MMTV, called Orf, is expressed on the surface of the B cell and binds to appropriate T-cell receptor V_β domains on CD4 T cells. The superantigen also has binding sites for MHC class II molecules, so that a complex between superantigen, MHC molecule, T-cell receptor, and CD4 is formed, activating the T cell. The T cell activates the B cell to divide, allowing viral replication within the B cell and subsequent infection of the mammary epithelium. If the T cells with appropriate V_β domains have been deleted previously because of the expression of a superantigen encoded by a defective endogenous MMTV genome (see Section 6-18), the infected B cell cannot activate any of the remaining T cells and therefore no B cells are stimulated to divide, blocking MMTV replication. Many different defective endogenous MMTV genomes are expressed in wild mouse populations, each deleting a characteristic V_β subset. Thus, individual mice are resistant to different MMTV strains. CD40L, CD40 ligand.

endogenous retroviruses have lost certain essential genes and are unable to produce virions but they have retained the genes encoding their superantigens, which are expressed on the cells of the host. Since these superantigens can induce clonal deletion in the thymus, the T cells carrying appropriate V_β domains are lost.

Why might it be beneficial to the mouse to lose a section of its repertoire? It has been proposed that removing the T cells that can be stimulated by a given superantigen might prevent infection with intact mouse mammary tumor viruses encoding the same superantigen. To test this, mice containing a transgenic MMTV genome were constructed. These mice express the MMTV superantigen and therefore delete T cells expressing V_β domains that bind to it. Since there are no T cells left that can be stimulated by the superantigen encoded by this strain of MMTV, B cells infected with the intact virus cannot be activated and this particular strain of MMTV, therefore, cannot be transmitted in these transgenic mice. Thus, in this example, the ability of a pathogen to elicit a response from the immune system is essential to its ability to cause disease. Mice containing different endogenous MMTV genomes delete different parts of their T-cell receptor repertoire, reducing the risk that whole mouse populations will be susceptible to a given mammary tumor virus. No human diseases dependent on such mechanisms have yet been described.

Summary.

Infectious agents can cause recurrent or persistent disease by avoiding normal host defense mechanisms or by subverting them to promote their own replication. There are many different ways to evade or subvert the immune response. Antigenic variation, latency, resistance to immune effector mechanisms, and suppression of the immune response all contribute to persistent and medically important infections. In some cases, the immune response is part of the problem; some pathogens use immune activation to spread infection, others would not cause disease if it were not for the immune response. Each of these mechanisms teaches us something about the nature of the immune response and its weaknesses, and each requires a different medical approach to prevent or to treat infection.

Inherited immunodeficiency diseases.

Immunodeficiencies occur when one or more components of the immune system is defective. The commonest cause of immune deficiency worldwide is malnutrition; however, in developed countries, most immunodeficiency diseases are inherited, and these are usually seen in the clinic as recurrent or overwhelming infections in very young children. Less commonly acquired immunodeficiencies with causes other than malnutrition can manifest later in life. While the pathogenesis of many of these acquired disorders has remained obscure, some are caused by known agents, such as drugs or irradiation which damage lymphocytes, or infection with HIV. By examining which infections accompany a particular inherited or acquired immunodeficiency, we can see which components of the immune system are important in the response to particular infectious agents. The inherited immunodeficiency diseases also reveal how interactions between different cell types contribute to the immune response and to the developmental sequence of T and B lymphocytes. Finally, these diseases can lead us to the defective gene, often revealing new information about the molecular basis of immune processes and providing the necessary information for diagnosis, genetic counseling, and gene therapy.

10-6   Inherited immunodeficiency diseases are caused by recessive gene defects.

Before the advent of antibiotic therapy, it is likely that most individuals with inherited immune defects died in infancy or early childhood because of their susceptibility to particular classes of pathogens (Fig. 10.8). Such deaths would not have been easy to identify, since many normal infants also died of infection. Thus, the first immunodeficiency disease was not described until 1952; since that time many inherited immunodeficiency diseases have been identified. Most of the gene defects that cause these inherited immunodeficiencies are recessive, and for this reason, many common immunodeficiencies are caused by mutations of genes on the X chromosome. Recessive defects cause disease only when both chromosomes are defective. As males have only one X chromosome, however, all males who inherit an X chromosome carrying a defective gene will manifest disease, whereas female carriers, having two X chromosomes, are perfectly healthy. Immunodeficiency diseases that affect many steps in B- and T-lymphocyte development have been described, as have defects in surface molecules that are important for T- or B-cell function. Defects in phagocytic cells, in complement, in cytokines, in cytokine receptors, and in molecules that mediate effector responses also occur (see Fig. 10.8). Thus immunodeficiency may be caused by defects either in the adaptive or the innate immune system. Individual examples of these diseases will be described in later sections.

More recently, the use of gene knock-out techniques in mice has allowed the creation of many immunodeficient states that are adding rapidly to our knowledge of the contribution of individual molecules to normal immune function. Nevertheless, human immunodeficiency disease is still the best source of insight into host defense in humans. The study of immunodeficiency provides the clearest evidence of the normal pathways of host defense against infectious disease. For example, as we will see later, deficiency in antibody, complement, or phagocytic function

Fig. 10.8 Human immunodeficiency syndromes. The specific gene defect, the consequence for the immune system, and the resulting disease susceptibilities are listed for some common and some rare human immunodeficiency syndromes. ADA, adenosine deaminase; PNP, purine nucleotide phosphorylase; TAP, transporters associated with antigen processing; WASP, Wiskott-Aldrich syndrome protein; EBV, Epstein-Barr virus; NK, natural killer.

Name of deficiency syndrome	Specific abnormality	Immune defect	Susceptibility
Severe combined immune deficiency	ADA deficiency	No T or B cells	General
	PNP deficiency	No T or B cells	General
	X-linked *scid*, γ_c chain deficiency	No T cells	General
	Autosomal *scid* DNA repair defect	No T or B cells	General
DiGeorge syndrome	Thymic aplasia	Variable numbers of T and B cells	General
MHC class I deficiency	TAP mutations	No CD8 T cells	Viruses
MHC class II deficiency	Lack of expression of MHC class II	No CD4 T cells	General
Wiskott-Aldrich syndrome	X-linked; defective WASP gene	Defective polysaccharide antibody responses	Encapsulated extracellular bacteria
Common variable immunodeficiency	Unknown; MHC-linked	Defective antibody production	Extracellular bacteria
X-linked agamma-globulinemia	Loss of Btk tyrosine kinase	No B cells	Extracellular bacteria, viruses
X-linked hyper-IgM syndrome	Defective CD40 ligand	No isotype switching	Extracellular bacteria
Selective IgA and/or IgG deficiency	Unknown; MHC-linked	No IgA synthesis	Respiratory infections
Phagocyte deficiencies	Many different	Loss of phagocyte function	Extracellular bacteria
Complement deficiencies	Many different	Loss of specific complement components	Extracellular bacteria especially *Neisseria* spp.
Natural killer (NK) cell defect	Unknown	Loss of NK function	Herpes viruses
X-linked lympho-proliferative syndrome	Unknown; X-linked	EBV-triggered immunodeficiency	EBV
Ataxia telangiectasia	Gene with PI-3 kinase homology	T cells reduced	Respiratory infections
Autoimmune lympho-proliferative disease	Mutant Fas	Failure of T- and B-cell apoptosis	Autoimmune disorders

each increases the risk of infection by certain pyogenic bacteria. This shows that the normal pathway of host defense against such bacteria is binding of antibody followed by fixation of complement, which allows uptake of opsonized bacteria by phagocytic cells. Breaking any one of the links in this chain of events leading to bacterial killing causes a similar immunodeficient state.

The study of immunodeficiency also teaches us about the redundancy of mechanisms of host defense against infectious disease. The first two humans to be discovered with hereditary deficiency of complement were healthy immunologists. This teaches us two lessons. The first is that there are multiple protective immune mechanisms against infection; for example, while there is abundant evidence that complement deficiency increases susceptibility to pyogenic infection, not every human with complement deficiency suffers from recurrent infections. The second lesson is about the phenomenon of **ascertainment artefact**. When an unusual observation is made in a patient with disease, there is a temptation to seek a causal link. However, no one would suggest that complement deficiency causes a genetic predisposition to becoming an immunologist. Complement deficiency was discovered in immunologists because they used their own blood in their experiments. If a particular measurement is only made in a group of patients with a particular disease, it is inevitable that the only abnormal results will be discovered in patients with that disease. This is an ascertainment artefact and emphasizes the importance of studying appropriate controls.

10-7 The main effect of low levels of antibody is an inability to clear extracellular bacteria.

Pyogenic or pus-forming bacteria have polysaccharide capsules which make them resistant to phagocytosis. Normal individuals can clear infections by such bacteria because antibody and complement opsonize the bacteria, making it possible for phagocytes to ingest and destroy them. The principal effect of deficiencies in antibody production is therefore failure to control this class of bacterial infection, although susceptibility to some viral infections, most notably those caused by enteroviruses, is also increased because of the importance of antibodies in neutralizing infectious viruses that enter the body through the gut (see Chapter 8).

The first description of an immunodeficiency disease was Ogden C. Bruton's account, in 1952, of the failure of a male child to produce antibody. As this defect is inherited in an X-linked fashion and is characterized by the absence of immunoglobulin in the serum, it was called **Bruton's X-linked agammaglobulinemia** (**XLA**). The absence of antibody can be detected using electrophoresis (see Section 2-9). Since then, many more diseases of antibody production have been described, most of them the consequence of failures in the development or activation of B lymphocytes.

The defective gene in XLA is now known to encode a protein tyrosine kinase known as Btk (Bruton's tyrosine kinase). This protein is expressed in polymorphonuclear neutrophilic leukocytes as well as in B cells, although only B cells are defective in these patients, in whom B-cell maturation halts at the pre-B-cell stage. Thus it is likely that Btk is required to couple the pre-B-cell receptor (which consists of heavy chains, surrogate light chains, and Igα and Igβ) to nuclear events that lead to pre-B-cell growth and differentiation. A homologous kinase called Itk has been found in T cells and is required for normal T-cell development. Defects in Btk are analogous to defects in Lck in T-cell development (see Section 6-8). In the mouse, Lck deficiency leads to the arrest of thymocyte development at the double-negative stage, after T-cell receptor β-chain gene rearrangement and cell-surface expression but before the rearrangement of the α-chain genes. Thus, there may be a cascade of tyrosine kinases, involving Lck and Itk in double-negative thymocytes, and Blk and Btk in pre-B cells, that is important for lymphocyte development. In both Lck and Btk deficiencies, some B or T cells mature despite the defect in the signaling molecule, suggesting that signals transmitted by these kinases promote rearrangement of light-chain or α-chain genes, respectively, but are not absolutely required.

Since the gene responsible for XLA is found on the X chromosome, it is possible to identify female carriers by analyzing X-chromosome inactivation in their B cells. During development, female cells randomly inactivate one of their two X chromosomes. Since the product of a normal *btk* gene is required for normal B-lymphocyte development, only cells in which the X chromosome carrying the normal allele of *btk* is active can develop into mature B cells (with a very few exceptions, see earlier). Thus, in female carriers of mutant *btk* genes, almost all B cells have the normal X chromosome as the active X. By contrast, the active X chromosomes in the T cells and macrophages of carriers are equally distributed between normal and *btk* mutants. This fact allowed female carriers of XLA to be identified even before the nature of *btk* was known. Non-random X inactivation only in B cells also demonstrates conclusively that the *btk* gene is required for normal B-cell development but not for the development of other cell types, and that Btk must act within B cells rather than on stromal cells or other cells required for B-cell development (Fig. 10.9).

Fig. 10.9 The product of the *btk* gene is important for B-cell development. In X-linked agammaglobulinemia (XLA), a protein tyrosine kinase called Btk, encoded on the X chromosome, is defective. In normal individuals, B-cell development proceeds through a stage in which the pre-B cell receptor consisting of μ:λ5:Vpre-B transduces a signal via Btk, triggering further B-cell development. In males with XLA, no signal can be transduced and although the pre-B-cell receptor is expressed, the B cells develop no further. In female mammals, including humans, one of the two X chromosomes in each cell is permanently inactivated early in development. Since the choice of which chromosome to inactivate is random, half of the pre-B cells in a carrier female express a wild-type *btk*, while half express the defective gene. None of the B cells that express *btk* from the defective chromosome can develop into mature B cells. Therefore, in the carrier, mature B cells always have the non-defective X chromosome active. This is in sharp contrast to all other cell types, which express the non-defective chromosome in only half of the population. Non-random X chromosome inactivation in a particular cell lineage is a clear indication that the product of the X-linked gene is required for the development of cells of that lineage. It is also sometimes possible to identify the stage at which the gene product is required, by detecting the point in development at which X-chromosome inactivation develops bias. Using this kind of analysis, one can identify carriers of X-linked traits such as XLA without needing to know the nature of the mutant gene.

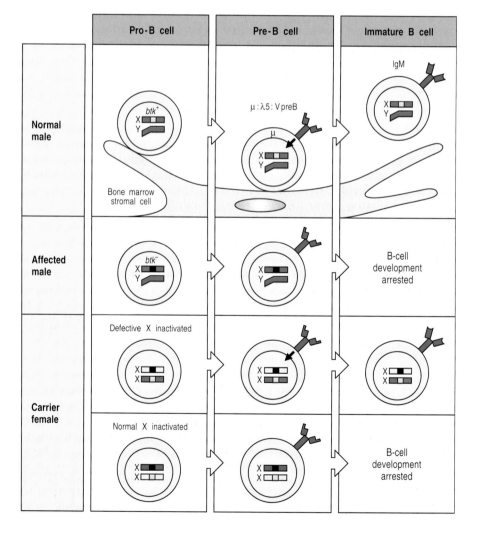

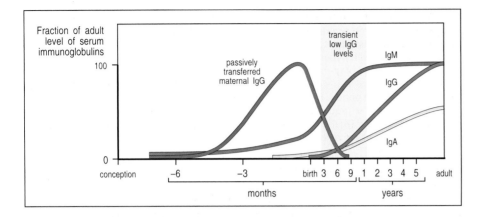

Fig. 10.10 Immunoglobulin levels in newborn infants fall to low levels around 6 months of age. Newborn babies have high levels of IgG, transported across the placenta from the mother during gestation. After birth, production of IgM starts almost immediately; production of IgG, however, does not begin for about 6 months, during which time the total level of IgG falls as the maternally acquired IgG is catabolized. Thus IgG levels are low from about the age of 3 months to 1 year, which may lead to susceptibility to disease. IgG levels fall further for longer in premature infants, resulting in a higher rate of infection because, at the time of birth, the level of transferred maternal IgG is lower and as the premature infant's immune system is less developed at birth, antibody production by the infant occurs at a later time after birth.

The commonest humoral immune defect is the transient deficiency in immunoglobulin production that occurs in the first 6–12 months of life. The newborn infant has initial antibody levels comparable with those of the mother, because of the transplacental transport of maternal IgG (see Chapter 8). As the transferred IgG is catabolized, antibody levels gradually decrease until the infant begins to produce useful amounts of its own IgG at about 6 months of age (Fig. 10.10). Thus, IgG levels are quite low between the ages of 3 months and 1 year and active IgG antibody responses are poor. In some infants, this can lead to a period of heightened susceptibility to infection. This is especially true for premature babies, who begin with lower levels of maternal IgG and also reach immune competence longer after birth.

The most common inherited form of immunoglobulin deficiency is selective IgA deficiency, which is seen in about 1 person in 800. Although no obvious disease susceptibility is associated with selective IgA defects, they are commoner in people with chronic lung disease than in the general population. This suggests that lack of IgA may result in a predisposition to lung infections with various pathogens and is consistent with the role of IgA in defense at the body's surfaces. The genetic basis of this defect is unknown but some data suggest that a gene of unidentified function mapping in the class III region of the MHC may be involved. A related syndrome called common variable immunodeficiency, in which there is generally a deficiency in IgG and IgA, also maps to the MHC region.

Low levels of antibody production lead to a susceptibility to infection with a fairly specific set of pathogens. People with pure B-cell defects resist many pathogens successfully. They cannot control infection with extracellular bacteria but these infections can be suppressed with antibiotics and periodic infusions with human immunoglobulin collected from a large pool of donors. Since there are antibodies to most pathogens in the immunoglobulin pool, it serves as a fairly successful shield against infection.

10-8   T-cell defects can result in low antibody levels.

Patients with **X-linked hyper-IgM syndrome** have normal B- and T-cell development and high serum levels of IgM but make very limited IgM antibody responses against T-cell dependent antigens and produce immunoglobulin isotypes other than IgM and IgD only in trace amounts. This makes them susceptible to infection with extracellular bacteria and certain opportunistic organisms such as *Pneumocystis carinii*. The molecular defect in this disease is in the CD40 ligand on activated T cells,

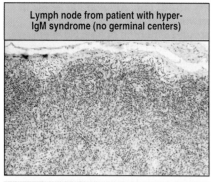

Lymph node from patient with hyper-IgM syndrome (no germinal centers)

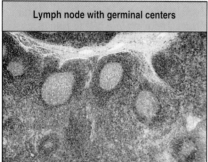

Lymph node with germinal centers

Fig. 10.11 Patients with X-linked hyper-IgM syndrome are unable to activate their B cells fully. Lymphoid tissues in patients with hyper-IgM syndrome are devoid of germinal centers (top panel), in comparison with a normal lymph node (bottom panel). B-cell activation by T cells is required both for isotype switching and for the formation of germinal centers, where extensive B-cell proliferation takes place. Patients with hyper-IgM syndrome have a mutation in the CD40 ligand gene, which lies on the X chromosome, and thus their T cells cannot fully activate their B cells. Only weak IgM responses are made to T-cell dependent antigens and serum immunoglobulin is predominantly IgM. Photographs courtesy of R Geha and A Perez-Atayde.

which cannot engage CD40; the B cells themselves are normal. We learned in Chapter 8 that CD40 ligand plays a critical role in the T-cell dependent activation of B-cell proliferation and these patients show that CD40 ligand is also essential for induction of the isotype switch and the formation of germinal centers (Fig. 10.11). The defects in cell-mediated immunity in these individuals may be due, at least in part, to the inability of their T cells to deliver an activating signal to macrophages by engaging the CD40 expressed on these cells (see Section 7-28). A defect in T-cell activation could also contribute to the profound immunodeficiency suffered by these patients, however, as studies on mice that lack CD40 ligand have revealed a failure of antigen-specific T cells to expand in response to primary immunization with antigen.

In XLA, the hunt for the cause of the disease led to a previously unidentified gene product. In the case of X-linked hyper-IgM syndrome, the gene for CD40 ligand was cloned independently and only then identified as the defective gene in this disorder. Thus, inherited immunodeficiencies can either lead us to new genes or help us to determine the roles of known genes in normal immune system function.

10-9 Defects in complement components cause defective humoral immune function and persistence of immune complexes.

Not surprisingly, the spectrum of infections associated with complement deficiencies overlaps substantially with that seen in patients with deficiencies in antibody production. Defects in the classical pathway and in C3 are associated with a wide range of pyogenic infections, emphasizing the important role of C4 and C3 as opsonins, promoting phagocytosis of bacteria (Fig. 10.12). In contrast, defects in the membrane-attack components of complement (C5–C9) have more limited effects and result exclusively in susceptibility to *Neisseria* spp. This indicates that host defense against these bacteria, which are capable of intracellular survival, is mediated by extracellular lysis by the membrane attack complex of complement.

The early components of the classical complement pathway are particularly critical for the elimination of immune complexes, which can cause significant pathology in autoimmune diseases such as systemic lupus erythematosus (see Chapter 12), and occasionally, in persistent infections. As we learned in Chapter 8, complement components attached to soluble immune complexes allow them to be transported, ingested, and degraded by cells bearing complement receptors. Transport is mediated by erythrocytes that capture immune complexes via the complement receptor CR1, which binds specifically to C4b and C3b. When this mechanism is inoperative, immune complexes are deposited in the tissues. Accumulating immune complexes activate phagocytes, causing inflammation and local tissue damage.

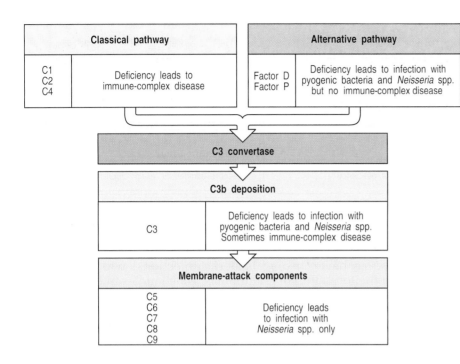

Fig. 10.12 Defects in complement components are associated with susceptibility to certain infections as well as accumulation of immune complexes. Defects in the early components of the alternative pathway lead to susceptibility to extracellular pathogens, and defects in the early components of the classical pathway affect removal of immune complexes via the complement receptor CR1, leading to immune complex disease. Finally, defects in the membrane-attack components are associated only with susceptibility to strains of *Neisseria* spp., the causative agents of meningitis and gonorrhea, implying that the effector pathway is important chiefly in defense against these organisms.

Deficiencies in control proteins that regulate complement activation can cause either immunodeficiency or autoimmune-like disease. People defective in properdin (factor P), which enhances the activity of the alternative pathway, have a heightened susceptibility to *Neisseria* spp. By contrast, patients lacking decay-accelerating factor (DAF) and CD59, which protect host cell surfaces from alternative pathway activation, destroy their own red blood cells. This results in the disease paroxysmal nocturnal hemoglobinuria, as we learned in Chapter 8. A more dramatic consequence arising from the loss of a regulatory protein is seen in patients with C1-inhibitor defects. These individuals fail to control the inappropriate activation of the classical pathway of complement activation and the uncontrolled cleavage of C2 allows the generation of a vasoactive fragment of C2a, causing fluid accumulation in the tissues and epiglottal swelling that may lead to suffocation. This syndrome is called **hereditary angioneurotic edema**.

10-10 | Phagocytic cell defects permit widespread bacterial infections.

The leukocyte integrins CD11a/CD18 (LFA-1), CD11b/CD18 (MAC-1/CR3), and CD11c/CD18 (CR4/gp150,95) are important for phagocytic cell adhesion, migration across blood vessel walls, and ingestion of bacteria opsonized with complement fragments (see Section 7-2). If these integrins are defective, phagocytes cannot get to sites of infection to ingest and destroy pathogens. Deficiencies have been identified in the leukocyte integrin common β2 subunit, CD18, which result in infections that are resistant to antibiotic treatment and persist despite an apparently effective cellular and humoral adaptive immune response. Neutropenia associated with chemotherapy, malignancy or aplastic anemia is associated with a similar spectrum of severe pyogenic bacterial infections.

Most of the other known defects in phagocytic cells affect their ability to kill intracellular and/or ingested extracellular bacteria (Fig. 10.13). In **chronic granulomatous disease**, phagocytes cannot produce the superoxide radical and their antibacterial activity is thereby seriously impaired. Several different genetic defects, affecting any one of the four constituent proteins of the NADPH oxidase system, can cause this. Patients

Fig. 10.13 Defects in phagocytic cells are associated with persistence of bacterial infection. Defects in the leukocyte integrins with a common β subunit (CD18) prevent phagocytic cell adhesion and migration to sites of infection. The respiratory burst is defective in chronic granulomatous disease, glucose-6-phosphate dehydrogenase (G6PD) deficiency and myeloperoxidase deficiency. In chronic granulomatous disease, infections persist because macrophage activation is defective, leading to chronic stimulation of CD4 T cells and hence to granulomas. Vesicle fusion in phagocytes is defective in Chediak-Higashi syndrome. These diseases illustrate the critical role of phagocytes in removing and killing pathogenic bacteria.

Type of defect / name of syndrome	Associated infectious or other diseases
Leukocyte adhesion (CD18) deficiency	Widespread pyogenic bacterial infections
Chronic granulomatous disease	Intra- and extra-cellular infection, granulomas
G6PD deficiency	Defective respiratory burst, chronic infection
Myeloperoxidase deficiency	Defective intracellular killing, chronic infection
Chediak-Higashi syndrome	Intra- and extra-cellular infection, granulomas

with this disease have chronic bacterial infections, which, in some cases, lead to the formation of granulomas. Deficiencies in the enzymes glucose-6-phosphate dehydrogenase and myeloperoxidase also impair intracellular killing and lead to a similar, although less severe, phenotype. Finally, in **Chediak-Higashi syndrome**, an unknown defect causes a failure to fuse lysosomes properly with phagosomes; the cells in these patients have enlarged granules and impaired intracellular killing.

10-11   Defects in T-cell function result in severe combined immunodeficiencies.

Although patients with B-cell defects can deal with most pathogens adequately, patients with defects in T-cell development are highly susceptible to a broad range of infectious agents. This demonstrates the central role of T cells in adaptive immune responses to virtually all antigens. As such patients make neither specific T-cell dependent antibody responses nor cell-mediated immune responses, and thus cannot develop protective immunity, such defects are called **severe combined immune deficiency (SCID)**.

There are several different defects that lead to the SCID phenotype. In X-linked severe combined immune deficiency, T cells fail to develop because of a mutation in the common γ chain of several cytokine receptors, including those for the interleukins IL-2, IL-4, IL-7, IL-9, and IL-15. We will examine this defect further in Section 10-12. Two defects in enzymes involved in purine degradation, **adenosine deaminase (ADA) deficiency** and **purine nucleotide phosphorylase (PNP) deficiency**, also give rise to T-cell deficiencies and a SCID phenotype. Both defects result in an accumulation of nucleotide metabolites that are particularly toxic to developing T cells. B cells are also somewhat compromised in these patients.

Recently, the molecular basis of **Wiskott-Aldrich syndrome (WAS)**, a disease that affects not only B and T lymphocytes but also platelets, has begun to emerge. It is caused by a defective gene on the X chromosome, encoding a protein called WAS protein (WASP). This protein has been shown to bind Cdc42, a small GTP-binding protein that is known to regulate the organization of the cytoskeleton and to be important for the effective collaboration of T and B cells. The WAS protein also has the capability of binding SH$_3$ domains—protein domains found on some proteins of intracellular signaling pathways—and may take part in other signaling pathways. It is expressed in thymus, spleen, and certain tumors of hematopoietic origin and is likely to be a key regulator of lymphocyte and platelet development and function.

One class of SCID individuals lack expression of all MHC class II gene products on their cells. This condition is referred to as the **bare lymphocyte syndrome**. Since the thymus also lacks MHC class II molecules CD4 T cells cannot be positively selected and therefore few develop. The antigen-presenting cells in these individuals also lack MHC class II molecules and so the few CD4 T cells that develop cannot be stimulated by antigen. In these individuals, MHC class I expression is normal and CD8 T cells develop normally. However, they suffer severe combined immunodeficiency, illustrating the central importance of CD4 T cells in adaptive immunity to most pathogens. The syndrome is caused by mutations in one of several different genes that regulate MHC class II gene expression rather than in the MHC genes themselves. At least five complementing gene defects have been defined in patients who fail to express MHC class II molecules, which implies that at least five different genes are required for normal MHC class II gene expression. One of these, named the **class II transactivator**, or **CIITA**, is known to be responsible for some cases, while a protein that binds to the MHC class II promoters, called RFX, is defective in others. An understanding of the other genes that cause this defect is still being sought.

A family showing almost complete absence of cell-surface MHC class I molecules has been described. These patients have normal levels of mRNA encoding MHC class I molecules and normal production levels of MHC class I proteins. The defect was shown to be similar to that of the TAP mutant cells we learned about in Section 4-7 and indeed, affected members of this family had mutations in a TAP gene. These people are immunodeficient owing to a lack of CD8 T cells.

An interesting mutant mouse strain called *scid* (because it has a severe combined B- and T-cell immune deficiency) has a defect in the enzyme DNA-dependent kinase, which binds to the end of the double-stranded breaks that occur during the process of antigen receptor gene rearrangement. Many DNA hairpin structures, which are formed when DNA rearrangement is initiated, have been found in T-cell receptor δ-chain genes of immature thymocytes of *scid* mice, and cells from *scid* mice can be rescued by transfection with the catalytic subunit of DNA-dependent protein kinase. Thus, it seems likely that DNA-dependent kinase is involved in resolving the hairpin structure (see Fig. 3.21). Only rare VJ or VDJ joints are seen in *scid* B and T cells, and most of these have abnormal features. These mice therefore produce very few mature B and T cells. Recently, similar abnormal DJ joints have been observed in pre-B cells of some patients with autosomal severe combined immunodeficiency and cells of such patients, like those of *scid* mice, are abnormally sensitive to ionizing radiation. Other patients who appear to have mutations of *RAG-1* or *RAG-2* genes, also show a SCID phenotype.

In patients with **DiGeorge syndrome** the thymic epithelium fails to develop normally. Without the proper inductive environment T cells cannot mature, and both T-cell dependent antibody production and cell-mediated immunity are absent. Such patients have some serum immunoglobulin and variable numbers of B and T cells. The severe combined immunodeficiency diseases abundantly illustrate the central role of T cells in virtually all adaptive immune responses. In many cases B-cell development is normal, yet the response to nearly all pathogens is profoundly suppressed.

| 10-12 | Defective T-cell signaling, cytokine production, or cytokine action can cause immunodeficiency. |

As we learned in Chapter 7, virtually all adaptive immune responses require the activation of antigen-specific T lymphocytes and their differentiation into cells that produce cytokines acting on specific cytokine receptors. Several gene defects have been described that interfere with these processes. Thus, patients who lack CD3γ chains have low levels of surface T-cell receptors and defective T-cell responses. Patients making low levels of mutant CD3ε chains are also deficient in T-cell activation. Patients who make a defective form of the cytosolic protein tyrosine kinase ZAP-70 (see Section 4-29) have more recently been described. Their CD4 T cells emerge from the thymus in normal numbers, whereas CD8 T cells are absent. However, the CD4 T cells that mature fail to respond to stimuli that normally activate via the T-cell receptor and the patients are thus very immunodeficient.

Another group of patients shows absence of IL-2 production upon receptor ligation, and these patients have a severe immunodeficiency; however, T-cell development is normal in these individuals, as it is in mice that have mutations in their IL-2 genes from gene knock-out (see Section 2-37). These IL-2-negative patients have heterogeneous defects; some of them fail to activate the transcription factor NF-AT (see Section 4-29), which induces transcription of several cytokine genes in addition to the IL-2 gene, and therefore presumably produce low levels of these cytokines as well. This may explain why their immunodeficiency is more profound than that of mice whose IL-2 gene has been disrupted; these mice can mount adaptive immune responses through an IL-2-independent pathway, possibly involving the cytokine IL-15, which shares many activities with IL-2. Nevertheless, mice lacking the ability to make IL-2 are susceptible to a variety of infectious agents.

There is an interesting contrast between patients deficient in IL-2 and those with X-linked severe combined immunodeficiency (X-linked SCID), which is caused by a defect in the γ chain of the IL-2 receptor. T cells in X-linked SCID patients fail to develop, while B cells appear reasonably normal. As mice and humans that lack IL-2 have normal T-cell development, the γ chain of the IL-2 receptor must be important in T-cell development for reasons unrelated to IL-2 binding or IL-2 responses. The recent demonstration that the IL-2 receptor γ chain is also part of other cytokine receptors, including the IL-7 receptor, may explain its role in early T-cell development. The γ chain appears to function in transducing the signal for this group of receptors and interacts with a kinase, JAK3 kinase, which has been shown to be defective in patients with an autosomally inherited immunodeficiency similar in phenotype to X-linked SCID.

As in all serious T-cell deficiencies, X-linked SCID patients do not make effective antibody responses to most antigens, although their B cells appear normal. However, since the gene defect is on the X chromosome, one can determine whether the lack of B-cell function is solely caused by the lack of T-cell help by examining X-chromosome inactivation (see Section 10-7) in B cells of unaffected carriers. Naive IgM-positive B cells have inactivated the defective X chromosome more often than the normal one, showing that B-cell development is affected by, but not wholly dependent on, the common γ chain. However, mature memory B cells that have switched to isotypes other than IgM, carry an inactive defective X chromosome in most cells. This may reflect the fact that the IL-2 receptor γ chain is also part of the IL-4 receptor. Thus, B cells that lack this chain will have defective IL-4 receptors and will not proliferate in T-cell dependent antibody responses. X-linked SCID is so severe that children who inherit it can survive only in a completely pathogen-free environment, unless given antibodies and successfully treated by bone-marrow engraftment. A famous case in Houston became known as the 'bubble baby' because of the plastic bubble in which he was enclosed to protect him from infection.

The production of defects in several cytokine and cytokine receptor genes in gene knock-out mice is rapidly increasing our understanding of the role of individual cytokines in immunity. Mice lacking transforming growth factor-β (TGF-β) die of overwhelming inflammatory disease, while mice lacking IFN-γ or the IFN-γ receptor succumb to infection with a range of intracellular pathogens, including *M. tuberculosis*. Several human families have recently been identified with children who are susceptible to early onset mycobacterial infections and have a homozygous deficiency of the IFN-γ receptor.

10-13 | Bone marrow transplantation or gene therapy may be useful to correct genetic defects.

It is frequently possible to correct the defects in lymphocyte development that lead to the SCID phenotype by replacing the defective component, generally by bone marrow transplantation. The major difficulties in these therapies result from MHC polymorphism. To be useful, the graft must share some MHC alleles with the host. As we learned in Section 6-14, the MHC alleles expressed by the thymic epithelium determine which T cells can be positively selected. When bone marrow cells are used to restore immune function to individuals with a normal thymic stroma, both the T cells and the antigen-presenting cells are derived from the graft. Therefore, unless the graft shares at least some MHC alleles with the recipient, the T cells that are selected on host thymic epithelium cannot be activated by graft-derived antigen-presenting cells (Fig. 10.14).

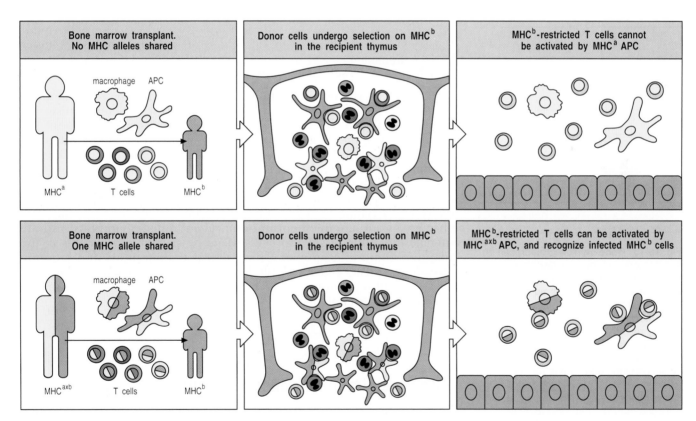

Fig. 10.14 Bone marrow donor and recipient must share at least some MHC molecules to restore immune function. If the bone marrow and the recipient thymus do not share any MHC alleles, T cells will mature in the thymus with receptors selected to recognize peptides presented by MHC molecules that are not expressed on the donor-derived antigen-presenting cells (APCs). These cells will not therefore be competent to mediate protective immunity (top panels). In the bottom panels, donor and recipient share the MHC^b allele, and T cells able to recognize MHC^b molecules are selected in the thymus. The antigen-presenting cells in the periphery can activate T cells that recognize MHC^b molecules; the activated T cells can then recognize infected MHC^b-bearing cells.

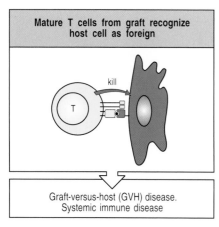

Graft-versus-host (GVH) disease. Systemic immune disease

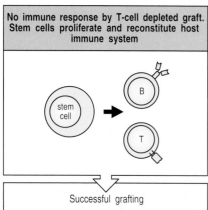

Successful grafting

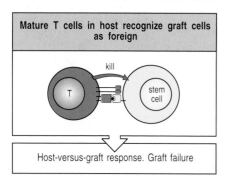

Host-versus-graft response. Graft failure

Fig. 10.15 Bone-marrow grafting can be used to correct immunodeficiencies caused by defects in lymphocyte maturation but two problems can arise. First, if there are mature T cells in the bone marrow, they can attack cells of the host by recognizing their MHC antigens, causing graft-versus-host disease (top panel). This can be prevented by T-cell depletion of the donor bone marrow (middle panel). Second, if the recipient has competent T cells, these may attack the bone marrow stem cells (bottom panel). This causes failure of the graft by the usual mechanism of transplant rejection (see Chapter 12).

There is also a danger that mature, post-thymic T cells in donor bone marrow may recognize the host as foreign and attack it, causing **graft-versus-host (GVH) disease** (Fig. 10.15). This can be overcome by depleting the donor bone marrow of mature T cells. In patients with the SCID phenotype, there is little problem with the host response to the graft, since the patient is immunodeficient.

Now that specific gene defects are being identified, a different approach to correcting these inherited immune deficiencies can be attempted. The strategy involves extracting a sample of the patients own bone marrow cells, inserting a normal copy of the defective gene into them, and returning them to the patient by transfusion. This approach, called **gene therapy**, should correct the gene defect. Moreover, in immunodeficient patients, it may be possible to re-infuse the bone marrow into the patient without the usual irradiation to suppress the recipient's bone marrow function. There is no risk of graft-versus-host immunity in this case, although it is possible that the host may respond to the replaced gene product and reject the engineered cells. Although this kind of approach is theoretically attractive, efficient transfer of genes into bone marrow stem cells is technically difficult and has been achieved only in mouse models. The few trials of gene therapy for correcting immunodeficiency, such as the treatment of a child with ADA deficiency at the National Institute of Health (NIH) in 1990, have used the patient's lymphocytes as the vehicle for gene introduction. However, because most lymphocytes are short-lived, the treatment has to be repeated regularly.

Summary.

Genetic defects can occur in almost any molecule involved in the immune response. These defects give rise to characteristic deficiency diseases, which, although rare, provide a great deal of information about the normal development and functioning of the immune system. Inherited immunodeficiencies illustrate the vital role played by the adaptive immune response, and in particular T cells, without which both cell-mediated and humoral immunity fail. They have provided information about the separate roles of B lymphocytes in humoral immunity, and the role of T lymphocytes in cell-mediated immunity the importance of phagocytes and complement in humoral and innate immunity and the specific functions of several cell-surface or signaling molecules in the adaptive immune response. There are also some inherited immune disorders whose causes we still do not understand. The study of these diseases will undoubtedly teach us more about the normal immune response and its control.

Acquired immune deficiency syndrome.

The first cases of the **acquired immune deficiency syndrome (AIDS)** were reported in 1981 but it is now clear that cases of the disease had been occurring unrecognized for about 4 years prior to its identification. The disease is characterized by susceptibility to infection with opportunistic pathogens, or the occurrence of an aggressive form of Kaposi's sarcoma or B-cell lymphoma, accompanied by a profound decrease in the number of CD4 T cells. As it appeared to be spread by contact with body fluids, it was early suspected to be caused by a new virus, and by 1983 the agent now known to be responsible for AIDS, called the **human immunodeficiency virus** (**HIV**), was isolated and identified. There are now known to be at least two types of HIV, HIV-1 and HIV-2, which share about 40% of their genome. HIV-2 is endemic in West Africa and is now spreading in India. Most AIDS worldwide, however, is caused by the more virulent HIV-1.

While the reason for the depletion of CD4 T cells in HIV and the issue of whether all HIV-infected patients will progress to overt disease remain controversial, accumulating evidence clearly implicates the growth of the virus and the immune response to it as the central keys to the puzzle of AIDS. HIV is now clearly a world pandemic and, while great strides are being made in understanding the pathogenesis and epidemiology of the disease, the number of infected people worldwide continues to grow at an alarming rate, presaging the death of many people from AIDS for many years to come (Fig. 10.16).

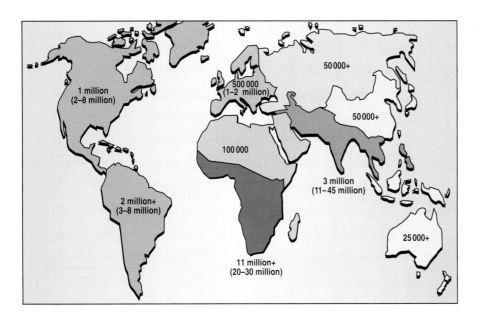

Fig. 10.16 HIV infection is spreading on all continents. The number of HIV-infected individuals is large (data are estimated total number of HIV infections by the end of 1994) and is increasing rapidly, especially in developing countries. Numbers in parentheses indicate the range of predictions for the total number of HIV infections from the beginning of the epidemic until the year 2000, in the major areas of infection.

10-14   Most individuals infected with HIV progress over time to AIDS.

Many viruses cause an acute but limited infection inducing lasting protective immunity. Others, such as herpes viruses, set up a latent infection that is not eliminated but is controlled adequately by an adaptive immune response. However, infection with HIV seems rarely, if ever, to lead to an immune response that can eliminate the virus. While the initial acute infection does seem to be controlled by the immune system, HIV continues to replicate rapidly and damages existing CD4 T cells all the time.

The initial infection with HIV generally occurs after transfer of bodily fluids from an infected person. The virus is carried in infected CD4 T cells and macrophages, and as a free virus in blood, semen, vaginal fluid, or milk. It is most commonly spread by sexual intercourse, contaminated needles used for intravenous drug delivery, and the therapeutic use of infected blood or blood products (although this last route of transmission has largely been eliminated in the developed world, where blood products are screened routinely for HIV). An important cause of virus transmission is from an infected mother to her baby at birth or through breast milk. In Africa, the perinatal transmission rate is approximately 25%, but this can largely be prevented by treating infected pregnant women with the drug zidovudine (AZT) (see Section 10-19). Mothers who are newly infected and breastfeed their infants transmit HIV 40% of the time, showing that HIV can also be transmitted in breast milk.

Primary infection with HIV is probably asymptomatic in most cases but sometimes causes a 'flu-like illness with an abundance of virus in the peripheral blood and a marked drop in the level of circulating CD4 T cells. This acute viremia is associated in virtually all patients with the activation of CD8 T cells, which kill HIV-infected cells, and subsequently by antibody production, or **seroconversion**. The cytotoxic T-cell response is thought to be important for controlling virus levels, which peak and then decline, as the CD4 T cell counts rebound to around 800 cells μl^{-1} (the normal value is 1200 cells μl^{-1}). At present, the best quantitative indicator of future disease is the level of virus that persists in the blood plasma once the symptoms of acute viremia have passed.

Fig. 10.17 Most HIV-infected individuals progress to AIDS over a period of years. The incidence of AIDS increases progressively with time after infection and is predicted to reach ~95% within 15 years, although data are only available for 12 years. Homosexuals and hemophiliacs are two of the groups at highest risk—homosexuals from sexually transmitted virus and hemophiliacs from infected human blood used to replace clotting factor VIII. Hemophiliacs are now protected by the screening of blood products and the use of recombinant factor VIII. Hemophiliacs who were over the age of 20 years at the time of infection and homosexual males progress to AIDS at the same rate, while younger hemophiliacs in some cases progress more rapidly. Neither homosexuals nor hemophiliacs who have not been infected with HIV show any evidence of AIDS. There are a few individuals who, while infected with HIV, appear not to have progressed to develop AIDS and may, in some way, be protected.

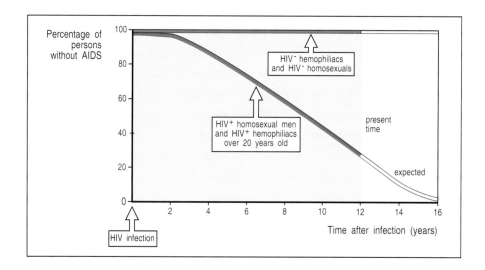

Most patients who are infected with HIV will eventually develop AIDS, after a period of apparent quiescence of the disease known as clinical latency or the asymptomatic period (Fig. 10.17). This period is not silent, however, for there is persistent replication of the virus, and a gradual decline in function and numbers of CD4 T cells until eventually patients have few CD4 T cells left. At this point, which can occur anywhere between 2 and 15 years or more after the primary infection, the period of clinical latency ends and opportunistic infections appear.

The typical course of an infection with HIV is illustrated in Fig. 10.18. However, it has become increasingly clear that the course of the disease can vary widely. Thus, while most people infected with HIV go on to develop AIDS and ultimately to die of opportunistic infection or cancer,

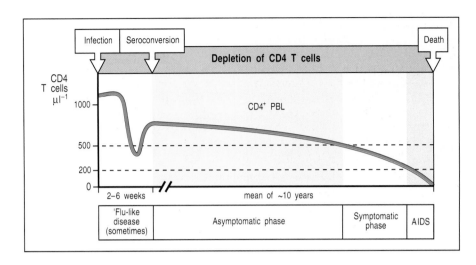

Fig. 10.18 The typical course of infection with HIV. The first few weeks are typified by an acute influenza-like viral illness, sometimes called seroconversion disease, with high titers of virus in the blood. An adaptive immune response follows, which controls the acute illness and largely restores levels of CD4 T cells (CD4$^+$ PBL) but does not eradicate the virus. Opportunistic infections and other symptoms become more frequent as the CD4 T-cell count falls, starting at around 500 cells μl^{-1}. The disease then enters the symptomatic phase. When CD4 T-cell counts fall below 200 cells μl^{-1} the patient is said to have AIDS. Note that CD4 T-cell counts are measured for clinical purposes in cells per microliter (μl^{-1}), rather than cells per milliliter (cells ml^{-1}) used elsewhere in this book.

this is not true of all individuals. One group comprises a small percentage of people who seroconvert, making antibodies to many HIV proteins, but who do not appear to have progressive disease, in that their CD4 T-cell counts and other measures of immune competence are maintained. These long-term non-progressors have unusually low levels of circulating virus and are being studied intensively to determine how they are able to control the infection with HIV. A second group consists of seronegative people who have been highly exposed to HIV, yet remain disease-free and virus-negative. Some of these individuals have specific cytotoxic lymphocytes and T$_H$1 lymphocytes directed against infected cells, which confirms that they have been exposed to HIV or possibly to non-infectious HIV antigens. Whether this immune response is responsible for clearing the infection is not clear, but it is a focus of considerable interest for the development and design of vaccines, which we discuss later. There is also evidence that some individuals are resistant to infection because they are genetically deficient in a chemokine receptor, CC-CKR-5, a co-receptor which allows the entry of HIV into macrophages and T cells.

Before going on to discuss in more detail the interactions of HIV with the immune system and the prospects for manipulating them, we must first describe the viral life cycle and the proteins on which it depends. Some of these proteins are the targets of the most successful drugs in use at present for the treatment of AIDS.

10-15   HIV is a retrovirus that infects CD4 T cells and macrophages.

HIV is an enveloped retrovirus. Each virus particle has two copies of an RNA genome, which are transcribed into DNA in the infected cell and integrated into the host cell chromosome. The RNA transcripts produced from the integrated viral DNA serve both as mRNA to direct the synthesis of the viral proteins and later as the RNA genomes of new viral particles, which escape from the cell by budding from the plasma membrane, each in a membrane envelope. The structure of the viral particle, or virion, is shown in Fig. 10.19.

HIV belongs to a group of retroviruses called the **lentiviruses**, from the Latin *lentus*, meaning slow, because of the gradual course of the

Fig. 10.19 The virion of human immunodeficiency virus (HIV). The virus illustrated is HIV-1. The other types of human immunodeficiency virus are similar in general structure. HIV-1 is the leading cause of AIDS. The reverse transcriptase, integrase, and viral protease enzymes are packaged in the virion and are shown schematically in the viral capsid. In reality, many molecules of these enzymes are contained in each virion. Some structural proteins of the virus have been omitted for simplicity. Photograph courtesy of H Gelderblom.

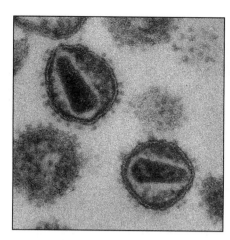

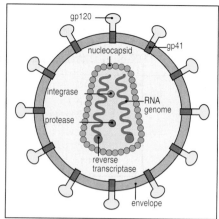

disease they cause. Although most of the cells producing HIV in AIDS patients are destroyed, it is still not clear whether this is a direct effect of the virus on the infected cell, or an indirect effect caused by the immune response to the virus. We shall return to this question later.

HIV enters cells by means of a complex of two noncovalently-associated viral glycoproteins, gp120 and gp41, in the viral envelope. The gp120 portion of the glycoprotein complex binds with high affinity to CD4 on the cell surface. This glycoprotein thereby draws the virus to CD4 T cells and to macrophages, which also express some CD4. The gp41 component then mediates fusion of the viral envelope with the plasma membrane of the cell, allowing the viral genome and associated viral proteins to enter the cytoplasm. Fusion and entry of the virus depends on the presence of a co-receptor in the membrane of the host cell. For laboratory strains of HIV, which are adapted for growth in T-cell lines and no longer able to infect macrophages, the co-factor has recently been identified as a G-protein-coupled receptor called LESTR (also called fusin) whose natural ligand is not known. This co-factor may also be used by primary HIV variants that induce cell-to-cell fusion of syncytia. Most isolates of HIV that are freshly derived from patients can infect macrophages as well as primary T cells however, and the co-receptor for these isolates has been shown to be a related seven-span receptor known as CC-CKR-5, which binds the CC chemokines RANTES, MIP-1α and MIP-1β (see Chapter 9). Since the ability to infect macrophages is determined by a loop of the gp120 envelope protein, which is thought to be exposed on binding to CD4, it seems likely that an interaction between this region of gp120 and one of these co-receptors is required for viral entry to take place.

Evidence is accumulating that macrophage-tropic isolates of HIV are preferentially transmitted by sexual contact and are the dominant viral phenotype found in newly infected individuals. Virus is disseminated from an initial reservoir of infected macrophages and there is evidence for an important role for mucosal lymphoid tissue in this process (see Section 10-21). Later in infection, the viral phenotype switches to a T-lymphocyte-tropic syncytium-inducing type, which is then followed by a rapid decline in CD4 count and progression to AIDS.

10-16   **Genetic deficiency of the macrophage chemokine co-receptor for HIV confers resistance to HIV infection *in vivo.***

Further evidence for the importance of chemokine receptors in HIV infection has come from studies in a small group of individuals with high risk exposure to HIV-1 but who remain seronegative. Lymphocytes and macrophages from these people were relatively resistant to macrophage-tropic HIV infection *in vitro* and were found to secrete high levels of RANTES, MIP-α and MIP-1β in response to inoculation with HIV. In other experiments, the addition of these chemokines to lymphocytes sensitive to HIV infection blocked their infection because of competition between the CC-chemokines, RANTES, MIP-1α, and MIP-1β and the virus for the CC-CKR-5 cell surface receptor.

The resistance of these rare individuals to HIV infection has now been explained by the discovery that they are homozygous for an allelic, non-functional variant of CC-CKR-5 which is caused by a 32 base-pair deletion from the coding region which leads to a frame shift and truncation of the translated protein. The gene frequency of this mutant allele in Caucasoid populations is quite high at .09 (meaning that approximately 10% of the Caucasoid population are heterozygous carriers of the allele and about 1% are homozygous). The mutant allele has not been found in Japanese or black Africans from Western or Central Africa. Studies of a large cohort of Caucasoid HIV positive patients showed no homozygotes for the mutant CC-CKR-5 allele and a 35% reduction in the frequency of hetero-zygotes compared with a matched population. This implied that even heterozygous deficiency of CC-CKR-5 may provide some protection against sexual transmission of HIV infection. These results provide a dramatic con-firmation of the experimental work suggesting that CC-CKR-5 is the major macrophage and T lymphocyte co-receptor for primary isolates of HIV and offers the possibility that primary infection may be blocked by therapeutic antagonists of the CC-CKR-5 receptor.

| 10-17 | **HIV RNA is transcribed by viral reverse transcriptase into DNA which integrates into the host cell genome.** |

One of the proteins that enters the cell with the viral genome is the viral reverse transcriptase, which transcribes the viral RNA into a comple-mentary DNA (cDNA) copy. The viral cDNA is then integrated into the host cell genome by the viral integrase, which also enters the cell with the viral RNA. The integrated cDNA copy is known as the **provirus**. The infectious cycle up to the integration of the provirus is shown in Fig. 10.20. HIV may, like other retroviruses, establish a latent infection in which the provirus remains quiescent, but it is not clear to what degree this occurs in HIV infection, as both the establishment of the provirus and its subsequent activation are favored by activation of the host cell. Furthermore, the viruses seen in infected individuals appear to be pro-duced, for the most part, by unbroken cycles of viral replication in newly infected cells.

The entire HIV genome consists of nine genes flanked by long terminal repeat sequences (LTR), which are required for integration of the provirus into the host cell DNA and contain binding sites for gene regu-latory proteins that control the expression of the viral genes. HIV shares with all other retroviruses three major genes, *gag*, *pol*, and *env*. The *gag* gene encodes the structural proteins of the viral core, the *pol* gene encodes the enzymes involved in viral replication and integration, and the *env* gene encodes the viral envelope glycoproteins. The *gag* and *pol* mRNAs are translated to give polyproteins—long polypeptide chains that are then cleaved by the viral protease (also encoded by *pol*) into individual functional proteins. The product of the *env* gene, gp160, has to be cleaved by a host-cell protease into gp120 and gp41, which are then assembled into the **viral envelope**. The other six genes encode

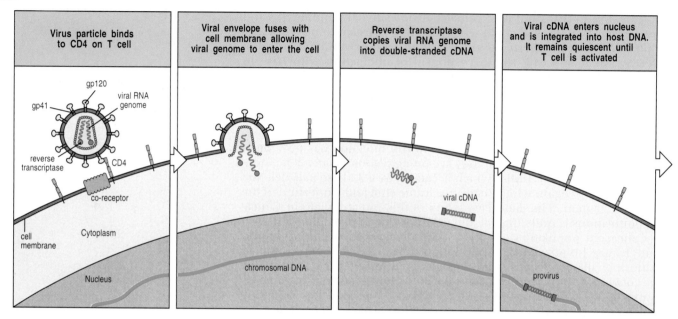

| Virus particle binds to CD4 on T cell | Viral envelope fuses with cell membrane allowing viral genome to enter the cell | Reverse transcriptase copies viral RNA genome into double-stranded cDNA | Viral cDNA enters nucleus and is integrated into host DNA. It remains quiescent until T cell is activated |

Fig. 10.20 The life cycle of HIV in CD4 T cells. The virus binds to CD4 using gp120:gp41, then mediates fusion with the target cell by a mechanism requiring the presence of a specific seven-span chemokine co-receptor at the surface of the cell.

Once in the cytoplasm, the RNA genome is reverse transcribed into double-stranded cDNA, which migrates to the nucleus and is integrated into the cell genome, where it is called a provirus.

proteins that affect viral replication and infectivity in various ways that we discuss in the next sections. The viral genes and the functions of their products are summarized in Fig. 10.21.

Fig. 10.21 The genes and proteins of HIV-1. Like all retroviruses, HIV-1 has an RNA genome flanked by long terminal repeats (LTR) involved in viral integration and in regulation of the viral genome. The genome can be read in three frames and several of the viral genes overlap in different reading frames. This allows the virus to encode many proteins in a small genome. The three main protein products, Gag, Pol, and Env, are synthesized by all infectious retroviruses. The known functions of the different genes and their products are listed. The products of *gag*, *pol* and *env* are known to be present in the mature viral particle, together with the viral RNA. The mRNAs for Tat and Rev proteins are produced by splicing of viral transcripts, so their genes are split in the viral genome. The other gene products affect the infectivity of the virus in various ways that are not fully understood.

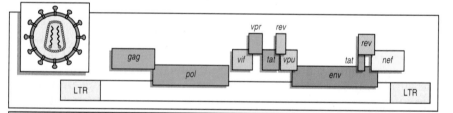

Gene		Gene product/function
gag	Group-specific antigen	Core protein
pol	Polymerase	Reverse transcriptase, protease, and integrase enzymes
env	Envelope	Transmembrane glycoproteins. gp120 binds CD4; gp41 is required for virus internalization
tat	Transactivator	Positive regulator of transcription
rev	Regulator of viral expression	Allows export of unspliced transcripts from nucleus
vif	Viral infectivity	Affects particle infectivity; helps assemble virions?
vpr	Viral protein R	Positive regulator of transcription. Augments virion production
vpu	Viral protein U	Unique to HIV-1. Downregulates CD4
nef	So-called negative-regulation factor	Augments viral replication *in vivo* and *in vitro*. Downregulates CD4

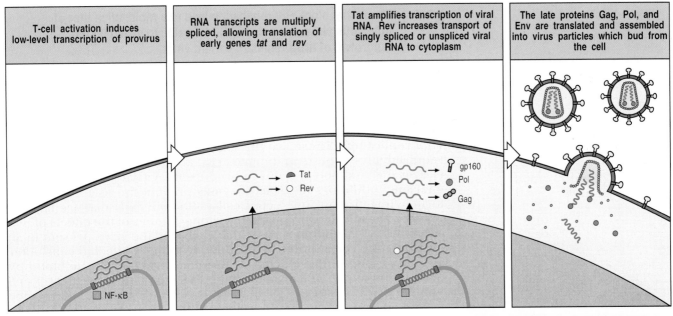

T-cell activation induces low-level transcription of provirus	RNA transcripts are multiply spliced, allowing translation of early genes *tat* and *rev*	Tat amplifies transcription of viral RNA. Rev increases transport of singly spliced or unspliced viral RNA to cytoplasm	The late proteins Gag, Pol, and Env are translated and assembled into virus particles which bud from the cell

10-18   Transcription of the HIV provirus depends on host-cell transcription factors induced upon activation of infected T cells.

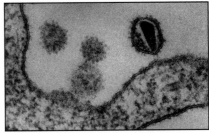

Fig. 10.22 Cells infected with HIV must be activated to replicate the virus. Activation of CD4 T cells induces the expression of the transcription factor NF-κB, which binds to the proviral LTR and initiates transcription of the HIV genome into RNA. The viral RNA encodes several regulatory proteins. Tat both enhances transcription from the provirus, and also binds to the RNA transcripts, stabilizing them in a form that can be translated. The protein Rev binds the RNA transcripts and transports them to the cytosol. The viral RNA also encodes the structural proteins that are required for the production of new viral particles. Early in the infectious cycle, levels of Rev are low and the transcript is retained in the nucleus and processed extensively: this produces mRNAs encoding the regulatory proteins, such as Tat, which are required for viral replication. Later, as levels of Rev increase, Rev acts to transport less extensively spliced and unspliced transcripts out of the nucleus. The spliced transcripts encode the structural proteins of the virus and the unspliced transcripts, which are the new viral genomes, are packaged with these to form many new virus particles. Photograph courtesy of H Gelderblom.

The production of infectious virus particles from an integrated HIV provirus is stimulated by a cellular transcription factor that is present in all activated T cells. Activation of CD4 T cells induces the transcription factor NF-κB, which binds to promoters not only in the cellular DNA but also in the viral LTR, thereby initiating transcription of viral RNA by the cellular RNA polymerase. This transcript is spliced in various ways to produce mRNAs for the viral proteins. At least two of the viral genes, *tat* and *rev*, encode proteins, **Tat** and **Rev** respectively, which promote viral replication in activated T cells. Tat is a potent transcriptional regulator that binds to an RNA sequence in the LTR known as the transcriptional activation region (TAR) and greatly enhances the rate of viral genome transcription.

The *rev* gene also has a complex function. It makes a protein that binds to a sequence called RRE in the RNA transcript of HIV, which controls delivery of the RNA to the cytoplasm. To express the Tat and Rev proteins, the viral transcripts must be spliced twice, while for other viral proteins only one splicing event is required. When the provirus is first activated, Rev levels are low, the transcripts are translocated slowly from the nucleus and thus multiple splicing events can occur. Later, when Rev levels have increased, the transcripts are translocated rapidly from the nucleus unspliced or only singly spliced. In the early stages, Tat is required to make multiple transcripts of the proviral genome. At later stages, the structural components of the viral core and envelope are needed, together with the reverse transcriptase, the integrase, and the viral protease, to make new viral particles. Complete, unspliced transcripts must also be exported from the nucleus for translation of *gag* and *pol*, and to be packaged with the proteins as the RNA genomes of the new virus particles (Fig. 10.22).

10-19 | **Drugs that block HIV replication lead to a rapid fall in titer of infectious virus and a rise in CD4 T cells, followed by the outgrowth of drug-resistant variant virus.**

Studies using drugs that are potent enough to block the cycle of HIV replication completely, indicate that the virus is replicating rapidly at all phases of infection, including the asymptomatic phase. Two viral proteins in particular have been the target of drugs aimed at arresting viral replication. These are the viral reverse transcriptase, which is required for synthesis of the provirus, and the viral protease, which cleaves the viral polyproteins to produce the virion proteins and viral enzymes. Inhibitors of these enzymes prevent the establishment of further infection in uninfected cells, although cells that are already infected can continue to produce virions. Studies of the effects of two of the protease inhibitors show that almost all the virus present in an individual's circulation is the product of recently infected cells. After as little as 2 days, these drugs can reduce viral titer in the blood by 100-fold or more. At the same time, there is a surge in CD4 T-cell numbers, which suggests that CD4 T cells are continuously being produced and just as rapidly being infected by HIV. These drugs thereby reveal that the viral load and CD4 T-cell numbers at any point in time represent a dynamic equilibrium between the rapid production of virus causing the destruction of CD4 T cells, and the clearance of virus and replacement of CD4 cells by the immune system. The studies also indicate that virus production from cells that were latently infected and subsequently activated, and virus production from long-lived chronically infected cells contribute less than 1% of the population of virions that are released into the blood (Fig. 10.23).

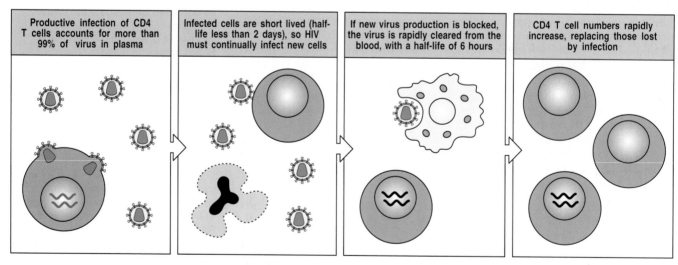

| Productive infection of CD4 T cells accounts for more than 99% of virus in plasma | Infected cells are short lived (half-life less than 2 days), so HIV must continually infect new cells | If new virus production is blocked, the virus is rapidly cleared from the blood, with a half-life of 6 hours | CD4 T cell numbers rapidly increase, replacing those lost by infection |

Fig. 10.23   Production and clearance of virus particles. In patients infected with HIV, there is continuous production of virus particles and continuous infection of new cells. Even in asymptomatic HIV-infected individuals, virus particles are continually being produced from productively infected CD4 T cells (first panel). If this new virus production is arrested, for example with drugs that block virus replication or interfere with the production of viral proteins, the infected cells die quickly—the half-life of these cells is around one and a half days (second panel). The virus itself disappears even more rapidly from the circulation, with a half-life of some 6 hours, being opsonized by antibody and complement and phagocytosed (third panel). The sustained production of viral particles in patients must therefore be due to a continuous process of infection of CD4 T cells. When HIV replication is arrested and new infections cease, the number of CD4 cells in the circulation increases rapidly, replacing those that have been lost to infection (fourth panel). Thus rather than being a static process, in which infected cells are removed slowly and the immune competence of the patient slowly declines, HIV appears to be a dynamic disease, in which infected cells die rapidly but are equally rapidly replaced with a fresh cohort of CD4 cells, which in turn become infected and thus sustain virus production.

These studies raise two questions. First, what is happening to all the virus that was in the blood originally: how is infectious virus removed so rapidly from the circulation? It seems most likely that infectious HIV particles are opsonized by specific antibody and removed by phagocytic cells of the mononuclear phagocytic system. Opsonized HIV particles may also be trapped on the surface of follicular dendritic cells, which are known to capture antigen:antibody complexes and retain them for prolonged periods (see Chapters 8 and 9). Second, what is the source of the new CD4 T cells that appear once treatment is started? It seems highly unlikely that these are the recent progeny of stem cells that have developed in the thymus, because CD4 T cells are not normally produced in large numbers from the thymus even at its maximum rate of production in adolescents. Some investigators believe that these cells are emerging from sites of sequestration and add little to the total numbers of CD4 T cells in the body, while others advocate their origin from mature CD4 T cells that replicate. Answers to both of these questions are now sought eagerly.

As the anti-viral drugs continue to be administered, the virus becomes resistant to their effects, probably because of the expansion of variants in the original viral population, which carry mutations conferring resistance. Resistance to some of the protease inhibitors appears after only a few days. Resistance to the reverse transcriptase inhibitor zidovudine, the drug most widely used for treating AIDS, takes months to develop. This is because resistance to zidovudine requires three or four mutations in the viral reverse transcriptase, whereas a single mutation can confer resistance to the protease inhibitors and other reverse transcriptase inhibitors. As a result of the relatively rapid appearance of resistance to all known anti-HIV drugs, successful drug treatment may depend upon the development of a range of anti-viral drugs that can be used in combination, thereby destroying the virus before any one strain has had a chance to accumulate all the necessary mutations to resist the entire cocktail.

10-20 | HIV accumulates many mutations in the course of infection in a single individual.

The rapid replication of HIV contributes to the very high mutation rate that generates the many variants of HIV that arise in a single infected patient in the course of infection. Replication of a retroviral genome depends upon two error-prone steps. Reverse transcriptase lacks the proofreading mechanisms associated with cellular DNA polymerases and the RNA genomes of retroviruses are therefore copied into DNA with relatively low fidelity; the transcription of the proviral DNA into RNA copies by the cellular RNA polymerase is a similarly low-fidelity process. A rapidly replicating persistent virus that is going through these two steps repeatedly in the course of an infection can thereby accumulate many mutations, and numerous variants of HIV, sometimes called quasi-species, are found within a single infected individual. This very high variability was first recognized in HIV and has since proved to be common to the other lentiviruses.

The generation of many mutants of HIV poses a problem for the design of vaccines aimed at eliciting neutralizing antibodies, and may also contribute to the failure of the immune system to contain the infection in the long term. In some cases, for example, variant peptides produced by the virus have been found to act as antagonists (see Section 4-30) for T cells responsive to the wild-type epitope, thus allowing both mutant and wild-type viruses to survive. Mutant peptides acting as antagonists have also been reported in hepatitis B virus infections, and similar mutant peptides may contribute to the persistence of some viral infections, especially where, as often happens, the immune response of an individual is dominated by T cells specific for a particular epitope.

10-21 | Replication of HIV has been observed in both lymphoid and mucosal tissue.

Although viral load is usually measured by detecting viral RNA in the blood, the highest viral load is in the lymph nodes, where most lymphocytes are found. Much of the viral RNA detected in lymph nodes is caused by virions trapped on the surface of dendritic follicular cells; however, productively infected cells can also be seen, usually in the paracortical T-cell area. The analysis of individual spleen white pulps show that some but not all contain virus, which appears to have expanded and diversified from one or few viral variants within each individual pulp. Viral replication may have originated from a latently infected memory CD4 T cell that became activated in response to antigen presentation in the lymph node. It could then have spread by rounds of replication in other activated CD4 T cells.

Active replication of HIV has also been observed at the mucosal surface of the enlarged adenoids removed from otherwise asymptomatic HIV-infected individuals. In this case, replication was detected by staining for a viral protein, p24, in giant dendritic cell syncytia found in the mucosal epithelium that surrounds the adenoid itself. Similar syncytia form when HIV is added to cultures of CD4 T cells and dendritic cells that have migrated out of normal skin explants, and these syncytia, which bear markers of both dendritic cells and T cells, are the source of the efficient HIV replication seen in these cultures. Studies of the relevance of these findings to HIV replication *in vivo* are still at an early stage, but the findings on HIV replication in the adenoid mucosa suggest that mucosal epithelia, which are constantly exposed to foreign antigens, provide a milieu in which HIV replication occurs readily. The T cells that migrate through the mucosa and epithelia and enter the lymph nodes, along with antigen-presenting cells via the afferent lymph, bear the phenotype of memory CD4 T cells; several studies have suggested that memory CD4 T cells are particularly susceptible to infection by HIV.

Macrophages, which are also infected by HIV, seem to be able to harbor replicating virus without necessarily being killed by it, and are believed to be an important reservoir of infection, as well as a means of spreading virus to other tissues such as the brain. Although the function of macrophages as antigen-presenting cells does not seem to be compromised by HIV infection, it is thought that the virus may cause abnormal patterns of cytokine secretion that could account for the wasting that commonly occurs in AIDS patients.

10-22 | An immune response controls but does not eliminate HIV.

Infection with HIV generates an adaptive immune response that contains the virus but usually cannot eliminate it. The time course of various elements in the adaptive immune response to HIV is shown, with the levels of infectious virus in plasma, in Fig. 10.24.

Seroconversion is the clearest evidence for an adaptive immune response to infection with HIV but the generation of T lymphocytes responding to infected cells is thought by most people to be central in controlling the infection. Both CD8 cytotoxic T cells and T_H1 cells specifically responsive to infected cells are associated with the decline in detectable virus after the initial infection. These T-cell responses are unable to clear the

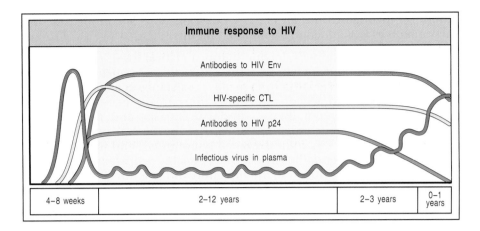

Fig. 10.24 The immune response to HIV. Infectious virus is present at relatively low levels in the peripheral blood of infected individuals during a prolonged asymptomatic phase but is replicated persistently in lymphoid tissues. During this period, CD4 T-cell counts gradually decline, although antibodies and CD8 cytotoxic T cells directed against the virus remain at high levels. Two different antibody responses are shown in the figure, one to the envelope protein (Env) of HIV, and one to the core protein p24. Eventually, the levels of antibody and HIV-specific cytotoxic T lymphocytes (CTLs) also fall, and there is a progressive increase of infectious HIV in the peripheral blood.

infection completely and may cause some pathology. Nonetheless, there is evidence that the virus is itself cytopathic, and T-cell responses that reduce viral spread should therefore, on balance, reduce the pathology of the disease.

Strong circumstantial evidence for destruction of infected cells by cytotoxic lymphocytes comes from studies of peripheral blood cells from infected individuals, in which cytotoxic T cells specific for viral peptides can be shown to kill infected cells *in vitro*. In one striking case, rapid progression of the disease was associated with the appearance of viruses expressing mutant peptides followed by the appearance of cytotoxic T cells capable of recognizing these mutant peptides and a rapid loss of CD4 T cells. CD8 T cells specific for HIV-infected cells in a given patient often have a single dominant Vβ-chain gene rearrangement that enables them to be identified. Using such a dominant Vβ rearrangement as a marker for HIV-specific cytotoxic cells, it has been possible to show that these cells have infiltrated infected splenic white pulps, suggesting that the splenic white pulps are sites where replication of HIV within infected CD4 T cells and elimination of infected cells by cytotoxic CD8 T cells occur simultaneously. Whatever the mechanism, the result of HIV infection in the lymphoid tissues is the gradual disruption of the lymphoid architecture, leading eventually to the destruction of the lymphoid follicles in the late stages of the disease.

10-23   HIV infection leads to low levels of CD4 T cells, increased susceptibility to opportunistic infection, and eventually to death.

The way in which HIV kills CD4 T cells is still being debated; the only fact on which all parties agree is that it does. There are probably three dominant mechanisms. First, there is evidence for direct viral killing of infected cells; second, there is increased susceptibility to the induction of apoptosis in infected cells; and third, there is killing of infected CD4 T cells by CD8 cytotoxic lymphocytes that recognize viral peptides.

In addition, the binding of CD4 by gp120 may damage CD4 T cells, even if they are not actually infected with HIV. There is some experimental support for this; CD4 T cells from HIV-infected patients are more susceptible to apoptosis driven by receptor crosslinking, and this effect can be replicated in normal CD4 T cells *in vitro* by crosslinking CD4 either with anti-CD4 or with gp120 complexed with anti-gp120. Moreover, memory CD4 T cells have been shown to be much more susceptible to

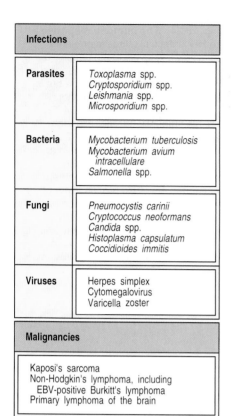

Infections	
Parasites	*Toxoplasma* spp. *Cryptosporidium* spp. *Leishmania* spp. *Microsporidium* spp.
Bacteria	*Mycobacterium tuberculosis* *Mycobacterium avium* *intracellulare* *Salmonella* spp.
Fungi	*Pneumocystis carinii* *Cryptococcus neoformans* *Candida* spp. *Histoplasma capsulatum* *Coccidioides immitis*
Viruses	Herpes simplex Cytomegalovirus Varicella zoster

Malignancies
Kaposi's sarcoma Non-Hodgkin's lymphoma, including   EBV-positive Burkitt's lymphoma Primary lymphoma of the brain

Fig. 10.25   A variety of opportunistic pathogens and cancers can kill AIDS patients. Infections are the major cause of death in AIDS, with respiratory infection with *Pneumocystis carinii* being the most prominent. Most of these pathogens require effective macrophage activation by CD4 T cells or effective cytotoxic T cells for host defense. Opportunistic pathogens are present in the normal environment but cause severe disease primarily in immunocompromised hosts, like AIDS patients and cancer patients. AIDS patients are also susceptible to several rare cancers, such as Kaposi's sarcoma and lymphomas, suggesting that immune surveillance by T cells may normally prevent such tumors (see Chapter 13).

inhibition through CD4 than naive T cells, perhaps accounting for the early effects of HIV infection on memory T cells.

When CD4 T-cell numbers decline below a critical level, cell-mediated immunity is lost, and infections with a variety of opportunistic infectious agents appear (Fig. 10.25). Typically, resistance is lost early to oral *Candida* spp. and to *Mycobacterium tuberculosis*, manifesting as an increased prevalence of thrush (oral candidiasis) and tuberculosis. Later, patients suffer from shingles, caused by the activation of latent herpes zoster, from EBV-induced B-cell lymphomas, and from Kaposi's sarcoma, a tumor of endothelial cells that probably represents a response both to cytokines produced in the infection and to a novel herpes virus called HHV8 that was recently identified in these lesions. *Pneumocystis carinii* pneumonia is an important cause of opportunistic infection. Finally, cytomegalovirus or infection with *Mycobacterium avium* complex are more prominent. It is important to note that not all patients with AIDS get all these infections or tumors, and there are other tumors and infections that are less prominent but still significant. Rather, this is a list of opportunistic infections and tumors, most of which are normally controlled by robust CD4 T-cell mediated immunity that wanes as the CD4 T cell counts drop toward zero (see Fig. 10.18).

10-24   Vaccination against HIV is an attractive solution but poses many difficulties.

The development of a safe and effective vaccine for the prevention of HIV infection and AIDS is an attractive goal but its development is fraught with difficulties that have not been faced in vaccination campaigns against other diseases. The first problem is that there is no exact animal model that can be used to test for successful vaccination against HIV, nor can the efficacy of vaccines be studied readily in humans. One model system is based on simian immunodeficiency virus (SIV), which is closely related to HIV and which infects macaques. SIV causes a closely similar disease to AIDS in Asian macaques such as the cynomolgus monkey, but does not cause disease in African macaques such as African green monkeys, with which it has probably co-existed for up to a million years. The variability of SIV infection between different species of monkeys emphasizes the potential difficulties in extrapolating the results of vaccine trials in macaques to trials in humans.

The second problem is that it is not clear what would be required to establish immunity to HIV. Whereas most infections elicit an immune response that can provide lasting protection, pathogens such as HIV that persist in spite of a vigorous immune response pose special problems. These are compounded in the case of HIV by the state of immunodeficiency that progressively results from the infection itself. This makes particularly interesting those rare patients who have been exposed often enough to make it virtually certain that they should have become infected but who have not developed the disease. These individuals are a focus of considerable interest to AIDS researchers but the explanation for their resistance to HIV is not yet clear. Some studies suggest that such people were initially infected by a mutant of HIV that lacks one or more gene products essential for establishing HIV infection, while others suggest a possible durable resistance to HIV infection based on CD8 T cells.

A further important question is the type of immunity one wishes to induce by vaccination. It seems likely that the most desirable type of response would be dominated by CD8 T cells and/or T$_H$1 cells. AIDS patients tend to produce cytokines typical of T$_H$2 cells, while CD4 T-cell responses to

HIV peptides in infected but still healthy individuals tend to be dominated by T_H1 cytokines. The accuracy and significance of this observation is still debated by AIDS researchers. In any case, methods have yet to be devised for designing vaccines that reliably elicit a desired type of immune response, as we discuss in Chapter 13.

Attempts have been made to design so-called subunit vaccines, which induce immunity to only some proteins in the virus, and one such vaccine has been made from the envelope protein gp120. However, when tested on chimpanzees, this vaccine proved to be specific to the precise strain of virus used to make it, and therefore useless in protection against natural infection.

Finally, there are difficult ethical issues in the development of a vaccine, as seems to be true of all aspects of this deadly disease. It would be unethical to conduct a vaccine trial without trying at the same time to minimize the exposure of a vaccinated population to the virus itself. However, the effectiveness of a vaccine can only be assessed in a population in which the exposure rate to the virus is high enough to assess whether vaccination is protective against infection. This means that initial vaccine trials may have to be conducted in countries where the incidence of infection is very high and public health measures have not yet succeeded in reducing the spread of HIV. An additional ethical problem is that any vaccine trial would need to have a placebo control and participants in any vaccine study would have to be fully informed that they may receive placebo rather than an active vaccine. These ethical and moral issues are a further impediment to the development of a new vaccine against HIV. Despite these experimental and ethical difficulties, there is reason to hope that the problem of HIV infection leading to AIDS will soon be met by a combination of several strategies. Therapy with a combination of anti-viral drugs, together with recombinant-derived chemokine analogs can be used for treatment, while a successful vaccine should ultimately be developed.

10-25   Prevention and education are one way in which the spread of HIV and AIDS can be controlled.

The one way in which we know we can protect against infection with HIV is by avoiding contact with bodily fluids, such as semen, blood, blood products, or milk, from people who are infected. Indeed, it has been demonstrated repeatedly that this precaution, simple enough in the developed world, is sufficient to prevent infection, as health care workers can take care of AIDS patients for long periods without sero-conversion or signs of infection.

For this strategy to work, however, two things are necessary. First, one must be able to test people at risk of infection with HIV periodically, so that they can take the kind of steps necessary to avoid passing the virus to others. For this to work, strict confidentiality is absolutely required. One intelligent suggestion to emerge from President Reagan's AIDS Advisory Group was that before anything could be accomplished in the fight against AIDS, the rights of HIV-infected people would have to be guaranteed in all aspects of life. This step, unfortunately, was never taken.

A barrier to the control of HIV is the reluctance of individuals to find out whether they are infected, especially as one of the consequences of a positive HIV test is stigmatization by society. As a result, infected individuals may unwittingly infect many others. Responsibility is at the heart of AIDS prevention, and a law guaranteeing the rights of people infected with HIV might go a long way to encouraging such behavior. The rights of HIV-infected people are protected in the Netherlands and Sweden. The problem in the less-developed nations, where elementary health precautions are also virtually impossible to establish, is more profound.

☐ Summary.

Infection with the human immunodeficiency virus (HIV) is the cause of acquired immune deficiency syndrome (AIDS). This worldwide epidemic is now spreading at an alarming rate, especially through heterosexual contact in less-developed countries. HIV is an enveloped retrovirus that replicates in cells of the immune system. Viral entry requires the presence of CD4 and a particular chemokine receptor, and the viral cycle is dependent on transcription factors found in activated T cells. Infection with HIV causes loss of CD4 T cells and an acute viremia that rapidly subsides as cytotoxic T-cell responses develop, but HIV infection is not eliminated by this immune response. HIV establishes a state of persistent infection in which the virus is continually replicating in newly infected cells, and responds only briefly to the anti-viral drugs developed to date. These anti-viral agents cause a rapid drop in virus levels and a rise in CD4 T-cell counts but virus variants resistant to the drug are rapidly selected, and former levels of virus production are regained. The use of a combination of drugs may be able to overcome this problem. The main effect of HIV infection is the destruction of CD4 T cells, but there is still no agreement about how they are destroyed, whether by a direct cytopathic effect of HIV infection, or indirectly by CD8 cytotoxic T cells, or both. As the CD4 T-cell counts wane, the body becomes progressively more susceptible to opportunistic infection with intracellular microbes. Eventually, most HIV-infected individuals develop AIDS and die; some people (3–7%), however, remain healthy for many years, with no apparent ill effects of infection. It is hoped that one can learn from such individuals ways in which infection with HIV can be controlled successfully. Analysis of such people appears to be one route to an effective vaccine for HIV.

☐ Summary to Chapter 10.

While most infections elicit protective immunity, most successful pathogens have developed some means of evading a fully effective immune response and some result in serious, persistent disease. In addition, some individuals have inherited deficiencies in different components of the immune system, making them highly susceptible to certain classes of infectious agents. Persistent infection and immunodeficiency illustrate the importance of effective host defense and present huge challenges for future immunological research. The human immunodeficiency virus (HIV) combines the characteristics of a persistent infectious agent with the ability to create immunodeficiency in its human host, a combination that is usually lethal to the patient. The key to fighting new pathogens like HIV is to develop more fully our understanding of the basic properties of the immune system and its role in combating infection.

General references.

Haynes, B.F., Pantaleo, G., and Fauci, A.S.: **Toward an understanding of the correlates of protective immunity to HIV infection.** *Science* 1996, **271**:324-328.

Mims, C.A.: *The Pathogenesis of Infectious Disease.* London, Academic Press, 1987.

Moller, G. (ed.): **Genetic basis of primary immunodeficiencies.** *Immunol. Rev.* 1994, **138**:1-221.

Moller, G. (ed.): **HIV and its receptors.** *Immunol. Rev.* 1994, **140**:1-171.

Rosen, F.S., Cooper, M.D., and Wedgwood, R.J.: **The primary immunodeficiencies.** *N. Engl. J. Med.* 1995, **333**:431-440.

Pantaleo, G., and Fauci, A.S.: **New concepts in the immunopathogenesis of HIV infection.** *Ann. Rev. Immunol.* 1995, **13**:487-512.

Section references.

10-1 Antigenic variation can allow pathogens to escape from immunity.

Borst, P.: **Molecular genetics of antigenic variation.** *Immunol. Today* 1991, **12**:A29-A33.

Clegg, S., Hancox, L.S., and Yeh, K.S.: **Salmonella typhimurium fimbrial phase variation and FimA expression.** *J. Bacteriol.* 1996, **178**:542-545.

Gorman, O.T., Bean, W.J., and Webster, R.G.: **Evolutionary processes in influenza viruses: divergence, rapid evolution, and stasis.** *Curr. Top. Microbiol. Immunol.* 1992, **176**:75-97.

Meyer, T.F.: **Evasion mechanisms of pathogenic Neisseriae.** *Behring. Inst. Mitt.* 1991, 194-199.

Pays, E., Vanhamme, L., and Berberof, M.: **Genetic controls for the expression of surface antigens in African trypanosomes.** *Ann. Rev. Microbiol.* 1994, **48**:25-52.

Seifert, H.S., Wright, C.J., Jerse, A.E., Cohen, M.S., and Cannon, J.G.: **Multiple gonococcal pilin antigenic variants are produced during experimental human infections.** *J. Clin. Invest.* 1994, **93**:2744-2749.

Shu, L.L., Bean, W.J., and Webster, R.G.: **Analysis of the evolution and variation of the human influenza A virus nucleoprotein gene from 1933 to 1990.** *J. Virol.* 1993, **67**:2723-2729.

Swanson, J., Belland, R.J., and Hill, S.A.: **Neisserial surface variation: how and why?** *Curr. Opin. Genet. Dev.* 1992, **2**:805-811.

Webster, R.G., Bean, W.J., Gorman, O.T., Chambers, T.M., and Kawaoka, Y.: **Evolution and ecology of influenza A viruses.** *Microbiol. Rev.* 1992, **56**:152-179.

Zhou, N., He, S., Zhang, T., Zou, W., Shu, L., Sharp, G.B., and Webster, R.G.: **Influenza infection in humans and pigs in southeastern China.** *Arch. Virol.* 1996, **141**:649-661.

10-2 Some viruses persist *in vivo* by ceasing to replicate until immunity wanes.

Bruggeman, C.A.: **Cytomegalovirus and latency: an overview.** *Virchows Arch. B. Cell Pathol. Incl. Mol. Pathol.* 1993, **64**:325-333.

Ehrlich, R.: **Selective mechanisms utilized by persistent and oncogenic viruses to interfere with antigen processing and presentation.** *Immunol. Res.* 1995, **14**:77-97.

Fraser, N.W. and Valyi Nagy, T.: **Viral, neuronal and immune factors which may influence herpes simplex virus (HSV) latency and reactivation.** *Microb. Pathog.* 1993, **15**:83-91.

Garcia Blanco, M.A., and Cullen, B.R.: **Molecular basis of latency in pathogenic human viruses.** *Science* 1991, **254**:815-820.

Ho, D.Y.: **Herpes simplex virus latency: molecular aspects.** *Prog. Med. Virol.* 1992, **39**:76-115.

Kadin, M.E.: **Pathology of Hodgkin's disease.** *Curr. Opin. Oncol.* 1994, **6**:456-463.

Steiner, I., and Kennedy, P.G.: **Molecular biology of herpes simplex virus type 1 latency in the nervous system.** *Mol. Neurobiol.* 1993, **7**:137-159.

10-3 Some pathogens resist destruction by host defense mechanisms or exploit them for their own purposes.

Alcami, A., and Smith, G.L.: **Cytokine receptors encoded by poxviruses: a lesson in cytokine biology.** *Immunol. Today* 1995, **16**:474-478.

Hall, B.F., and Joiner, K.A.: **Strategies of obligate intracellular parasites for evading host defences.** *Immunol. Today* 1991, **12**:A22-A27.

Joiner, K.A.: **Vacuolar membranes surrounding intracellular pathogens: where do they come from and what do they do?** *Infect. Agents Dis.* 1993, **2**:215-219.

Nocton, J.J., and Steere, A.C.: **Lyme disease.** *Adv. Intl. Med.* 1995, **40**:69-117.

Smith, G.L.: **Virus strategies for evasion of the host response to infection.** *Trends Microbiol.* 1994, **2**:81-88.

10-4 Immunosuppression or inappropriate immune responses can contribute to persistent disease.

Bloom, B.R., Modlin, R.L., and Salgame, P.: **Stigma variations: observations on suppressor T cells and leprosy.** *Ann. Rev. Immunol.* 1992, **10**:453-488.

Fleischer, B.: **Superantigens.** *APMIS* 1994, **102**:3-12.

Rott, O. and Fleischer, B.: **A superantigen as virulence factor in an acute bacterial infection.** *J. Infect. Dis.* 1994, **169**:1142-1146.

Salgame, P., Abrams, J.S., Clayberger, C., Goldstein, H., Convit, J., Modlin, R.L., and Bloom, B.R.: **Differing lymphokine profiles of functional subsets of human CD4 and CD8 T cell clones.** *Science* 1991, **254**:279-282.

10-5 Immune responses can contribute directly to pathogenesis.

Golovkina, T.V., Dudley, J.P., Jaffe, A.B., and Ross, S.R.: **Mouse mammary tumor viruses with functional superantigen genes are selected during** *in vivo* **infection.** *Proc. Natl. Acad. Sci.* 1995, **92**:4828-4832.

Openshaw, P.J.: **Immunity and immunopathology to respiratory syncytial virus. The mouse model.** *Am. J. Resp. Crit. Care Med.* 1995, **152**:S59-S62.

Openshaw, P.J.: **Immunopathological mechanisms in respiratory syncytial virus disease.** *Springer Semin. Immunopath.* 1995, **17**:187-201.

Zinkernagel, R.M., Haenseler, E., Leist, T., Cerny, A., Hengartner, H., and Althage, A.: **T cell-mediated hepatitis in mice infected with lymphocytic choriomeningitis virus. Liver cell destruction by H-2 class I-restricted virus-specific cytotoxic T cells as a physiological correlate of the 51Cr-release assay** *J. Exp. Med* .1986, **164**:1075-1092.

10-6 Inherited immunodeficiency diseases are caused by recessive gene defects.

Conley, M.E.: **Molecular approaches to analysis of X-linked immunodeficiencies.** *Ann. Rev. Immunol.* 1992, **10**:215-238.

Conley, M.E.: **Primary immunodeficiencies: a flurry of new genes.** *Immunol. Today* 1995, **16**:313-315.

Fischer, A.: **Primary T-cell immunodeficiencies.** *Curr. Opin. Immunol.* 1993, **5**:569-578.

Fischer, A.: **Inherited disorders of lymphocyte development and function.** *Curr. Opin. Immunol.* 1996, **8**:445-447.

Hammarstrom, L., Gillner, M., and Smith, C.I.: **Molecular basis for human immunodeficiencies.** *Curr. Opin. Immunol.* 1993, **5**:579-584.

10-7	The main effect of low levels of antibody is an inability to clear extracellular bacteria.

Bruton, O.C.: **Agammaglobulinemia.** *Pediatrics* 1952, **9**:722-728.

Fuleihan, R., Ramesh, N., and Geha, R.S.: **X-linked agammaglobulinemia and immunoglobulin deficiency with normal or elevated IgM: immunodeficiencies of B cell development and differentiation.** *Adv. Immunol.* 1995, **60**:37-56.

Khan, W.N., Sideras, P., Rosen, F.S., and Alt, F.W.: **The role of Bruton's tyrosine kinase in B-cell development and function in mice and man.** *Ann. N. Y. Acad. Sci.* 1995, **764**:27-38.

Ochs, H.D. and Wedgwood, R.J.: **IgG subclass deficiencies.** *Ann. Rev. Med.* 1987, **38**:325-340.

Preud'homme, J.L. and Hanson, L.A.: **IgG subclass deficiency.** *Immunodefic. Rev.* 1990, **2**:129-149.

Truedsson, L., Baskin, B., Pan, Q., Rabbani, H., Vorechovsky, I., Smith, C.I.E., and Hammarstrom, L.: **Genetics of IgA deficiency.** *APMIS* 1995, **103**:833-842.

Vetrie, D., Vorechovsky, I., Sideras, P., Holland, J., Davies, A., Flinter, F., Hammarstrom, L., Kinnon, C., Levinsky, R., Bobrow, M., Edvard Smith. C.I., and Bentley, D.R.: **The gene involved in X-linked agammaglobulinaemia is a member of the src family of protein-tyrosine kinases.** *Nature* 1993, **361**:226-233.

10-8	T-cell defects can result in low antibody levels.

Allen, R.C., Armitage, R.J., Conley, M.E., Rosenblatt, H., Jenkins, N.A., Copeland, N.G., Bedell, M.A., Edelhoff, S., Disteche, C.M., Simoneaux, D.K., Fanslow, W.C., Belmont, J., and Spriggs, M.K.: **CD40 ligand gene defects responsible for X-linked hyper-IgM syndrome.** *Science* 1993, **259**:990-993.

DiSanto, J.P., Bonnefoy, J.Y., Gauchat, J.F., Fischer, A., and de Saint Basile, G.: **CD40 ligand mutations in X-linked immunodeficiency with hyper-IgM.** *Nature* 1993, **361**:541-543.

Korthauer, U., Graf, D., Mages, H.W., Briere, F., Padayachee, M., Malcolm, S., Ugazio, A.G., Notarangelo, L.D., Levinsky, R.J., and Kroczek, R.A.: **Defective expression of T-cell CD40 ligand causes X-linked immunodeficiency with hyper-IgM.** *Nature* 1993, **361**:539-541.

10-9	Defects in complement components cause defective humoral immune function and persistence of immune complexes.

Colten, H.R., and Rosen, F.S.: **Complement deficiencies.** *Ann. Rev. Immunol.* 1992, **10**:809-834.

Lachmann, P.J., Walport, M.J.: **Deficiency of the effector mechanisms of the immune response and autoimmunity.** In Whelan J (Ed.) *Ciba Foundation Symposium 129: Autoimmunity and Autoimmune Diseases.* Wiley, Chichester 1987:149-171.

Morgan, B.P., and Walport, M.J.: **Complement deficiency and disease.** *Immunol. Today* 1991, **12**:301-306.

10-10	Phagocytic cell defects permit widespread bacterial infections.

Barbosa, M.D.F.S., Nguyen, Q.A., Tchernev, V.T., Ashley, J.A., Detter, J.C., Blaydes, S.M., Brandt, S.J., Chotai, D., Hodgman, C., Solari, R.C.E., Lovett, M., and Kingsmore, S.F.: **Identification of the homologous beige and Chediak Higashi syndrome genes** *Nature* 1996, **382**:262-265.

Fischer, A., Lisowska Grospierre, B., Anderson, D.C., and Springer, T.A.: **Leukocyte adhesion deficiency: molecular basis and functional consequences.** *Immunodefic. Rev.* 1988, **1**:39-54.

Jackson, S.H., Gallin, J.I., and Holland, S.M.: **The p47phox mouse knock-out model of chronic granulomatous disease.** *J. Exp. Med.* 1995, **182**:751-758.

Rotrosen, D. and Gallin, J.I.: **Disorders of phagocyte function.** *Ann. Rev. Immunol.* 1987, **5**:127-150.

10-11	Defects in T-cell function result in severe combined immunodeficiencies.

Bosma, M.J., and Carroll, A.M.: **The SCID mouse mutant: definition, characterization, and potential uses.** *Ann. Rev. Immunol.* 1991, **9**:323-350.

Douhan, J., Hauber, I., Eibl, M.M., and Glimcher, L.H.: **Genetic evidence for a new type of major histocompatibility complex class II combined immunodeficiency characterized by a dyscoordinate regulation of HLA-D alpha and beta chains.** *J. Exp. Med.* 1996, **183**:1063-1069.

Grusby, M.J., and Glimcher, L.H.: **Immune responses in MHC class II-deficient mice.** *Ann. Rev. Immunol.* 1995, **13**:417-435.

Hirschhorn, R.: **Adenosine deaminase deficiency: molecular basis and recent developments.** *Clin. Immunol. Immunopath.* 1995, **76**:S219-S227.

Kara, C.J., and Glimcher, L.H.: *In vivo* **footprinting of MHC class II genes: bare promoters in the bare lymphocyte syndrome.** *Science* 1991, **252**:709-712.

Kara, C.J., and Glimcher, L.H.: **Promoter accessibility within the environment of the MHC is affected in class II-deficient combined immunodeficiency.** *EMBO J.* 1993, **12**:187-193.

Kirchhausen, T., and Rosen, F.S.: **Disease mechanisms: unravelling Wiskott-Aldrich syndrome.** *Curr. Biol.* 1996, **6**:676-678.

Kolluri, R., Tolias, K.F., Carpenter, C.L., Rosen, F.S., and Kirchhausen, T.: **Direct interaction of the Wiskott-Aldrich syndrome protein with the GTPase Cdc42.** *Proc. Natl. Acad. Sci.* 1996, **93**:5615-5618.

Roth, D.B., Menetski, J.P., Nakajima, P.B., Bosma, M.J., and Gellert, M.: **V(D)J recombination: broken DNA molecules with covalently sealed (hairpin) coding ends in scid mouse thymocytes.** *Cell* 1992, **70**:983-991.

10-12	Defective T-cell signaling, cytokine production, or cytokine action can cause immunodeficiency.

Arnaiz Villena, A., Timon, M., Corell, A., Perez Aciego, P., Martin Villa, J.M., and Regueiro, J.R.: **Brief report: primary immunodeficiency caused by mutations in the gene encoding the CD3-gamma subunit of the T-lymphocyte receptor.** *N. Engl. J. Med.* 1992, **327**:529-533.

Castigli, E., Pahwa, R., Good, R.A., Geha, R.S., and Chatila, T.A.: **Molecular basis of a multiple lymphokine deficiency in a patient with severe combined immunodeficiency.** *Proc. Natl. Acad. Sci.* 1993, **90**:4728-4732.

Chatila, T., Wong, R., Young, M., Miller, R., Terhorst, C., and Geha, R.S.: **An immunodeficiency characterized by defective signal transduction in T lymphocytes.** *N. Engl. J. Med.* 1989, **320**:696-702.

Chatila, T., Castigli, E., Pahwa, R., Pahwa, S., Chirmule, N., Oyaizu, N., Good, R.A., and Geha, R.S.: **Primary combined immunodeficiency resulting from defective transcription of multiple T-cell lymphokine genes.** *Proc. Natl. Acad. Sci.* 1990, **87**:10033-10037.

DiSanto, J.P., Keever, C.A., Small, T.N., Nicols, G.L., O'Reilly, R.J., and Flomenberg, N.: **Absence of interleukin 2 production in a severe combined immunodeficiency disease syndrome with T cells**. *J. Exp. Med.* 1990, **171**:1697-1704.

DiSanto, J.P., Rieux Laucat, F., Dautry Varsat, A., Fischer, A., and de Saint Basile, G.: **Defective human interleukin 2 receptor gamma chain in an atypical X chromosome-linked severe combined immunodeficiency with peripheral T cells**. *Proc. Natl. Acad. Sci.* 1994, **91**:9466-9470.

Leonard, W.J.: **The defective gene in X-linked severe combined immunodeficiency encodes a shared interleukin receptor subunit: implications for cytokine pleiotropy and redundancy**. *Curr. Opin. Immunol.* 1994, **6**:631-635.

Leonard, W.J.: **The molecular basis of X linked severe combined immunodeficiency**. *Ann. Rev. Med.* 1996, **47**:229-239.

Noguchi, M., Nakamura, Y., Russell, S.M., Ziegler, S.F., Tsang, M., Cao, X., and Leonard, W.J.: **Interleukin-2 receptor gamma chain: a functional component of the interleukin-7 receptor**. *Science* 1993, **262**:1877-1880.

Noguchi, M., Yi, H., Rosenblatt, H.M., Filipovich, A.H., Adelstein, S., Modi, W.S., McBride, O.W., and Leonard, W.J.: **Interleukin-2 receptor gamma chain mutation results in X-linked severe combined immunodeficiency in humans**. *Cell* 1993, **73**:147-157.

Russell, S.M., Keegan, A.D., Harada, N., Nakamura, Y., Noguchi, M., Leland, P., Friedmann, M.C., Miyajima, A., Puri, R.K., Paul, W.E., and et al, : **Interleukin-2 receptor gamma chain: a functional component of the interleukin-4 receptor**. *Science* 1993, **262**:1880-1883.

Soudais, C., de Villartay, J.P., Le Deist, F., Fischer, A., and Lisowska Grospierre, B.: **Independent mutations of the human CD3-epsilon gene resulting in a T cell receptor/CD3 complex immunodeficiency**. *Nat. Genet.* 1993, **3**:77-81.

Weinberg, K. and Parkman, R.: **Severe combined immunodeficiency due to a specific defect in the production of interleukin-2**. *N. Engl. J. Med.* 1990, **322**:1718-1723.

10-13 | **Bone marrow transplantation or gene therapy may be useful to correct genetic defects.**

Blaese, R.M., Culver, K.W., Miller, A.D., Carter, C.S., Fleisher, T., Clerici, M., Shearer, G., Chang, L., Chiang, Y., Tolstoshev, P., Greenblatt, J.J., Rosenberg, S.A., Klein, H., Berger, M., Mullen, C.A., Ramsey, W.J., Muul, L., Morgan, R.A., and Anderson, W.F.: **T lymphocyte-directed gene therapy for ADA- SCID: initial trial results after 4 years**. *Science* 1995, **270**:475-480.

Buckley, R.H., Schiff, S.E., Sampson, H.A., Schiff, R.I., Markert, M.L., Knutsen, A.P., Hershfield, M.S., Huang, A.T., Mickey, G.H., and Ward, F.E.: **Development of immunity in human severe primary T cell deficiency following haploidentical bone marrow stem cell transplantation**. *J. Immunol.* 1986, **136**:2398-2407.

Cournoyer, D., and Caskey, C.T.: **Gene therapy of the immune system**. *Ann. Rev. Immunol.* 1993, **11**:297-329.

Kohn, D.B., Weinberg, K.I., Nolta, J.A., Heiss, L.N., Lenarsky, C., Crooks, G.M., Hanley, M.E., Annett, G., Brooks, J.S., El Khoureiy, A., Lawrence, K., Wells, S., Moen, R.C., Bastian, J., Williams-Herman, D.E., Elder, M., Wara, D., Bowen, T., Herschfield, M.S., Mullen, C.A., Blaese, R.M., and Parkman, R.: **Engraftment of gene-modified umbilical cord blood cells in neonates with adenosine deaminase deficiency**. *Nat. Med.* 1995, **1**:1017-1023.

Morgan, R.A. and Anderson, W.F.: **Human gene therapy**. *Ann. Rev. Biochem.* 1993, **62**:191-217.

10-14 | Most individuals infected with HIV progress over time to AIDS.

Baltimore, D.: **Lessons from people with nonprogressive HIV infection**. *N. Engl. J. Med.* 1995, **332**:259-260.

Cao, Y., Qin, L., Zhang, L., Safrit, J., and Ho, D.D.: **Virologic and immunologic characterization of long-term survivors of human immunodeficiency virus type 1 infection**. *N. Engl. J. Med.* 1995, **332**:201-208.

Darby, S.C., Ewart, D.W., Giangrande, P.L.F., Spooner, R.J.D., and Rizza, C.R.: **Importance of age at infection with HIV 1 for survival and development of AIDS in UK haemophilia population**. *Lancet* 1996, **347**:1573-1579.

Fang, G., Burger, H., Grimson, R., Tropper, P., Nachman, S., Mayers, D., Weislow, O., Moore, R., Reyelt, C., Hutcheon, N., Baker, D., and Weiser, B.: **Maternal plasma human immunodeficiency virus type 1 RNA level: a determinant and projected threshold for mother-to-child transmission**. *Proc. Natl. Acad. Sci.* 1995, **92**:12100-12104.

Kirchhoff, F., Greenough, T.C., Brettler, D.B., Sullivan, J.L., and Desrosiers, R.C.: **Brief report: absence of intact nef sequences in a long-term survivor with nonprogressive HIV-1 infection**. *N. Engl. J. Med.* 1995, **332**:228-232.

Pantaleo, G., Menzo, S., Vaccarezza, M., Graziosi, C., Cohen, O.J., Demarest, J.F., Montefiori, D., Orenstein, J.M., Fox, C., Schrager, L.K., Margolick, J.B., Buchbinder, S., Giorgi, J.V., amd Fauci, A.S.: **Studies in subjects with long-term nonprogressive human immunodeficiency virus infection**. *N. Engl. J. Med.* 1995, **332**:209-216.

Peckham, C. and Gibb, D.: **Mother-to-child transmission of the human immunodeficiency virus**. *N. Engl. J. Med.* 1995, **333**:298-302.

Wang, W.K., Essex, M., McLane, M.F., Mayer, K.H., Hsieh, C.C., Brumblay, H.G., Seage, G., and Lee, T.H.R.: **Pattern of gp120 sequence divergence linked to a lack of clinical progression in human immunodeficiency virus type 1 infection**. *Proc. Natl. Acad. Sci.* 1996, **93**:6693-6697.

10-15 | HIV is a retrovirus that infects CD4 T cells and macrophages.

Bleul, C.C., Farzan, M., Choe, H., Parolin, C., Clark-Lewis, I., Sodroski, J., and Springer, T.A.R.: **The lymphocyte chemoattractant SDF 1 is a ligand for LESTR/fusin and blocks HIV 1 entry**. *Nature* 1996, **382**:829-833.

Deng, H.K., Liu, R., Ellmeier, W., Choe, S., Unutmaz, D., Burkhart, M., DiMarzio, P., Marmon, S., Sutton, R.E., Hill, C.M., Davis, C.B., Peiper, S.C., Schall, T.J., Littmann, D.R.R., and Landau, N.R.: **Identification of a major co receptor for primary isolates of HIV 1**. *Nature* 1996, **381**:661-666.

Doranz, B.J., Rucker, J., Yi, Y.J., Smyth, R.J., Samson, M., Peiper, S.C., Parmentier, M., Collman, R.G., and Doms, R.W.: **A dual tropic primary HIV 1 isolate that uses fusin and the beta chemokine receptors CKR 5, CKR 3, and CKR 2B as fusion cofactors**. *Cell* 1996, **85**:1149-1158.

Dragic, T., Litwin, V., Allaway, G.P., Martin, S.R., Huang, Y.X., Nagashima, K.A., Cayanan, C., Maddon, P.J., Koup, R.A.R., Moore, J.P., and Paxton, W.A.: **HIV 1 entry into CD4(+) cells is mediated by the chemokine receptor CC CKR 5**. *Nature* 1996, **381**:667-673.

Oberlin, E., Amara, A., Bachelerie, F., Bessia, C., Virelizier, J.L., Arenzanaseisdedos, F.R., Schwartz, O., Heard, J.M., Clarklewis, I., Legler, D.F., Loetscher, M., Baggiolini, M., and Moser, B.: **The CXC chemokine SDF 1 is the ligand for LESTR/fusin and prevents infection by T cell line adapted HIV 1**. *Nature* 1996, **382**:833-835.

10-16 | Genetic deficiency of the macrophage chemokine co-receptor for HIV confers resistance to HIV infection *in vivo*.

Liu, R., Paxton, W.A., Choe, S., Ceradini, D., Martin, S.R., Horuk, R., Macdonald, M.E., Stuhlmann, H., Koup, R.A., and Landau, N.R.: **Homozygous** defect in HIV 1 coreceptor accounts for resistance of some multiply exposed individuals to HIV 1 infection. *Cell* 1996, **86**:367-377.

Samson, M., Libert, F., Doranz, B.J., Rucker, J., Liesnard, C., Farber, C.M., Saragosti, S., Lapoumeroulie, C., Cognaux, J., Forceille, C., Muyldermans, G., Verhofstede, C., Burtonboy, G., Georges, M., Imai, T., Rana, S., Yi, Y.J., Smyth, R.J., Collman, R.G., Doms, R.W., Vassart, G., and Parmentier, M.R.: **Resistance to HIV 1 infection in Caucasian individuals bearing mutant alleles of the CCR 5 chemokine receptor gene.** *Nature* 1996, **382**:722-725.

10-17   HIV RNA is transcribed by viral reverse transcriptase into DNA which integrates into the host cell genome.

Andrake, M.D., and Skalka, A.M.R.: **Retroviral integrase, putting the pieces together.** *J.Biol.Chem.* 1995, **271**:19633-19636.

Baltimore, D.: **The enigma of HIV infection.** *Cell* 1995, **82**:175-176.

McCune, J.M.: **Viral latency in HIV disease.** *Cell* 1995, **82**:183-188.

10-18   Transcription of the HIV provirus depends on host-cell transcription factors induced upon activation of infected T cells.

Trono, D.: **HIV accessory proteins: leading roles for the supporting cast.** *Cell* 1995, **82**:189-192.

10-19   Drugs that block HIV replication lead to a rapid fall in titer of infectious virus and a rise in CD4 T cells, followed by the outgrowth of drug-resistant variant virus.

Carpenter, C.C.J., Fischl, M.A., Hammer, S.M., Hirsch, M.S., Jacobsen, D.M., Katzenstein, D.A., Montaner, J.S.G., Richman, D.D., Saag, M.S., Schooley, R.T., Thompson, M.A., Vella, S., Yeni, P.G., and Volberding, P.A.: **Antiretroviral therapy for HIV infection in 1996: recommendations of an international panel.** *JAMA* 1995, **276**:146-154.

Condra, J.H., Schleif, W.A., Blahy, O.M., Gabryelski, L.J., Graham, D.J., Quintero, J.C., Rhodes, A., Robbins, H.L., Roth, E., Shivaprakash, M., Titus, D., Yang, T., Teppler, H., Squires, K.E., Deutsch, P.J., and Emini, E.A.: **In vivo emergence of HIV-1 variants resistant to multiple protease inhibitors.** *Nature* 1995, **374**:569-571.

Moutouh, L., Corbeil, J., and Richman, D.D.: **Recombination leads to the rapid emergence of HIV 1 dually resistant mutants under selective drug pressure.** *Proc. Natl. Acad. Sci.* 1996, **93**:6106-6111.

Wei, X., Ghosh, S.K., Taylor, M.E., Johnson, V.A., Emini, E.A., Deutsch, P., Lifson, J.D., Bonhoeffer, S., Nowak, M.A., Hahn, B.H., Saag, M.S., and Shaw, G.M.: **Viral dynamics in human immunodeficiency virus type 1 infection.** *Nature* 1995, **373**:117-122.

10-20   HIV accumulates many mutations in the course of infection in a single individual.

Coffin, J.M.: **HIV population dynamics** *in vivo*: **implications for genetic variation, pathogenesis, and therapy.** *Science* 1995, **267**:483-489.

10-21   Replication of HIV has been observed in both lymphoid and mucosal tissue.

Cameron, P., Pope, M., Granellipiperno, A., and Steinman, R.M.: **Dendritic cells and the replication of HIV 1.** *J. Leuk. Biol.* 1996, **59**:158-171.

Dianzani, F., Antonelli, G., Riva, E., Uccini, S., and Visco, G.: **Plasma HIV viremia and viral load in lymph nodes.** *Nat. Med.* 1996, **2**:832-833.

Glushakova, S., Baibakov, B., Margolis, L.B., and Zimmerberg, J.: **Infection of human tonsil histocultures: a model for HIV pathogenesis.** *Nat. Med.* 1995, **1**:1320-1322.

Heath, S.L., Tew, J.G., Szakal, A.K., and Burton, G.F.: **Follicular dendritic cells and human immunodeficiency virus infectivity.** *Nature* 1995, **377**:740-744.

Pantaleo, G., Graziosi, C., Butini, L., Pizzo, P.A., Schnittman, S.M., Kotler, D.P., and Fauci, A.S.: **Lymphoid organs function as major reservoirs for human immunodeficiency virus.** *Proc. Natl. Acad. Sci. 1991,* **88**:9838-9842.

10-22   An immune response controls but does not eliminate HIV.

Autran, B., Hadida, F., and Haas, G.: **Evolution and plasticity of CTL responses against HIV.** *Curr. Opin. Immunol.* 1996, **8**:546-553.

Bevan, M.J., and Braciale, T.J.: **Why can't cytotoxic T cells handle HIV?** *Proc. Natl. Acad. Sci. 1995,* **92**:5765-5767.

Moss, P.A., Rowland Jones, S.L., Frodsham, P.M., McAdam, S., Giangrande, P., McMichael, A.J., and Bell, J.I.: **Persistent high frequency of human immunodeficiency virus-specific cytotoxic T cells in peripheral blood of infected donors.** *Proc. Natl. Acad. Sci. 1995,* **92**:5773-5777.

Rowland Jones, S., Sutton, J., Ariyoshi, K., Dong, T., Gotch, F., McAdam, S., Whitby, D., Sabally, S., Gallimore, A., Corrah, T., Takiguchi, M., Schultz, T., McMichael, A., Whittle, H.: **HIV-specific cytotoxic T-cells in HIV-exposed but uninfected Gambian women.** *Nat. Med.* 1995, **1**:59-64.

Sattentau, Q.J.: **Neutralization of HIV 1 by antibody.** *Curr. Opin. Immunol.* 1996, **8**:540-545.

10-23   HIV infection leads to low levels of CD4 T cells, increased susceptibility to opportunistic infection, and eventually to death.

Ho, D.D., Neumann, A.U., Perelson, A.S., Chen, W., Leonard, J.M., and Markowitz, M.: **Rapid turnover of plasma virions and CD4 lymphocytes in HIV-1 infection.** *Nature* 1995, **373**:123-126.

Katlama, C. and Dickinson, G.M.: **Update on opportunistic infections.** *AIDS* 1993, **7 Suppl 1**:S185-S194.

Kedes, D.H., Operskalski, E., Busch, M., Kohn, R., Flood, J., and Ganem, D.R.: **The seroepidemiology of human herpesvirus 8 (Kaposis sarcoma associated herpesvirus): distribution of infection in KS risk groups and evidence for sexual transmission.** *Nature Med.* 1996, **2**:918-924.

Kolesnitchenko, V., Wahl, L.M., Tian, H., Sunila, I., Tani, Y., Hartmann, D.P., Cossman, J., Raffeld, M., Orenstein, J., Samelson, L.E., and Cohen, D.I.: **Human immunodeficiency virus 1 envelope-initiated G2-phase programmed cell death.** *Proc. Natl. Acad. Sci. 1995,* **92**:11889-11893.

Pantaleo, G., and Fauci, A.S.: **Apoptosis in HIV infection.** *Nat. Med.* 1995, **1**:118-120.

Zhong, W.D., Wang, H., Herndier, B., and Ganem, D.R.: **Restricted expression of Kaposi sarcoma associated herpesvirus (human herpesvirus 8) genes in Kaposi sarcoma.** *Proc. Natl. Acad. Sci.* 1996, **93**:6641-6646.

10-24   Vaccination against HIV is an attractive solution but poses many difficulties.

Fast, P.E., Mathieson, B.J., and Schultz, A.M.: **Efficacy trials of AIDS vaccines: how science can inform ethics.** *Curr. Opin. Immunol.* 1994, **6**:691-697.

Girard, M.P., and Shearer, G.M.: **AIDS 92/93. Vaccines and immunology: overview.** *AIDS* 1993, **7 Suppl 1**:S115-S116.

MacQueen, K.M., Buchbinder, S., Douglas, J.M., Judson, F.N., McKirnan, D.J., and Bartholow, B.: **The decision to enroll in HIV vaccine efficacy trials:**

concerns elicited from gay men at increased risk for HIV infection. *AIDS Res. Hum. Retroviruses.* 1994, **10 Suppl 2**:S261-S264.

Miller, C.J., and McGhee, J.R.: **Progress towards a vaccine to prevent sexual transmission of HIV**. *Nat. Med.* 1996, **2**:751-752.

Salk, J., Bretscher, P.A., Salk, P.L., Clerici, M., and Shearer, G.M.: **A strategy for prophylactic vaccination against HIV**. *Science* 1993, **260**:1270-1272.

10-25   **Prevention and education are one way in which the spread of HIV and AIDS can be controlled.**

Decosas, J.: **Fighting AIDS or responding to the epidemic: can public health find its way?** *Lancet* 1994, **343**:1145-1146.

Decosas, J., Kane, F., Anarfi, J.K., Sodji, K.D., and Wagner, H.U.: **Migration and AIDS**. *Lancet* 1995, **346**:826-828.

Decosas, J., and Finlay, J.: **International AIDS aid: the response of development aid agencies to the HIV/AIDS pandemic**. *AIDS* 1993, **7 Suppl 1**:S281-S286.

Dowsett, G.W.: **Sustaining safe sex: sexual practices, HIV and social context**. *AIDS* 1993, **7 Suppl 1**:S257-S262.

Kimball, A.M., Berkley, S., Ngugi, E., and Gayle, H.: **International aspects of the AIDS/HIV epidemic**. *Ann. Rev. Public Health* 1995, **16**:253-282.

Nelson, K.E., Celentano, D.D., Eiumtrakol, S., Hoover, D.R., Beyrer, C., Suprasert, S., Kuntolbutra, S., and Khamboonruang, C.: **Changes in sexual behavior and a decline in HIV infection among young men in Thailand**. *N. Engl. J. Med.* 1996, **335**:297-303.

Weniger, B.G., and Brown, T.: **The march of AIDS through Asia**. *N. Engl. J. Med.* 1996, **335**:343-345.

Allergy and Hypersensitivity

Allergic reactions occur when an individual who has produced IgE antibody in response to an innocuous antigen, or **allergen**, subsequently encounters the same allergen. This triggers the activation of IgE-binding mast cells in the exposed tissue, leading to a series of responses that are characteristic of **allergy**. As we learned in Chapter 8, there are circumstances in which IgE mediates protective immunity, especially in response to parasitic worms, which are prevalent in underdeveloped countries. In more advanced countries, however, IgE responses to innocuous antigens predominate, and allergy is one of the most prevalent diseases (Fig. 11.1). Allergic reactions to common environmental antigens affect up to half the population in North America and Europe and, although rarely life-threatening, cause much distress and lost time from school and work. Owing to their medical importance in industrialized societies, much more is known about the pathophysiology of IgE-mediated immune responses than about their physiology.

Fig. 11.1 IgE-mediated reactions to extrinsic antigens. All IgE-mediated responses involve mast-cell degranulation, but the symptoms experienced by the patient can be very different depending on whether the allergen is injected, inhaled, or eaten, and depending also on the dose of the allergen (see also Fig. 11.12).

IgE-mediated allergic reactions			
Syndrome	Common allergens	Route of entry	Response
Systemic anaphylaxis	Drugs Serum Venoms Peanuts	Intravenous (either directly or following rapid absorption)	Edema, Increased vascular permeability Tracheal occlusion Circulatory collapse Death
Wheal-and-flare	Insect bites Allergy testing	Subcutaneous	Local increase in blood flow and vascular permeability
Allergic rhinitis (hay fever)	Pollens (ragweed, timothy, birch) Dust-mite feces	Inhaled	Edema of nasal mucosa Irritation of nasal mucosa
Bronchial asthma	Pollens Dust-mite feces	Inhaled	Bronchial constriction Increased mucus production Airway inflammation
Food allergy	Shellfish Milk Eggs Fish Wheat	Oral	Vomiting Diarrhea Pruritis (itching) Urticaria (hives) Anaphylaxis (rarely)

The term allergy was originally defined by Clemens Von Pirquet as 'an altered capacity of the body to react to a foreign substance', which was an extremely broad definition that included all immunological reactions. Allergy is now defined in a much more restricted manner as 'disease following an immune response to an otherwise innocuous antigen'. Allergy is a member of a class of immune responses that have been termed **hypersensitivity reactions**; these are harmful immune responses that produce tissue injury and may cause serious disease. Hypersensitivity reactions were classified into four types by Gell and Coombs (Fig. 11.2). Allergy is usually equated with type I, or immediate-type hypersensitivity reactions mediated by IgE, and will be used in this sense here.

In this chapter, we will first consider the mechanisms that favor the switching of the humoral immune response to the production of IgE. We will then describe the pathophysiological consequences of ligation by antigen of IgE bound by the high-affinity Fcε receptor (FcεRI) on mast cells. Finally, we will consider the causes and consequences of other types of immunological hypersensitivity reactions.

The production of IgE.

A **type I hypersensitivity reaction** is triggered by antigens cross-linking preformed IgE antibody that is bound to FcεRI on mast-cell surfaces. Basophils and activated eosinophils also express FcεRI. The factors that lead to an antibody response that is dominated by IgE are still being worked out. Here, we shall describe our current understanding of these processes, before turning to the question of how IgE mediates allergic reactions.

	Type I	Type II	Type III	Type IV	
Immune reactant	IgE antibody, T$_H$2 cells	IgG antibody	IgG antibody	T cells	
Antigen	Soluble antigen	Cell- or matrix-associated antigen	Soluble antigen	Soluble antigen	Cell-associated antigen
Effector mechanism	Mast-cell activation	Complement, FcR$^+$ cells (phagocytes, NK cells)	Complement Phagocytes	Macrophage activation	Cytotoxicity
Example of hypersensitivity reaction	Allergic rhinitis, asthma, systemic anaphylaxis	Some drug allergies (eg penicillin)	Serum sickness, Arthus reaction	Contact dermatitis, tuberculin reaction	Contact dermatitis

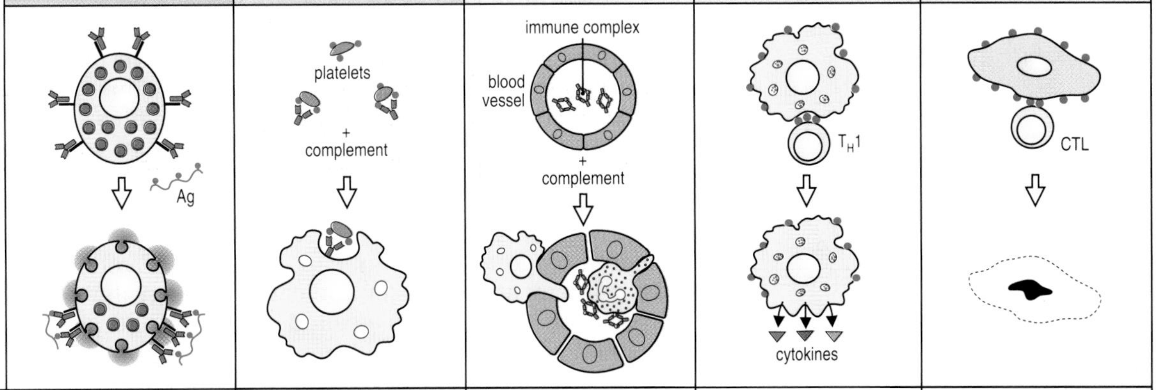

Fig. 11.2 There are four types of immune-mediated hypersensitivity reactions causing tissue damage. Types I–III are antibody-mediated and are distinguished by the different types of antigens recognized and the different classes of antibody involved. Type I responses are mediated by IgE, which induces mast-cell activation, while types II and III are mediated by IgG, which can engage complement-mediated and phagocytic effector mechanisms to varying degrees, depending on the subtype of IgG and the nature of the antigen involved. Type II responses are directed against cell-surface antigens and lead to cell-specific tissue damage, whereas type III responses are directed against soluble or matrix antigens, and the tissue damage involved is caused by responses triggered by immune complexes. Type IV hypersensitivity reactions are T-cell mediated, and can be subdivided into two classes: in the first class, tissue damage is caused by activation of inflammatory responses by T$_H$1 cells, mediated mainly by macrophages; and in the second, damage is caused directly by cytotoxic T cells (CTL).

11-1   **Allergens are a class of antigen that evoke an IgE response and are often delivered transmucosally at low dose.**

There are certain antigens and routes of antigen presentation to the immune system that favor the production of IgE. As we learned in Chapter 8, T$_H$2 cells can switch the antibody isotype from IgM to IgE as well as to IgG2 and IgG4 (human) or IgG1 and IgG3 (mouse). Antigens that selectively evoke T$_H$2 cells that drive an IgE response are known as allergens.

Much human allergy is caused by a limited number of inhaled protein allergens that reproducibly elicit IgE production in some individuals. Since we inhale many different proteins that do not induce IgE production, this has led researchers to ask what is unusual about the proteins that are common allergens. Although we still do not understand this completely, some general principles have emerged (Fig. 11.3).

It seems likely that transmucosal presentation of very low doses of allergen is particularly efficient at inducing T$_H$2-driven IgE responses. IgE antibody production requires IL-4-producing T$_H$2 cells and can be inhibited by T$_H$1 cells that produce interferon-γ (IFN-γ) (see Fig. 8.7). We have also learned (see Section 9-19) that the low doses at which

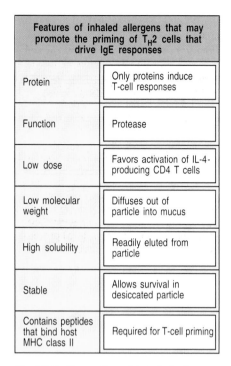

Features of inhaled allergens that may promote the priming of T_H2 cells that drive IgE responses	
Protein	Only proteins induce T-cell responses
Function	Protease
Low dose	Favors activation of IL-4-producing CD4 T cells
Low molecular weight	Diffuses out of particle into mucus
High solubility	Readily eluted from particle
Stable	Allows survival in desiccated particle
Contains peptides that bind host MHC class II	Required for T-cell priming

Fig. 11.3 Properties of inhaled allergens.

allergens enter the body across mucosal surfaces can favor activation of T_H2 cells over T_H1 cells. The dominant antigen-presenting cell type in the respiratory mucosa is a cell with characteristics similar to Langerhans' cells (see Chapters 7 and 9). These cells very efficiently take up and process protein antigens, a step that is accompanied by cellular activation. This in turn induces their migration to regional lymph nodes and differentiation into cells that are highly co-stimulatory in a manner that favors T_H2 differentiation.

11-2 Enzymes are frequent triggers of allergy.

Many parasites invade their hosts by secretion of proteolytic enzymes that break down connective tissue and allow the parasite access to host tissues. It has been proposed that these enzymes are particularly active at promoting T_H2 responses. This idea receives some support from the many examples of allergens that are enzymes. The major allergen of the house dust mite, *Dermatophagoides pteronyssimus*, responsible for allergy in up to 20% of the North American population, is a cysteine protease homologous to papain. Papain itself, derived from the papaya fruit, is used as a meat tenderizer and causes allergy in workers preparing the enzyme. Such allergies are called industrial allergies, and an analogous industrial allergy is the asthma caused by inhalation of the bacterial enzyme subtilisin, the 'biological' component of certain laundry detergents. Injection of enzymatically active papain (but not inactivated papain) into mice stimulates an IgE response. A closely related enzyme, chymopapain, is used in medicine to chemically destroy intervertebral disks in patients with sciatica; the major although rare complication of this procedure is anaphylaxis, an acute systemic response to allergens (see Section 11-10). However, it is not universally the case that allergens are enzymes; by complete contrast, two allergens identified from filarial worms are enzyme inhibitors. Although the amino acid sequences of many protein allergens derived from plants have been identified, their functions are presently obscure.

Most allergens are relatively small, highly soluble proteins that are inhaled in desiccated particles such as pollen grains or mite feces. The allergen elutes from the particle because it is readily soluble and diffuses into the mucosa. Allergens are typically presented to the immune system at very low doses. It has been estimated that the maximum exposure of a person to common pollen allergens in ragweed (*Artemisia artemisiifolia*) cannot exceed 1 μg per year! Yet many people develop irritating and even life-threatening T_H2-driven IgE antibody responses to these minute doses of allergen. It is important to note that only a fraction of people who are exposed to these substances make IgE antibody to them. The host factors that influence which individuals will respond to allergens are considered in Section 11-4.

11-3 Class switching to IgE in B lymphocytes is favored by specific accessory signals.

IgE production requires cytokines that are released by T_H2 cells, in particular IL-4. T_H2 cells, in turn, arise when naive T cells first encounter antigen in the presence of IL-4. The importance of IL-4 in driving IgE production is seen in mice lacking a functional IL-4 gene: the major abnormality associated with this defect appears to be a reduced synthesis of IgE. In mice, the early production of IL-4 has been shown to be the result of activation of a small subset of CD4 T cells with unusual properties (Fig. 11.4). These cells, the NK1.1[+] subset, express T-cell receptors made

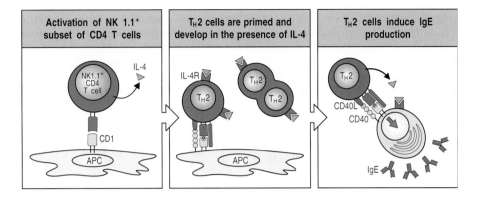

Fig. 11.4 IgE class switching in B cells is initiated by T_H2 cells, which develop in the presence of an early burst of IL-4. IL-4 is secreted early in some immune responses by a small subset of CD4 T cells (NK1.1⁺ CD4 T cells), which interact with antigen-presenting cells bearing the non-classical MHC class I-like molecule, CD1. Naive T cells being primed by their first encounter with antigen are driven to differentiate into T_H2 cells in the presence of this early burst of IL-4. These effector T_H2 cells interact with antigen-specific B lymphocytes and stimulate switching of the antibody isotype to IgE, by secreting IL-4 and expressing CD40L. These same signals drive B-cell proliferation and thereby IgE production.

up of a restricted set of β chains and an invariant α chain, and develop in response to CD1, an MHC class I-like molecule found in humans as well as mice. Evidence for the development of these cells in response to CD1 derives from their absence in mice that cannot express CD1 molecules because of engineered defects in their β₂-microglobulin genes. The invariant T-cell receptor α chain expressed by these cells is encoded in a single V_α gene segment and a single J_α gene segment; similar cells in humans are also specific for the homolog of mouse CD1, called CD1d, and use the homologous V_α and J_α gene segments. These T cells produce IL-4 almost immediately upon encountering their CD1 ligand, which is expressed on cortical thymocytes and on Langerhans' cells and other antigen-presenting cells. In mice, CD1-specific T cells are the only known source of early IL-4: mice lacking β₂-microglobulin fail to make early IL-4 and are deficient in IgE production.

The early exposure of naive CD4 T cells to IL-4 produced in this way drives them to differentiate into T_H2 cells and inhibits T_H1 development. Once T_H2 cells are primed, they can deliver several molecular signals that favor class switching in B lymphocytes to the production of IgE antibody (see Fig. 11.4). Ligation of the T-cell receptor stimulates expression of CD40 ligand (CD40L) on the T_H2 cell surface, which interacts with CD40 on B cells. A second accessory signal is the production of IL-4 by the activated T_H2 cell, which in turn ligates the IL-4 receptor on B lymphocytes; recent studies show that IL-13 can also have this effect on B cells by interaction with a receptor that shares some properties with the IL-4 receptor. The combination of these signals drives productive class switching to IgE and B-cell proliferation.

The IgE response, once initiated, may be further amplified by basophils, mast cells, and eosinophils, which are also capable of driving IgE production (Fig. 11.5). All three cell types express the FcεRI, although eosinophils

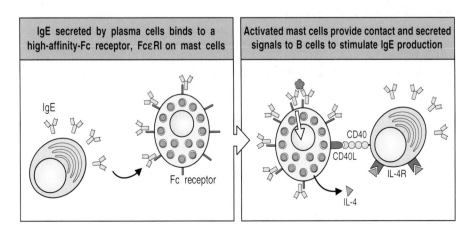

Fig. 11.5 IgE production is amplified following ligation by antigen of IgE bound to mast cells. IgE secreted by B lymphocytes binds to the high-affinity IgE receptor on mast cells, basophils, and activated eosinophils. Isotype switching and production of IgE by B cells can be amplified by these cells, which express CD40L and secrete IL-4 in response to ligation of surface-bound IgE by antigen. This may occur *in vivo* at the site of allergen-triggered inflammation, for example in bronchial-associated lymphoid aggregates.

only express it when activated. When these specialized granulocytes are activated by antigen crosslinking of their FcεRI-bound IgE, they can express cell-surface CD40L and secrete IL-4, driving class switching and IgE production by B cells in a manner similar to T$_H$2 cells. The interaction between these specialized granulocytes and B cells may occur at the site of the allergic reaction, as B cells are observed to form germinal centers at inflammatory foci.

11-4 **Genetic factors contribute to the preferential priming of T$_H$2 cells and IgE-mediated allergy.**

Up to 40% of people in western populations show an exaggerated tendency to mount IgE responses to a wide variety of common environmental antigens. This state is called **atopy** and appears to be influenced by several genetic loci. Atopic individuals have higher total levels of IgE measured in the circulation and higher eosinophil levels than their normal counterparts. They are more susceptible to allergic diseases such as hay fever and asthma. On the basis of family linkage studies, loci on chromosomes 11q and 5q have been implicated as containing genes that may be important in determining the presence of atopy, and candidate genes that might affect IgE responses are found in these areas. The candidate gene on chromosome 11 encodes the β subunit of the high-affinity IgE receptor, while on chromosome 5 there is a cluster of tightly linked genes that includes those encoding IL-3, IL-4, IL-5, IL-9, IL-13, and GM-CSF. These cytokines play important roles in IgE isotype switching, eosinophil survival, and mast-cell proliferation. Of particular note, a polymorphism in the IL-4 promoter region is associated with raised IgE levels in atopic subjects and directs elevated expression of a reporter gene in experimental systems. It is too early to know whether this polymorphism plays an important role in the complex genetics of atopy.

A second type of inherited variation in IgE responses is linked to the MHC class II region and affects responses to specific allergens. Many studies have shown that specific IgE production to individual allergens is associated with particular HLA class II alleles, implying that particular MHC:peptide combinations may favor a strong T$_H$2 response. As an example, IgE responses to several ragweed pollen allergens are particularly associated with haplotypes containing the MHC class II allele, DRB1*1501. Many individuals are therefore generally predisposed to make T$_H$2 responses and specifically predisposed to respond to some allergens more than others. However, allergies to common drugs such as penicillin show no association with MHC class II and the presence or absence of atopy.

Summary.

Allergic reactions are the result of the production of specific IgE antibody to common, innocuous antigens. Allergens are antigens that commonly provoke an IgE antibody response. Such antigens normally enter the body at very low doses by diffusion across mucosal surfaces, and trigger a T$_H$2 response. Naive allergen-specific T cells are induced to develop into T$_H$2 cells in the presence of an early burst of IL-4, which appears to be derived from a specialized subset of T cells. The allergen-specific T$_H$2 cells drive allergen-specific B cells to produce IgE. The IgE binds to the high-affinity receptor for IgE on mast cells, basophils, and activated eosinophils. IgE production can be amplified by these cells because upon activation they produce IL-4 and CD40L. The production of IgE is influenced by host genetic factors. Once IgE is produced in response to an allergen, re-exposure to the allergen triggers an allergic response by mechanisms to which we now turn.

Effector mechanisms in allergic reactions.

Allergic reactions are triggered when allergens crosslink preformed IgE bound to the high-affinity FcεRI on mast cells. Mast cells line the body surfaces and serve to alert the immune system to local infection. In allergy, they have the unfortunate ability to provoke very unpleasant allergic reactions to innocuous antigens which are not associated with invading pathogens that need to be expelled. Mast cells act by releasing stored mediators by granule exocytosis, and also by synthesizing leukotrienes and cytokines (Fig. 11.6). The consequences of IgE-mediated mast-cell activation depend on the dose of antigen and its route of entry, ranging from the irritating sniffles of hay fever when pollen is inhaled, to the life-threatening circulatory collapse that occurs in systemic anaphylaxis. The immediate allergic reaction caused by mast-cell degranulation is followed by a more sustained inflammation, known as the late-phase response. This involves the recruitment of other effector cells, notably T$_H$2 lymphocytes, eosinophils, and basophils, which contribute significantly to the immunopathology of an allergic response.

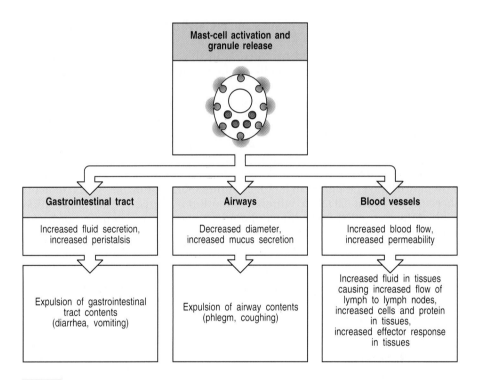

Fig. 11.6 **Mast cells secrete an extensive range of cytokines and mediators of inflammation.** Mast-cell products can be divided into two categories: first, those molecules, both preformed and rapidly synthesized, that mediate acute inflammatory events following mast-cell activation; and second, cytokines and lipid mediators, which induce a late-phase chronic inflammatory response with influx and activation of T$_H$2 lymphocytes, monocytes, eosinophils, and neutrophils. There is some overlap between mediators that induce acute and chronic inflammatory responses, particularly among the lipid mediators, which have rapid effects causing smooth muscle contraction, increased vascular permeability, and mucus secretion, and also induce influx and activation of leukocytes, which contribute to the late-phase response.

11-5 | **Most IgE is cell-bound and engages effector mechanisms of immunity by different pathways from other antibody isotypes.**

Most antibodies are found in body fluids and engage effector cells through receptors specific for their Fc constant regions only after binding specific antigen through their variable domains. IgE is an exception, however, as it is captured by high-affinity receptors specific for the IgE Fc region in the absence of bound antigen. This means that IgE is mostly found fixed in the tissues on mast cells that bear this receptor, as well as on circulating basophils and activated eosinophils. The mast cells are highly specialized leukocytes, located prominently as resident cells in mucosal and epithelial tissues, where they are well-placed to guard against invading pathogens (see Sections 8-20 and 8-21), as well as in subendothelial regions in connective tissue. The ligation of cell-bound IgE by antigen triggers activation of these cells at the site of antigen entry into the tissues. The release of inflammatory lipid mediators, cytokines, and chemokines at sites of IgE-triggered reactions results in the recruitment of eosinophils and basophils to augment the type I response.

There are two types of IgE-binding Fc receptor. The first, **FcεRI**, is a high-affinity receptor of the immunoglobulin superfamily, which mediates the binding of IgE to mast cells, basophils, and activated eosinophils (see Chapter 8). This molecule transduces the signal that activates these cells following crosslinking of cell-bound IgE. The second IgE receptor, **CD23**, is a structurally unrelated molecule that binds IgE with low affinity. CD23 is widely distributed on cells, including B cells, activated T cells, monocytes, eosinophils, platelets, follicular dendritic cells, and some thymic epithelial cells. This receptor was thought to play a crucial role in regulation of IgE antibody levels; however, a mouse strain in which the CD23 gene was deleted by homologous recombination (see Section 2-37) shows no major abnormality in the development of polyclonal IgE responses. However, CD23 deficient mice did not show antigen-specific Ig-mediated enhancement of antibody responses. This demonstrates a role for CD23 on antigen presenting cells in the capture of antigen by specific IgE.

11-6   Mast cells reside in tissues and orchestrate allergic reactions.

Mast cells were described by Ehrlich in the mesentery of rabbits and named *Mastzellen* ('fattened cells'). Like basophils, mast cells have granules rich in acidic molecules that take up basic dyes. However, in spite of this resemblance, and the similar range of mediators stored in these basophilic granules, the mast cells are derived from a different myeloid lineage from basophils and eosinophils. Mast cells are located in tissues, mainly in the vicinity of small blood vessels and postcapillary venules. They home to tissues as agranular cells and their final differentiation with granule formation occurs after they have arrived in the tissues. The major mast-cell growth factor is stem-cell factor (SCF), which acts on its receptor, c-Kit (CD117), which is encoded by a proto-oncogene. Mice with defective c-Kit lack differentiated mast cells and studies of these mice have shown that IgE-mediated inflammatory responses are almost exclusively mast-cell dependent.

Mast cells express FcεRI constitutively on their surface and they are activated when antigens crosslink FcεRI-bound IgE. Degranulation occurs within seconds, releasing a variety of preformed mediators (see Figs. 8.29 and 11.11). Among these are histamine, a short-lived vasoactive amine which causes an immediate increase in local blood flow and permeability, mast-cell chymase, tryptase, and serine esterases that may in turn activate matrix metalloproteinases, which collectively break down tissue matrix proteins. TNF-α is also stored in mast-cell granules and is released in large amounts on mast-cell activation. This causes endothelial activation with upregulation of the expression of adhesion molecules, which promotes the influx of inflammatory leukocytes and lymphocytes.

Chemokines, lipid mediators known as leukotrienes, and further cytokines such as IL-4, are synthesized upon activation and act to sustain the inflammatory response. Thus, the IgE-mediated activation of mast cells orchestrates an important inflammatory cascade which is amplified by the recruitment of eosinophils, basophils, and T$_H$2 lymphocytes. The physiological importance of this is as a host defense mechanism, as we learned in Chapter 8. However, the acute and chronic inflammatory reactions triggered by mast-cell activation can also have important pathophysiological consequences, as seen in the diseases associated with allergic responses to environmental antigens.

11-7   **Eosinophils and basophils are specialized granulocytes that release toxic mediators in IgE-mediated responses.**

Eosinophils are bone marrow-derived granulocytic leukocytes, so named because their granules, which contain arginine-rich basic proteins, are colored bright orange by the acidic stain eosin (Fig. 11.7). Only very small numbers of these cells are normally present in the circulation; the majority of eosinophils reside in tissues, especially in the respiratory, gut, and urogenital subepithelium, implying a likely role for these cells in defense against invading organisms. The effector functions of eosinophils are of two types. First, they release highly toxic granule proteins and free radicals, which can kill microorganisms and parasites but which can also cause significant tissue damage in allergic reactions. Second, they produce molecules including prostaglandins, leukotrienes, and cytokines, which amplify the inflammatory response by recruiting and activating further eosinophils, leukocytes, and epithelial cells (Fig. 11.8).

Important regulatory mechanisms inhibit the inappropriate activation and degranulation of eosinophils, which could otherwise be very harmful to the host. The first level of control regulates the production of eosinophils by the bone marrow, which remain low in the absence of infection or other immune stimulation. When T_H2 cells are activated, cytokines such as IL-5 are released, which increase the production of eosinophils in the bone marrow and promote their release into the circulation. However, transgenic animals over-expressing IL-5 show eosinophilia in the circulation but not in tissues. This demonstrates that a second level of control on eosinophil activity regulates the migration of eosinophils from the circulation into tissues. The key molecules for this response are products of the chemokine family of genes (see Chapter 9). The majority

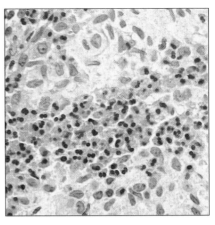

Fig. 11.7 Eosinophils can be detected readily in tissue sections by their bright orange coloration. A dense infiltrate of eosinophils is seen infiltrating a Langerhans' cell histiocytosis. Photograph courtesy of T Krausz.

Class of product	Examples	Biological effects
Enzyme	Eosinophil peroxidase	Toxic to targets by catalyzing halogenation Triggers histamine release from mast cells
	Eosinophil collagenase	Remodeling of connective tissue matrix
Toxic protein	Major basic protein	Toxic to parasites and mammalian cells Triggers histamine release from mast cells
	Eosinophil cationic protein	Toxic to parasites Neurotoxin
	Eosinophil-derived neurotoxin	Neurotoxin
Cytokine	IL-3, IL-5, GM-CSF	Amplify eosinophil production by bone marrow Cause eosinophil activation
Chemokine	IL-8	Promote influx of leukocytes
Lipid mediators	Leukotrienes C4 and D4	Smooth muscle contraction Increased vascular permeability Mucus secretion
	Platelet-activating factor	Chemotactic to leukocytes Amplifies production of lipid mediators Neutrophil, eosinophil, and platelet activation

Fig. 11.8 Eosinophils secrete a range of highly toxic granule proteins and other mediators of inflammation.

of chemokines cause chemotaxis of several types of leukocytes; one of the newest members of this family of molecules shows specific activity for eosinophils and has been named **eotaxin**.

The third level of eosinophil regulation is control of their state of activation. In the basal state, eosinophils do not express high-affinity IgE receptors and have a high threshold for release of their granule contents. Following cytokine and chemokine activation, these thresholds drop, FcεRI is expressed, and the numbers of surface complement and Fcγ receptors increase. The consequence of these changes is that the eosinophil is primed to express effector activity.

The potential for eosinophils to cause tissue injury to the host is illustrated by rare hypereosinophilic syndromes. These are sometimes seen in association with T-cell lymphomas in which unregulated IL-5 secretion drives a dramatic blood eosinophilia. The clinical manifestations of hypereosinophilia are damage to the endocardium (Fig. 11.9) and nerves, leading to heart failure and neuropathy, both thought to be caused by the toxic effects of eosinophil granule proteins.

In a local allergic reaction, mast-cell degranulation and T_H2 activation cause activated eosinophils to accumulate in large numbers. Their continued presence is characteristic of chronic allergic inflammation and they are thought to be the chief contributors to the tissue damage that occurs.

Basophils are bone marrow-derived granulocytes, which share a common stem-cell precursor with eosinophils. Basophil growth factors are very similar to those for eosinophils and include IL-3, IL-5, and GM-CSF. There is evidence for reciprocal control of the maturation of the stem-cell population into basophils or eosinophils. For example, TGF-β in the presence of IL-3 suppresses eosinophil and enhances basophil differentiation. Basophils are normally present in very low numbers in the circulation and appear to play a similar role to eosinophils in host defense against parasitic disease. Like eosinophils, they are recruited to the sites of allergic reactions. Basophils express FcεRI on the cell surface and, on activation, they release toxic mediators from their basophilic granules which give them their name.

Eosinophils, mast cells, and basophils can interact with each other. Eosinophil degranulation causes the release of **major basic protein**, which in turn causes mast cell and basophil degranulation. This effect is augmented by the presence of any of the cytokines, IL-3, IL-5, or GM-CSF, which affect eosinophil and basophil growth, differentiation, and activation.

Fig. 11.9 Hypereosinophilia can cause injury to the endocardium. The left hand panel shows a section of the endocardium from a patient with hypereosinophilic syndrome. There is an organized fibrous exudate and the underlying endocardium is thickened by fibrous tissue. Although there are large numbers of circulating eosinophils, these cells are not seen in the injured endocardium, which is thought to be damaged by granules released from circulating eosinophils. The panel on the right shows two partially degranulated eosinophils (center) surrounded by erythrocytes in a peripheral blood film. Photographs courtesy of D Swirsky and T Krausz.

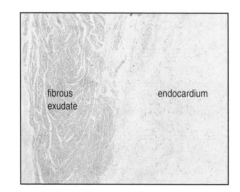

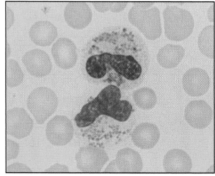

| 11-8 | **Allergic reactions following ligation of IgE on mast cells may be divided into an immediate and a late response.** |

The inflammatory response following IgE-mediated mast-cell activation occurs as an **immediate reaction**, starting within seconds, and a late reaction, which takes up to 8–12 hours to develop. These reactions can be distinguished clinically (Fig. 11.10). The immediate reaction follows from the activity of histamine, prostaglandins, and other preformed or rapidly synthesized toxic molecules, which cause a rapid increase in vascular permeability and the contraction of smooth muscle. The second, **late-phase reaction** is caused by the induced synthesis and release of mediators including leukotrienes, chemokines, and cytokines from the activated mast cells (Fig. 11.11). Although this reaction is clinically less dramatic than the immediate response, it is associated with a second phase of smooth muscle contraction and sustained edema.

The late-phase reaction is an important cause of much more serious long-term morbidity, as for example in chronic asthma. This is because the late reaction induces the recruitment of inflammatory leukocytes, including especially eosinophils and T$_{\text{H}}$2 lymphocytes, to the site of the allergen-triggered mast-cell response. This can easily convert into a chronic inflammatory response if antigen persists, allowing allergen-specific T$_{\text{H}}$2 cells to promote eosinophilia and IgE production.

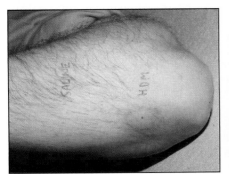
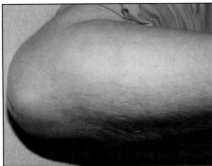
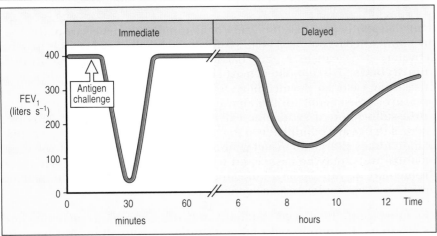

Fig. 11.10 Allergic reactions can be divided into an immediate- and a late-phase response. A wheal-and-flare allergic reaction develops within a minute or two of superficial injection of antigen into the epidermis and lasts for up to 30 minutes. The reaction to an intracutaneous injection of house dust mite antigen is shown in the upper left panel and is labeled HDM; the area labeled saline shows the absence of any response to a control injection of saline solution. A more widespread edematous response, as shown in the upper right panel develops approximately 8 hours later and may persist for some hours. An asthmatic response in the lungs with narrowing of the airways caused by constriction of bronchial smooth muscle can be measured as a fall in the forced expired volume of air in one second (FEV$_1$). This immediate response (see bottom panel), following inhalation of antigen, peaks within minutes and then subsides, but 8 hours after antigen challenge, there is a late-phase response that also results in a fall in the FEV$_1$. The immediate response is caused by the direct effects on blood vessels and smooth muscle of rapidly metabolized mediators such as histamine released by mast cells. The late-phase response is caused by the effects of an influx of inflammatory leukocytes attracted by chemokines and other mediators released by mast cells during and following the immediate response. Photographs courtesy of A B Kay.

Fig. 11.11 **Molecules synthesized and released by mast cells upon stimulation by antigen binding to IgE.** Mast cells release a wide variety of biologically active proteins and other chemical mediators. The lipid mediators derive from membrane phospholipids, which are cleaved to release the precursor molecule arachidonic acid. This molecule can be modified by two pathways, to give rise to prostaglandins, thromboxanes, and leukotrienes. Important products of mast cells are the leukotrienes, which sustain inflammatory responses in the tissues. This is especially true of the leukotriene molecules C4, D4, and E4. Many anti-inflammatory drugs are inhibitors of arachidonic acid metabolism. Aspirin, for example, is an inhibitor of cyclo-oxygenase and blocks the production of prostaglandins.

Class of product	Examples	Biological effects
Enzyme	Tryptase, chymase, cathepsin G, carboxypeptidase	Remodeling of connective tissue matrix
Toxic mediators	Histamine, heparin	Toxic to parasites Increase vascular permeability Cause smooth muscle contraction
Cytokine	IL-4, IL-13	Stimulate and amplify T_H2 cell response
	IL-3, IL-5, GM-CSF	Promote eosinophil production and activation
	TNF-α (stored pre-formed in granules)	Promote inflammation, stimulate cytokine production by many cell types, activate endothelium
Lipid mediators	Leukotrienes C4 and D4	Smooth muscle contraction Increased vascular permeability Mucus secretion
	Platelet-activating factor	Chemotactic to leukocytes Amplifies production of lipid mediators Neutrophil, eosinophil, and platelet activation

11-9 The clinical effects of allergic reactions vary according to the site of mast-cell activation.

When re-exposure to allergen triggers an allergic reaction, the effects are focused on the site at which mast-cell degranulation occurs. In the immediate response, the preformed mediators released are short-lived, and their potent effects on blood vessels and smooth muscles are therefore confined to the immediate vicinity of the activated mast cell. The more sustained effects of the late-phase response are also focused on the site of initial allergen-triggered activation, and the particular anatomy of this site may determine how readily the inflammation produced can be resolved. Thus the clinical syndrome produced by an allergic reaction depends critically on three variables: the amount of allergen-specific IgE antibody present; the route by which the allergen is introduced; and its dose (Fig. 11.12).

11-10 The degranulation of mast cells in the walls of blood vessels following systemic absorption of allergen may cause generalized cardiovascular collapse.

If an allergen is given systemically or is rapidly absorbed from the gut, the connective tissue mast cells associated with all blood vessels may be activated. This causes a very dangerous syndrome called **systemic anaphylaxis**. Disseminated mast-cell activation causes a widespread increase in vascular permeability, leading to a catastrophic loss of blood pressure, constriction of the airways, and epiglottal swelling that may cause suffocation, a syndrome called **anaphylactic shock**. This can occur if drugs are administered to allergic people, or after an insect bite in individuals allergic to insect venom. Some foods, for example peanuts or brazil nuts, may be associated with systemic anaphylaxis. This syndrome may be rapidly fatal but can usually be controlled by immediate injection of epinephrine (see Section 11-14).

The most frequent allergic reactions to drugs occur with penicillin and its relatives. In people with IgE antibodies to penicillin, intravenous

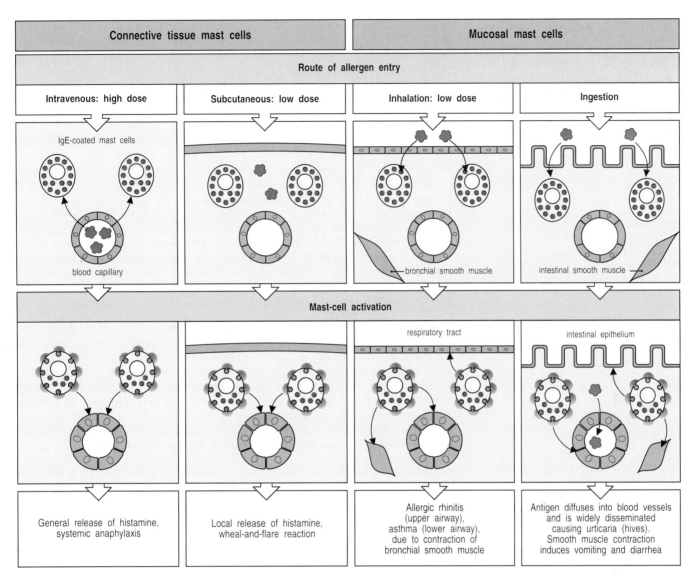

Fig. 11.12 The dose and route of allergen administration determines the type of IgE-mediated allergic reaction that results. There are two main classes of mast cells: those associated with blood vessels, called connective tissue mast cells; and those found in submucosal layers, called mucosal mast cells. In an allergic individual, all of these are loaded with IgE directed against specific allergens. The overall response to an allergen then depends on which mast cells are activated. Allergen in the bloodstream activates connective tissue mast cells throughout the body, resulting in systemic release of histamine and other mediators. Subcutaneous administration of allergen activates only local connective tissue mast cells, leading to a local inflammatory reaction. Inhaled allergen, penetrating across epithelia, activates mainly mucosal mast cells, causing smooth muscle contraction in the lower airways, which leads to bronchoconstriction and difficulty in expelling inhaled air. Mucosal mast-cell activation also increases the local secretion of mucus by epithelial cells and causes irritation. Similarly, ingested allergen penetrates across gut epithelia, causing vomiting due to smooth muscle contraction; the food allergen is also disseminated in the bloodstream, causing urticaria (hives).

administration can cause anaphylaxis and even death. Great care should taken to avoid giving drugs to patients with a past history of allergy to the same drug, or one that is closely related structurally. Penicillin acts as a hapten (see Section 8-2); it is a small molecule with a highly reactive β-lactam ring, crucial for its antibiotic activity. This ring reacts with amino groups on host proteins to form covalent conjugates. When penicillin is ingested or injected, it forms conjugates with self proteins, and these penicillin-modified self peptides may provoke a T_H2 response in some individuals. These T_H2 cells then activate penicillin-binding B cells to produce IgE antibody to the penicillin hapten. Thus, penicillin acts both as the B-cell antigen and, by modifying self peptides, as the T-cell antigen. When penicillin is injected intravenously into allergic individuals, the penicillin-modified proteins crosslink IgE molecules on the mast cells to cause anaphylaxis.

11-11   Exposure of the airways to allergens is associated with the development of rhinitis and asthma.

Inhalation is the most common route for allergen entry. Many people have mild allergies to inhaled antigens, manifesting as sneezing and a runny nose. This is called **allergic rhinitis** or hay fever, and results from activation of mucosal mast cells beneath the nasal epithelium by allergens that diffuse across the mucous membrane of the nasal passages. Allergic rhinitis is characterized by local edema leading to nasal obstruction, a nasal discharge, which is typically rich in eosinophils, and irritation of the nose from histamine release. A similar reaction to airborne allergens deposited on the conjunctiva of the eye is called allergic conjunctivitis. These reactions are annoying but cause little lasting damage.

A more serious syndrome is **allergic asthma**, which is triggered by allergen-induced activation of submucosal mast cells in the lower airways. This leads, within seconds, to bronchial constriction and increased fluid and mucus secretion, making breathing more difficult by trapping inhaled air in the lungs. Patients with allergic asthma often need treatment and asthmatic attacks can be life-threatening. An important feature of asthma is chronic inflammation of the airways (Fig. 11.13), characterized morphologically by the continued presence of increased T_H2 lymphocytes, eosinophils, neutrophils, and other leukocytes (Fig. 11.14).

Although allergic asthma is initially driven by a response to a specific allergen, the subsequent chronic inflammation appears to be perpetuated even in the apparent absence of further exposure to allergen, and factors other than re-exposure to antigen may then trigger subsequent

Acute responses		Chronic response
Inflammatory mediators cause increased mucus secretion and smooth muscle contraction causing airway obstruction	Recruitment of cells from the circulation	Chronic response mediated by cytokines and eosinophil products

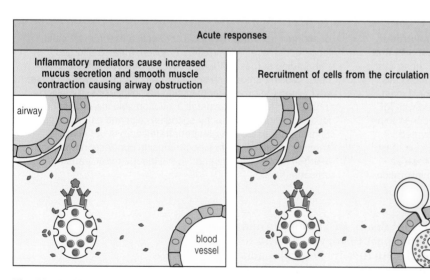
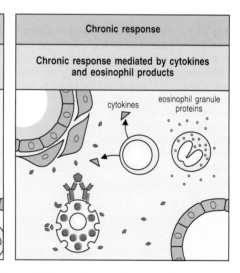

Fig. 11.13 Allergic asthma is characterized by T_H2-mediated chronic inflammation of the airways. T_H2 lymphocytes specific for peptides derived from allergens secrete cytokines that cause B cells to switch to IgE production and also activate eosinophils. Crosslinking of specific IgE on the surface of mast cells by inhaled allergen triggers them to secrete inflammatory mediators, causing bronchial smooth muscle contraction and an influx of inflammatory cells. Activated mast cells also augment eosinophil activation and degranulation, which causes further tissue injury and influx of inflammatory cells. The end result is chronic inflammation, which may then cause irreversible damage to the airways.

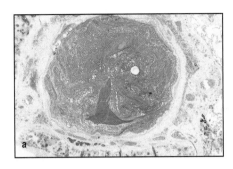 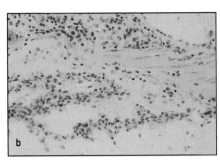

Fig. 11.14 Morphological evidence of chronic inflammation in the airways of an asthmatic patient. Panel a shows a section through a bronchus of a patient who died of asthma; there is almost total occlusion of the airway by a mucus plug. In panel b, a close-up view of the bronchial wall shows injury to the epithelium lining the bronchus, accompanied by a dense inflammatory infiltrate that includes eosinophils, neutrophils, and lymphocytes. Photographs courtesy of T Krausz.

asthmatic attacks. For example, the airways of asthmatics characteristically show hyper-responsiveness to environmental chemical irritants such as cigarette smoke and sulfur dioxide. Disease may be exacerbated further by a T_H2-dominated local immune response to bacterial or viral respiratory tract infections.

11-12 | Skin allergy is manifest as urticaria or chronic eczema.

The same dichotomy between immediate and delayed responses is seen in cutaneous allergic responses. The skin forms an effective barrier to the entry of most allergens. However, this barrier can be breached by local injection of small amounts of allergen into the skin, for example by a stinging insect. This causes a localized allergic reaction. Local mast-cell activation in the skin leads immediately to a local increase in vascular permeability, which causes extravasation of fluid. The mast-cell activation also stimulates a nerve axon reflex, causing vasodilation of surrounding cutaneous blood vessels. The resulting skin lesion is called a **wheal-and-flare reaction**. About 8 hours later, a more widespread and sustained edematous response appears in some individuals as a consequence of the late-phase response (see Fig. 11.10).

Allergists take advantage of the immediate response to test for allergy by injecting minute amounts of potential allergens intracutaneously. Although the reaction following administration of antigen by injection is usually very localized, there is a small risk of induction of systemic anaphylaxis following intracutaneous injection of allergen. Another standard test for allergy is to measure specific IgE antibody levels to a particular allergen in a sandwich ELISA (see Section 2-7).

A more prolonged allergic response is seen mainly in atopic children. They develop a chronic skin rash called **eczema**, due to a chronic inflammatory response similar to that seen in the bronchial walls of patients with asthma. The etiology of eczema is not well understood and it usually clears in adolescence, unlike rhinitis and asthma, which may persist throughout life.

11-13 | Allergy to foods can cause symptoms limited to the gut but also commonly causes systemic reactions.

When an allergen is eaten, two types of allergic response are seen. Activation of mucosal mast cells associated with the gastrointestinal tract can lead to transepithelial fluid loss and smooth muscle contraction, generating vomiting and diarrhea. For reasons that are not understood, connective tissue mast cells in the deeper layers of the skin are also activated, presumably by IgE binding to the ingested and absorbed allergen borne by the blood. Histamine released by activated mast cells in these sites produces **urticaria** or hives—large, itchy red swellings beneath the skin. This is a common reaction when penicillin is ingested by an allergic patient.

11-14 Allergy may be treated by inhibition of the effector pathways activated by antigen crosslinking of cell-surface IgE or by inhibiting IgE production.

The approaches to the treatment and prevention of allergy are set out in Fig. 11.15. The most desirable approach is to shift the antibody response away from an IgE-dominated response towards one dominated by IgG, which can prevent the allergen from activating IgE-mediated effector pathways. A technique to achieve this, known as **desensitization**, has been used in clinical practice for many years. Patients are injected with escalating doses of allergen, starting with tiny amounts. This immunization schedule appears gradually to divert an IgE-dominated response, driven by T_H2 cells, to one driven by T_H1 cells, with the consequent downregulation of IgE production. Recent evidence shows that desensitization is also associated with a reduction in the numbers of mast cells at the site of the allergic reaction.

An alternative and still experimental approach is to vaccinate with peptides derived from common allergens. This procedure induces T-cell anergy *in vivo* by downregulation of expression of the TCR:CD3 complex without triggering IgE-mediated responses, because IgE can only recognize the intact antigen. A major difficulty with this approach is that individual peptide responses are restricted by specific MHC class II alleles and therefore different allergen-derived peptides may be recognized by allergen-specific T cells in individuals expressing different MHC class II alleles. This may present a problem in the outbred human population which expresses a wide variety of polymorphic MHC class II products.

The signaling pathways that enhance the IgE response are potential targets for therapy in allergic disease. Inhibitors of IL-4, IL-5, and IL-13 might reduce IgE responses, although redundancy between some of the activities of these cytokines might make this approach difficult in practice. An alternative approach is to use the cytokines that promote T_H1-type responses. IFN-γ, IFN-α, IL-10, IL-12, and TGF-β have each been shown to reduce IL-4-stimulated IgE synthesis *in vitro* and IFN-γ and IFN-α reduce IgE synthesis *in vivo*.

Fig. 11.15 Approaches to the treatment of allergy. Possible methods of inhibiting allergic reactions are shown. Two approaches are in regular clinical use. The first is the injection of specific antigen in desensitization regimes, which are believed to divert the immune response to the allergen from a T_H2 to a T_H1 type. The second approach is the use of specific inhibitors to block the effects or synthesis of mast cell inflammatory mediators.

Step affected	Mechanism	Specific approach
T_H2 activation	Reverse T_H2/T_H1 balance	Injection of specific antigen or peptides
Activation of B cell to produce IgE	Block co-stimulation Inhibit T_H2 cytokines	Inhibit CD40L Inhibit IL-4 or IL-13
Mast-cell activation	Inhibit effects of IgE binding to mast cell	Blockade of IgE receptor
Mediator action	Inhibit effects of mediators on specific receptors Inhibit synthesis of specific mediators	Antihistamine drugs Cyclo-oxygenase inhibitors eg aspirin

A third approach to the treatment of IgE-mediated disease is to target the high-affinity IgE receptor. An effective competitor for IgE binding to this receptor would block access of IgE with harmful specificities to the surfaces of mast cells, basophils, and eosinophils. Candidate molecules as inhibitors include modified IgE Fc constructs lacking variable regions.

The fourth approach is to block the effector pathways of the allergic response, with the aim of limiting the inflammatory response that follows the activation of cells induced by crosslinking of surface IgE by antigen. This is the mainstay of therapy at present. Epinephrine is an effective inhibitor of anaphylactic reactions by stimulating the reformation of endothelial tight junctions, promoting the relaxation of constricted bronchial smooth muscle, and stimulating the heart. Antihistamines that block the H1 receptor reduce the urticaria following histamine release from cutaneous mast cells and eosinophils. Systemic or local corticosteroids (see Chapter 13) may be needed to suppress the chronic inflammatory changes seen in asthma, rhinitis, or eczema.

Summary.

The allergic response to innocuous antigens reflects the pathophysiological aspect of a response that may have been selected over evolutionary time for its physiological role in protecting hosts against helminthic parasites. It is triggered by IgE antibody bound to the high-affinity mast cell IgE receptor FcεRI. Mast cells are strategically distributed beneath the mucosal surfaces of the body and in connective tissue. The resulting inflammation can be divided into early events, characterized by rapidly dispersed mediators like histamine, and later events that involve leukotrienes, cytokines, and chemokines, which recruit and activate particularly eosinophils, but also basophils. The late phase of this response can evolve into chronic inflammation, which is most clearly seen in allergic asthma.

Hypersensitivity diseases.

In the first part of this chapter we have seen how IgE mediates allergic reactions, also known as type I hypersensitivity. Immunological responses mediated by IgG antibodies or specific T cells can also cause adverse hypersensitivity reactions. Although these effector arms of the immune response normally participate in protective immunity to infection, they occasionally react with non-infectious antigens to produce acute or chronic hypersensitivity reactions. We shall describe common examples of such reactions in this last part of this chapter.

11-15 Innocuous antigens can cause type II hypersensitivity reactions in susceptible individuals by binding to the surfaces of circulating blood cells.

Antibody-mediated destruction of red blood cells (hemolytic anemia) or platelets (thrombocytopenia) is an uncommon side-effect associated with the intake of some drugs, such as the antibiotic penicillin, the anti-cardiac arrhythmia drug, quinidine, or the anti-hypertensive agent, methyldopa. This is an example of a **type II hypersensitivity reaction** in which the drug binds to the cell surface and serves as a target for anti-drug antibodies, which initiate complement activation on the cell surface (see Fig. 11.2). The anti-drug antibodies are only made in a minority of individuals whose susceptibility to develop such antibodies is not understood. The combination of cell-bound antibody and complement trigger clearance of the cell from the circulation, predominantly by tissue macrophages in the spleen, which bear Fcγ and complement receptors.

11-16 Systemic immune complex-mediated disease may follow the administration of large quantities of poorly catabolized antigens.

Type III hypersensitivity reactions arise when the antigen is soluble. The pathology is caused by the deposition of antigen:antibody aggregates or **immune complexes** in certain tissue sites. Immune complexes are generated in every antibody response. The pathogenic potential of immune complexes is determined, in part, by their size. Larger aggregates fix complement and are readily cleared from the circulation by the mononuclear phagocytic system, while the small complexes that form at antigen excess (see Fig. 2.13) tend to deposit in blood vessel walls, and it is here that they cause tissue damage by ligation of Fc and complement receptors on leukocytes, which in turn cause tissue injury.

A local **type III hypersensitivity reaction** can be triggered in the skin of sensitized individuals possessing IgG antibodies directed against the sensitizing antigen. When antigen is injected into the skin, IgG antibody that has diffused into the tissues forms immune complexes locally. The immune complexes bind Fc receptors on leukocytes and also activate complement, releasing C5a, which creates a local inflammatory response with increased vascular permeability. The enhanced vascular permeability allows fluid and cells, especially polymorphonuclear leukocytes, to enter the site from the local vessels. This reaction, called an **Arthus reaction** (Fig. 11.16), is absent in mice lacking expression of

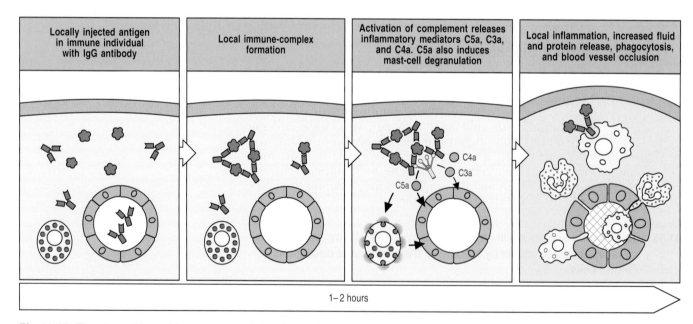

| Locally injected antigen in immune individual with IgG antibody | Local immune-complex formation | Activation of complement releases inflammatory mediators C5a, C3a, and C4a. C5a also induces mast-cell degranulation | Local inflammation, increased fluid and protein release, phagocytosis, and blood vessel occlusion |

1–2 hours

Fig. 11.16 The deposition of immune complexes in local tissues causes a local inflammatory response known as an Arthus reaction (type III hypersensitivity reaction). In individuals who have already made IgG antibody to allergen, allergen injected into the skin forms immune complexes with IgG antibody that has diffused out of the capillaries. Since the dose of antigen is low, the immune complexes are only formed close to the site of injection, where they activate Fcγ receptor-bearing cells and complement. As a result, inflammatory cells invade the site, and blood vessel permeability and blood flow are increased. Platelets also accumulate at the site, ultimately leading to vessel occlusion.

the γ chain common to all Fc receptors, showing the primary importance of Fc receptors on leukocytes in triggering inflammatory responses.

Systemic injection of large quantities of a poorly catabolized foreign antigen may cause a type III hypersensitivity reaction which is known as **serum sickness**. This term described the illness that followed the administration of therapeutic horse antiserum. In the pre-antibiotic era, immune horse serum was often used to treat pneumococcal pneumonia. Specific antibodies in the horse serum would help the patient to clear the infection. In much the same way, anti-venin (serum from horses immunized with snake venoms) is still used today as a source of neutralizing antibodies to treat people suffering from the bites of poisonous snakes.

Serum sickness follows 7–10 days after the injection of the horse serum, a time interval which corresponds with the time for a primary immune response against the foreign antigen. The clinical features of serum sickness are chills, fevers, rash, arthritis, and sometimes glomerulonephritis. Urticaria is a prominent feature of the rash, implying a role for histamine derived from mast-cell degranulation.

The immunopathological basis of serum sickness is illustrated in Fig. 11.17. The onset of disease coincides with the development of antibodies, which form immune complexes with the antigen throughout the body. These immune complexes fix complement and bind and activate all leukocyte types bearing Fc and complement receptors, which in turn cause widespread tissue injury. The formation of immune complexes causes clearance of the foreign antigen and for this reason, serum sickness is a self-limiting disease. Serum sickness following a second dose of horse antiserum follows the kinetics of a secondary antibody response and the onset of disease occurs typically within a day or two. Serum sickness is nowadays seen following the use of anti-lymphocyte globulin, used as an immunosuppressive agent in transplant recipients (see Chapter 13), and also rarely after the administration of streptokinase, a bacterial enzyme that is used as a thrombolytic agent to treat patients with a myocardial infarction or heart attack.

A similar type of immunopathological response is seen in response to soluble antigens in two other situations in which antigen persists. The first is when an adaptive antibody response fails to clear an infectious agent, for example in subacute bacterial endocarditis or in chronic viral hepatitis. In this situation, the multiplying bacteria or viruses are continuously generating new antigen in the presence of a persistent antibody response, which fails to eliminate the organism. Immune complex disease ensues, with injury to small blood vessels in many organs including the skin, kidneys, and nerves. Immune complexes also form in autoimmune diseases such as systemic lupus erythematosus where, because the antigen persists, the deposition of immune complexes continues, and serious disease can result (see Section 12-6).

Some inhaled allergens provoke IgG rather than IgE antibody responses, perhaps because they are present at much higher levels in inhaled air. When a person is re-exposed to high doses of such inhaled antigens, immune complexes form in the alveolar wall of the lung. This leads to the accumulation of fluid, protein, and cells in the alveolar wall, slowing blood–gas interchange and compromising lung function. This type of reaction occurs in certain occupations such as farming, where exposure to hay dust or mold spores is repetitive. The disease that results is therefore called **farmer's lung**. It can lead to permanent damage to the alveolar membranes if exposure is sustained.

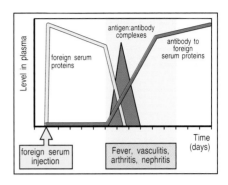

Fig. 11.17   Serum sickness is a classical example of a transient immune-complex-mediated syndrome. An injection of a foreign protein or proteins, in this case derived from horse serum, leads to an antibody response. These antibodies form immune complexes with the circulating foreign proteins. These complexes are deposited in small vessels and activate complement and phagocytes, inducing fever, and the symptoms of vasculitis, nephritis, and arthritis. All these effects are transient and resolve when the foreign protein is cleared.

<table>
<tr><td>11-17</td><td>Delayed-type hypersensitivity reactions are mediated by T$_H$1 cells and CD8 cytotoxic T cells.</td></tr>
</table>

Unlike the immediate hypersensitivity reactions, which are mediated by antibodies, **delayed-type hypersensitivity** or **type IV hypersensitivity reactions** are mediated by specific T cells. Such effector T cells function in essentially the same way as during a response to an infectious pathogen, as described in Chapter 7. Diseases in which type IV hypersensitivity responses predominate are shown in Fig. 11.18. These responses are clearly caused by T cells, since they can be seen in agammaglobulinemic individuals. Such responses can also be transferred between experimental animals using pure T cells or cloned T-cell lines.

The prototypic delayed-type hypersensitivity reaction is an artefact of modern medicine, the tuberculin test (see Section 2-30). This is a way of determining whether an individual has previously been infected with *Mycobacterium tuberculosis*. When small amounts of a protein from *M. tuberculosis* are injected into subcutaneous tissue, a T-cell mediated local inflammatory reaction evolves over 24–72 hours in individuals who have previously responded to this pathogen. The response is mediated by T$_H$1 cells, which enter the site of antigen injection, recognize complexes of peptide:MHC class II on antigen-presenting cells, and release inflammatory cytokines that increase local blood vessel permeability, bringing fluid and protein into the tissue and recruiting accessory cells to the site (Figs. 11.19 and 11.20). Each of these phases takes several hours and so the mature response appears only 24–48 hours after challenge.

Very similar reactions are observed in several cutaneous hypersensitivity responses. For instance, the rash produced by poison ivy is caused by a T-cell response to a chemical in the poison ivy leaf called pentadeca-catechol. This compound binds covalently to host proteins. The modified self proteins are then cleaved into modified self peptides, which may bind to self MHC class II molecules where they can be recognized by T$_H$1 cells. When specifically sensitized T cells recognize these complexes, they can produce extensive inflammation. As the chemical is delivered by contact with the skin, this is called a **contact hypersensitivity reaction**. The compounds that cause such reactions must be chemically active so that they can form stable complexes with host proteins.

Fig. 11.18 Type IV responses in allergy. These reactions are mediated by T cells and all take some time to develop. They can be grouped into three syndromes, according to the route by which antigen passes into the body.

Type IV hypersensitivity reactions are mediated by antigen-specific effector T cells		
Syndrome	Antigen	Consequence
Delayed-type hypersensitivity	Proteins: Insect venom Mycobacterial proteins (tuberculin, lepromin)	Local skin swelling: Erythema Induration Cellular infiltrate Dermatitis
Contact hypersensitivity	Haptens: Pentadecacatechol (poison ivy) DNFB Small metal ions: Nickel Chromate	Local epidermal reaction: Erythema Cellular infiltrate Contact dermatitis
Gluten-sensitive enteropathy (celiac disease)	Gliadin	Villous atrophy in small bowel Malabsorption

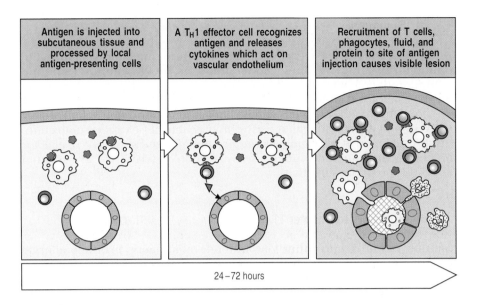

| Antigen is injected into subcutaneous tissue and processed by local antigen-presenting cells | A T$_H$1 effector cell recognizes antigen and releases cytokines which act on vascular endothelium | Recruitment of T cells, phagocytes, fluid, and protein to site of antigen injection causes visible lesion |

24–72 hours

Fig. 11.19 The time course of a delayed-type hypersensitivity reaction. The first phase involves uptake, processing, and presentation of the antigen by local antigen-presenting cells. In the second phase, T$_H$1 cells that were primed by a previous exposure to the antigen migrate to the site of injection and become activated. Since these specific cells are rare, and since there is no inflammation to attract cells to the site, it may take several hours for a T cell of the correct specificity to arrive. These cells release mediators that activate local endothelial cells, recruiting an inflammatory cell infiltrate dominated by macrophages and causing accumulation of fluid and protein. At this point, the lesion becomes apparent.

Some insect proteins also elicit delayed-type hypersensitivity responses. However, the early phases of the host reaction to an insect bite are often IgE-mediated or the result of the direct effects of insect venoms. Finally, some unusual delayed-type hypersensitivity responses to divalent cations have been observed, for example to nickel, which may alter the conformation or peptide binding of MHC class II molecules.

Type IV hypersensitivity reactions can also involve CD8 T cells, which damage tissues mainly by cell-mediated cytotoxicity. Some chemicals, including pentadecacatechol, are soluble in lipid and can therefore cross the cell membrane and modify intracellular proteins. These modified proteins generate modified peptides within the cytosol, which are translocated into the endoplasmic reticulum and delivered to the cell surface by MHC class I molecules. These are recognized by CD8 T cells, which can cause damage either by killing the eliciting cell or by secreting cytokines such as IFN-γ.

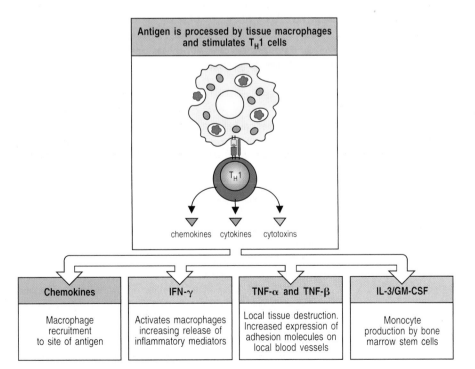

Antigen is processed by tissue macrophages and stimulates T$_H$1 cells

chemokines   cytokines   cytotoxins

Chemokines	IFN-γ	TNF-α and TNF-β	IL-3/GM-CSF
Macrophage recruitment to site of antigen	Activates macrophages increasing release of inflammatory mediators	Local tissue destruction. Increased expression of adhesion molecules on local blood vessels	Monocyte production by bone marrow stem cells

Fig. 11.20 The delayed-type (type IV) hypersensitivity response is directed by cytokines released by T$_H$1 cells stimulated by antigen. Antigen in the local tissues is processed by antigen-presenting cells and presented on MHC class II molecules. Antigen-specific T$_H$1 cells can recognize the antigen locally at the site of injection, and release chemokines and cytokines that recruit macrophages to the site of antigen deposition. Antigen presentation by the newly recruited macrophages then amplifies the response. T cells may also affect local blood vessels through release of TNF-β and TNF-α, and stimulate the production of macrophages through the release of IL-3 and GM-CSF. Finally, T$_H$1 cells activate macrophages through release of IFN-γ and TNF-α, and kill macrophages and other sensitive cells through release of TNF-β or by expression of the Fas ligand.

Summary.

Hypersensitivity diseases reflect normal immune mechanisms directed to innocuous antigens. They can be mediated by IgG antibodies bound to modified cell surfaces, or by complexes of antibodies bound to poorly catabolized antigens, as occurs in serum sickness. Hypersensitivity reactions mediated by T cells can be activated by modified self proteins, or by injected proteins such as the mycobacterial extract, tuberculin. These T-cell mediated responses require the induced synthesis of effector molecules and develop more slowly, which is why they are termed delayed-type hypersensitivity.

Summary to Chapter 11.

Immune responses to otherwise innocuous antigens produce allergic or hypersensitive reactions upon re-exposure to the same antigen. Most allergies involve the production of IgE antibody to common environmental allergens. Some people are intrinsically prone to making IgE antibodies against many allergens, and such people are said to be atopic. IgE production is driven by antigen-specific T_H2 cells, which are initially primed in the presence of a burst of IL-4 released by specialized T cells early in the immune response. The IgE produced binds to the high-affinity IgE receptor FcεRI on mast cells, basophils, and activated eosinophils. Physiologically, this provides front-line defense against pathogens but, in advanced societies, the IgE bound to mast cells triggers allergic reactions. Antibodies of other isotypes and specific effector T cells contribute to hypersensitivity to other antigens.

General references.

Geha, R.S.: **Regulation of IgE synthesis in humans**. *J. Allergy. Clin. Immunol.* 1992, **90**:143-150.

Maggi, E. and Romagnani, S.: **Role of T cells and T-cell-derived cytokines in the pathogenesis of allergic diseases**. *Ann. N. Y. Acad. Sci.* 1994, **725**:2-12.

Middleton, E., Jr., Reed, C.E., Ellis, E.F., Adkinson, N.F., Yunginger, J.W., Busse, W.W.: *Allergy: Principles and Practice,,* 4th edn. St Louis. Mosby, 1993.

Paul, W.E., Seder, R.A., and Plaut, M.: **Lymphokine and cytokine production by Fc epsilon RI⁺ cells**. *Adv. Immunol.* 1993, **53**:1-29.

Rosen, F.S.: **Urticaria, angioedema, and anaphylaxis**. *Pediatr. Rev.* 1992, **13**:387-390.

Scharenberg, A.M. and Kinet, J.P.: **Allergy. Is localized immunoglobulin E synthesis the problem?** *Curr. Biol.* 1994, **4**:140-142.

Sutton, B.J. and Gould, H.J.: **The human IgE network**. *Nature* 1993, **366**:421-428.

Section references.

11-1 Allergens are a class of antigen that evoke an IgE response and are often delivered transmucosally at low dose.

O'Hehir, R.E., Garman, R.D., Greenstein, J.L., and Lamb, J.R.: **The specificity and regulation of T-cell responsiveness to allergens**. *Ann. Rev. Immunol.* 1991, **9**:67-95.

Parronchi, P., Macchia, D., Piccinni, M.P., Biswas, P., Simonelli, C., Maggi, E., Ricci, M., Ansari, A.A., and Romagnani, S.: **Allergen- and bacterial antigen-specific T-cell clones established from atopic donors show a different profile of cytokine production**. *Proc. Natl. Acad. Sci.* 1991, **88**:4538-4542.

Romagnani, S.: **Regulation of the development of type 2 T-helper cells in allergy**. *Curr. Opin. Immunol.* 1994, **6**:838-846.

Sertl, K., Takemura, T., Tschachler, E., Ferrans, V.J., Kaliner, M.A., and Shevach, E.M.: **Dendritic cells with antigen-presenting capability reside in airway epithelium, lung parenchyma, and visceral pleura**. *J. Exp. Med.* 1986, **163**:436-451.

11-2 Enzymes are frequent triggers of allergy.

Creticos, P.S., Reed, C.E., Norman, P.S., Khoury, J., Adkinson, N.F.,Jr., Buncher, C.R., Busse, W.W., Bush, R.K., Gadde, J., Li, J.T., Richerson, H.B., Rosenthal, R.R., Solomon, W.R., Steinberg, P., and Yunginger, J.W.: **Ragweed immunotherapy in adult asthma**. *N. Engl. J. Med.* 1996, **334**:501-506.

Garraud, O., Nkenfou, C., Bradley, J.E., Perler, F.B., and Nutman, T.B.: **Identification of recombinant filarial proteins capable of inducing polyclonal and antigen-specific IgE and IgG4 antibodies**. *J. Immunol.* 1995, **155**:1316-1325.

Grammer, L.C. and Patterson, R.: **Proteins: chymopapain and insulin**. *J. Allergy Clin. Immunol.* 1984, **74**:635-640.

Hewitt, C.R., Brown, A.P., Hart, B.J., and Pritchard, D.I.: **A major house dust mite allergen disrupts the immunoglobulin E network by selectively cleaving CD23: innate protection by antiproteases**. *J. Exp. Med.* 1995, **182**:1537-1544.

Thomas, W.R.: **Mite allergens groups I-VII. A catalogue of enzymes**. *Clin. Exp. Allergy* 1993, **23**:350-353.

11-3 Class switching to IgE in B lymphocytes is favored by specific accessory signals.

Aoki, I., Kinzer, C., Shirai, A., Paul, W.E., and Klinman, D.M.: **IgE receptor-positive non-B/non-T cells dominate the production of interleukin-4 and interleukin-6 in immunized mice.** *Proc. Natl. Acad. Sci.* 1995, **92**:2534-2538.

Burd, P.R., Thompson, W.C., Max, E.E., and Mills, F.C.: **Activated mast cells produce interleukin-13.** *J. Exp. Med.* 1995, **181**:1373-1380.

Gauchat, J.F., Henchoz, S., Mazzei, G., Aubry, J.P., Brunner, T., Blasey, H., Life, P., Talabot, D., Flores Romo, L., Thompson, J., and et al, : **Induction of human IgE synthesis in B cells by mast cells and basophils.** *Nature* 1993, **365**:340-343.

Gauchat, J.F., Henchoz, S., Fattah, D., Mazzei, G., Aubry, J.P., Jomotte, T., Dash, L., Page, K., Solari, R., Aldebert, D., and et al, : **CD40 ligand is functionally expressed on human eosinophils.** *Eur. J. Immunol.* 1995, **25**:863-865.

Keegan, A.D., Johnston, J.A., Tortolani, P.J., McReynolds, L.J., Kinzer, C., O'Shea, J.J., and Paul, W.E.: **Similarities and differences in signal transduction by interleukin-4 and interleukin-13: analysis of Janus kinase activation.** *Proc. Natl. Acad. Sci.* 1995, **92**:7681-7685.

Life, P., Aubry, J.P., Estoppey, S., Schnuriger, V., and Bonnefoy, J.Y.: **CD28 functions as an adhesion molecule and is involved in the regulation of human IgE synthesis.** *Eur. J. Immunol.* 1995, **25**:333-339.

Vercelli, D. and Geha, R.S.: **Regulation of IgE synthesis: from the membrane to the genes.** *Springer Semin. Immunopath.* 1993, **15**:5-16.

Yoshimoto, T., Bendelac, A., Watson, C., Hu Li, J., and Paul, W.E.: **Role of NK1.1$^+$ T cells in a TH2 response and in immunoglobulin E production.** *Science* 1995, **270**:1845-1847.

Yoshimoto, T., Bendelac, A., Hu Li, J., and Paul, W.E.: **Defective IgE production by SJL mice is linked to the absence of CD4$^+$, NK1.1$^+$ T cells that promptly produce interleukin 4.** *Proc. Natl. Acad. Sci.* 1995, **92**:11931-11934.

11-4 Genetic factors contribute to the preferential priming of T$_H$2 cells and IgE-mediated allergy.

Howell, W.M. and Holgate, S.T.: **HLA genetics and allergic disease.** *Thorax* 1995, **50**:815-818.

Marsh, D.G., Neely, J.D., Breazeale, D.R., Ghosh, B., Freidhoff, L.R., Ehrlich Kautzky, E., Schou, C., Krishnaswamy, G., and Beaty, T.H.: **Linkage analysis of IL-4 and other chromosome 5q31.1 markers and total serum immunoglobulin E concentrations.** *Science* 1994, **264**:1152-1156.

Marsh, D.G., Neely, J.D., Breazeale, D.R., Ghosh, B., Freidhoff, L.R., Schou, C., and Beaty, T.H.: **Genetic basis of IgE responsiveness: relevance to the atopic diseases.** *Intl. Arch. Allergy Immunol.* 1995, **107**:25-28.

Postma, D.S., Bleecker, E.R., Amelung, P.J., Holroyd, K.J., Xu, J., Panhuysen, C.I., Meyers, D.A., and Levitt, R.C.: **Genetic susceptibility to asthma—bronchial hyperresponsiveness coinherited with a major gene for atopy.** *N. Engl. J. Med.* 1995, **333**:894-900.

Shirakawa, T., Li, A., Dubowitz, M., Dekker, J.W., Shaw, A.E., Faux, J.A., Ra, C., Cookson, W.O., and Hopkin, J.M.: **Association between atopy and variants of the beta subunit of the high-affinity immunoglobulin E receptor.** *Nat. Genet.* 1994, **7**:125-129.

11-5 Most IgE is cell-bound and engages effector mechanisms of immunity by different pathways from other antibody isotypes.

Adamczewski, M. and Kinet, J.P.: **The high-affinity receptor for immunoglobulin E.** *Chem. Immunol.* 1994, **59**:173-190.

Bonnefoy, J.Y., Aubry, J.P., Gauchat, J.F., Graber, P., Life, P., Flores Romo, L., and Mazzei, G.: **Receptors for IgE.** *Curr. Opin. Immunol.* 1993, **5**:944-949.

Delespesse, G., Sarfati, M., Wu, C.Y., Fournier, S., and Letellier, M.: **The low-affinity receptor for IgE.** *Immunol. Rev.* 1992, **125**:77-97.

Fujiwara, H., Kikutani, H., Suematsu, S., Naka, T., Yoshida, K., Tanaka, T., Suemura, M., Matsumoto, N., Kojima, S., and et al, : **The absence of IgE antibody-mediated augmentation of immune responses in CD23-deficient mice.** *Proc. Natl. Acad. Sci.* 1994, **91**:6835-6839.

Metzger, H.: **The receptor with high affinity for IgE.** *Immunol. Rev.* 1992, **125**:37-48.

Scharenberg, A.M. and Kinet, J.P.: **Initial events in FcεRI signal transduction.** *J. Allergy Clin. Immunol.* 1994, **94**:1142-1146.

Scharenberg, A.M. and Kinet, J.P.: **Early events in mast cell signal transduction.** *Chem. Immunol.* 1995, **61**:72-87.

Stief, A., Texido, G., Sansig, G., Eibel, H., Le Gros, G., and van der Putten, H.: **Mice deficient in CD23 reveal its modulatory role in IgE production but no role in T and B cell development.** *J. Immunol.* 1994, **152**:3378-3390.

11-6 Mast cells reside in tissues and orchestrate allergic reactions.

Austen, K.F.: **The Paul Kallos Memorial Lecture. From slow-reacting substance of anaphylaxis to leukotriene C4 synthase.** *Intl. Arch. Allergy Immunol.* 1995, **107**:19-24.

Galli, S.J.: **New concepts about the mast cell.** *N. Engl. J. Med.* 1993, **328**:257-265.

Galli, S.J., Tsai, M., and Wershil, B.K.: **The c-kit receptor, stem cell factor, and mast cells. What each is teaching us about the others.** *Am. J. Pathol.* 1993, **142**:965-974.

Galli, S.J., Zsebo, K.M., and Geissler, E.N.: **The kit ligand, stem cell factor.** *Adv. Immunol.* 1994, **55**:1-96.

Valent, P. and Bettelheim, P.: **Cell surface structures on human basophils and mast cells: biochemical and functional characterization.** *Adv. Immunol.* 1992, **52**:333-423.

11-7 Eosinophils and basophils are specialized granulocytes that release toxic mediators in IgE-mediated responses.

Capron, M., Truong, M.J., Aldebert, D., Gruart, V., Suemura, M., Delespesse, G., Tourvieille, B., and Capron, A.: **Eosinophil IgE receptor and CD23.** *Immunol. Res.* 1992, **11**:252-259.

Collins, P.D., Marleau, S., Griffiths Johnson, D.A., Jose, P.J., and Williams, T.J.: **Cooperation between interleukin-5 and the chemokine eotaxin to induce eosinophil accumulation in vivo.** *J. Exp. Med.* 1995, **182**:1169-1174.

Gleich, G.J., Adolphson, C.R., and Leiferman, K.M.: **The biology of the eosinophilic leukocyte.** *Ann. Rev. Med.* 1993, **44**:85-101.

Gounni, A.S., Lamkhioued, B., Delaporte, E., Dubost, A., Kinet, J.P., Capron, A., and Capron, M.: **The high-affinity IgE receptor on eosinophils: from allergy to parasites or from parasites to allergy?** *J. Allergy Clin. Immunol.* 1994, **94**:1214-1216.

Parker, C.W.: **Lipid mediators produced through the lipoxygenase pathway.** *Ann. Rev. Immunol.* 1987, **5**:65-84.

Schroeder, J.T., Kagey Sobotka, A., and Lichtenstein, L.M.: **The role of the basophil in allergic inflammation.** *Allergy* 1995, **50**:463-472.

Seminario, M.C. and Gleich, G.J.: **The role of eosinophils in the pathogenesis of asthma.** *Curr. Opin. Immunol.* 1994, **6**:860-864.

Thomas, L.L.: **Basophil and eosinophil interactions in health and disease.** *Chem. Immunol.* 1995, **61**:186-207.

Wardlaw, A.J., Moqbel, R., and Kay, A.B.: **Eosinophils: biology and role in disease.** *Adv. Immunol.* 1995, **60**:151-266.

11-8 Allergic reactions following ligation of IgE on mast cells may be divided into an immediate and a late response.

Charlesworth, E.N., Kagey Sobotka, A., Schleimer, R.P., Norman, P.S., and Lichtenstein, L.M.: **Prednisone inhibits the appearance of inflammatory mediators and the influx of eosinophils and basophils associated with the cutaneous late-phase response to allergen**. *J. Immunol.* 1991, **146**:671-676.

Guo, C.B., Liu, M.C., Galli, S.J., Bochner, B.S., Kagey Sobotka, A., and Lichtenstein, L.M.: **Identification of IgE-bearing cells in the late-phase response to antigen in the lung as basophils**. *Am. J. Resp. Cell Mol. Biol.* 1994, **10**:384-390.

Liu, M.C., Hubbard, W.C., Proud, D., Stealey, B.A., Galli, S.J., Kagey Sobotka, A., Bleecker, E.R., and Lichtenstein, L.M.: **Immediate and late inflammatory responses to ragweed antigen challenge of the peripheral airways in allergic asthmatics. Cellular, mediator, and permeability changes**. *Am. Rev. Resp. Dis.* 1991, **144**:51-58.

Varney, V.A., Hamid, Q.A., Gaga, M., Ying, S., Jacobson, M., Frew, A.J., Kay, A.B., and Durham, S.R.: **Influence of grass pollen immunotherapy on cellular infiltration and cytokine mRNA expression during allergen-induced late-phase cutaneous responses**. *J. Clin. Invest.* 1993, **92**:644-651.

Werfel, S., Massey, W., Lichtenstein, L.M., and Bochner, B.S.: **Preferential recruitment of activated, memory T lymphocytes into skin chamber fluids during human cutaneous late-phase allergic reactions**. *J. Allergy Clin. Immunol.* 1995, **96**:57-65.

11-9 The clinical effects of allergic reactions vary according to the site of mast-cell activation.

Anderson, J.A.: **Allergic reactions to drugs and biological agents**. *JAMA* 1992, **268**:2844-2857.

11-10 The degranulation of mast cells in the walls of blood vessels following systemic absorption of allergen may cause generalized cardiovascular collapse.

Bochner, B.S. and Lichtenstein, L.M.: **Anaphylaxis** . *N. Engl. J. Med.* 1991, **324**:1785-1790.

Dombrowicz, D., Flamand, V., Brigman, K.K., Koller, B.H., and Kinet, J.P.: **Abolition of anaphylaxis by targeted disruption of the high affinity immunoglobulin E receptor alpha chain gene**. *Cell* 1993, **75**:969-976.

Fernandez, M., Warbrick, E.V., Blanca, M., and Coleman, J.W.: **Activation and hapten inhibition of mast cells sensitized with monoclonal IgE anti-penicillin antibodies: evidence for two-site recognition of the penicillin derived determinant**. *Eur. J. Immunol.* 1995, **25**:2486-2491.

Kemp, S.F., Lockey, R.F., Wolf, B.L., and Lieberman, P.: **Anaphylaxis. A review of 266 cases**. *Arch. Intl. Med.* 1995, **155**:1749-1754.

Martin, T.R., Galli, S.J., Katona, I.M., and Drazen, J.M.: **Role of mast cells in anaphylaxis. Evidence for the importance of mast cells in the cardiopulmonary alterations and death induced by anti-IgE in mice**. *J. Clin. Invest.* 1989, **83**:1375-1383.

Oettgen, H.C., Martin, T.R., Wynshaw Boris, A., Deng, C., Drazen, J.M., and Leder, P.: **Active anaphylaxis in IgE-deficient mice**. *Nature* 1994, **370**:367-370.

Reisman, R.E.: **Insect stings**. *N. Engl. J. Med.* 1994, **331**:523-527.

11-11 Exposure of the airways to allergens is associated with the development of rhinitis and asthma.

Arm, J.P. and Lee, T.H.: **The pathobiology of bronchial asthma**. *Adv. Immunol.* 1992, **51**:323-382.

Badhwar, A.K. and Druce, H.M.: **Allergic rhinitis**. *Med. Clin. North Am.* 1992, **76**:789-803.

Bochner, B.S., Undem, B.J., and Lichtenstein, L.M.: **Immunological aspects of allergic asthma**. *Ann. Rev. Immunol.* 1994, **12**:295-335.

Corrigan, C.J. and Kay, A.B.: **T cells and eosinophils in the pathogenesis of asthma**. *Immunol. Today* 1992, **13**:501-507.

Drazen, J.M., Arm, J.P., and Austen, K.F.: **Sorting out the cytokines of asthma**. *J. Exp. Med.* 1996, **183**:1-5.

Huang, S.K., Xiao, H.Q., Kleine Tebbe, J., Paciotti, G., Marsh, D.G., Lichtenstein, L.M., and Liu, M.C.: **IL-13 expression at the sites of allergen challenge in patients with asthma**. *J. Immunol.* 1995, **155**:2688-2694.

Kaliner, M. and Lemanske, R.: **Rhinitis and asthma**. *JAMA* 1992, **268**:2807-2829.

Naclerio, R.M., Baroody, F.M., Kagey Sobotka, A., and Lichtenstein, L.M.: **Basophils and eosinophils in allergic rhinitis**. *J Allergy. Clin. Immunol.* 1994, **94**:1303-1309.

11-12 Skin allergy is manifest as urticaria or chronic eczema.

Leung, D.Y.: **Immune mechanisms in atopic dermatitis and relevance to treatment**. *Allergy Proc.* 1991, **12**:339-346.

Ring, J., Bieber, T., Vieluf, D., Kunz, B., and Przybilla, B.: **Atopic eczema, Langerhans cells and allergy**. *Intl. Arch. Allergy Appl. Immunol.* 1991, **94**:194-201.

11-13 Allergy to foods can cause symptoms limited to the gut but also commonly causes systemic reactions.

Ewan, P.W.: **Clinical study of peanut and nut allergy in 62 consecutive patients: new features and associations**. *BMJ* 1996, **312**:1074-1078.

Nordlee, J.A., Taylor, S.L., Townsend, J.A., Thomas, L.A., and Bush, R.K.: **Identification of a Brazil-nut allergen in transgenic soybeans**. *N. Engl. J. Med.* 1996, **334**:688-692.

Opper, F.H. and Burakoff, R.: **Food allergy and intolerance**. *Gastroenterologist* 1993, **1**:211-220.

11-14 Allergy may be treated by inhibition of the effector pathways activated by antigen crosslinking of cell-surface IgE or by inhibiting IgE production.

O'Hehir, R.E. and Lamb, J.R.: **Strategies for modulating immunoglobulin E synthesis**. *Clin. Exp. Allergy.* 1992, **22**:7-10.

Kinet, J.P., Blank, U., Brini, A.8, Jouvin, M.H., Kuster, H., Mejan, O., and Ra, C.: **The high-affinity receptor for immunoglobulin E: a target for therapy of allergic diseases**. *Intl. Arch. Allergy Appl. Immunol.* 1991, **94**:51-55.

Lee, T.H., O'Hickey, S.P., Jacques, C., Hawksworth, R.J., Arm, J.P., Christie, P., Spur, B.W., and Crea, A.E.: **Sulphidopeptide leukotrienes in asthma**. *Adv. Prostagl. Thrombox. Leukot. Res.* 1991, **21A**:415-419.

Pauwels, R.A., Joos, G.F., and Kips, J.C.: **Leukotrienes as therapeutic target in asthma**. *Allergy* 1995, **50**:615-622.

Platts Mills, T.A.: **Allergen-specific treatment for asthma: III**. *Am. Rev. Resp. Dis.* 1993, **148**:553-555.

Yeo, A. and Lamb, J.R.: **Manipulating the immune response in allergic disease: targeting CD4+ T cells**. *Trends Biotechnol.* 1995, **13**:186-190.

11-15 Innocuous antigens can cause type II hypersensitivity reactions in susceptible individuals by binding to the surfaces of circulating blood cells.

Greinacher, A., Potzsch, B., Amiral, J., Dummel, V., Eichner, A., and Mueller Eckhardt, C.: **Heparin-associated thrombocytopenia: isolation of the antibody and characterization of a multimolecular PF4-heparin complex as the major antigen**. *Thromb. Haemost.* 1994, **71**:247-251.

Murphy, W.G. and Kelton, J.G.: **Immune haemolytic anaemia and thrombocytopenia: drugs and autoantibodies.** *Biochem. Soc. Trans.* 1991, **19**:183-186.

Petz, L.D.: **Drug-induced autoimmune hemolytic anemia.** *Transf. Med. Rev.* 1993, **7**:242-254.

Petz, L.D. and Mueller Eckhardt, C.: **Drug-induced immune hemolytic anemia.** *Transfusion* 1992, **32**:202-204.

Salama, A., Santoso, S., and Mueller Eckhardt, C.: **Antigenic determinants responsible for the reactions of drug-dependent antibodies with blood cells.** *Br. J. Haematol.* 1991, **78**:535-539.

11-16	Systemic immune complex-mediated disease may follow the administration of large quantities of poorly-catabolized antigens.

Bielory, L., Gascon, P., Lawley, T.J., Young, N.S., and Frank, M.M.: **Human serum sickness: a prospective analysis of 35 patients treated with equine anti-thymocyte globulin for bone marrow failure.** *Medicine. Baltimore 1988,* **67**:40-57.

Cochrane, C.G. and Koffler, D.: **Immune complex disease in experimental animals and man.** *Adv. Immunol.* 1973, **16**:185-264.

Davies, K.A., Mathieson, P., Winearls, C.G., Rees, A.J., and Walport, M.J.: **Serum sickness and acute renal failure after streptokinase therapy for myocardial infarction.** *Clin. Exp. Immunol.* 1990, **80**:83-88.

Lawley, T.J., Bielory, L., Gascon, P., Yancey, K.B., Young, N.S., and Frank, M.M.: **A prospective clinical and immunologic analysis of patients with serum sickness.** *N. Engl. J. Med. 1984,* **311**:1407-1413.

Schifferli, J.A., Ng, Y.C., and Peters, D.K.: **The role of complement and its receptor in the elimination of immune complexes.** *N. Engl. J. Med.* 1986, **315**:488-495.

Theofilopoulos, A.N. and Dixon, F.J.: **Immune complexes in human diseases: a review.** *Am. J. Pathol.* 1980, **100**:529-594.

11-17	Delayed-type hypersensitivity reactions are mediated by T_H1 cells and CD8 cytotoxic T cells.

Bernhagen, J., Bacher, M., Calandra, T., Metz, C.N., Doty, S.B., Donnelly, T., and Bucala, R.: **An essential role for macrophage migration inhibitory factor in** the tuberculin delayed-type hypersensitivity reaction. *J. Exp. Med.* 1996, **183**: 277-282.

Ishii, N., Sugita, Y., Nakajima, H., Tanaka, S., and Askenase, P.W.: **Elicitation of nickel sulfate ($NiSO_4$)-specific delayed-type hypersensitivity requires early-occurring and early-acting, $NiSO_4$-specific DTH-initiating cells with an unusual mixed phenotype for an antigen-specific cell.** *Cell. Immunol.* 1995, **161**:244-255.

Kalish, R.S., Wood, J.A., and LaPorte, A.: **Processing of urushiol (poison ivy) hapten by both endogenous and exogenous pathways for presentation to T cells** *in vitro. J. Clin. Invest.* 1994, **93**:2039-2047.

Larsen, C.G., Thomsen, M.K., Gesser, B., Thomsen, P.D., Deleuran, B.W., Nowak, J., Skodt, V., Thomsen, H.K., Deleuran, M., Thestrup Pedersen, K., and et al, : **The delayed-type hypersensitivity reaction is dependent on IL-8. Inhibition of a tuberculin skin reaction by an anti-IL-8 monoclonal antibody.** *J. Immunol.* 1995, **155**:2151-2157.

Muller, G., Saloga, J., Germann, T., Schuler, G., Knop, J., and Enk, A.H.: **IL-12 as mediator and adjuvant for the induction of contact sensitivity** *in vivo. J. Immunol.* 1995, **155**:4661-4668.

Immune Responses in the Absence of Infection

12

We have learned in preceding chapters that the adaptive immune response is a critical component of host defense against infection and therefore essential for normal health. Unfortunately, adaptive immune responses are also sometimes elicited by antigens not associated with infectious agents, and this may cause serious disease. These responses are essentially identical to adaptive immune responses to infectious agents; only the antigens differ. In Chapter 11, we saw how responses to certain environmental antigens cause allergic diseases and other hypersensitivity reactions. In this chapter we will examine responses to two particularly important categories of antigen: responses to self tissue antigens, called **autoimmunity**, which can lead to **autoimmune diseases** characterized by tissue damage; and responses to transplanted organs that lead to **graft rejection**. We will examine these disease processes and the mechanisms that lead to the undesirable adaptive immune responses that are their root cause.

Autoimmunity: responses to self antigens.

Autoimmune disease occurs when a specific adaptive immune response is mounted against self antigens. The normal consequence of an adaptive immune response against a foreign antigen is the clearance of the antigen from the body. Virus-infected cells, for example, are destroyed by cytotoxic T cells, while soluble antigens are cleared by formation of immune complexes, which are taken up by cells of the mononuclear phagocytic system, such as macrophages. However, when a sustained immune response develops against self antigens, it is usually impossible for immune effector mechanisms to eliminate the antigen completely. The consequence is that the effector pathways of immunity cause chronic inflammatory injury to tissues, which may prove lethal. The mechanisms of tissue damage in autoimmune diseases are essentially the same as those that operate in protective immunity and in allergy (Fig. 12.1).

Fig. 12.1 Autoimmune diseases classified by the mechanism of tissue damage. All the mechanisms outlined in Fig. 11.2 except type I responses also occur in autoimmune diseases. Some additional autoimmune diseases in which the antigen is a cell-surface receptor are listed later in Fig. 12.9.

Some common autoimmune diseases classified by immunopathogenic mechanism		
Syndrome	Autoantigen	Consequence
Type II antibody to cell-surface or matrix antigens		
Autoimmune hemolytic anemia	Rh blood group, I antigen	Destruction of red blood cells by complement and phagocytes, anemia
Autoimmune thrombocytopenia purpura	Platelet integrin GpIIb:IIIa	Abnormal bleeding
Goodpasture's syndrome	Non-collagenous domain of basement membrane collagen type IV	Glomerulonephritis Pulmonary hemorrhage
Pemphigus vulgaris	Epidermal cadherin	Blistering of skin
Acute rheumatic fever	Streptococcal cell wall antigens, antibodies cross-react with cardiac muscle	Arthritis, myocarditis, late scarring of heart valves
Type III immune-complex disease		
Mixed essential cryoglobulinemia	Rheumatoid factor IgG complexes (with or without hepatitis C antigens)	Systemic vasculitis
Systemic lupus erythematosus	DNA, histones, ribosomes, snRNP, scRNP	Glomerulonephritis, vasculitis, arthritis
Type IV T-cell mediated disease		
Insulin-dependent diabetes mellitus	Pancreatic β-cell antigen	β-cell destruction
Rheumatoid arthritis	Unknown synovial joint antigen	Joint inflammation and destruction
Experimental autoimmune encephalomyelitis (EAE), multiple sclerosis	Myelin basic protein, proteolipid protein	Brain invasion by CD4 T cells, paralysis

It is believed that autoimmunity is initiated by responses involving T cells. Cytotoxic T-cell responses and inappropriate activation of macrophages can cause extensive tissue damage, while inappropriate T-cell help can initiate a harmful antibody response to self antigens. Autoimmune responses are a natural consequence of the open repertoires of both B-cell and T-cell receptors that allows them to recognize any pathogen, since such receptors will also include those reactive to self antigens. It is not known what triggers autoimmunity but both environmental and genetic factors, especially MHC genotype, are clearly important. Transient autoimmune responses are common but it is only when they are sustained and cause lasting tissue damage that they attract medical attention. In this section, we shall examine the nature of autoimmune responses and how autoimmunity leads to tissue damage. In the last section of this chapter, we shall examine the mechanisms by which autoimmune responses are initiated.

12-1 Specific adaptive immune responses to self antigens can cause autoimmune disease.

It was realized early in the study of immunity that the powerful effector mechanisms used in host defense could, if turned against the host, lead to severe tissue damage; Ehrlich termed this *horror autotoxicus*. Normal individuals do not mount sustained adaptive immune responses to their own antigens and, although transient responses to damaged self tissues occur, these rarely cause additional tissue damage. However, while self tolerance is the general rule, sustained immune responses to self tissues occur, and these autoimmune responses cause the severe tissue damage that Ehrlich predicted.

In experimental animals, autoimmune disease can be induced artificially by mixing tissues with strong adjuvants containing bacteria (see Section 2-4) and injecting them into a genetically identical animal. This shows that autoimmunity involves a specific, adaptive immune response to self antigens and forms the basis for our understanding of how autoimmune disease arises. In humans, autoimmunity usually arises spontaneously; that is, we do not know what events initiated the immune response to self that leads to the autoimmune disease. However, as we shall learn in the last section of this chapter, there is a strong association between infection and the onset of autoimmunity, suggesting that infectious agents play a critical role in the process.

Although anyone can, in principle, develop an autoimmune disease, it seems that some individuals are more at risk than others of developing particular diseases. We shall first consider those factors that contribute to susceptibility.

12-2 Susceptibility to autoimmune diseases is controlled by environmental and genetic factors, especially MHC genes.

The best evidence in humans that there are disease susceptibility genes for autoimmunity comes from family studies and especially from studies of twins. A semiquantitative technique for measuring what proportion of the susceptibility to a particular disease arises from genetic factors is to compare the incidence of disease in monozygotic and dizygotic twins. If a disease shows a high concordance in all twins this could be caused by shared genetic or environmental factors. This is because both monozygotic and dizygotic twins tend to be brought up in similarly shared environmental conditions. However, if the high concordance is restricted to monozygotic rather than dizygotic twins, then genetic factors are likely to be more important than environmental factors. Studies with twins have been undertaken for several human diseases in which autoimmunity plays an important role, including insulin-dependent diabetes mellitus, rheumatoid arthritis, multiple sclerosis, and systemic lupus erythematosus. In each case, around 20% of pairs of monozygotic twins show disease concordance, compared with less than 5% of dizygotic twins. These results show an important role for both inherited and environmental factors in the induction of autoimmune disease. In addition to these findings in humans, certain inbred mouse strains reliably develop particular spontaneous or experimentally induced autoimmune diseases. These findings have led to an extensive search for genes that determine susceptibility to autoimmune disease.

To date, the most consistent association for susceptibility to autoimmune disease has been with the MHC genotype. Many human autoimmune diseases show HLA-linked disease associations (Fig. 12.2) and these have been defined more exactly as HLA genotyping has become more precise (see Section 2-27). For example, the association between insulin-dependent diabetes mellitus, and the DR3 and DR4 alleles—initially discovered by HLA typing using antibodies—is now known to be between the disease and the DQβ MHC genotype, which is linked closely to DR3 and DR4. The normal DQβ amino acid sequence has an aspartic acid at position 57, whereas in Caucasoid populations, patients with diabetes most often have valine, serine, or alanine at that position (Fig. 12.3); mice that develop spontaneous diabetes also have a serine at this position in the homologous MHC class II molecule. In most autoimmune diseases, susceptibility is linked most closely with MHC class II alleles but in some cases MHC class I alleles are involved.

Fig. 12.2 Associations of HLA genotype and of sex with susceptibility to autoimmune disease. The 'relative risk' for an HLA allele in an autoimmune disease is calculated by comparing the observed number of patients carrying the HLA allele with the number that would be expected, given the prevalence of the HLA allele in the general population. HLA-DR genes are tightly linked to HLA-DQ genes and it is the latter that are the relevant disease susceptibility genes for insulin-dependent diabetes mellitus (see Section 2-26). Some diseases show a significant bias in the sex ratio; this is taken to imply that sex hormones are involved in pathogenesis. Consistent with this, the difference in the sex ratio in these diseases is greatest between the menarche and the menopause, when levels of such hormones are highest.

Associations of HLA genotype with susceptibility to autoimmune disease			
Disease	HLA allele	Relative risk	Sex ratio (♀:♂)
Ankylosing spondylitis	B27	87.4	0.3
Acute anterior uveitis	B27	10.04	<0.5
Goodpasture's syndrome	DR2	15.9	~1
Multiple sclerosis	DR2	4.8	10
Graves' disease	DR3	3.7	4–5
Myasthenia gravis	DR3	2.5	~1
Systemic lupus erythematosus	DR3	5.8	10–20
Insulin-dependent diabetes mellitus	DR3 and DR4	3.2	~1
Rheumatoid arthritis	DR4	4.2	3
Pemphigus vulgaris	DR4	14.4	~1
Hashimoto's thyroiditis	DR5	3.2	4–5

Fig. 12.3 Amino acid changes in the sequence of an MHC class II protein correlate with susceptibility to and protection from diabetes. The sequence of HLA-DQβ₁ contains an aspartic acid at position 57 in most people; in Caucasoid populations, patients with insulin-dependent diabetes mellitus (IDDM) more often have valine, serine, or alanine at this position instead, as well as other differences. Asp 57, shown in red on the backbone structure of the DQβ chain forms a salt bridge (shown in green) to an arginine residue (shown in pink, middle panel) in the adjacent α chain (gray). The change to an uncharged residue (for example, alanine, shown in yellow in the bottom panel) disrupts this salt bridge, altering the stability of the DQ molecule. In mice, the non-obese diabetic (NOD) strain, which develops spontaneous diabetes, shows a similar replacement of serine for aspartic acid at position 57 of the homologous I-Aβ chain, and NOD mice transgenic for β chains with Asp 57 have a marked reduction in diabetes incidence. Photographs courtesy of C Thorpe.

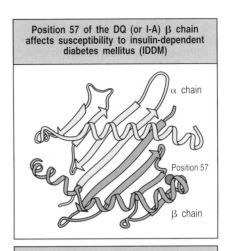

Position 57 of the DQ (or I-A) β chain affects susceptibility to insulin-dependent diabetes mellitus (IDDM)

α chain

Position 57

β chain

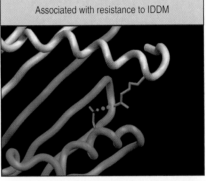

Associated with resistance to IDDM

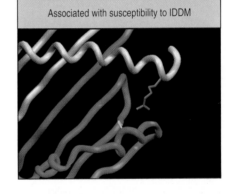

Associated with susceptibility to IDDM

The association of MHC genotype with autoimmune disease is not surprising, since all autoimmune responses involve T cells, and the ability of T cells to respond to a particular antigen depends on MHC genotype. However, this simple model for the way that MHC genotype determines susceptibility to autoimmune disease has not been proven. Susceptibility might be determined by differences in the ability of different allelic variants of MHC molecules to present autoantigenic peptides to autoreactive T cells but this remains hypothetical. Identification of the autoantigenic peptides and a demonstration that they bind selectively to MHC molecules associated with the disease would help to answer this question. We need to find out whether the binding of a particular autoantigenic peptide to a particular MHC molecule is an essential factor in susceptibility or simply a trait that is linked to the true susceptibility locus. MHC class I alleles are also linked to susceptibility to diabetes, in which the autoimmunity appears to involve both CD4 and CD8 T cells. An alternative and not necessarily mutually exclusive hypothesis for the association of MHC and susceptibility is that certain MHC molecules and their associated self peptides drive positive selection of developing thymocytes, some of which are specific for antigens that are at this time hidden from the immune system. Since these same peptides cannot drive T-cell deletion, the potentially self-reactive T cells are not deleted from the repertoire.

The association of MHC genotype with disease is assessed initially by comparing the frequency of different alleles in patients with their frequency in the normal population. For insulin-dependent diabetes mellitus, this approach demonstrated an association between disease susceptibility and the MHC class II alleles HLA-DR3 and HLA-DR4, which are linked tightly to HLA-DQ (Fig. 12.4). In addition, such studies showed that the MHC class II allele HLA-DR2 has a dominant protective effect; individuals carrying HLA-DR2, even in association with one of the susceptibility alleles, rarely develop diabetes. Another way of determining whether MHC genes are important in autoimmune disease is to study the families of affected patients. In family studies, it has been shown that two siblings affected with the same autoimmune disease are far more likely than expected to share the same MHC haplotypes (Fig. 12.5).

However, MHC genotype alone does not determine whether a person develops disease. Identical twins, sharing all of their genes, are far more likely to develop the same autoimmune disease than MHC-identical siblings, demonstrating that genetic factors other than the MHC also affect disease susceptibility. Recent studies of the genetics of autoimmune diabetes in humans and mice have shown that there are several independently segregating disease susceptibility loci in addition to the MHC.

Fig. 12.4 Population studies show linkage of insulin-dependent diabetes mellitus (IDDM) susceptibility to HLA genotype. The prevalence of diabetes in individuals varies enormously with HLA genotype. Prevalence here is relative to prevalence of diabetes in the population as a whole, which is one person in 300 in North America. Diabetes is clearly more frequent in people who express HLA-DR3 or DR4, and greatest when both DR3 and DR4 are expressed together; these alleles are linked tightly to HLA-DQ alleles that are associated with susceptibility to IDDM.

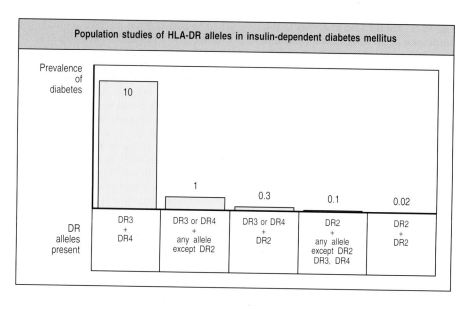

There is evidence that several other families of genes may play an important role in increasing susceptibility to autoimmune disease. In humans, inherited homozygous deficiency of the early proteins (C1, C4, or C2) of the classical pathway of complement is very strongly associated with the development of systemic lupus erythematosus (SLE). The mechanism of this association is unknown but may involve the abnormal processing of immune complexes in the absence of a functional classical pathway of complement fixation. In mice, abnormalities in the genes encoding proteins involved in the regulation of lymphocyte apoptosis, including Fas (CD95) and Fas ligand (CD95 ligand), are strongly associated with the development of SLE and this is considered further in Section 12-6. There is preliminary evidence that inherited variation in the level of expression of certain cytokines such as TNF-α may also increase susceptibility to autoimmune disease.

A further very important additional factor in disease susceptibility is the hormonal status of the patient. Many autoimmune diseases show a strong sex bias (see Fig. 12.2). Where a bias towards disease in one sex is observed in experimental animals, castration usually normalizes disease

Fig. 12.5 Family studies show strong linkage of susceptibility to insulin-dependent diabetes mellitus (IDDM) with HLA genotype. In families in which two or more siblings have IDDM, it is possible to compare the HLA genotypes of affected siblings. Affected siblings share two HLA alleles much more frequently than would be expected if the HLA genotype did not influence disease susceptibility.

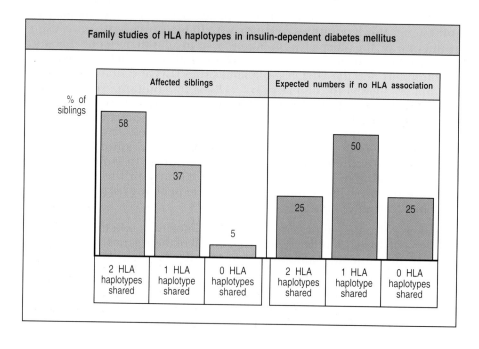

incidence between the two sexes. Furthermore, many autoimmune diseases that are more common in females show peak incidence in the years of active childbearing, when maximal production of the female sex hormones estrogen and progesterone occurs. A thorough understanding of how these genetic and hormonal factors contribute to disease susceptibility may allow us to prevent the autoimmune response.

12-3 | Either antibody or T cells can cause tissue damage in autoimmune disease.

Autoimmune diseases are mediated by sustained adaptive immune responses specific for self antigens. Tissue injury results because the antigen is an intrinsic component of the body and consequently the effector mechanisms of the immune system are directed at self tissues. Also, because the adaptive immune response is incapable of removing the offending autoantigen from the body, the immune response persists, and there is a constant supply of new autoantigen, which amplifies the response. The mechanisms of tissue injury in autoimmunity may be classified according to the same scheme adopted for hypersensitivity reactions (see Fig. 11.2). The specific antigen or group of antigens against which the autoimmune response is directed and the mechanism by which the antigen-bearing tissue is damaged, together determine the pathology and clinical expression of the disease (see Fig. 12.1).

Type I IgE-mediated autoimmune responses do not appear to play a major role in autoimmune disease. Asthma and eosinophilia (see Chapter 11) are found in a rare autoimmune vasculitis (an inflammatory disease of blood vessels), known as Churg-Strauss vasculitis. IgE responses to self tissues have been suggested as a cause of intrinsic asthma, a late-onset form of asthma with no identified extrinsic allergenic precipitator; however, the involvement of IgE autoantibodies has not been proven in this or any other autoimmune disease.

Autoimmunity causing tissue injury by mechanisms analogous to type II hypersensitivity reactions is quite common. In this form of autoimmunity, IgG or IgM responses to autoantigens located on cell surfaces or extracellular matrix cause the tissue damage. In **autoimmune hemolytic anemia**, for instance, antibodies to self antigens on red blood cells trigger red blood cell destruction (Fig. 12.6). There are two mechanisms of red cell destruction. The first is lysis of autoantibody-sensitized red cells by complement. The second is accelerated clearance from the circulation of red cells with bound antibody by interaction with Fc receptors on cells of the reticuloendothelial system, which occurs particularly in the spleen.

Lysis of nucleated cells by complement is less common because these cells are better defended by complement regulatory proteins (see Section 8-31), making them resistant to lysis, and by exocytosis or endocytosis of parts of the cell membrane bearing the membrane-attack complex. In **autoimmune thrombocytopenic purpura**, autoantibodies to the GpIIb:IIIa fibrinogen receptor on platelets cause thrombocytopenia (a depletion of platelets), which may in turn cause hemorrhage. Autoantibodies to neutrophils cause neutropenia, which increases susceptibility to pyogenic infection. In all of these cases, accelerated clearance of autoantibody-sensitized cells is the cause of their depletion from the blood. One therapeutic approach to this type of autoimmunity is removal of the spleen, the organ in which the main clearance of red cells, platelets, and leukocytes occurs.

Fig. 12.6 Antibodies specific for cell surface antigens can destroy cells (type II hypersensitivity). For example, in autoimmune hemolytic anemia, antibody-coated cells can be destroyed by one of three mechanisms: red cells coated with IgG autoantibodies are cleared predominantly by uptake on Fc receptor-bearing macrophages in the fixed mononuclear phagocytic system, (left panel). This uptake occurs mainly in the spleen; red cells coated with IgM autoantibodies fix C3 and are cleared by CR1- and CR3-bearing macrophages in the fixed mononuclear phagocytic system (right panel); the binding of certain rare autoantibodies, which fix complement extremely efficiently, cause intravascular hemolysis mediated by the membrane-attack complex (not shown).

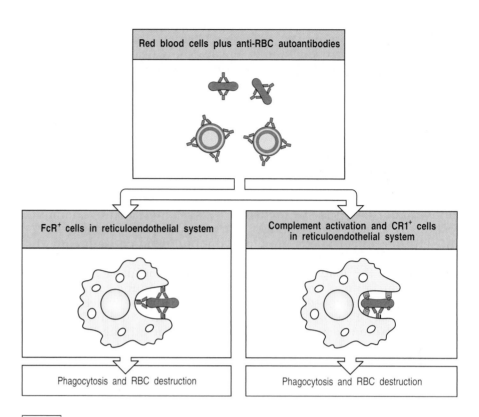

Red blood cells plus anti-RBC autoantibodies

FcR⁺ cells in reticuloendothelial system

Complement activation and CR1⁺ cells in reticuloendothelial system

Phagocytosis and RBC destruction

Phagocytosis and RBC destruction

12-4 | The fixation of sub-lytic doses of complement to cells in tissues stimulates a powerful inflammatory response.

The binding of IgG and IgM autoantibodies to cells in tissues causes inflammatory injury by different mechanisms. Most cells in tissues are fixed in place and cells of the inflammatory system must therefore travel to them. Traveling cells of the mononuclear phagocytic system bearing Fc and C3 receptors may bind and be activated by cells bearing autoantibodies and fixed complement fragments. Although nucleated cells are relatively resistant to lysis by complement, as described above, the binding of small amounts of the membrane-attack complex of complement provides a powerful activating stimulus. Depending on the type of cell binding the membrane-attack complex, interaction with sub-lytic doses of complement may cause cytokine release, generation of a respiratory burst, and the mobilization of membrane phospholipids, with the generation of arachidonic acid—the precursor to prostaglandins and leukotrienes. Chemoattractants such as leukotriene B4 and the complement component C5a are generated following complement activation in tissues that specifically attract and activate inflammatory leukocytes. Tissue injury may then result from the products of activated leukocytes and by antibody-dependent cellular cytotoxicity mediated by natural killer (NK) cells (see Section 8-19). A probable example of this type of autoimmunity is **Hashimoto's thyroiditis**, in which autoantibodies to tissue-specific antigens such as thyroid peroxidase and thyroglobulin are found at extremely high levels for prolonged periods. In this disease, direct T-cell-mediated cytotoxicity is probably also important, as discussed later.

12-5 | Autoantibodies to receptors cause disease by stimulating or blocking receptor function.

A special class of type II hypersensitivity reaction occurs when the autoantibody binds to a cell-surface receptor. Antibody binding to a receptor can either stimulate the receptor or block its stimulation by its

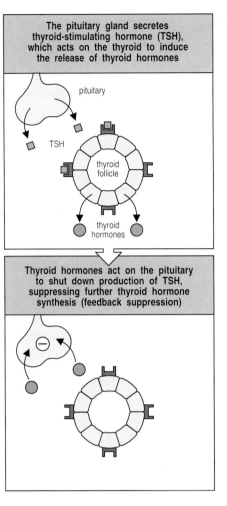

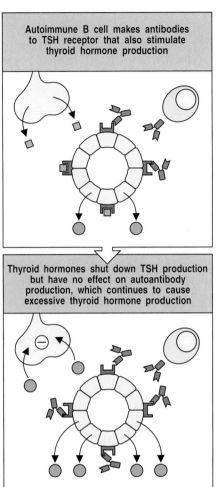

Fig. 12.7   Feedback regulation of thyroid hormone production is disrupted in Graves' disease. Graves' disease is caused by antibodies specific for the receptor for thyroid-stimulating hormone (TSH). Normally, thyroid hormones are produced in response to TSH and limit their own production by inhibiting the production of TSH by the pituitary (left panels). In Graves' disease, the autoantibodies are agonists for the TSH receptor and therefore stimulate production of thyroid hormones (right panels). The thyroid hormones inhibit TSH production in the normal way but do not affect production of the autoantibody; the excessive thyroid hormone production induced in this way causes hyperthyroidism.

natural ligand. In **Graves' disease**, autoantibody to the thyroid-stimulating hormone receptor on thyroid cells stimulates the production of excessive thyroid hormone. The production of thyroid hormone is normally controlled by feedback regulation; high levels of thyroid hormone inhibit release of thyroid-stimulating hormone by the pituitary but of course do not inhibit autoantibody production. Thus, in Graves' disease, feedback inhibition fails, and the patients become hyperthyroid (Fig. 12.7).

In **myasthenia gravis**, autoantibodies to the α chain of the nicotinic acetylcholine receptor, found at neuromuscular junctions, can block neuromuscular transmission. The antibodies are believed to drive the internalization and intracellular degradation of acetylcholine receptors (Fig. 12.8). Patients with myasthenia gravis develop progressive weakness

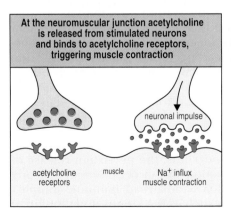

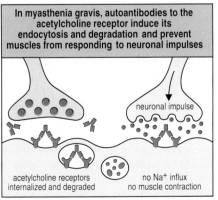

Fig. 12.8   Autoantibodies inhibit receptor function in myasthenia gravis. Myasthenia gravis is caused by antibodies to the α subunit of the receptor for acetylcholine, which is involved in neuromuscular transmission. These antibodies bind to the receptor without activating it and also cause receptor internalization and degradation. As the number of receptors on the muscle is decreased, the muscle becomes less responsive to acetylcholine released by motor neurons.

Fig. 12.9 Autoimmune diseases caused by autoantibodies to cell-surface receptor molecules. These antibodies produce different effects depending on whether they are agonists, which stimulate, or antagonists, which inhibit the receptor. Note that different autoantibodies to the insulin receptor can either stimulate or inhibit signaling.

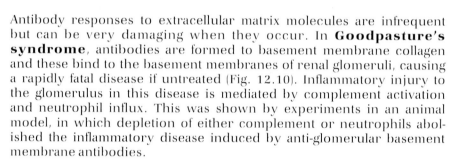

Diseases mediated by antibodies to cell-surface receptors		
Syndrome	**Antigen**	**Consequence**
Graves' disease	Thyroid-stimulating hormone receptor	Hyperthyroidism
Myasthenia gravis	Acetylcholine receptor	Progressive weakness
Insulin-resistant diabetes	Insulin receptor (antagonist)	Hyperglycemia, ketoacidosis
Hypoglycemia	Insulin receptor (agonist)	Hypoglycemia

and may eventually die as a result of their autoimmune disease. Diseases caused by autoantibodies that act as agonists or antagonists for cell-surface receptors are listed in Fig. 12.9.

12-6   Autoantibodies to extracellular antigens cause inflammatory injury by mechanisms akin to type II or type III hypersensitivity reactions.

Antibody responses to extracellular matrix molecules are infrequent but can be very damaging when they occur. In **Goodpasture's syndrome**, antibodies are formed to basement membrane collagen and these bind to the basement membranes of renal glomeruli, causing a rapidly fatal disease if untreated (Fig. 12.10). Inflammatory injury to the glomerulus in this disease is mediated by complement activation and neutrophil influx. This was shown by experiments in an animal model, in which depletion of either complement or neutrophils abolished the inflammatory disease induced by anti-glomerular basement membrane antibodies.

A much more common disease, affecting as many as one in 500 African-American or Asian women living in westernized societies, is **systemic lupus erythematosus (SLE)**. This disease is characterized by chronic IgG antibody production directed at ubiquitous self antigens present in all nucleated cells. As a result of the widespread distribution of autoantigen, many organs are affected. SLE is therefore classified as a **systemic autoimmune disease**, as opposed to the **tissue-** or **organ-specific autoimmune diseases** such as Graves' disease, which affect only one organ or tissue.

Immune complexes are produced whenever there is an antibody response to a soluble antigen. Normally, these are cleared efficiently by red blood cells bearing complement receptors and by phagocytes of the mononuclear phagocytic system that have both complement and Fc receptors, and such complexes cause little tissue damage. This system may, however, fail in three circumstances. The first follows the injection of large amounts of antigen, leading to the formation of large amounts of immune complexes that overwhelm the normal clearance mechanisms. As we learned in Section 11-16, injection of large amounts of serum proteins causes serum sickness, a transient disease that lasts only until the immune complexes have been cleared. The second example is seen in chronic infections such as bacterial endocarditis, where the immune response to bacteria lodged on a cardiac valve is incapable of clearing infection. In bacterial endocarditis, the persistent release of bacterial antigens from the valve infection in the presence of a strong antibacterial antibody response causes widespread immune complex injury to small blood vessels in organs such as the kidney and the skin.

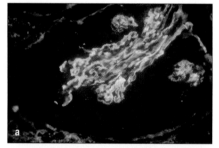

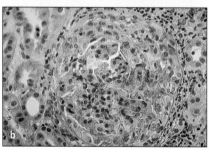

Fig. 12.10 Autoantibodies reacting with glomerular basement membrane cause the inflammatory glomerular disease Goodpasture's syndrome. Linear deposition of antibody on the basement membrane is shown by direct immunofluorescence in the top panel. The autoantibody causes local activation of complement and influx of neutrophils. Staining of a glomerulus by hematoxylin and eosin in the bottom panel shows that the glomerulus is compressed by formation of a crescent of proliferating mononuclear cells within the Bowman's capsule and there is an influx of neutrophils into the glomerular tuft. Photographs courtesy of M Thompson and D Evans.

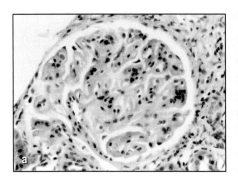 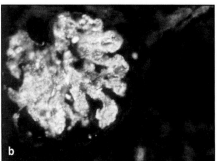 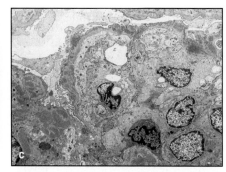

Fig. 12.11 Deposition of immune complexes in the renal glomerulus causes renal failure in systemic lupus erythematosus (SLE). The deposition of immune complexes in SLE causes thickening of the glomerular basement membrane, as shown in panel a. In panel b, such kidney sections have been stained with fluorescent anti-immunoglobulin (see Section 2-13) revealing immunoglobulin in the basement membrane deposits. By electron microscopy, as shown in panel c, dense protein deposits are seen between the glomerular basement membrane and the renal podocytes. Polymorphonuclear neutrophilic leukocytes are also present, attracted by the deposited immune complexes. Photographs courtesy of M Kashgarian.

The third type of failure to clear immune complexes is seen in SLE. In this disease, a wide range of autoantibodies is produced to common cellular constituents. The main antigens are three intracellular nucleoprotein particles—the nucleosome, the spliceosome, and a small cytoplasmic ribonucleoprotein complex containing two proteins known as Ro and La (named after the first two letters of the surnames of the two patients in which autoantibodies against these proteins were discovered). In SLE, large quantities of antigen are available, so large numbers of small immune complexes are produced continuously and deposited in the walls of small blood vessels in the renal glomerulus (Fig. 12.11), joints, and other organs. This leads to complement fixation and the activation of phagocytic cells; the consequent tissue damage releases more nucleoprotein complexes, which in turn form more immune complexes. Eventually, the inflammation induced in small blood vessel walls, especially in the kidney and brain, can cause sufficient damage to kill the patient.

12-7 Environmental co-factors may influence the expression of autoimmune disease.

The presence of an autoantibody is not sufficient to cause the expression of autoimmune disease. For disease to occur, the autoantigen must be available for binding by the autoantibody. Two examples illustrate how the availability of autoantigens and the resulting expression of disease may be modulated by environmental co-factors. As we have just seen, in untreated Goodpasture's disease autoantibodies to the α_3 chain of type IV collagen typically cause a fatal glomerulonephritis. Type IV collagen is distributed widely in basement membranes throughout the body, including those of the alveoli of the lung, the renal glomeruli and the cochlea of the inner ear. All patients with Goodpasture's disease develop glomerulonephritis, about 40% develop pulmonary hemorrhage, but none become deaf. This pattern of disease expression was explained when it was discovered that pulmonary hemorrhage was found almost exclusively only in those patients who smoked cigarettes. What differs between basement membrane in glomeruli, alveoli, and the cochlea is the availability of the antigen to antibodies. The major function of glomerular basement membrane is the filtration of plasma and the endothelium lining glomerular capillaries is fenestrated to allow access of plasma to the basement membrane. Glomerular basement membrane is therefore immediately accessible to circulating autoantibodies. In the

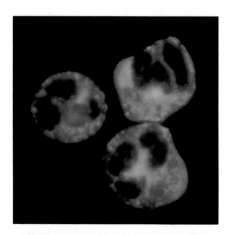

Fig. 12.12 Serum from patients with Wegener's granulomatosis contains autoantibodies reactive with neutrophil cytoplasmic granules. Normal neutrophils with permeabilized cell membranes have been incubated with serum from a patient with Wegener's granulomatosis. IgG antibodies in the serum reactive with cytoplasmic granules are detected by addition of fluorescein-conjugated antibodies to IgG. Photograph courtesy of C Pusey.

alveoli, in contrast, the basement membrane separates alveolar epithelial cells from capillary endothelial cells, which are joined by tight junctions. Injury to the endothelial lining of pulmonary capillaries is therefore necessary before antibodies can gain access to the basement membrane. Cigarette smoke stimulates an inflammatory response in the lungs, which damages alveolar capillaries and exposes the autoantigen to antibody. Finally, in the inner ear, the cochlear basement membrane appears to remain inaccessible to autoantibodies at all times.

A second example of the importance of environmental influences on the expression of autoimmunity is the effect of infection on the vasculitis associated with **Wegener's granulomatosis**. This disease, which is characterized by a severe necrotizing vasculitis, is strongly associated with the presence of autoantibodies to a granule proteinase of neutrophils, known as anti-neutrophil cytoplasmic antigen (commonly abbreviated as ANCA) (Fig. 12.12). The autoantigen is proteinase-3, an abundant serine proteinase of neutrophil granules. Although there is a general correlation between the levels of ANCA and the expression of disease, it is quite common to find patients with high levels of ANCA who remain asymptomatic. If such an individual develops an infection, however, this frequently induces a severe flare-up of the vasculitis.

It is thought that resting neutrophils do not express proteinase-3 on the cell surface, which means that in the absence of infection the antigen is inaccessible to anti-proteinase-3 autoantibodies. Following infection, a variety of cytokines cause neutrophil activation, with translocation of proteinase-3 to the cell surface. Anti-proteinase-3 antibodies can now bind neutrophils and stimulate degranulation and release of free radicals. In parallel, activation of vascular endothelial cells by the infection causes the expression of vascular adhesion molecules, such as E-selectin, which promote binding of activated neutrophils to vessel walls with resultant injury. In this way a variety of non-specific infections can cause an exacerbation of an autoimmune disease.

12-8 The pattern of inflammatory injury in autoimmunity may be modified by anatomical constraints.

We have seen that the distribution of organ injury in Goodpasture's syndrome may be explained by the accessibility of the α_3 chain of type IV collagen to autoantibodies and that environmental factors may influence the availability of antigen in different organs. Another example of how the expression of autoimmune inflammation may be modified by anatomical factors is seen in **membranous glomerulonephritis**. In this disease, patients develop heavy proteinuria (the excretion of protein in the urine), which may cause life-threatening depletion of plasma protein levels. Biopsy of an affected kidney reveals evidence of deposition of antibody and complement beneath the basement membrane of the glomerulus but, in contrast to Goodpasture's disease, there is no significant influx of inflammatory cells. The autoantigen in this disease has not been characterized. However, an excellent animal model of membranous glomerulonephritis is **Heymann's nephritis**, in which autoantibodies to a glycoprotein on the surface of tubular epithelial cells are induced by injection of tubular epithelial tissue. In this disease, proteinuria can be abolished by depletion of any of the proteins of the membrane-attack complex of complement but is unaltered by depletion of neutrophils. Thus, antibodies deposited beneath the glomerular basement membrane in this disease cause tissue injury by activation of complement but the glomerular basement membrane acts as a complete barrier to inflammatory leukocytes.

In other autoimmune diseases, high levels of autoantibodies to intracellular antigens may be found in the absence of any evidence of antibody-induced inflammation. One such example is a rare myositis (inflammation of muscle) associated with pulmonary fibrosis. Some patients with this disease develop high levels of autoantibodies reactive with aminoacyl-tRNA synthetases, the intracellular enzymes responsible for charging tRNAs with amino acids. Addition of these autoantibodies to cell-free extracts *in vitro* stops translation and protein synthesis completely. However, there is no evidence that these antibodies cause any injury *in vivo*, where it is unlikely that they can enter living cells. In this disease, the autoantibody is thought to be a marker of a particular pattern of tissue injury, possibly stimulated by an unknown infectious agent, and does not contribute to the immunopathology of the myositis.

12-9 | **The mechanism of autoimmune tissue damage can often be determined by adoptive transfer.**

To classify a disease as autoimmune one must show that an adaptive immune response to a self antigen causes the observed pathology. Initially, the demonstration that antibodies to the affected tissue could be detected in the serum of patients suffering from various diseases was taken as evidence that the diseases had an autoimmune basis. However, such autoantibodies are also found when tissue damage is caused by trauma or infection. This suggests that autoantibodies can result from, rather than be the cause of, tissue damage. Thus, one must show that the observed autoantibodies are pathogenic before classifying a disease as autoimmune.

It is often possible to transfer disease to experimental animals through the transfer of autoantibodies, causing pathology similar to that seen in the patient from whom the antibodies were obtained (Fig. 12.13). However, this does not always work, presumably because of species differences in autoantigen structure. Antibody transfer of autoimmune disease can also be observed in newborn babies of diseased mothers (Fig. 12.14). When babies are exposed to IgG autoantibodies transferred across the placenta, they will often manifest pathology similar to the mother's. These symptoms disappear rapidly as the antibody is catabolized. The process can be speeded up by a complete exchange of the infant's blood or plasma (plasmapheresis).

12-10 | **T cells specific for self antigens can cause direct tissue injury and play a role in sustained autoantibody responses.**

Immune T cells specific for self peptide:self MHC complexes can cause local inflammation by activating macrophages or can damage tissue cells directly. Diseases in which this mechanism is likely to be important include **rheumatoid arthritis** and **multiple sclerosis**. Affected tissues in patients with these diseases are heavily infiltrated by T lymphocytes and

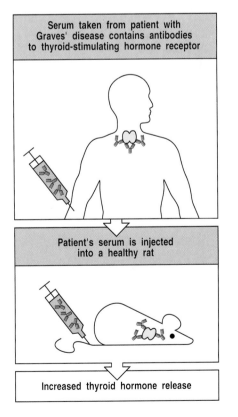

Serum taken from patient with Graves' disease contains antibodies to thyroid-stimulating hormone receptor

Patient's serum is injected into a healthy rat

Increased thyroid hormone release

Fig. 12.13 Serum from some patients with autoimmune disease can transfer the same disease to experimental animals. When the autoantigen is well conserved between humans and mice or rats, the transfer of antibody from an affected human can cause the same symptoms in an experimental animal. For example, antibody from patients with Graves' disease frequently produces thyroid activation in rats.

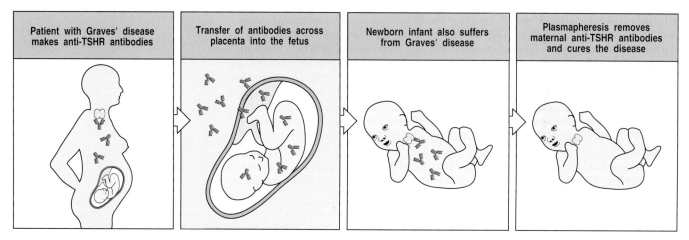

| Patient with Graves' disease makes anti-TSHR antibodies | Transfer of antibodies across placenta into the fetus | Newborn infant also suffers from Graves' disease | Plasmapheresis removes maternal anti-TSHR antibodies and cures the disease |

Fig. 12.14 Antibody-mediated autoimmune diseases can appear in the infants of affected mothers as a consequence of transplacental antibody transfer. In pregnant women, IgG antibodies cross the placenta and accumulate in the fetus before birth (see Fig. 8.20). Babies born to mothers with IgG-mediated autoimmune disease therefore frequently show symptoms similar to the mother in the first few weeks of life. Fortunately, this causes little lasting damage as the symptoms disappear along with the maternal antibody. In Graves' disease, the symptoms are caused by antibodies to the thyroid-stimulating hormone receptor (TSHR). Children of mothers making thyroid-stimulating antibody are born with hyperthyroidism, but this can be corrected by replacing the plasma with normal plasma, thus removing the maternal antibody.

by activated macrophages. These autoimmune diseases are mediated by specifically reactive T cells, which are also required to sustain all autoantibody responses.

It is much more difficult to demonstrate the existence of autoimmune T cells than it is to demonstrate the presence of autoantibodies. First, autoimmune human T cells cannot be used to transfer disease to experimental animals because T-cell recognition is MHC-restricted and animals have different MHC alleles from humans. Second, it is difficult to identify the antigen recognized by a T cell; for example, autoantibodies can be used to stain self tissues to reveal the distribution of the autoantigen, whereas T cells cannot. Nevertheless, there is strong evidence for involvement of autoreactive T cells in several autoimmune diseases. **Insulin-dependent diabetes mellitus (IDDM)** is a disease in which the insulin-producing β cells of the pancreatic islets are selectively destroyed by specific T cells. When such diabetic patients are transplanted with half a pancreas from an identical twin donor, the β cells in the grafted tissue are rapidly and selectively destroyed by CD8 T cells. Recurrence of disease can be prevented by the immunosuppressive drug cyclosporin A (see Chapter 13), which inhibits T-cell activation. Progress towards identifying such autoimmune T cells and proving that they cause disease will be discussed in Section 12-12.

12-11   Autoantibodies can be used to identify the target of the autoimmune process.

Once autoantibodies have been shown to be required for pathogenesis, they can be used to purify the autoantigen so that it can be identified. This approach is particularly useful if the autoantibody causes disease in animals from which large amounts of tissue can be obtained. Autoantibodies can also be used to examine the distribution of the target antigen in cells and tissues by immunohistology, often providing clues to the pathogenesis of the disease.

The identification of a critical autoantigen may also lead to the identification of the CD4 T cells responsible for autoantibody production. As we learned in Chapter 8, CD4 T cells selectively activate those B cells that bind epitopes that are physically linked to the peptide recognized by the T cell. It follows that autoantibodies can be used to purify proteins or protein complexes that should contain the peptide recognized by the autoreactive CD4 T cell. For example, in myasthenia gravis the autoantibodies that cause disease bind mainly to the α chain of the acetylcholine receptor. CD4 T cells that recognize peptide fragments of this receptor subunit can also be found in patients with myasthenia gravis. Thus, both autoreactive B cells and autoreactive T cells are required for this disease (Fig. 12.15).

The same phenomenon is seen in SLE. Tissue damage in this disease is caused by immune complexes of autoantibodies directed against a variety of nucleoprotein antigens (see Section 12-6). Interestingly, these antibodies show a high degree of somatic mutation, and the B cells that produce them can be shown to have undergone extensive clonal expansion; these properties are characteristic of antibodies formed in response to chronic stimulation of B cells by antigen and specific CD4 T cells. This strongly suggests that the autoantibodies in SLE must be produced in response to autoantigens that contain peptides recognized by specific autoreactive CD4 T cells. Furthermore, the autoantibodies in any one individual tend to bind all constituents of a particular nucleoprotein particle. This is explained readily by the presence in individual patients of CD4 T cells that are specific for a peptide constituent of this particle. A B cell whose receptor binds any component of the particle will process and present this peptide to these autoreactive T cells and receive help from them (Fig. 12.16). This accounts for the observed characteristics of the autoantibody response as well as the clustering of autoantibody specificities in individual patients.

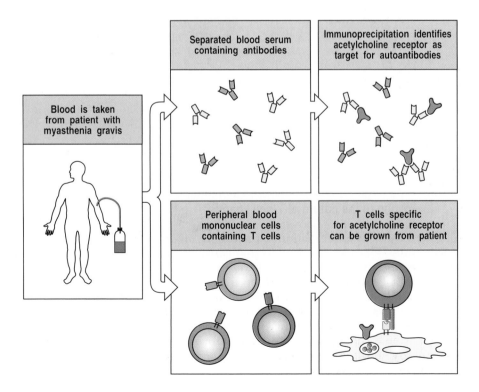

Fig. 12.15 Autoantibodies can be used to identify both the B- and T-cell epitopes of some autoantigens. In myasthenia gravis, autoantibodies immunoprecipitate the α chain of the acetylcholine receptor from lysates of skeletal muscle cells (top panels). This suggests that the same patients should also have CD4 T cells that respond to a peptide of the acetylcholine receptor. To investigate this, T cells from myasthenia gravis patients have been isolated and grown in the presence of the acetylcholine receptor plus antigen-presenting cells of the correct MHC type—T cells specific for epitopes of the α chain of the acetylcholine receptor can indeed be identified (bottom panels).

Blood is taken from patient with myasthenia gravis

Separated blood serum containing antibodies

Immunoprecipitation identifies acetylcholine receptor as target for autoantibodies

Peripheral blood mononuclear cells containing T cells

T cells specific for acetylcholine receptor can be grown from patient

Fig. 12.16 Autoreactive helper T cells of one specificity can drive the production of autoantibodies with several different specificities. In systemic lupus erythematosus, patients frequently produce autoantibodies to all of the components of a nucleosome, or all of the components of a ribosome, instead of producing autoantibodies to some components of each of these particles. This occurs because all the autoreactive B cells are receiving help from a single clone of autoreactive helper T cells specific for a peptide of one of the proteins that make up the particle. Since B cells internalize and process particles that contain the antigen they recognize, any B cell specific for any protein or nucleic acid within the particle can receive help from a T cell that recognizes a peptide derived from a protein found in the particle. For example, if a patient has a helper T cell specific for a peptide of the histone protein H1, any B cell that recognizes any antigen in a nucleosome can present histone peptides to that T cell and be activated by it. Thus, a single autoreactive helper T cell could give a diverse antibody response. However, B cells able to bind ribosomes cannot present the H1 peptide and so will not be activated to produce anti-ribosomal antibodies (bottom panels). In other patients, responses focusing on ribosomes or small nuclear ribonucleoproteins (snRNPs) are observed, reflecting the existence of different helper T cells specific for peptides derived from those particles.

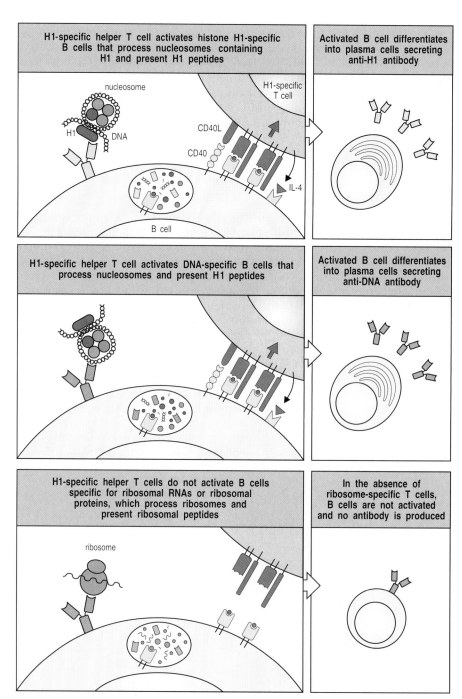

12-12   The target of T-cell mediated autoimmunity is difficult to identify owing to the nature of T-cell ligands.

Although there is good evidence for the involvement of T cells in many autoimmune diseases, the T cells that cause particular diseases are hard to isolate, and their targets are difficult to identify. In part, this is because one cannot grow the specific T cells needed to identify the autoantigenic peptide without supplying them with their specific antigen in the first place. It is also difficult to assay the T cells for their ability to cause disease, since any assay requires target cells of the same MHC genotype as the patient. This problem becomes more tractable in animal models. Since many autoimmune diseases in animals are induced by immunization with self tissue, the nature of the autoantigen can be determined by fractionating an extract of the tissue and testing the fractions for their ability to induce disease. It is also possible to clone T-cell lines that will transfer the disease from an affected animal to another animal with the same MHC genotype.

This has made it possible to identify the autoantigens involved in many experimental autoimmune diseases; they are commonly single peptides that bind to specific MHC molecules. The peptide antigen, when made immunogenic, is able to elicit the entire disease spectrum in animals of the appropriate MHC genotype. An example of an experimental autoimmune disease that illustrates this is **experimental allergic encephalomyelitis** (**EAE**), which can be induced in certain susceptible strains of mice and rats by injection of CNS tissue together with Freund's complete adjuvant. Further analysis of this experimental autoimmune disease, which resembles multiple sclerosis, showed that injection of purified components of myelin, notably myelin basic protein (MBP), with adjuvant could induce EAE. Disease can be transferred to syngeneic animals using cloned T-cell lines derived from animals with EAE. Many of these cloned T-cell lines are stimulated by peptides of MBP, which is found in the myelin sheath that surrounds nerve cell axons in the brain and spinal cord. When animals with the appropriate MHC allele are immunized with this peptide, active disease results (Fig. 12.17). Activated T cells specific for myelin basic protein have also been identified in patients with multiple sclerosis. Although it has not yet been proved that these cells cause the demyelination in multiple sclerosis, this finding suggests that animal models may provide clues to the identity of autoantigenic proteins in human disease.

In a variety of inflammatory autoimmune diseases, it appears that self antigens are presented to T_H1 cells. One example is experimental allergic encephalomyelitis, which is caused by T_H1, but not T_H2, cells specific for myelin basic protein, as shown by the ability of specific clones of T_H1, but not T_H2, cells to cause disease on adoptive transfer. Although myelin basic protein is an intracellular protein, it is processed for presentation by the vesicular pathway and thus its peptides are presented by MHC class II molecules. Rheumatoid arthritis may be caused by T_H1 cells

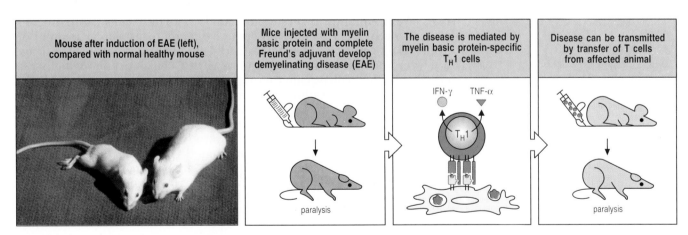

| Mouse after induction of EAE (left), compared with normal healthy mouse | Mice injected with myelin basic protein and complete Freund's adjuvant develop demyelinating disease (EAE) | The disease is mediated by myelin basic protein-specific T_H1 cells | Disease can be transmitted by transfer of T cells from affected animal |

Fig. 12.17 T cells specific for myelin basic protein mediate inflammation of the brain in experimental autoimmune encephalomyelitis (EAE). This disease is produced in experimental animals by injecting them with isolated spinal cord homogenized in complete Freund's adjuvant. It causes a progressive paralysis that affects first the tail and hind limbs (as shown in the mouse on the left of the photograph, compared with a healthy mouse on the right) before progressing to forelimb paralysis and eventual death. The disease is caused by T_H1 cells specific for a protein in myelin called myelin basic protein (MBP); immunization with MBP alone can also cause disease and cloned MBP-specific T_H1 cells can transfer the disease to naive recipients provided that the recipients carry the correct MHC allele. In this system it has therefore proved possible to identify the peptide:MHC complex recognized by the T_H1 clones that transfer disease.

Fig. 12.18 Selective destruction of pancreatic β cells in insulin-dependent diabetes mellitus (IDDM) indicates that the autoantigen is produced in β cells and recognized on their surface. In IDDM, there is highly specific destruction of insulin-producing β cells in the pancreatic islets of Langerhans, sparing other islet cell types (α and δ). This is shown schematically in the upper panels. In the lower panels, islets from normal (left) and diabetic (right) mice are stained for insulin (brown), which shows the β cells, and glucagon (black), which shows the α cells. Note the lymphocytes infiltrating the islet in the diabetic mouse (right) and the selective loss of the β cells (brown) while the α cells (black) are spared. The characteristic morphology of the islet is also disrupted with the loss of the β cells. It is likely that cytotoxic CD8 T cells are responsible for β-cell destruction; they probably recognize peptides derived from β cell-specific proteins presented by MHC class I molecules. However, the autoantigen in insulin-dependent diabetes mellitus has not yet been identified. Photographs courtesy of I Visintin.

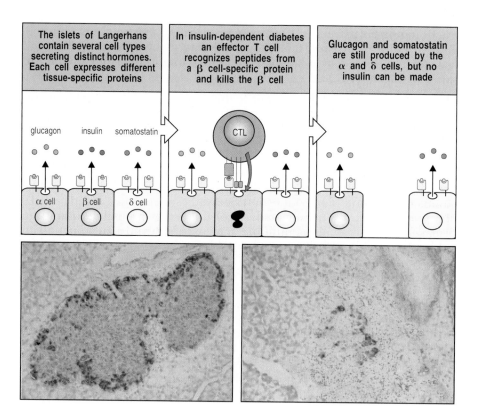

specific for an antigen present in joints, which triggers them to release lymphokines that initiate local inflammation within the joint. This causes swelling, accumulation of polymorphonuclear leukocytes and macrophages, and damage to cartilage, leading to the destruction of the joint. Rheumatoid arthritis is a complex disease and also involves antibodies, often including an IgM anti-IgG autoantibody called **rheumatoid factor**. Some of the tissue damage in this disease is caused by the resultant IgM:IgG immune complexes.

Identification of autoantigenic peptides is particularly difficult in the case of autoimmune diseases mediated by CD8 T cells. Autoantigens recognized by CD4 T cells can come from any extracellular protein or from cells ingested by phagocytes and degraded in intracellular vesicles; however, autoantigens recognized by CD8 T cells must be made by the target cells themselves (see Chapter 4). Therefore, one can use cellular extracts to identify the autoantigen recognized by autoimmune CD4 T cells but intact cells from the target tissue of the patient must be used to study autoimmune CD8 T cells that cause tissue damage. Conversely, the pathogenesis of the disease can itself give clues to the identity of the antigen in some CD8 T-cell mediated diseases. For example, in insulin-dependent diabetes mellitus, the insulin-producing β cells of the pancreatic islets of Langerhans appear to be specifically targeted and destroyed by CD8 T cells. It is likely therefore that a protein unique to β cells is the source of the peptide that is recognized by the pathogenic CD8 T cells (Fig. 12.18).

CD4 T cells also seem to be involved in insulin-dependent diabetes mellitus, consistent with the linkage of disease susceptibility to particular MHC class II alleles, as discussed earlier in this chapter (see Figs. 12.4 and 12.5). Identifying the autoantigen recognized by T cells in these diseases is an important goal. Not only may it help us to understand disease pathogenesis but it may also result in several innovative approaches to treatment (see Chapter 13).

Summary.

To define a disease as autoimmune, the tissue damage must be shown to be caused by an adaptive immune response to self antigens. Autoimmune diseases can be caused by autoantibodies or by autoimmune T cells, and tissue damage may result from direct attack on the cells bearing the antigen, from immune-complex formation, or from local inflammation. Autoimmune diseases caused by antibodies that bind to cellular receptors, causing either excess activity or inhibition of receptor function, fall into a special class. T cells may be involved directly in inflammation or cellular destruction, and they are also required to sustain autoantibody responses. The most convincing proof that the immune response is causal in autoimmunity is transfer of disease by transferring the active component of the immune response to an appropriate recipient. However, this is often not practicable. The current challenge is to identify the autoantigens recognized by T cells in autoimmunity, and to use this information to control the activity of these T cells, or to prevent their activation in the first place. The deeper, more important question is how the autoimmune response is induced. This issue is most commonly studied by examining the response to non-self tissues in transplantation experiments. We will therefore examine the immune response to grafted tissues in the next section before turning to the problem of how tolerance is maintained normally and why responses occur in autoimmune disease.

Transplant rejection: responses to alloantigens.

The transplantation of tissues to replace diseased organs is now an important medical therapy. In most cases, adaptive immune responses to the grafted tissues are the major impediment to successful transplantation. In blood transfusion, which is the earliest and still the commonest tissue transplant, blood must be matched for ABO and Rh blood group antigens to avoid the rapid destruction of mismatched red blood cells by antibodies (see Fig. 2.9). Since there are only four major ABO types and two Rh blood types, this is relatively easy. However, when tissues containing nucleated cells are transplanted, T-cell responses to the highly polymorphic MHC molecules almost always trigger a response against the grafted organ. Matching the MHC type of donor and recipient increases the success rate of grafts, but perfect matching is possible only when donor and recipient are related and, in these cases, genetic differences at other loci still trigger rejection. In this section, we will examine the immune response to tissue grafts, and ask why such responses do not reject the one foreign tissue graft that is tolerated routinely, the mammalian fetus.

12-13 | The rejection of grafts is an immunological response mediated primarily by T cells.

The basic rules of tissue grafting were first elucidated using skin transplanted between inbred strains of mice. Skin can be grafted with 100% success between different sites on the same animal or person (an **autograft**), or between genetically identical animals or people (a **syngeneic graft**). However, when skin is grafted between unrelated or **allogeneic** individuals (an **allograft**), the graft is initially accepted

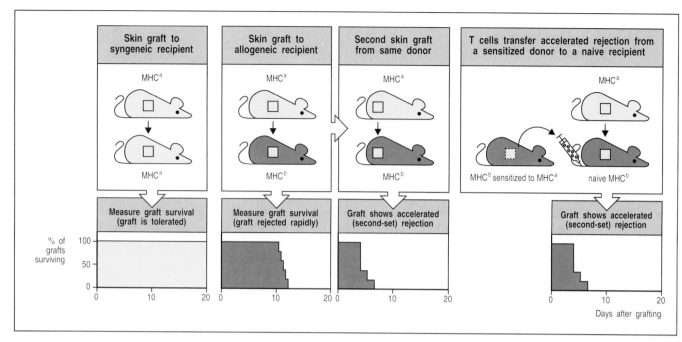

Fig. 12.19 Skin graft rejection is the result of a T-cell mediated anti-graft response. Grafts that are syngeneic are permanently accepted (left panels) but grafts differing at the MHC are rejected around 10–14 days after grafting (first-set rejection). When a mouse is grafted for a second time with skin from the same donor, it rejects the second graft faster (center panels). This is called a second-set rejection and the accelerated response is MHC-specific; skin from a second donor of the same MHC type is rejected equally fast, while skin from an MHC-different donor is rejected in a first-set pattern (not shown). Naive mice that are given T cells from a sensitized donor behave as if they had already been grafted (right panels).

but is then rejected about 11–15 days after grafting (Fig. 12.19). This response is called a **first-set rejection** and is quite consistent. It depends on a recipient T-cell response, since skin grafted onto *nude* mice, which lack T cells, is not rejected. The ability to reject skin can be restored to *nude* mice by the adoptive transfer of normal T cells.

When a recipient that has previously rejected a graft is regrafted with skin from the same donor, the second graft is rejected more rapidly (6–8 days) in a **second-set rejection** (see Fig. 12.19). Skin from a third-party donor grafted onto the same recipient at the same time does not show this faster response but follows a first-set rejection course. The rapid course of second-set rejection can be transferred to normal or irradiated recipients by transferring T cells from the initial recipient, showing that graft rejection is caused by a specific immunological reaction.

Immune responses are a major barrier to effective tissue transplantation, destroying grafted tissue by an adaptive immune response to its foreign proteins. These responses may be mediated by cytotoxic CD8 T cells, by T$_H$1 cells, or by both. Antibodies may also contribute to second-set rejection of tissue grafts.

12-14 | Matching donor and recipient at the MHC improves the outcome of transplantation.

When donor and recipient differ at the MHC, the immune response is directed at the non-self MHC molecule or molecules expressed by the graft. Once a recipient has rejected a graft of a particular MHC type, any further graft bearing the same non-self MHC molecule will be rapidly rejected in a second-set response. As we learned in Chapter 4, the frequency of T cells specific for any non-self MHC molecule is high, making differences at MHC loci the most potent trigger of the rejection of initial grafts; indeed, the major histocompatibility complex was originally named because of this central role in graft rejection.

Once it became clear that recognition of non-self MHC molecules is a major determinant of graft rejection, a considerable amount of effort was put into MHC matching between recipient and donor. Although HLA matching significantly improves the success rate of clinical organ transplantation it does not in itself prevent rejection reactions. There are two main reasons for this. First, HLA typing is imprecise, owing to the polymorphism and complexity of the human MHC; unrelated individuals who type as HLA-identical using antibodies to MHC proteins rarely have identical MHC genotypes (see Section 2-27). However, this should not be a problem with HLA-identical siblings; because siblings inherit their MHC genes as a haplotype, one sibling in four should be truly HLA-identical (see Fig. 2.43). Nevertheless, grafts between HLA-identical siblings are invariably rejected, albeit more slowly, unless donor and recipient are identical twins. This rejection is the result of minor histocompatibility antigens, which will be discussed in the next section.

Thus, unless donor and recipient are identical twins, all graft recipients must be given immunosuppressive drugs to prevent rejection. Indeed, the current success of clinical transplantation of solid organs is more the result of advances in immunosuppressive therapy, discussed in Chapter 13, than of improved tissue matching. The limited supply of cadaveric organs, coupled with the urgency of identifying a recipient once a donor becomes available, means that accurate matching of tissue types is achieved only rarely.

12-15 | In MHC-identical grafts, rejection is caused by non-self peptides bound to graft MHC molecules.

When donor and recipient are identical at the MHC but differ at other genetic loci, graft rejection is not so rapid (Fig. 12.20). The genetic polymorphisms responsible for rejection of MHC-identical grafts are therefore

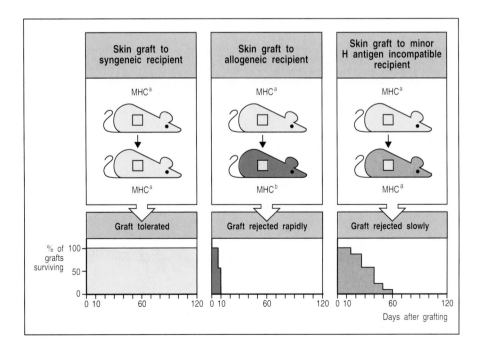

Fig. 12.20 Even complete matching at the MHC does not ensure graft survival. Although syngeneic grafts are not rejected (left panels), MHC-identical grafts from donors that differ at other loci (minor H antigen loci) are rejected (right panels), albeit more slowly than MHC-disparate grafts (center panels).

termed **minor histocompatibility antigens or minor H antigens**. Responses to single minor H antigens are much less potent than responses to MHC differences because the frequency of responding T cells is much lower; indeed, minor H antigen-specific T cells need to be primed *in vivo* before they can be detected in a mixed lymphocyte culture. However, most inbred mouse strains that are identical at MHC differ at multiple minor H antigen loci, so grafts between them are still uniformly and relatively rapidly rejected. The cells that respond to minor H antigens are generally CD8 T cells, implying that most minor H antigens are peptides bound to self MHC class I molecules. However, peptides bound to self MHC class II molecules can also participate in the response to MHC-identical grafts

Minor H antigens are now known to be peptides derived from polymorphic proteins that are presented by MHC molecules on the graft (Fig. 12.21). Virtually any protein made by a cell has the potential to produce peptides that are recognized as minor H antigens. One set of proteins that induce minor H responses are encoded on the male-specific Y chromosome; these are known collectively as H-Y. Since these Y-chromosome specific genes are not expressed in females, female anti-male minor H responses occur; however, male anti-female responses are not seen, since both males and females express X-chromosome genes. One H-Y antigen has recently been identified in the mouse as a peptide of eight amino acids encoded by a Y-chromosome gene, *Smcy*. An X-chromosome homolog of *Smcy*, called *Smcx*, does not contain this peptide sequence, which is therefore expressed uniquely in males.

The response to minor H antigens is in every way analogous to the response to viral infection but this response only eliminates infected cells. As all cells in the graft express the minor H antigen, the entire graft is destroyed in such responses, just as analogous responses to tissue-specific peptides can destroy an entire tissue in autoimmunity. Thus, even though MHC genotype may be matched exactly, polymorphism in any protein may elicit potent T-cell responses that will destroy the entire graft. It is no wonder that successful transplantation requires the use of potent immunosuppressive drugs.

Fig. 12.21 Minor H antigens are peptides derived from polymorphic cellular proteins bound to MHC class I molecules. Self proteins are digested routinely by proteasomes within the cell's cytosol, and peptides derived from them are delivered to the rough endoplasmic reticulum where they can bind to MHC class I molecules and be delivered to the cell surface (left panel; see also Section 4-7). If any polymorphic protein differs between the graft donor and the recipient, it may give rise to a peptide that can be recognized by T cells as non-self and elicit an immune response (right panel).

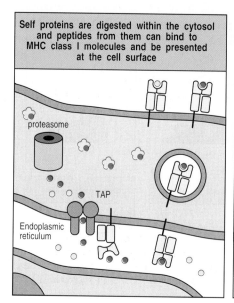

Self proteins are digested within the cytosol and peptides from them can bind to MHC class I molecules and be presented at the cell surface

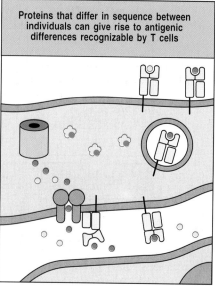

Proteins that differ in sequence between individuals can give rise to antigenic differences recognizable by T cells

Antibodies reacting with endothelium cause hyperacute graft rejection.

Antibody responses are also an important potential cause of graft rejection. Alloantibodies to blood group antigens and polymorphic MHC antigens can cause rapid rejection of transplanted organs in a complement-dependent reaction that may occur within minutes. This type of reaction is known as **hyperacute graft rejection**. Most grafts that are transplanted routinely in clinical medicine are vascularized organ grafts linked directly to the recipient's circulation. In some cases, the recipient may already have circulating antibodies to donor graft antigens, which were produced in response to a previous transplant or a blood transfusion. Such antibodies can cause very rapid rejection of vascularized grafts, since they react with antigens on the vascular endothelial cells of the graft and initiate the complement and clotting cascades, blocking the vessels of the graft and causing its immediate death. Such grafts become engorged and purple-colored from hemorrhage of blood, which becomes deoxygenated (Fig. 12.22). This problem can be avoided by **cross-matching** donor and recipient. Cross-matching, as in blood transfusion, involves determining whether the recipient has antibodies that react with the white blood cells of the donor. If antibodies of this type are found, they are a serious contraindication to transplantation, as they lead to near-certain hyperacute rejection.

A very similar problem prevents the routine use of animal organs—**xenografting**—in transplantation. If xenogeneic grafts could be used, it would avoid a major barrier to organ replacement therapy, namely, the severe shortage of donor organs. Pigs have been selected as a potential source species for xenografting as they are a similar size to humans and are readily farmed. Most humans have antibodies that react with endothelial cell antigens of other species such as pigs. When pig xenografts are placed in humans, these antibodies trigger hyperacute rejection by reacting with endothelial cell antigens and initiating the complement and clotting cascades. Hyperacute rejection is even more of a problem in the case of xenografts because complement regulatory proteins such as CD59, DAF (CD55), and MCP (CD46) (see Section 8-31) show species specificity; the complement regulatory proteins of the xenogeneic endothelial cells cannot protect them from attack by human complement. A recent step towards the development of xenotransplantation has been the development of transgenic pigs expressing human DAF. Preliminary experiments have shown prolonged survival of organs transplanted from these pigs into recipient cynomolgus monkeys, under cover of heavy immunosuppression. However, hyperacute rejection is only the first barrier faced by a xenotransplanted organ. Conventional T-lymphocyte-mediated graft rejection mechanisms may be extremely difficult to overcome using present immunosuppressive regimes.

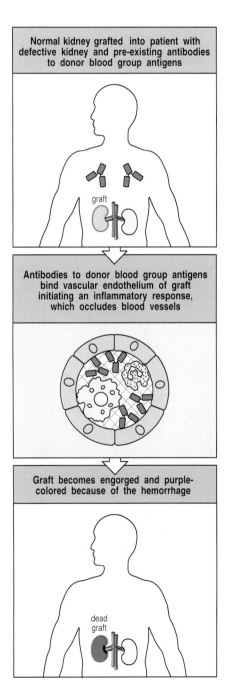

Normal kidney grafted into patient with defective kidney and pre-existing antibodies to donor blood group antigens

graft

Antibodies to donor blood group antigens bind vascular endothelium of graft initiating an inflammatory response, which occludes blood vessels

Graft becomes engorged and purple-colored because of the hemorrhage

dead graft

Fig. 12.22 Antibody to donor graft antigens can cause acute graft rejection. In some cases, recipients have antibodies to donor antigens. When the donor organ is grafted into such recipients, these antibodies bind to vascular endothelium, initiating the complement and clotting cascades. Blood vessels in the graft become obstructed by clots and leak, causing hemorrhage of blood into the graft. This becomes engorged and turns purple from the presence of de-oxygenated blood.

Tissue transplanted	5 year graft survival*	No. of grafts in USA (1992)
Kidney	80–90%	9736
Liver	40–50%	3064
Heart	70%	2172
Lung	30–40%	535
Cornea	>90%	N/A
Bone marrow	80%	N/A

Fig. 12.23 Tissues commonly transplanted in clinical medicine. All grafts except corneal and some bone marrow grafts require long-term immunosuppression. The number of organ grafts performed in the USA in 1992 is shown. *The 5 year survival values are an average; closer matching between donor and recipient generally gives better survival.

12-17   A variety of organs are transplanted routinely in clinical medicine.

Although the immune response makes organ transplantation difficult, there are few alternative therapies for organ failure. Three major advances have made it possible to use organ transplantation routinely in the clinic. First, the technical skill to carry out organ replacement surgery has been mastered by many people. Second, networks of transplantation centers have been organized to ensure that the few healthy organs that are available are HLA-typed and so matched with the most suitable recipient. Third, the use of potent immunosuppressive drugs, especially cyclosporin A and FK-506 to inhibit T-cell activation (see Chapter 13), has increased graft survival rates dramatically. Fig. 12.23 lists the different organs that are transplanted in the clinic. Some of these operations are performed routinely with a very high success rate. By far the most frequently transplanted organ is the kidney, the organ first successfully transplanted between identical twins in the 1950s. Transplantation of the cornea is the most successful; this tissue is a special case, as it is not vascularized, and corneal grafts between unrelated people are usually successful even without immunosuppression (see Section 12-23).

There are, however, many problems other than graft rejection associated with organ transplantation. First, donor organs are difficult to obtain; this is especially a problem when the organ involved is a vital one, such as the heart or liver. Moreover, as there is no supportive therapy that would allow survival, the time available to find a suitable donor organ is limited. Second, the disease that destroyed the patient's organ may also destroy the graft. Third, the immunosuppression required to prevent graft rejection increases the risk of cancer and infection. Finally, the procedure is very costly. All of these problems need to be addressed before clinical transplantation can become commonplace. The problems most amenable to scientific solution are the development of more effective means of immunosuppression and the induction of graft-specific tolerance.

12-18   The fetus is an allograft that is tolerated repetitively.

All of the transplants discussed so far are artefacts of modern medical technology. However, one tissue that is repeatedly grafted and repeatedly tolerated is the mammalian fetus. The fetus carries paternal MHC and minor H antigens that differ from those of the mother (Fig. 12.24), and yet a mother can bear many children expressing the same non-self MHC proteins derived from the father. The mysterious lack of rejection of the fetus has puzzled generations of reproductive immunologists and no comprehensive explanation has yet emerged. One problem is that acceptance of the fetal allograft is so much the norm that it is difficult to study the mechanism that prevents rejection; if the mechanism for rejecting the fetus is rarely activated, how can one analyze the mechanisms that control it?

Various hypotheses have been advanced to account for the tolerance normally shown to the fetus. It has been proposed that, for some reason, the fetus is simply not recognized as foreign in the first place. There is evidence against this hypothesis, since women who have borne several children usually have antibodies directed at the father's MHC proteins; indeed, this is the best source of antibodies for human MHC typing. However, the placenta, which is a fetus-derived tissue, appears to sequester the fetus away from the mother's T cells. The trophoblast cells that form the outer layer of the placenta in contact with maternal tissues do not express classical MHC proteins, perhaps due to

Fig. 12.24 The fetus is an allograft that is not rejected. Although the fetus carries MHC molecules derived from the father, and other foreign antigens, it is not rejected. Even when the mother bears several children to the same father, no sign of immunological rejection is seen.

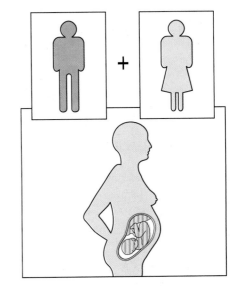

a transcriptional inhibitor. The outer layer of the trophoblast, the syncytiotrophoblast derived from the trophoectoderm layer of the blastocyst, displays a non-classical, non-polymorphic HLA class I molecule. We do not yet know whether this molecule can display peptides to T cells and whether it plays any role in protecting the fetus from immunological attack by the mother.

It is likely that fetal tolerance is a multifactorial process. The trophoblast does not act as an absolute barrier between mother and fetus, and fetal blood cells may cross the placenta and be detected in the maternal circulation, albeit in very low numbers. There is direct evidence from experiments in mice of specific T-cell tolerance against paternal MHC alloantigens. Pregnant female mice whose T cells bear a transgenic receptor specific for a paternal alloantigen showed reduced expression of this T-cell receptor. During pregnancy, these mice lost the ability to control the growth of an experimental tumor bearing the same paternal MHC alloantigen. After pregnancy, tumor growth was controlled and the level of the T-cell receptor increased. This experiment demonstrates that the maternal immune system must have been exposed to paternal MHC alloantigens.

A further factor that may contribute to maternal tolerance to the fetus is the secretion of cytokines at the feto-maternal interface. Both uterine epithelium and trophoblast secrete cytokines, including transforming growth factor-β (TGF-β), IL-4, and IL-10. This is a cytokine pattern that tends to promote T$_H$2 responses (see Chapter 9). Induction or injection of cytokines such as IFN-γ and IL-12, which promote T$_H$1 responses in experimental animals, promote fetal resorption, the equivalent of spontaneous abortion in humans.

The fetus is thus tolerated for two main reasons: it occupies a site protected by a non-immunogenic tissue barrier, and it promotes an immuno-suppressive response in the mother. We shall see in Section 12-23 that several sites in the body have these characteristics and allow prolonged acceptance of foreign tissue grafts. They are usually called immunologically privileged sites.

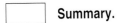 **Summary.**

Clinical transplantation is now an everyday reality, its success built on MHC matching, immunosuppressive drugs, and technical skill. However, even accurate MHC matching does not prevent graft rejection; any genetic difference between host and donor may encode a protein whose peptides are presented as minor H antigens by MHC molecules on the grafted tissue, and responses to these can lead to rejection. As we lack the ability to suppress the response to the graft specifically without compromising host defense, most transplants require generalized immunosuppression of the recipient, which may cause significant toxicity and increases the risk of cancer and infection. The fetus is a natural allograft that must be accepted or the species will not survive; it almost always is. Tolerance to the fetus may hold the key to specific graft tolerance, or it may be a special case not applicable to organ replacement therapy.

Fig. 12.25 An autoantigenic peptide will be presented at different levels on different MHC molecules. Peptides bind to different MHC molecules with varying affinities; in this example, the peptide binds well to MHC^a, less well to MHC^b, and poorly to all other MHC types. The graph shows the number of cells expressing a given density of antigen:MHC complex. For MHC^a, most cells express high levels of the complex, and reactive T-cell clones are therefore deleted in the thymus or anergized in the periphery. For MHC^b, and for all other MHC types, few thymic cells express levels of antigen:MHC complex above the tolerance threshold, and therefore T cells whose receptors could recognize this self peptide mature. However, on all MHC haplotypes other than MHC^b, the peptide is presented so poorly on tissue cells that even T cells with receptors that can recognize the peptide do not respond. Only MHC^b presents the peptide at an intermediate level so that significant levels of the peptide:MHC^b complex are present in the periphery. Normally this would not cause problems, since the peptide would not normally be presented on cells that carry co-stimulatory molecules. However, if the autoreactive T-cell clones are activated inappropriately, they may be able to attack self cells bearing the peptide:MHC^b complex. It is probably rare for a peptide to be presented at this intermediate level by any of the MHC molecules in the population. This situation probably arises most frequently when the antigen is expressed selectively in a tissue rather than ubiquitously, since tissue-specific antigens are less likely to induce clonal deletion in the thymus.

Tolerance and response to self and non-self tissues.

Tolerance to self is acquired by clonal deletion or inactivation of developing lymphocytes, and its loss leads to autoimmune disease, which is fortunately a rare occurrence. Tolerance to antigens expressed by grafted tissues can be induced artificially, but it is very difficult to establish once a full repertoire of functional lymphocytes has been produced, which occurs in fetal life in humans and around the time of birth in mice. We have already discussed the two important mechanisms of self tolerance, clonal deletion by ubiquitous self antigens, and clonal inactivation by tissue-specific antigens presented in the absence of co-stimulatory signals (see Chapters 5–7). These processes were first discovered by studying tolerance to non-self, where the absence of tolerance could be studied in the form of graft rejection. In this section, we shall consider tolerance to self and tolerance to non-self as two aspects of the same basic mechanism. We also examine the instances where tolerance to self or non-self is lost, in an attempt to understand the related phenomena of autoimmunity and graft rejection.

12-19   **Autoantigens are not so abundant that they induce clonal deletion or anergy but are not so rare as to escape recognition entirely.**

We saw in Chapter 6 that clonal deletion removes T cells that recognize ubiquitous self antigens and in Chapter 7 that antigens expressed abundantly in the periphery induce anergy or clonal deletion in lymphocytes that encounter them on tissue cells. Most self proteins are expressed at levels that are too low to serve as targets for T-cell recognition on any cell type and thus cannot serve as autoantigens. It is likely that only rare proteins contain peptides that are presented by a given MHC molecule at a level that is sufficient for effector T-cell recognition but too low to induce tolerance (Fig. 12.25). The nature of such peptides will vary depending on the MHC genotype of the individual, since MHC polymorphism profoundly affects peptide binding (see Section 4-17). T cells able to recognize these rare antigens will be present in the individual but will not normally be activated; they are said to be in a state of **immunological ignorance**. Most autoimmunity is likely to reflect the activation of such immunologically ignorant cells.

Autoimmunity is unlikely to reflect the failure of the main mechanisms of tolerance, clonal deletion and clonal inactivation, because these are such efficient processes. For example, clonal deletion of developing lymphocytes mediates tolerance to self MHC molecules. If such tolerance were not induced, the reactions to self tissues would be similar to those seen in graft-versus-host disease (see Section 10-13). To estimate the impact of clonal deletion on the developing T-cell repertoire, we should remember that the frequency of T cells able to respond to any set of non-self MHC molecules can be as high as 5% (see Section 4-19), yet responses to self MHC antigens are not detected in naturally self-tolerant individuals. Moreover, mice given bone marrow cells from a foreign donor at birth, before significant numbers of mature T cells have appeared, can be rendered fully and permanently tolerant to the bone marrow donor's tissues, provided that the bone marrow donor's cells continue to be produced so as to induce tolerance in each new cohort of developing T cells (Fig. 12.26). This experiment, performed by Medawar, validated Burnet's prediction that developing lymphocytes with an open repertoire of receptors must be purged of self-reactive cells before they achieve functional maturity; it won them a Nobel Prize.

Fig. 12.26 Tolerance to allogeneic skin can be established in bone marrow chimeric mice. In normal mice, T cells that would respond to peptides borne by self antigen-presenting cells (APCs) are negatively selected in the thymus, while T cells reactive to non-self MHC molecules mature, allowing the mouse to reject allogeneic skin grafts. If mice are injected with allogeneic bone marrow at birth (top panel) before they achieve immune competence, they become chimeric, with T cells and APCs deriving from both host and donor bone marrow stem cells. T cells developing in these mice are negatively selected on APCs of both host and donor (middle panel), so that mature T cells are tolerant to the MHC molecules of the bone marrow donor. This allows the chimeric mouse to accept skin derived from the bone marrow donor. Such acquired tolerance is specific, since skin from an unrelated or 'third party' donor is rejected normally (bottom panel). This tolerance lasts only while the recipient is chimeric; if donor bone marrow ceases to produce APCs, then tolerance is lost as new T cells develop, and the mice acquire the ability to reject donor skin.

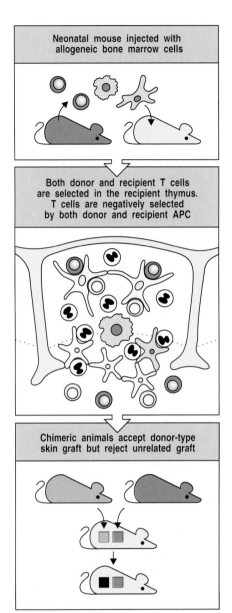

Clonal deletion reliably removes all T cells that can mount aggressive responses against self MHC molecules; autoimmune diseases, which involve rare T-cell responses to a particular self peptide bound to a self MHC molecule, are therefore unlikely to reflect a general failure in clonal deletion. Rather, the lymphocytes that mediate autoimmune responses appear not to be subject to clonal deletion, and such autoreactive cells are present in all of us. They do not normally cause autoimmunity because they are only activated under special circumstances. Similar arguments apply to the idea that autoimmunity is caused by a random failure in the mechanisms responsible for anergy. Therefore it seems unlikely that naturally occurring autoimmune diseases arise because of a failure in these mechanisms of ensuring self-tolerance.

A striking demonstration that autoreactive T cells can be present in healthy individuals comes from a strain of mice carrying transgenes encoding an autoreactive T-cell receptor specific for a peptide of myelin basic protein bound to self MHC class II molecules. The autoreactive receptor is present on every T cell, and yet the mice are healthy unless their T cells are activated. We will discuss these mice further in Section 12-23. As the level of the specific peptide:MHC class II complex is low except in the central nervous system, a site not visited by naive T cells, the autoreactive T cells remain in a state of immunological ignorance. When these T cells are activated, for example by deliberate immunization as in experimental allergic encephalomyelitis, they migrate into all the tissues, including the central nervous system, where they can recognize their myelin basic protein:MHC class II ligand. This triggers cytokine production by the activated T cells, causing inflammation in the brain and the destruction of myelin and neurons that ultimately cause the symptoms of paralysis in this disease.

It is likely that only a small fraction of proteins will be able to serve as autoantigens, since if a self protein is abundant, naive T cells specific for its peptides will be deleted or rendered anergic, while many proteins will be expressed at levels too low to be detected by T cells (see Fig. 12.25). It has been estimated that we can make approximately 10^5 proteins of average length 300 amino acids, capable of generating about 3×10^7 distinct self peptides. Since MHC molecules are rarely expressed at levels above 10^5 molecules per cell, and since the MHC molecules on a cell must bind 10–100 identical peptides for T-cell recognition to occur, fewer than 10 000 self peptides (<1/3000) can be presented by a given MHC molecule at levels detectable by T cells. Many of these will be presented at a high enough level to induce tolerance. Therefore, most self peptides will be presented at levels that are too low to induce tolerance in naive

T cells by any mechanism, and will also be displayed on tissue cells at levels insufficient for recognition by armed effector T cells and thus cannot serve as autoantigens. However, as shown in Fig. 12.25, a few peptides may fail to induce tolerance, yet are present at high enough levels for recognition by effector T cells. This argument leaves aside the crucial issue of how such effector T cells are activated, which we shall consider in a later section (see Section 12-25).

If the idea that only a few peptides can act as autoantigens is correct, then it is not surprising that there are relatively few distinct autoimmune syndromes, and that all individuals with a particular autoimmune disease tend to recognize the same antigen. If all antigens could give rise to autoimmunity, one would expect that different individuals with the same disease might recognize different antigens on the target tissue, which does not appear to be the case. Finally, since the level of auto-antigenic peptide presented is determined by polymorphic residues in MHC molecules that govern the affinity of peptide binding, this idea could also explain the association of autoimmune diseases with particular MHC genotypes (see Fig. 12.2).

12-20   The induction of a tissue-specific response requires expression of co-stimulator activity on antigen-presenting cells.

As we learned in Chapter 7, only professional antigen-presenting cells that express co-stimulatory activity can initiate clonal expansion of T cells—an essential step in all adaptive immune responses, including graft rejection and presumably, autoimmunity. In tissue grafts, it is the donor antigen-presenting cells in the graft that stimulate the host T cells, initiating the response that leads to graft rejection. If the grafted tissue is depleted of antigen-presenting cells by treatment with antibodies or by prolonged incubation, rejection occurs only after a much longer time. The normal route for sensitization to a graft appears to involve the antigen-presenting cells leaving the graft and migrating to regional lymph nodes (Fig. 12.27); when the site of grafting lacks lymphatic drainage, no response against the graft results. Thus, to induce an efficient immune response,

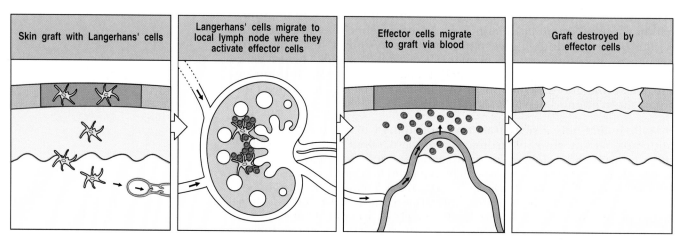

| Skin graft with Langerhans' cells | Langerhans' cells migrate to local lymph node where they activate effector cells | Effector cells migrate to graft via blood | Graft destroyed by effector cells |

Fig. 12.27 The initiation of graft rejection normally involves migration of donor antigen-presenting cells from the graft to local lymph nodes. Here they encounter recirculating T cells, some of which are specific for graft antigens, stimulating these T cells to divide. The resulting activated effector T cells migrate via the thoracic duct to the blood and home to the grafted tissue, which they rapidly destroy. Destruction is highly specific for donor-derived cells, suggesting it is mediated by direct cytotoxicity and not by non-specific inflammatory processes.

antigen-presenting cells bearing both graft antigens and co-stimulatory activity must travel to regional lymph nodes. Here, they are examined by large numbers of host T cells and can activate those that have specific receptors. This clearly reflects the way that responses to infection are normally induced (see Section 9-16).

Although grafts depleted of antigen-presenting cells are tolerated for long periods of time, such grafts are eventually rejected. This process appears to involve host antigen-presenting cells. Interestingly, when grafts that are MHC-identical to the host but mismatched at minor H antigens are depleted of antigen-presenting cells, they are rejected more rapidly than similarly depleted grafts that are MHC-different from the host but identical at minor H antigens. This suggests that host antigen-presenting cells pick up proteins from the graft and present their peptides, including those that contain minor H antigens, to MHC-restricted host T cells. As MHC-different grafts present different peptides and lack self MHC molecules, they may evade this type of response. These MHC-different grafts are rejected by inflammation, probably triggered when host T cells recognize graft peptides presented by host antigen-presenting macrophages, rather than by the direct attack of cytotoxic T cells on cells of the graft. These experiments also show that the co-stimulation needed to induce a response to the non-self MHC molecules on the graft cannot be delivered separately by host antigen-presenting cells. The ability of professional antigen-presenting cells to pick up antigens in tissues and initiate graft rejection is important, as it may play a role in the initiation of autoimmune tissue damage as well. However, the mechanism by which graft antigens are presented is not currently understood.

12-21   In the absence of co-stimulation, tolerance is induced.

As discussed in Section 7-4, T-cell activation requires that one cell express both peptide:MHC and co-stimulatory molecules; in the absence of co-stimulation, specific antigen recognition leads to anergy or deletion of mature T cells (see Section 7-10). For instance, expression of foreign antigens in peripheral tissues is not sufficient to induce autoimmunity, but co-expression of antigen and B7 in the same target tissue will do so. As B7 expression on peripheral tissue cells is not by itself a sufficient stimulus for autoimmunity, it is clear that the loss of tolerance to self tissues requires both a suitable target antigen (see Section 12-19) and co-stimulation expressed by one cell. As tissue cells are not known to express B7 or other co-stimulatory molecules, tolerance to self tissues is the norm.

From these experiments, it seems likely that autoimmunity results when an antigen-presenting cell that has co-stimulatory activity picks up a tissue-specific antigen. Once an autoantigen is expressed on a cell with co-stimulatory potential, T cells specific for the autoantigen may become activated and can home to the tissues, where they produce tissue damage.

A second level at which autoimmune responses to tissue cells may be controlled is that armed effector T cells kill only a limited number of antigen-expressing tissue cells if these lack co-stimulatory activity; after killing a few targets, the effector cell dies. Thus, not only can responses not be initiated in the absence of co-stimulatory activity, they also cannot be sustained in its absence. Thus, in addition to the question of how autoimmunity is avoided, we must ask why does it ever occur? How are responses to self initiated, and how are they sustained? It is thought that one trigger for autoimmunity is infection (see Section 12-25).

12-22 | Dominant immune suppression can be demonstrated in models of tolerance and can affect the course of autoimmune disease.

In some models of tolerance, it can be demonstrated that specific T cells play an active role in suppressing the activity of other T cells that are capable of causing tissue damage. Tolerance in these cases is dominant in that it can be transferred by T cells, which are usually called **suppressor T cells**. Furthermore, depletion of the suppressor T cells leads to aggravated responses to self or graft antigens. Although it is clear that these phenomena of immune suppression exist, the mechanisms responsible have been the subject of much controversy. Here, we will examine the phenomenon in three animal models.

In a skin graft rejection model, neonatal rats can be rendered tolerant to allogeneic grafts by injection of allogeneic bone marrow. The tolerance induced is highly specific and can be transferred to normal adult recipient rats. This shows that tolerance in this model is dominant and active, as the lymphocytes of the recipient are prevented from mediating graft rejection by the transferred cells. Transfer requires cells of both the allogeneic donor and the original tolerized host. Depletion of either cell type abolishes the transfer of tolerance.

This finding is reminiscent of the studies of Medawar on tolerance in neonatal bone marrow chimeric mice discussed in Section 12-19. In both cases, even injection of massive numbers of normal syngeneic lymphocytes, which would react vigorously against the foreign cells in the normal environment of the cell donor, did not break tolerance. Tolerance could only be broken with cells that had been immunized before transfer; such cells probably break tolerance by killing the allogeneic donor cells. Thus, an active host response prevents graft rejection in this model. Since the tolerance is specific for cells of the original donor, the suppression must also be specific.

In the mouse model for insulin-dependent diabetes, transfer of certain islet-specific T-cell clones can prevent the destruction of pancreatic β cells by autoreactive cytotoxic T cells. This suggests that the islet-specific T cells can suppress the activity of autoaggressive T cells in an antigen-dependent manner. There are interesting hints that such cells naturally affect the course of the autoimmune response that causes diabetes; β-cell destruction in humans occurs over a period of several years before diabetes is manifest, yet when new islets are transplanted from an identical twin into his or her diabetic sibling, they are destroyed within a few weeks. This suggests that, in the normal course of the disease, specific cells protect the β cells from attack by effector T cells and the disease therefore progresses slowly. It may be that after the host islets have been destroyed, these protective mechanisms decline in activity, but that the effector cells responsible for β-cell destruction do not.

If specific suppression of autoimmune responses could be elicited at will, autoimmunity would not be a problem. While this has not yet been documented in human autoimmunity, experimental studies in which tissue antigens are fed to mice have shown some protective effects, and early studies of this procedure in humans have also shown benefits. Feeding with specific antigen is known to elicit a local immune response in the intestinal mucosa, while responses to the same antigen given subsequently by a systemic route are suppressed (see Section 2-3). This has been exploited in experimental autoimmune diseases by feeding proteins from target tissues to mice; mice fed insulin are protected from diabetes, while mice fed myelin basic protein are resistant to experimental allergic encephalomyelitis (Fig. 12.28).

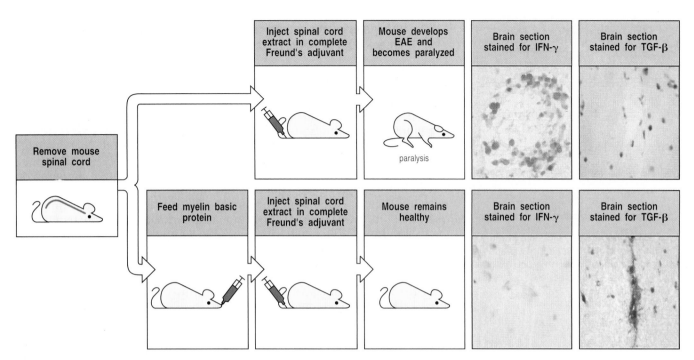

Fig. 12.28 Antigen given orally can lead to protection against autoimmune disease. The autoimmune disease experimental allergic encephalomyelitis (EAE) is induced in mice by immunizing them with spinal cord in complete Freund's adjuvant (top panels); the disease is caused by T_H1 cells specific for myelin basic protein (MBP). When mice are first fed with MBP, later immunization with spinal cord or MBP fails to induce the disease. T_H1 cells that produce IFN-γ are found in the brains of diseased mice (upper left photograph, where the brown staining reveals the presence of IFN-γ). These T cells are presumably responsible for the damage that results in paralysis. Note that cells expressing TGF-β are not seen in diseased mice (upper right photograph). In orally tolerized mice, IFN-γ-producing cells are absent (lower left photograph) while TGF-β-producing T cells are found in the brain in place of the autoaggressive T_H1 cells (lower right photograph, the brown stain in this case reveals the presence of TGF-β), and presumably protect the brain from autoimmune attack. Photographs courtesy of S Khoury, W Hancock, and H Weiner.

This disease is normally caused by T_H1 cells that produce IFN-γ in response to myelin basic protein; in mice fed this protein, CD4 T cells that produce cytokines such as TGF-β and IL-4 are found in the brain instead. TGF-β, in particular, suppresses the function of inflammatory T_H1 lymphocytes. In both these cases, the protection appears to be tissue- rather than antigen-specific. Thus, feeding insulin protects against diabetes, yet insulin is not thought to be the target of autoimmune attack on the β cells. Likewise, feeding myelin basic protein will protect against experimental allergic encephalomyelitis elicited by other brain antigens. Feeding with antigen may induce the production of T cells producing TGF-β and IL-4 because these cytokines are also required for IgA production to antigens ingested in food. If feeding with antigen works as a clinical therapy, it would have the advantage over treatments with immunosuppressive drugs that it does not alter the general immune competence of the host.

Like human diabetes, multiple sclerosis is a chronic relapsing disease with acute episodes followed by periods of quiescence. This again suggests a balance between autoimmune and protective T cells, which may alter at different stages of the disease. However, it remains to be proven whether the specific suppressive cells discussed in this section exist naturally and contribute to self tolerance, or whether they only arise upon artificial stimulation or in response to autoimmune attack. Nevertheless, as they can play an active, dominant role in self tolerance, they are particularly attractive targets for immunotherapy of autoimmune disease.

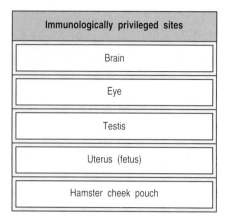

Immunologically privileged sites
Brain
Eye
Testis
Uterus (fetus)
Hamster cheek pouch

Fig. 12.29 Some body sites are immunologically privileged. Tissue grafts placed in these sites often last indefinitely and antigens placed in these sites do not elicit destructive immune responses.

12-23 **Antigens in immunologically privileged sites do not induce immune attack but can serve as targets.**

Tissue grafts placed in some sites in the body do not elicit immune responses. For instance, the brain and the anterior chamber of the eye are sites in which tissues can be grafted without inducing graft rejection. Such locations in the body are termed **immunologically privileged sites** (Fig. 12.29). It was originally believed that immunological privilege arose from the failure of antigens to leave privileged sites and induce responses. However, subsequent studies have shown that antigens do leave immunologically privileged sites, and that these antigens do interact with T cells; however, instead of eliciting a destructive immune response, they induce tolerance or a response that is not destructive to the tissue. Immunologically privileged sites appear to be unusual in two ways. First, the communication between the privileged site and the body is atypical in that extracellular fluid in these sites does not pass through conventional lymphatics, although proteins placed in these sites do leave them and can have immunological effects. Second, humoral factors, presumably cytokines, which affect the behavior of the immune response are produced in privileged sites and leave them together with antigens. The cytokine TGF-β appears to be particularly important in this regard and antigens mixed with TGF-β appear to induce T-cell responses that do not damage tissues, such as T$_H$2 rather than T$_H$1 responses.

Paradoxically, it is often the antigens sequestered in immunologically privileged sites that are the targets of autoimmune attack; for example, multiple sclerosis is directed at brain autoantigens such as myelin basic protein and is one of the most prevalent autoimmune diseases. As we have already seen, experimental allergic encephalomyelitis is induced in some strains of rats and mice upon immunization with spinal cord or myelin basic protein in adjuvant. It is therefore clear that this antigen does not induce deletional tolerance and anergy. As we saw in Section 12-19, mice transgenic for a T-cell receptor specific for myelin basic protein carry this autoreactive receptor on most of their T cells, yet develop normally. These T cells are readily activated by the appropriate peptide of the protein; nevertheless, the mice do not become diseased unless they are deliberately immunized with myelin basic protein, in which case they become acutely sick, show severe infiltration of the brain with specific T$_H$1 cells, and often die. The non-transgenic littermates have a milder, transient illness. Thus, at least some antigens expressed in immunologically privileged sites induce neither tolerance nor activation, but if activation is induced elsewhere they may become targets for autoimmune attack. It seems plausible that T cells specific for antigens that are sequestered in immunologically privileged sites are more likely to remain in the state of immunological ignorance described in Section 12-19. This is further shown in the eye disease **sympathetic ophthalmia** (Fig. 12.30). If one eye is ruptured by a blow or other trauma, an autoimmune response to eye proteins can occur although it happens only rarely. Once the response is induced, it often attacks both eyes. Immunosuppression and removal of the damaged eye, the source of antigen, is frequently required to preserve vision in the undamaged eye.

It is not surprising that effector T cells can enter immunologically privileged sites: such sites can become infected and effector cells must be able to enter these sites during infection. As we learned in Chapter 9, effector T cells enter most or all tissues after activation, but accumulations of cells are only seen when antigen is recognized in the site, triggering the production of cytokines that alter tissue barriers.

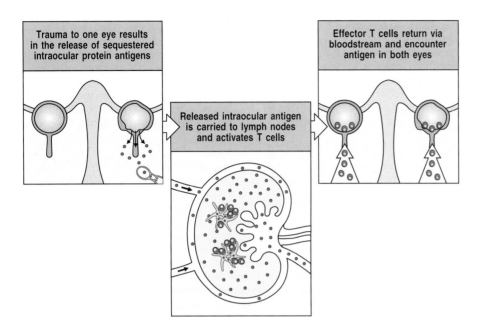

Fig. 12.30 **Damage to an immunologically privileged site can induce an autoimmune response.** In the disease sympathetic ophthalmia, trauma to one eye releases the sequestered eye antigens into the surrounding tissues, making them accessible to T cells. The effector cells elicited attack the traumatized eye, and also infiltrate and attack the healthy eye. Thus, although the sequestered antigens do not induce a response by themselves, if a response is induced elsewhere they can serve as targets for attack.

The testes are immunologically privileged sites that retain their privilege even when relocated by transplantation to other sites in the body. This implies that properties intrinsic to testicular tissue rather than a physical barrier preventing access by cells of the immune system may be important in determining its privileged nature. Recent experiments have shown that testicular tissue expresses high levels of Fas ligand and this protects the tissue from attack by T cells, which are killed through ligation of Fas. Testis derived from mice genetically deficient in Fas ligand has lost its immunological privilege, and can be rejected by T cells. This discovery offers a potential therapeutic strategy to reduce graft rejection by engineering high expression of Fas ligand in the graft, provided that the cells themselves cannot be induced to express Fas. Such cells could also be resistant to killing by pathogen-specific cytotoxic T cells, so such organs could provide a source of infected cells from which pathogens could not be cleared.

12-24   B cells with receptors specific for peripheral autoantigens are held in check by a variety of mechanisms.

When B-cell antigen receptors are first expressed in the bone marrow, receptors specific for self molecules are produced because of the random generation of the repertoire. If a self molecule is expressed in the bone marrow in an appropriate form, clonal deletion and receptor editing can remove all of these self-reactive B cells while they are still immature (see Sections 5-10 and 5-11). There are, however, many self molecules available only in the periphery, whose expression is restricted to particular organs, such as thyroglobulin (the precursor of thyroxine), which is expressed only in the thyroid. Therefore back-up mechanisms exist to ensure that B cells reactive to these self molecules do not cause autoimmune disease. When a mature B cell in the periphery encounters self molecules that bind its receptor, four mechanisms have been proposed to explain the observed non-reactivity. Failure of each of these mechanisms could lead to autoimmunity.

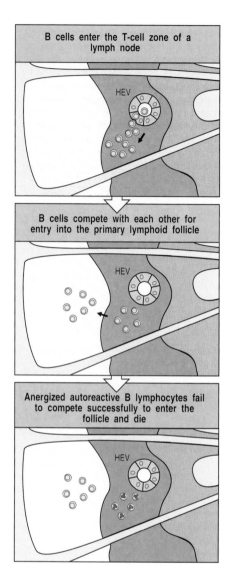

B cells enter the T-cell zone of a lymph node

HEV

B cells compete with each other for entry into the primary lymphoid follicle

HEV

Anergized autoreactive B lymphocytes fail to compete successfully to enter the follicle and die

HEV

Fig. 12.31 Autoreactive B cells do not compete effectively in peripheral lymphoid tissue to enter primary lymphoid follicles. In the top panel, B cells are seen entering the T-cell zone of a lymph node through high endothelial venules (HEVs) with reactivity for foreign antigen (yellow) and anergized autoreactive cells (gray). The anergized cells fail to compete with B lymphocytes that have specificity for foreign antigens for exit from the T-cell zone and entry into primary follicles (middle panel). The autoreactive B cells fail to receive survival signals and undergo apoptosis *in situ* in the T-cell zone (bottom panel).

First, B cells that recognize a self antigen arrest their migration in the T-cell zone of peripheral lymphoid tissues (Fig. 12.31), just like B cells that bind a foreign antigen (see Chapter 8). However, unlike the response to foreign antigens, in which armed CD4 T cells are present, no such cells exist for self antigens. This prevents the B cells migrating out of the T-cell zones into the follicles; instead the trapped B cells undergo apoptosis. An example of this in normal humans is the existence of circulating B lymphocytes expressing anti-thyroglobulin activity which, because of a lack of T-cell help specific for this self antigen, do not make autoantibodies against thyroglobulin.

A second mechanism for inactivation of autoreactive B cells in the periphery is the induction of B-cell anergy by downregulation of surface IgM expression and partial inhibition of the linked B-cell signaling pathways (Fig. 12.32). B-cell anergy can also be induced by exposure to soluble circulating antigen; if mice are inoculated intravenously with protein solutions from which all trace of aggregates has been rigorously removed in order to eliminate multivalent complexes, their peripheral B cells can be inactivated.

A third mechanism is the induction of apoptosis in mature autoreactive B cells. This mechanism is dependent on the presence of T cells that are specific for the self antigen and that express Fas ligand. Although negative selection in the thymus usually eliminates such T cells, when an autoreactive T cell is activated, it is able to kill autoreactive B cells in a Fas-dependent manner (see Fig. 12.32). The importance of this mechanism

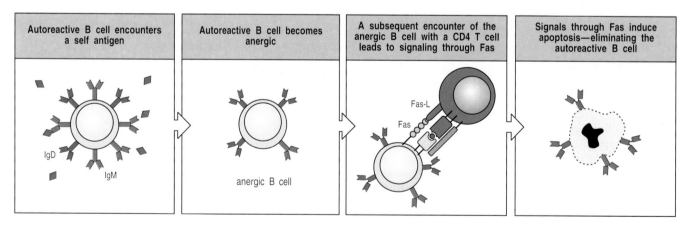

Autoreactive B cell encounters a self antigen

IgD

IgM

Autoreactive B cell becomes anergic

anergic B cell

A subsequent encounter of the anergic B cell with a CD4 T cell leads to signaling through Fas

Fas-L

Fas

Signals through Fas induce apoptosis—eliminating the autoreactive B cell

Fig. 12.32 Peripheral B lymphocyte anergy. An autoreactive B lymphocyte encounters its soluble autoantigen in the periphery (first panel), which leads to the development of B-cell anergy. This is shown in the second panel, and is characterized by reduction in both the expression of surface IgM and of the signaling pathways following ligation of surface immunoglobulin. A further mechanism to maintain peripheral B-cell tolerance is shown in the two panels on the right. If an anergized, self-reactive B lymphocyte encounters a T cell that is specific for a self peptide from the relevant autoantigen, T-cell surface Fas ligand binds to Fas (CD95) on the B-lymphocyte surface. In the absence of the normal pathways of co-stimulation the anergized B lymphocytes show enhanced sensitivity to apoptosis following ligation of Fas by Fas ligand on the T cell.

Fig. 12.33 Elimination of autoreactive B lymphocytes in germinal centers. During the process of somatic hypermutation in germinal centers, depicted in the top panel, autoreactive antibody specificities may arise. Ligation of these antibody receptors by soluble autoantigen induces apoptosis of the autoreactive B lymphocyte by signaling through the B-cell antigen receptor.

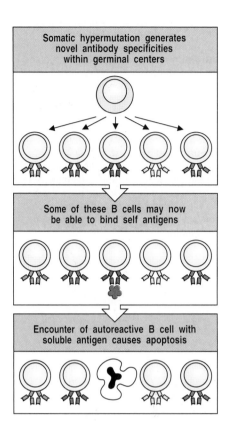

is nicely illustrated by the consequences of having mutant genes for Fas or Fas ligand. Mice and humans deficient in Fas or Fas ligand develop severe autoimmune disease associated with the overproduction of lymphocytes.

Finally, there is evidence for a distinct mechanism for dealing with B cells that develop self-reactive specificities as a result of somatic hypermutation during a response to a foreign antigen (Fig. 12.33). At a crucial phase at the height of the germinal center reaction, encounter with a large dose of soluble antigen causes a wave of apoptosis in germinal center B cells within a few hours. This mechanism is also defective in mice mutant for Fas or Fas ligand.

All these mechanisms re-emphasize the fact that the mere existence in the body of some B lymphocytes with receptor specificities directed against self is not in itself harmful. Before an immune response may be initiated they need to receive effective help, the B-cell antigen receptors must be ligated, and their intracellular signaling machinery must be set to respond normally.

12-25 Autoimmunity could be triggered by infection in a variety of ways.

Human autoimmune diseases often appear gradually, making it difficult to find out how the process is initiated. Nevertheless, there is a strong suspicion that infections can trigger autoimmune disease in genetically susceptible individuals. Indeed, many experimental autoimmune diseases are induced by mixing tissue cells with adjuvants that contain bacteria. For example, to induce experimental allergic encephalomyelitis (see Fig. 12.28), it is necessary to emulsify the spinal cord or myelin basic protein used for immunization in complete Freund's adjuvant, which includes killed *Mycobacterium tuberculosis* (see Section 2-4); however, when the mycobacteria are omitted from the adjuvant, not only is no disease elicited but the animals become refractory to disease induction with antigen in complete Freund's adjuvant, and T cells can transfer this resistance to syngeneic recipients (Fig. 12.34). There are several other systems in which infection is important in the induction of disease; for example, the transgenic mice that express a T-cell receptor specific for myelin basic protein (see Sections 12-19 and 12-23) often develop spontaneous autoimmunity if they become infected. One possible mechanism for this loss of tolerance is that the infectious agents induce co-stimulatory activity on cells expressing low levels of peptides from myelin basic protein, thus activating the autoreactive T cells.

It has also been suggested that autoimmunity may be initiated by a mechanism known as **molecular mimicry**, in which antibodies or T cells generated in the response to an infectious agent cross-react with self antigens. To show that infectious agents can trigger responses that have the capacity to destroy tissues, mice were made transgenic for a viral nuclear protein driven by the insulin promoter, so that the protein was expressed only in pancreatic β cells. As the amount of protein

Fig. 12.34 Bacterial adjuvants are required to induce experimental autoimmune disease. Mice immunized with spinal-cord homogenate in complete Freund's adjuvant, which contains large numbers of *Mycobacterium tuberculosis* organisms, get experimental allergic encephalomyelitis (EAE). Mice immunized with the same antigen in incomplete Freund's adjuvant, which lacks the *M. tuberculosis*, not only do not become diseased but are actually protected from subsequent disease induction. Moreover, T cells from these mice can transfer protection from disease to naive, syngeneic recipients.

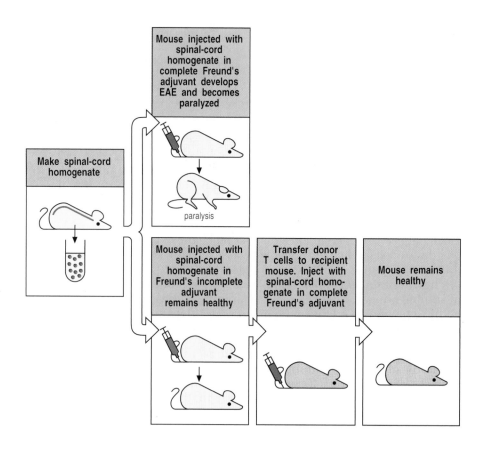

expressed was low, the T cells that recognized the viral protein remained ignorant, that is, they were neither tolerant to the viral protein nor activated by it, and the animals showed no sign of disease. However, if they were infected with the live virus, they responded by making cytotoxic CD8 T cells specific for the viral protein, and these armed CD8 cytotoxic T cells could destroy the β cells, causing diabetes (Fig. 12.35). Recent work suggests that the immune response to natural infection occasionally elicits T cells that cause autoimmune disease by recognizing cross-reacting self peptides.

Fig. 12.35 Virus infection can break tolerance to a transgenic viral protein expressed in pancreatic β cells. Mice that express a protein from the lymphocytic choriomeningitis virus (LCMV) in pancreatic β cells do not respond to the protein and therefore do not get diabetes. However, if the transgenic mice are infected with LCMV, a potent anti-viral cytotoxic T-cell response is elicited, and this kills the β cells, leading to diabetes. It is thought that infectious agents may sometimes elicit T-cell responses that cross-react with self peptides (a process known as molecular mimicry) and that this could cause autoimmune disease in a similar way.

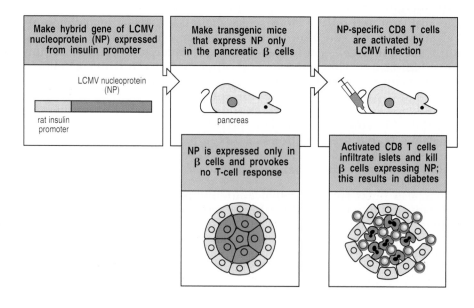

In antibody-mediated autoimmunity, it is clear that molecular mimicry can operate; microbial antigens can elicit antibody responses that react not only with the pathogen but also with host antigens that are similar in structure. This type of response occurs after infection with some *Streptococcus* species that elicit antibodies that cross-react with kidney, joint, and heart antigens to produce pathology. However, such responses are usually transient and do not lead to sustained auto-antibody production, since the helper T cells are specific for the microbe and not for self proteins. Host proteins that complex with bacteria can induce a similar transient response; in this case, the antibody response is not cross-reactive but the bacterium is acting as a carrier, allowing B cells that express an autoreactive receptor to receive inappropriate T-cell help. These and some other mechanisms that could allow an infectious agent to break tolerance are summarized in Fig. 12.36. All of these mechanisms can be shown to act in experimental systems, and some evidence supports their importance in human autoimmune disease as well.

The argument that autoimmunity may be initiated by infection is strengthened by the fact that there are several human autoimmune diseases in which a prior infection with a specific agent or class of agents leads to a particular disease (Fig. 12.37). Again, disease susceptibility in these cases is determined largely by MHC genotype. However, in most autoimmune diseases there is still no firm evidence that a particular infectious agent is associated with onset of the disease; this may be partly because it often takes many years for a patient with an autoimmune disease to show noticeable symptoms.

Mechanism	Disruption of cell or tissue barrier	Infection of antigen-presenting cell	Binding of pathogen to self protein	Molecular mimicry	Superantigen
Effect	Release of sequestered self antigen; activation of non-tolerized cells	Induction of co-stimulator activity	Pathogen acts as carrier to allow anti-self response	Production of cross-reactive antibodies or T cells	Polyclonal activation of autoreactive T cells
Example	Sympathetic ophthalmia	Effect of adjuvants: induction of EAE	? Interstitial nephritis	Rheumatic fever ? Diabetes ? Multiple sclerosis	? Rheumatoid arthritis

Fig. 12.36 There are several ways in which infectious agents could break self tolerance. Since some antigens are sequestered from the circulation, either behind a tissue barrier or within the cell, it is possible that an infection that breaks cell and tissue barriers may expose hidden antigens (first panel). A second possibility is that the local inflammation in response to an infectious agent may trigger expression of MHC molecules and co-stimulators on tissue cells, inducing an autoimmune response (second panel). In some cases, infectious agents may bind to self proteins. Since the infectious agent induces a helper T-cell response, any B cell that recognizes the self protein will also receive help. Such responses should be self-limiting once the infectious agent is eliminated, since at this point the T-cell help will no longer be provided (third panel). Infectious agents may induce either T- or B-cell responses that can cross-react with self antigens. This is termed molecular mimicry (fourth panel). T-cell polyclonal activation by a bacterial superantigen could overcome clonal anergy, allowing an autoimmune process to begin (fifth panel). There is little evidence for most of these mechanisms in human autoimmune disease (see text).

Fig. 12.37 Association of infection with autoimmune diseases. Several autoimmune diseases occur after specific infections and are presumably triggered by the infection. The case of post-streptococcal disease is best known but is now rare since effective antibiotic therapy of Group A streptococcal infection usually prevents post-infection complications. Most of these post-infection autoimmune diseases also show susceptibility linked to MHC.

Associations of infection with immune-mediated tissue damage		
Infection	HLA association	Consequence
Group A *Streptococcus*	?	Rheumatic fever (carditis, polyarthritis)
Chlamydia trachomatis	HLA-B27	Reiter's syndrome (arthritis)
Shigella flexneri, Salmonella typhimurium, Salmonella enteritidis, Yersinia enterocolitica, Campylobacter jejuni	HLA-B27	Reactive arthritis
Borrelia burgdorferi	HLA-DR2, DR4	Chronic arthritis in Lyme disease

Summary.

Tolerance to self is a normal state that is maintained chiefly by clonal deletion of developing T and B cells and clonal deletion or inactivation of mature, peripheral T and B cells. In addition, some antigens are ignored by the immune system, many by being present in immunologically privileged sites. When the state of self tolerance is disrupted, perhaps by infection, autoimmunity can result. The process of clonal deletion sets limits on the kinds of autoimmune diseases that can occur; indeed, only antigens that do not trigger clonal deletion in the thymus, either because they are not abundant enough or because they are tissue-specific and not expressed in the thymus, are candidate autoantigens. Tolerance to non-self can be acquired by mimicking the mechanisms responsible for tolerance to self. A third mechanism for self tolerance, dominant suppression, has been noted in several experimental systems of autoimmunity and graft rejection; if this mechanism could be understood, it is possible that it could be used to prevent both graft rejection and autoimmunity, which are closely related problems.

Summary to Chapter 12.

The response to non-infectious antigens causes three types of medical problem: allergy, the subject of Chapter 11, and autoimmunity and graft rejection, the subjects of this chapter. These responses have many features in common because all use the normal mechanisms of the adaptive immune response to produce symptoms and pathology. What is unique to these syndromes is their initiation and the nature of the antigens recognized, not the underlying nature of the response itself. For each of these undesirable categories of response, the question is how to control them without adversely affecting protective immunity to infection. The answer may lie in a more complete understanding of the regulation of the immune response, especially the suppressive mechanisms that appear to be important in tolerance. The deliberate control of the immune response is examined further in the next chapter.

General references.

Andre, I., Gonzalez, A., Wang, B., Katz, J., Benoist, C., and Mathis, D.: **Checkpoints in the progression of autoimmune disease: lessons from diabetes models.** *Proc. Natl. Acad. Sci. 1996,* **93**:2260-2263.

Charlton, B., Auchincloss, H., Jr., and Fathman, C.G.: **Mechanisms of transplantation tolerance.** *Ann. Rev. Immunol.* 1994, **12**:707-734.

Moller, G. (ed.): **Models of autoimmunity.** *Immunol. Rev.* 1993, **118**:1-310.

Moller, G. (ed.): **Peripheral T-cell immunological tolerance.** *Immunol. Rev.* 1993, **133**:1-240.

Moller, G. (ed.): **Chronic graft rejection.** *Immunol. Rev.* 1993, **134**:1-116.

Moller, G. (ed.): **Xenotransplantation** *Immunol. Rev.* 1994, **141**:1-276.

Moller, G. (ed.): **Chronic autoimmune diseases** *Immunol. Rev.* 1995, **144**:1-314.

Mueller, R. and Sarvetnick, N.: **Transgenic/knockout mice—tools to study autoimmunity.** *Curr. Opin. Immunol.* 1995, **7**:799-803.

Romagnani, S.: **Lymphokine production by human T cells in disease states.** *Ann. Rev. Immunol.* 1994, **12**:227-257.

Steinman, L.: **Escape from "horror autotoxicus": pathogenesis and treatment of autoimmune disease.** *Cell* 1995, **80**:7-10.

Steinman, L.: **A few autoreactive cells in an autoimmune infiltrate control a vast population of nonspecific cells: a tale of smart bombs and the infantry.** *Proc. Natl. Acad. Sci. 1996,* **93**:2253-2256.

Tan, E.M.: **Autoantibodies in pathology and cell biology.** *Cell* 1991, **67**:841-842.

Section references.

12-1 Specific adaptive immune responses to self antigens can cause autoimmune disease.

Martin, R., McFarland, H.F., and McFarlin, D.E.: **Immunological aspects of demyelinating diseases.** *Ann. Rev. Immunol.* 1992, **10**:153-187.

Naparstek, Y. and Plotz, P.H.: **The role of autoantibodies in autoimmune disease.** *Ann. Rev. Immunol.* 1993, **11**:79-104.

12-2 Susceptibility to autoimmune diseases is controlled by environmental and genetic factors, especially MHC genes.

Gautam, A.M., Lock, C.B., Smilek, D.E., Pearson, C.I., Steinman, L., and McDevitt, H.O.: **Minimum structural requirements for peptide presentation by major histocompatibility complex class II molecules: implications in induction of autoimmunity.** *Proc. Natl. Acad. Sci. 1994,* **91**:767-771.

Merriman, T.R. and Todd, J.A.: **Genetics of autoimmune disease.** *Curr. Opin. Immunol.* 1995, **7**:786-792.

Todd, J.A. and Steinman, L.: **The environment strikes back.** *Curr. Opin. Immunol.* 1993, **5**:863-865.

Todd, J.A.: **Genetic analysis of type 1 diabetes using whole genome approaches.** *Proc. Natl. Acad. Sci.* 1995, **92**:8560-8565.

Vyse, T.J. and Todd, J.A.: **Genetic analysis of autoimmune disease.** *Cell* 1996, **85**:311-318.

Waksman, B.H.: **Multiple sclerosis. More genes versus environment.** *Nature* 1995, **377**:105-106.

Wicker, L.S., Todd, J.A., and Peterson, L.B.: **Genetic control of autoimmune diabetes in the NOD mouse.** *Ann. Rev. Immunol.* 1995, **13**:179-200.

12-3 Either antibody or T cells can cause tissue damage in autoimmune disease.

Kiefel, V., Santoso, S., and Mueller Eckhardt, C.: **Serological, biochemical, and molecular aspects of platelet autoantigens.** *Semin. Hematol.* 1992, **29**:26-33.

Silberstein, L.E.: **Natural and pathologic human autoimmune responses to carbohydrate antigens on red blood cells.** *Springer Semin. Immunopath.* 1993, **15**:139-153.

12-4 The fixation of sub-lytic doses of complement to cells in tissues stimulates a powerful inflammatory response.

Couser, W.G.: **Pathogenesis of glomerulonephritis.** *Kidney Intl. Suppl.* 1993, **42**:S19-S26.

Hansch, G.M.: **The complement attack phase: control of lysis and non-lethal effects of C5b-9.** *Immunopharmacol.* 1992, **24**:107-117.

Jennette, J.C. and Falk, R.J.: **The pathology of vasculitis involving the kidney.** *Am. J. Kidney Dis.* 1994, **24**:130-141.

Rapoport, B.: **Pathophysiology of Hashimoto's thyroiditis and hypothyroidism.** *Ann. Rev. Med* 1991, **42**:91-96.

Rother, K., Hansch, G.M., and Rauterberg, E.W.: **Complement in inflammation: induction of nephritides and progress to chronicity.** *Intl. Arch. Allergy Appl. Immunol.* 1991, **94**:23-37.

Shin, M.L. and Carney, D.F.: **Cytotoxic action and other metabolic consequences of terminal complement proteins.** *Prog. Allergy* 1988, **40**:44-81.

12-5 Autoantibodies to receptors cause disease by stimulating or blocking receptor function.

Bahn, R.S. and Heufelder, A.E.: **Pathogenesis of Graves' ophthalmopathy.** *N. Engl. J. Med.* 1993, **329**:1468-1475.

Feldmann, M., Dayan, C., Grubeck Loebenstein, B., Rapoport, B., and Londei, M.: **Mechanism of Graves thyroiditis: implications for concepts and therapy of autoimmunity.** *Intl. Rev. Immunol.* 1992, **9**:91-106.

McLachlan, S.M. and Rapoport, B.: **Recombinant thyroid autoantigens: the keys to the pathogenesis of autoimmune thyroid disease.** *J. Intl. Med.* 1993, **234**:347-359.

Newsom Davis, J. and Vincent, A.: **Antibody-mediated neurological disease.** *Curr. Opin. Neurobiol.* 1991, **1**:430-435.

Vincent, A., Newsom Davis, J., Wray, D., Shillito, P., Harrison, J., Betty, M., Beeson, D., Mills, K., Palace, J., Molenaar, P., et al.: **Clinical and experimental observations in patients with congenital myasthenic syndromes.** *Ann. N. Y. Acad. Sci.* 1993, **681**:451-460.

12-6 Autoantibodies to extracellular antigens cause inflammatory injury by mechanisms akin to type II or type III hypersensitivity reactions.

Hardin, J.A. and Craft, J.E.: **Patterns of autoimmunity to nucleoproteins in patients with systemic lupus erythematosus.** *Rheum. Dis. Clin. North Am.* 1987, **13**:37-46.

Kelly, P.T. and Haponik, E.F.: **Goodpasture syndrome: molecular and clinical advances.** *Med. Baltimore* 1994, **73**:171-185.

Kotzin, B.L.: **Systemic lupus erythematosus.** *Cell* 1996, **85**:303-306.

Mamula, M.J.: **Lupus autoimmunity: from peptides to particles.** *Immunol. Rev.* 1995, **144**:301-314.

Tan, E.M.: **Antinuclear antibodies: diagnostic markers for autoimmune diseases and probes for cell biology.** *Adv. Immunol.* 1989, **44**:93-151.

Turner, N., Mason, P.J., Brown, R., Fox, M., Povey, S., Rees, A., and Pusey, C.D.: Molecular cloning of the human Goodpasture antigen demonstrates it to be the alpha 3 chain of type IV collagen. J. Clin. Invest. 1992, 89:592-601.

12-7   Environmental co-factors may influence the expression of autoimmune disease.

Donaghy, M. and Rees, A.J.: Cigarette smoking and lung haemorrhage in glomerulonephritis caused by autoantibodies to glomerular basement membrane. Lancet 1983, 2:1390-1393.

Kallenberg, C.G., Brouwer, E., Weening, J.J., and Tervaert, J.W.: Anti-neutrophil cytoplasmic antibodies: current diagnostic and pathophysiological potential. Kidney Intl. 1994, 46:1-15.

Pinching, A.J., Rees, A.J., Russell, B.A., Lockwood, C.M., Mitchison, R.S., and Peters, D.K.: Relapses in Wegener's granulomatosis: the role of infection. BMJ 1980, 281:836-838.

Rees, A.J., Lockwood, C.M., and Peters, D.K.: Enhanced allergic tissue injury in Goodpasture's syndrome by intercurrent bacterial infection. BMJ 1977, 2:723-726.

12-8   The pattern of inflammatory injury in autoimmunity may be modified by anatomical constraints.

Cavallo, T.: Membranous nephropathy. Insights from Heymann nephritis . Am. J. Pathol. 1994, 144:651-658.

Couser, W.G. and Abrass, C.K.: Pathogenesis of membranous nephropathy. Ann. Rev. Med 1988, 39:517-530.

Plotz, P.H., Rider, L.G., Targoff, I.N., Raben, N., O'Hanlon, T.P., and Miller, F.W.: NIH conference. Myositis: immunologic contributions to understanding cause, pathogenesis, and therapy. Ann. Intl. Med. 1995, 122:715-724.

Salant, D.J., Quigg, R.J., and Cybulsky, A.V.: Heymann nephritis: mechanisms of renal injury. Kidney Intl. 1989, 35:976-984.

Tan, E.M.: Do autoantibodies inhibit function of their cognate antigens in vivo? Arthritis Rheum. 1989, 32:924-925.

Targoff, I.N.: Immune mechanisms in myositis. Curr. Opin. Rheumatol. 1990, 2:882-888.

12-9   The mechanism of autoimmune tissue damage can often be determined by adoptive transfer.

Bottazzo, G.F. and Doniach, D.: Autoimmune thyroid disease. Ann. Rev. Med. 1986, 37:353-359.

Gossage, A.A. and Munro, D.S.: The pathogenesis of Graves' disease. Clin. Endocrinol. Metab. 1985, 14:299-330.

Lindstrom, J., Shelton, D., and Fujii, Y.: Myasthenia gravis. Adv. Immunol. 1988, 42:233-284.

McFarland, H.F.: Significance of autoreactive T cells in diseases such as multiple sclerosis using an innovative primate model. J. Clin. Invest. 1994, 94:921-922.

Vernet der Garabedian, B., Lacokova, M., Eymard, B., Morel, E., Faltin, M., Zajac, J., Sadovsky, O., Dommergues, M., Tripon, P., and Bach, J.F.: Association of neonatal myasthenia gravis with antibodies against the fetal acetylcholine receptor. J Clin. Invest. 1994, 94:555-559.

Willcox, N.: Myasthenia gravis. Curr. Opin. Immunol. 1993, 5:910-917.

Zamvil, S., Nelson, P., Trotter, J., Mitchell, D., Knobler, R., Fritz, R., and Steinman, L.: T-cell clones specific for myelin basic protein induce chronic relapsing paralysis and demyelination. Nature 1985, 317:355-358.

12-10   T cells specific for self antigens can cause direct tissue injury and play a role in sustained autoantibody responses.

Baekkeskov, S., Aanstoot, H.J., Christgau, S., Reetz, A., Solimena, M., Cascalho, M., Folli, F., Richter Olesen, H., DeCamilli, P., and Camilli, P.D.: Identification of the 64K autoantigen in insulin-dependent diabetes as the GABA-synthesizing enzyme glutamic acid decarboxylase. Nature 1990, 347:151-156.

Feldmann, M., Brennan, F.M., and Maini, R.N.: Rheumatoid arthritis. Cell 1996, 85:307-310.

Moss, P.A., Rosenberg, W.M., and Bell, J.I.: The human T cell receptor in health and disease. Ann. Rev. Immunol. 1992, 10:71-96.

Nepom, G.T.: Glutamic acid decarboxylase and other autoantigens in IDDM. Curr. Opin. Immunol. 1995, 7:825-830.

Tisch, R. and McDevitt, H.: Insulin-dependent diabetes mellitus. Cell 1996, 85:291-297.

12-11   Autoantibodies can be used to identify the target of the autoimmune process.

James, J.A., Gross, T., Scofield, R.H., and Harley, J.B.: Immunoglobulin epitope spreading and autoimmune disease after peptide immunization: Sm B/B'-derived PPPGMRPP and PPPGIRGP induce spliceosome autoimmunity. J. Exp. Med. 1995, 181:453-461.

Topfer, F., Gordon, T., and McCluskey, J.: Intra- and inter-molecular spreading of autoimmunity involving the nuclear self-antigens La (SS-B) and Ro (SS-A). Proc. Natl. Acad. Sci. 1995, 92:875-879.

Mamula, M.J. and Janeway, C.A.,Jr.: Do B cells drive the diversification of immune responses? Immunol. Today 1993, 14:151-152.

Mamula, M.J. and Craft, J.: The expression of self antigenic determinants: implications for tolerance and autoimmunity. Curr. Opin. Immunol. 1994, 6:882-886.

Protti, M.P., Manfredi, A.A., Horton, R.M., Bellone, M., and Conti Tronconi, B.M.: Myasthenia gravis: recognition of a human autoantigen at the molecular level. Immunol. Today. 1993, 14:363-368.

12-12   The target of T-cell mediated autoimmunity is difficult to identify owing to the nature of T-cell ligands.

Bell, R.B. and Steinman, L.: Trimolecular interactions in experimental autoimmune demyelinating disease and prospects for immunotherapy. Semin. Immunol. 1991, 3:237-245.

Hafler, D.A. and Weiner, H.L.: Immunologic mechanisms and therapy in multiple sclerosis. Immunol. Rev. 1995, 144:75-107.

Steinman, L.: Multiple sclerosis: a coordinated immunological attack against myelin in the central nervous system. Cell 1996, 85:299-302.

Tisch, R. and McDevitt, H.O.: Antigen-specific immunotherapy: is it a real possibility to combat T-cell-mediated autoimmunity? Proc. Natl. Acad. Sci. 1994, 91:437-438.

Tisch, R., Yang, X.D., Singer, S.M., Liblau, R.S., Fugger, L., and McDevitt, H.O.: Immune response to glutamic acid decarboxylase correlates with insulitis in non-obese diabetic mice. Nature 1993, 366:72-75.

Wraith, D.C., Smilek, D.E., Mitchell, D.J., Steinman, L., and McDevitt, H.O.: Antigen recognition in autoimmune encephalomyelitis and the potential for peptide-mediated immunotherapy. Cell 1989, 59:247-255.

12-13   The rejection of grafts is an immunological response mediated primarily by T cells.

Hayry, P., Isoniemi, H., Yilmaz, S., Mennander, A., Lemstrom, K., Raisanen Sokolowski, A., Koskinen, P., Ustinov, J., Lautenschlager, I., Taskinen, E., Krogerus, L., Aho, P., and Paavonen, T.: Chronic allograft rejection. Immunol. Rev. 1993, 134:33-81.

Lafferty, K.J.: **A contemporary view of transplantation tolerance: an immunologist's perspective**. *Clin. Transplant.* 1994, **8**:181-187.

Lechler, R., Gallagher, R.B., and Auchincloss, H.: **Hard graft? Future challenges in transplantation**. *Immunol. Today* 1991, **12**:214-216.

Lee, R.S. and Auchincloss, H.,Jr.: **Mechanisms of tolerance to allografts**. *Chem. Immunol.* 1994, **58**:236-258.

Rosenberg, A.S. and Singer, A.: **Cellular basis of skin allograft rejection: an in vivo model of immune-mediated tissue destruction**. *Ann. Rev. Immunol.* 1992, **10**:333-358.

Shi, C., Lee, W.S., He, Q., Zhang, D., Fletcher, D.L.,Jr., Newell, J.B., and Haber, E.: **Immunologic basis of transplant-associated arteriosclerosis**. *Proc. Natl. Acad. Sci.* 1996, **93**:4051-4056.

12-14 Matching donor and recipient at the MHC improves the outcome of transplantation.

Benichou, G., Takizawa, P.A., Olson, C.A., McMillan, M., and Sercarz, E.E.: **Donor major histocompatibility complex (MHC) peptides are presented by recipient MHC molecules during graft rejection**. *J. Exp. Med.* 1992, **175**:305-308.

Martin, S. and Dyer, P.A.: **The case for matching MHC genes in human organ transplantation** *Nat. Genet.* 1993, **5**:210-213.

Matas, A.J.: **Is MHC matching as a primary criterion in kidney allocation justified?** *Nat. Genet.* 1993, **5**:210-213.

Opelz, G., Wujciak, T., Mytilineos, J., and Scherer, S.: **Revisiting HLA matching for kidney transplantation**. *Transplant. Proc.* 1993, **25**:173-175.

Opelz, G. and Wujciak, T.: **The influence of HLA compatibility on graft survival after heart transplantation. The Collaborative Transplant Study**. *N. Engl. J. Med.* 1994, **330**:816-819.

Opelz, G. and Wujciak, T.: **Cadaveric kidneys should be allocated according to the HLA match**. *Transplant. Proc.* 1995, **27**:93-99.

Tay, G.K., Witt, C.S., Christiansen, F.T., Charron, D., Baker, D., Herrmann, R., Smith, L.K., Diepeveen, D., Mallal, S., McCluskey, J., Lester, S., Loiseau, P., Teisserenc, H., Chapman, J., Tait, B., and Dawkins, R.L.: **Matching for MHC haplotypes results in improved survival following unrelated bone marrow transplantation**. *Bone Marrow Transplant.* 1995, **15**:381-385.

12-15 In MHC-identical grafts, rejection is caused by non-self peptides bound to graft MHC molecules.

Auchincloss, H.,Jr., Lee, R., Shea, S., Markowitz, J.S., Grusby, M.J., and Glimcher, L.H.: **The role of "indirect" recognition in initiating rejection of skin grafts from major histocompatibility complex class II-deficient mice**. *Proc. Natl. Acad. Sci.* 1993, **90**:3373-3377.

den Haan, J.M., Sherman, N.E., Blokland, E., Huczko, E., Koning, F., Drijfhout, J.W., Skipper, J., Shabanowitz, J., Hunt, D.F., Engelhard, V.H., and Goulmy, E.: **Identification of a graft versus host disease-associated human minor histocompatibility antigen**. *Science* 1995, **268**:1476-1480.

Scott, D.M., Ehrmann, I.E., Ellis, P.S., Bishop, C.E., Agulnik, A.I., Simpson, E., and Mitchell, M.J.: **Identification of a mouse male-specific transplantation antigen, H-Y**. *Nature* 1995, **376**:695-698.

Warrens, A.N., Lombardi, G., and Lechler, R.I.: **Presentation and recognition of major and minor histocompatibility antigens**. *Transpl. Immunol.* 1994, **2**:103-107.

12-16 Antibodies reacting with endothelium cause hyperacute graft rejection.

Dorling, A. and Lechler, R.I.: **Prospects for xenografting**. *Curr. Opin. Immunol.* 1994, **6**:765-769.

Kaufman, C.L., Gaines, B.A., and Ildstad, S.T.: **Xenotransplantation**. *Ann. Rev. Immunol.* 1995, **13**:339-367.

Kissmeyer Nielsen, F., Olsen, S., Petersen, V.P., and Fjeldborg, O.: **Hyperacute rejection of kidney allografts, associated with pre-existing humoral antibodies against donor cells**. *Lancet* 1966, **2**:662-665.

Sharma, A., Okabe, J., Birch, P., McClellan, S.B., Martin, M.J., Platt, J.L., and Logan, J.S.: **Reduction in the level of Gal(alpha1,3)Gal in transgenic mice and pigs by the expression of an alpha(1,2)fucosyltransferase**. *Proc. Natl. Acad. Sci.* 1996, **93**:7190-7195.

Steele, D.J. and Auchincloss, H.,Jr.: **Xenotransplantation**. *Ann. Rev. Med.* 1995, **46**:345-360.

Williams, G.M., Hume, D.M., Hudson, R.P.,Jr., Morris, P.J., Kano, K., and Milgrom, F.: **"Hyperacute" renal-homograft rejection in man**. *N. Engl. J. Med.* 1968, **279**:611-618.

12-17 A variety of organs are transplanted routinely in clinical medicine.

Murray, J.E.: **Human organ transplantation: background and consequences**. *Science* 1992, **256**:1411-1416.

12-18 The fetus is an allograft that is tolerated repetitively.

Flanagan, J.R., Murata, M., Burke, P.A., Shirayoshi, Y., Appella, E., Sharp, P.A., and Ozato, K.: **Negative regulation of the major histocompatibility complex class I promoter in embryonal carcinoma cells**. *Proc. Natl. Acad. Sci.* 1991, **88**:3145-3149.

Hunt, J.S.: **Immunobiology of pregnancy**. *Curr. Opin. Immunol.* 1992, **4**:591-596.

Hunt, J.S. and Orr, H.T.: **HLA and maternal-fetal recognition**. *FASEB J.* 1992, **6**:2344-2348.

Loke, Y.W. and King, A.: **Recent developments in the human maternal-fetal immune interaction**. *Curr. Opin. Immunol.* 1991, **3**:762-766.

Wood, G.W.: **Is restricted antigen presentation the explanation for fetal allograft survival?** *Immunol. Today* 1994, **15**:15-18.

12-19 Autoantigens are not so abundant that they induce clonal deletion or anergy, but are not so rare as to escape recognition entirely.

Billingham, R.E., Brent, L., and Medawar, P.B.: **Actively acquired tolerance of foreign cells**. *Nature* 1953, **172**:603-606.

Brent, L.: **Tolerance: past, present, and future**. *Transplant. Proc.* 1991, **23**:2056-2060.

Brent, L.: **Medawar Prize Lecture: tolerance and graft-vs-host disease: two sides of the same coin**. *Transplant. Proc.* 1995, **27**:12-14.

Goverman, J., Woods, A., Larson, L., Weiner, L.P., Hood, L., and Zaller, D.M.: **Transgenic mice that express a myelin basic protein-specific T cell receptor develop spontaneous autoimmunity**. *Cell* 1993, **72**:551-560.

Katz, J.D., Wang, B., Haskins, K., Benoist, C., and Mathis, D.: **Following a diabetogenic T cell from genesis through pathogenesis**. *Cell* 1993, **74**:1089-1100.

12-20 The induction of a tissue-specific response requires expression of co-stimulator activity on antigen-presenting cells.

Guerder, S., Picarella, D.E., Linsley, P.S., and Flavell, R.A.: **Costimulator B7-1 confers antigen-presenting-cell function to parenchymal tissue and in conjunction with tumor necrosis factor alpha leads to autoimmunity in transgenic mice**. *Proc. Natl. Acad. Sci.* 1994, **91**:5138-5142.

Lafferty, K.J., Prowse, S.J., Simeonovic, C.J., and Warren, H.S.: **Immunobiology of tissue transplantation: a return to the passenger leukocyte concept**. *Ann. Rev. Immunol.* 1983, **1**:143-173.

| 12-21 | In the absence of co-stimulation, tolerance is induced. |

Hammerling, G.J., Schonrich, G., Ferber, I., and Arnold, B.: **Peripheral tolerance as a multi-step mechanism.** *Immunol. Rev.* 1993, **133**:93-104.

Lenschow, D.J. and Bluestone, J.A.: **T cell co-stimulation and** *in vivo* **tolerance.** *Curr. Opin. Immunol.* 1993, **5**:747-752.

Liu, Y., and Janeway, C.A. Jr.: **Interferon-γ plays a critical role in induced cell death of effector T cell: A possible third mechanism of self tolerance.** *J. Exp. Med.* 1990, **172**:1735-1739.

| 12-22 | Dominant immune suppression can be demonstrated in models of tolerance and can affect the course of autoimmune disease. |

Miller, J.F. and Flavell, R.A.: **T-cell tolerance and autoimmunity in transgenic models of central and peripheral tolerance.** *Curr. Opin. Immunol.* 1994, **6**:892-899.

Olsson, T.: **Critical influences of the cytokine orchestration on the outcome of myelin antigen-specific T-cell autoimmunity in experimental autoimmune encephalomyelitis and multiple sclerosis.** *Immunol. Rev.* 1995, **144**:245-268.

Qin, S., Cobbold, S.P., Pope, H., Elliott, J., Kioussis, D., Davies, J., and Waldmann, H.: **"Infectious" transplantation tolerance.** *Science* 1993, **259**:974-977.

Reich, E.P., Scaringe, D., Yagi, J., Sherwin, R.S., and Janeway, C.A.,Jr.: **Prevention of diabetes in NOD mice by injection of autoreactive T-lymphocytes.** *Diabetes* 1989, **38**:1647-1651.

Ridgway, W.M., Weiner, H.L., and Fathman, C.G.: **Regulation of autoimmune response.** *Curr. Opin. Immunol.* 1994, **6**:946-955.

Tian, J., Atkinson, M.A., Clare Salzler, M., Herschenfeld, A., Forsthuber, T., Lehmann, P.V., and Laufman, D.L.: **Nasal administration of glutamate decarboxylase (GAD65) peptides induces T$_H$2 responses and prevents murine insulin-dependent diabetes.** *J. Exp. Med.* 1996, **183**:1561-1567.

| 12-23 | Antigens in immunologically privileged sites do not induce immune attack but can serve as targets. |

Bellgrau, D., Gold, D., Selawry, H., Moore, J., Franzusoff, A., and Duke, R.C.: **A role for CD95 ligand in preventing graft rejection.** *Nature* 1995, **377**:630-632.

Gery, I. and Streilein, J.W.: **Autoimmunity in the eye and its regulation.** *Curr. Opin. Immunol.* 1994, **6**:938-945.

Streilein, J.W.: **Unraveling immune privilege.** *Science* 1995, **270**:1158-1159.

Williams, G.A., Mammolenti, M.M., and Streilin, J.W.: **Studies on the induction of anterior chamber-associated immune deviation (ACAID). III Induction of ACAID depends upon intraocular transforming growth factor-β.** *Eur. J. Immunol.* 1992, **22**:165-173.

| 12-24 | B cells with receptors specific for peripheral autoantigens are held in check by a variety of mechanisms. |

Goodnow, C.C., Cyster, J.G., Hartley, S.B., Bell, S.E., Cooke, M.P., Healy, J.I., Akkaraju, S., Rathmell, J.C., Pogue, S.L., and Shokat, K.P.: **Self-tolerance checkpoints in B lymphocyte development.** *Adv. Immunol.* 1995, **59**:279-368.

Goodnow, C.C.: **Balancing immunity and tolerance: deleting and tuning lymphocyte repertoires.** *Proc. Natl. Acad. Sci.* 1996, **93**:2264-2271.

Rathmell, J.C., Cooke, M.P., Ho, W.Y., Grein, J., Townsend, S.E., Davis, M.M., and Goodnow, C.C.: **CD95 (Fas)-dependent elimination of self-reactive B cells upon interaction with CD4$^+$ T cells.** *Nature* 1995, **376**:181-184.

Shokat, K.M. and Goodnow, C.C.: **Antigen-induced B-cell death and elimination during germinal-centre immune responses.** *Nature* 1995, **375**:334-338.

| 12-25 | Autoimmunity could be triggered by infection in a variety of ways. |

Brocke, S., Veromaa, T., Weissman, I.L., Gijbels, K., and Steinman, L.: **Infection and multiple sclerosis: a possible role for superantigens?** *Trends. Microbiol.* 1994, **2**:250-254.

Gianani, R. and Sarvetnick, N.: **Viruses, cytokines, antigens, and autoimmunity.** *Proc. Natl. Acad. Sci.* 1996, **93**:2257-2259.

Moens, U., Seternes, O.M., Hey, A.W., Silsand, Y., Traavik, T., Johansen, B., and Rekvig, O.P.: **In vivo expression of a single viral DNA-binding protein generates systemic lupus erythematosus-related autoimmunity to double-stranded DNA and histones.** *Proc. Natl. Acad. Sci.* 1995, **92**:12393-12397.

Ohashi, P.S., Oehen, S., Buerki, K., Pircher, H., Ohashi, C.T., Odermatt, B., Malissen, B., Zinkernagel, R.M., and Hengartner, H.: **Ablation of "tolerance" and induction of diabetes by virus infection in viral antigen transgenic mice.** *Cell* 1991, **65**:305-317.

Rocken, M., Urban, J.F., and Shevach, E.M.: **Infection breaks T-cell tolerance.** *Nature* 1992, **359**:79-82.

Steinhoff, U., Burkhart, C., Arnheiter, H., Hengartner, H., and Zinkernagel, R.: **Virus or a hapten-carrier complex can activate autoreactive B cells by providing linked T help.** *Eur. J. Immunol.* 1994, **24**:773-776.

Wucherpfennig, K.W. and Strominger, J.L.: **Molecular mimicry in T cell-mediated autoimmunity: viral peptides activate human T cell clones specific for myelin basic protein.** *Cell* 1995, **80**:695-705

Manipulation of the Immune Response

Most of this book has been concerned with the mechanisms whereby the immune system successfully protects us from disease. In the preceding three chapters, however, we have seen examples of the failure of immunity to some important infections, and conversely, in the case of allergy and autoimmunity, how inappropriate immune responses can themselves cause disease. We have also discussed the problems arising from immune responses to grafted tissues.

In this chapter, we shall consider the ways in which the immune system may be manipulated or controlled, both to suppress unwanted immune responses in autoimmunity, allergy and allograft rejection, and to stimulate protective immune responses to some of the diseases that, at present, largely elude the immune system. It has long been felt that it should be possible to deploy the powerful and specific mechanisms of natural immunity to destroy tumors, and we shall discuss the present state of progress toward that goal. In the final section of the chapter, we discuss present vaccination strategies and how a more rational approach to the design and development of vaccines promises to increase their efficacy and widen their scope.

Extrinsic regulation of unwanted immune responses.

The unwanted immune responses that occur in autoimmune disease, transplant rejection, and allergy present slightly different problems, and the approach to developing effective treatment is correspondingly different for each. We have already discussed the treatment of allergy in Chapter 11: the problems in this case are due to the production of IgE, and the goals are, accordingly, to treat the adverse consequences of an IgE response, or to induce the production of IgG to the allergenic antigens instead of IgE. In autoimmune disease and graft rejection the problem is an immune response to tissue antigens, and its goal is to downregulate the response to avoid damage to the tissues or disruption of their function. From the point of view of management, the single most important difference between allograft rejection and autoimmunity is that allografts are a deliberate surgical intervention and the immune response to them can be foreseen, whereas autoimmune responses are not detected until they are already established. Effective treatment of an established immune response is much harder to achieve than prevention of a response before it has had a chance to develop, and autoimmune diseases are generally harder to control than a *de novo* immune response to an allograft. The relative difficulty of suppressing established immune responses is seen in animal models of autoimmunity, in which methods able to prevent the induction of autoimmune disease generally fail to halt established disease.

Current treatments for immunological disorders are nearly all empirical in origin, using immunosuppressive drugs identified by screening large numbers of natural and synthetic compounds. The drugs currently used to suppress the immune system may be divided into three categories: first, powerful anti-inflammatory drugs of the corticosteroid family such as **prednisone**; second, cytotoxic drugs such as **azathioprine** and **cyclophosphamide**; and third, fungal and bacterial derivatives, such as **cyclosporin A**, **FK506** (**tacrolimus**) and **rapamycin**, which inhibit signaling events within T lymphocytes. These drugs are all very broad in their actions and inhibit protective functions of the immune system, as well as harmful ones. Opportunistic infection is therefore a common complication of immunosuppressive drug therapy. The ideal immunosuppressive agent would be one that targets the specific part of the adaptive immune response responsible for causing tissue injury. Paradoxically, antibodies themselves, by virtue of their exquisite specificity, may offer the best possibility for the therapeutic inhibition of specific immune responses. We shall also consider experimental approaches to controlling specific immune responses by manipulating the local cytokine environment or by manipulating antigen so as to divert the response from a pathogenic pathway to an innocuous one. We have discussed briefly how this can occur in infections with *Mycobacterium leprae* (see Section 7-29).

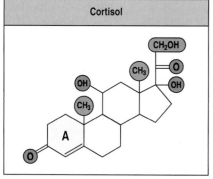

Cortisol

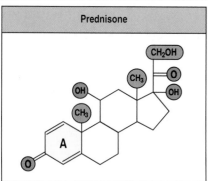

Prednisone

Fig. 13.1 The structure of the anti-inflammatory corticosteroid drug, prednisone. Prednisone is a synthetic analog of the natural adrenocorticosteroid, cortisol. Introduction of the 1,2 double bond in the A ring increases the anti-inflammatory potency approximately four-fold compared with cortisol, without modifying the sodium-retaining activity of the compound.

13-1 Corticosteroids are powerful anti-inflammatory drugs that alter the transcription of many genes.

Corticosteroid drugs are powerful anti-inflammatory agents that are used widely to suppress the harmful effects of immune responses of autoimmune or allergic origin, as well as those induced by graft rejection, where other measures are insufficient or have failed. Corticosteroids are pharmacological derivatives of members of the glucocorticoid family of steroid hormones (Fig. 13.1), which act through intracellular

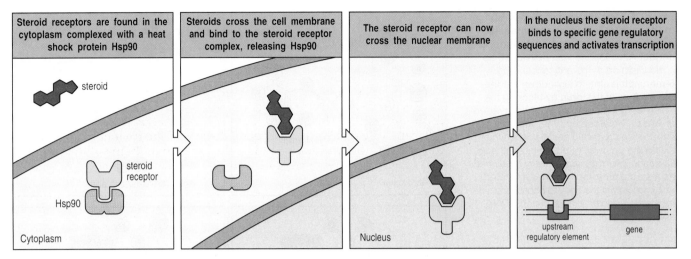

| Steroid receptors are found in the cytoplasm complexed with a heat shock protein Hsp90 | Steroids cross the cell membrane and bind to the steroid receptor complex, releasing Hsp90 | The steroid receptor can now cross the nuclear membrane | In the nucleus the steroid receptor binds to specific gene regulatory sequences and activates transcription |

Fig. 13.2 Mechanisms of steroid action. Corticosteroids are lipid-soluble compounds that enter cells by diffusing across the plasma membrane and bind to their receptors in the cytosol. The binding of corticosteroid to the receptor displaces a dimer of a heat-shock protein named Hsp90, exposing the DNA-binding region of the receptor, which then enters the nucleus and binds to specific DNA sequences in the promoter regions of steroid-responsive genes. The effects of corticosteroids are mediated by modulation of the transcription of a wide variety of genes.

receptors that are expressed in almost every cell of the body to regulate the transcription of specific genes. Their mechanism of action is illustrated in Fig. 13.2.

The expression of as many as 1% of genes may be regulated by glucocorticoids, which may either upregulate or, less commonly, down-regulate responsive genes. The pharmacological effects of corticosteroid drugs result from exposure of the glucocorticoid receptors to supraphysiological concentrations of ligand. The abnormally high level of ligation of glucocorticoid receptors causes exaggerated glucocorticoid-mediated responses, which have both beneficial and toxic effects.

Given the large number of genes regulated by corticosteroids, it is hardly surprising that the effects of steroid therapy are very complex. The beneficial effects are anti-inflammatory and are summarized in Fig. 13.3; however there are also many adverse effects, including fluid retention, weight gain, diabetes, bone mineral loss and thinning of the skin. The use of corticosteroids to control disease requires a careful balance between helping the patient by reducing the inflammatory manifestations of disease and avoiding harm from the toxic side-effects of the drug. For this reason, corticosteroids used in transplant recipients and to treat inflammatory autoimmune and allergic disease are often administered in combination with other drugs in an effort to keep the dose and toxic effects to a minimum. In the case of autoimmunity and allograft rejection, corticosteroids are commonly combined with cytotoxic immunosuppressive drugs.

| 13-2 | **Cytotoxic drugs cause immunosuppression by killing dividing cells and have serious side-effects.** |

The two cytotoxic drugs most commonly used as immunosuppressants are azathioprine and cyclophosphamide (Fig. 13.4). Both interfere with DNA synthesis and have their major pharmacological action on dividing tissues. They were developed originally to treat cancer and, following observations that they were cytotoxic to dividing lymphocytes, were found to be immunosuppressive as well. The use of these compounds is limited by a range of toxic effects on tissues in the body, which have in common the property of continuous cell division. These effects include

Corticosteroid therapy	
Activity	**Effect**
↑ IL-1, TNF-α, GM-CSF ↓ IL-3, IL-4, IL-5, IL-8	↓ Inflammation ↓ caused by cytokines
↓ NOS	↓ NO
↓ Phospholipase A₂ ↓ Cyclo-oxygenase type2 ↑ Lipocortin-1	↓ Prostaglandins ↓ Leukotrienes
↓ Adhesion molecules	Reduced emigration of leukocytes from vessels
Induction of endonucleases	Induction of apoptosis in lymphocytes and eosinophils

Fig. 13.3 Anti-inflammatory effects of corticosteroid therapy. Corticosteroids regulate the expression of many genes, with a net anti-inflammatory effect. First, they reduce the production of inflammatory mediators including cytokines, prostaglandins and nitric oxide. Second, they inhibit inflammatory cell migration to sites of inflammation by inhibiting the expression of the adhesion molecules. Third, corticosteroids promote the death by apoptosis of leukocytes and lymphocytes.

Fig. 13.4 The structure and metabolism of the cytotoxic immunosuppressive drugs azathioprine and cyclophosphamide. Azathioprine was developed as a modification of the anticancer drug 6-mercaptopurine to slow down the the metabolism of this drug by blocking the reactive thiol group. It is slowly converted *in vivo* to 6-mercaptopurine, which is then metabolised to 6-thioinosinic acid, which blocks the pathway of purine biosynthesis. Cyclophosphamide was similarly developed as a stable pro-drug, which is activated enzymatically in the body to phosphoramide mustard, a powerful and unstable DNA alkylating agent.

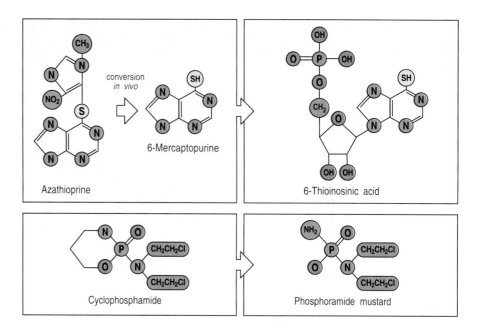

decreased immune function, as well as anemia, leukopenia, thrombocytopenia, damage to intestine epithelium, hair loss, and fetal death or injury. As a result of these toxic effects, they are used at high doses only when the aim is to eliminate all dividing lymphocytes, as in the treatment of some recipients of bone marrow transplants. They are used at lower doses, and in combination with other drugs such as corticosteroids, to treat unwanted immune responses.

Azathioprine is a purine antagonist that interferes in the synthesis of nucleic acids and is toxic to dividing cells. It is metabolized to 6-thioinosinic acid, which competes with inosine monophosphate, thereby blocking the synthesis of adenosine monophosphate and guanosine monophosphate and thus inhibiting DNA synthesis. It is less toxic than cyclophosphamide, which is metabolized to phosphoramide mustard, which alkylates DNA. Cyclophosphamide is a member of the nitrogen mustard family of compounds, which were originally developed as chemical weapons. With this pedigree goes a range of highly toxic effects including inflammation of and hemorrhage from the bladder, known as hemorrhagic cystitis, and induction of bladder neoplasia.

13-3   Cyclosporin A, FK506 (tacrolimus), and rapamycin are powerful immunosuppressive agents that interfere with T-cell signaling.

There are now relatively non-toxic alternatives to the cytotoxic drugs used for immunosuppression in transplant patients. The systematic study of products from bacteria and fungi has led to the development of a large array of important medicines including two immunosuppressive drugs **cyclosporin A**, a cyclic decapeptide derived from a soil fungus from Norway, *Tolypocladium inflatum*, and **FK506**, now known as **tacrolimus**, a macrolide compound from the filamentous bacteria *Streptomyces tsukabaensis*, found in Japan. These compounds are not made in mammalian cells and are too complex to be made synthetically (macrolides are compounds that contain a many-membered lactone ring to which is attached one or more de-oxy sugars). They exert their pharmacological effects by binding to members of a family of intracellular proteins known as the immunophilins, forming complexes that interfere with signaling pathways important for the clonal expansion of lymphocytes.

Immunological effects of cyclosporin A and tacrolimus	
Cell type	Effects
T lymphocyte	Reduced expression of IL-2, IL-3, IL-4, GM-CSF, TNF-α. Reduced proliferation following decreased IL-2 production. Reduced Ca^{2+}-dependent exocytosis of granule-associated serine esterases. Inhibition of antigen-driven apoptosis.
B lymphocyte	Inhibition of proliferation secondary to reduced cytokine production by T lymphocytes. Inhibition of proliferation following ligation of surface immunoglobulin. Induction of apoptosis following B-cell activation.
Granulocyte	Reduced Ca^{2+}-dependent exocytosis of granule-associated serine esterases.

Fig. 13.5 Cyclosporin A and tacrolimus inhibit lymphocyte and some granulocyte responses.

Cyclosporin A and tacrolimus block T-cell proliferation by reducing the expression of several cytokine genes that are normally induced on T-cell activation (Fig. 13.5). These include IL-2, whose synthesis by T lymphocytes is an important growth signal for T cells. These drugs inhibit T-cell proliferation in response to either specific antigens or allogeneic cells and are used extensively in medical practice to prevent rejection of allogeneic organ grafts. Although the major immunosuppressive effects of both drugs are probably the result of T-cell proliferation, they have a large variety of other immunological effects (see Fig. 13.5) some of which may turn out to be important pharmacologically.

Cyclosporin A and tacrolimus are effective but they are not free from problems. First, as with the cytotoxic agents, they affect all immune responses indiscriminately. The only way of controlling their immunosuppressive action is by varying the dose; at the time of grafting, high doses are required but, once a graft is established, the dose can be reduced to allow useful protective immune responses while maintaining adequate suppression of the residual response to the grafted tissue. This is a difficult balance that is not always achieved successfully. Furthermore, as the immunophilins are found in many cells, it is to be expected that these drugs will have effects on many other tissues. Cyclosporin A and tacrolimus are both toxic to kidneys and other organs. Finally, treatment with these drugs is expensive, since they are complex natural products that must be taken indefinitely. Thus, there is room for improvement on these compounds and better and less expensive analogs are being sought. Nevertheless, at present, they are the drugs of choice in clinical transplantation, and they are also being tested in a variety of autoimmune diseases, especially those that, like graft rejection, are mediated by T cells.

13-4 | Immunosuppressive drugs are valuable probes of intracellular signaling pathways in lymphocytes.

The mechanism of action of cyclosporin A and tacrolimus is now fairly well understood. Each binds to a different group of immunophilins: cyclosporin A to the cyclophilins and tacrolimus to the FK-binding proteins (FKBP). These immunophilins are peptidyl-prolyl *cis-trans* isomerases but their isomerase activity does not seem to be relevant to the immunosuppressive activation of the drugs that bind them. Rather, the immunophilin:drug complexes bind and inhibit the Ca^{2+}-activated serine/threonine phosphatase **calcineurin**. Calcineurin is activated when intracellular calcium ion levels rise following T-cell receptor binding and dephosphorylates the cytosolic component of the transcription factor NF-AT, NF-ATc, allowing it to migrate to the nucleus where it pairs with a second nuclear component, NF-ATn, and induces transcription of the IL-2 gene (see Sections 4-29 and 7-9) (Fig. 13.6).

So far it is unclear why calcineurin binds to these two complexes of drug and immunophilin. It is tempting to speculate that there are endogenous equivalents for cyclosporin A and FK506 that perform similar regulatory functions but, to date, none has been discovered. Physiological roles for each of the members of the immunophilin families also remain to be uncovered.

Fig. 13.6 Cyclosporin A and FK506 inhibit T-cell activation by interfering with the serine/threonine-specific phosphatase calcineurin. Signaling via T-cell receptor-associated tyrosine kinases (see Section 4-28) leads to increased synthesis of the nuclear component of the nuclear factor of activated T cells (NF-ATn), as well as increasing the concentration of calcium in the cytoplasm (left panels). The calcium binds to calcineurin and thereby activates it to dephosphorylate the cytoplasmic component of NF-AT, NF-ATc. Once dephosphorylated, the active NF-ATc migrates to the nucleus to form a complex with NF-ATn; the NF-AT complex can then induce transcription of genes required for T-cell activation, including the IL-2 gene. When cyclosporin A (CsA) or FK506 are present, they form complexes with their immunophilin targets, cyclophilin (CyP) and FK-binding protein (FKBP), respectively (right panels). The complex of cyclophilin with cyclosporin A can bind to calcineurin, blocking its ability to activate NF-ATc. The complex of FK506 with FKBP binds to calcineurin at the same site, also blocking its activity.

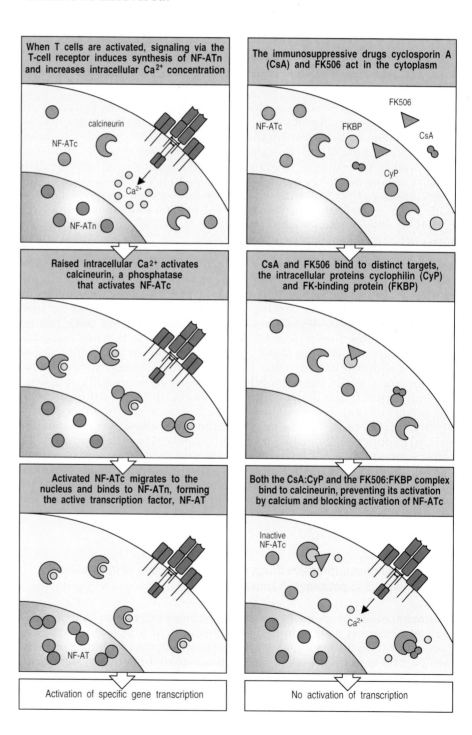

When T cells are activated, signaling via the T-cell receptor induces synthesis of NF-ATn and increases intracellular Ca^{2+} concentration

The immunosuppressive drugs cyclosporin A (CsA) and FK506 act in the cytoplasm

Raised intracellular Ca^{2+} activates calcineurin, a phosphatase that activates NF-ATc

CsA and FK506 bind to distinct targets, the intracellular proteins cyclophilin (CyP) and FK-binding protein (FKBP)

Activated NF-ATc migrates to the nucleus and binds to NF-ATn, forming the active transcription factor, NF-AT

Both the CsA:CyP and the FK506:FKBP complex bind to calcineurin, preventing its activation by calcium and blocking activation of NF-ATc

Activation of specific gene transcription

No activation of transcription

of the cytokine environment. In animal experiments, anti-cytokine antibodies (or recombinant cytokines) at the time of immunization with an autoantigen can sometimes divert a pathogenic immune response. However, modification of an ongoing immune response is much harder to achieve using this approach, although there have been some examples of success in animal experiments, as we shall see in later sections.

13-9 Controlled administration of antigen can be used to manipulate the nature of an antigen-specific response.

When the target antigen of an unwanted response is identified, it is possible to manipulate the response using antigen rather than antibodies. This is because the way in which antigen is presented to the immune system affects the nature of the response, and the induction of one type of response to an antigen may inhibit a pathogenic response to the same antigen.

As mentioned in Chapter 11, this principle has been applied with some success in treating allergies caused by an IgE response to very low doses of antigen. Repeated treatment of allergic individuals with higher doses of allergen appears to divert this response to one dominated by T cells that favor the production of IgG and IgA antibodies that are thought to **desensitize** the patient by binding the low levels of allergen normally encountered and preventing it from binding to IgE.

In the case of T-cell mediated autoimmune disease, there has been considerable interest in using peptide antigens to suppress pathogenic responses. The type of CD4 T-cell response induced by a peptide depends on the way it is presented to the immune system. For instance, peptides given orally tend to prime T_H2 T cells that make IL-4 or T cells that make predominantly TGF-β without activating T_H1 cells or inducing a great deal of systemic antibody. These mucosal immune responses have relatively little pathogenic potential. This approach has been used to generate a non-pathogenic response that protects against induced disease in two animal models of autoimmune disease. Experimental autoallergic encephalomyelitis (EAE) is induced by injection of myelin basic protein in complete Freund's adjuvant and resembles multiple sclerosis, while collagen arthritis is similarly induced by injection of collagen type II and has features in common with rheumatoid arthritis. Oral administration of myelin basic protein or type II collagen inhibits the development of disease in animals and has some beneficial effects in reducing the activity of pre-established disease. Trials using this approach in humans with multiple sclerosis or rheumatoid arthritis have found marginal therapeutic effects. Intravenous delivery of peptides can also inhibit inflammatory responses stimulated by the same peptide presented in a different context. When a soluble peptide is given intravenously, it binds preferentially to MHC class II molecules on resting B cells and tends to induce anergy in T_H1 cells. Thus, careful choice of the dose or structure of antigen, or its route of administration, may allow us to control the type of response that results.

One drawback of this approach, even if it can be effective in manipulating established immune responses, is that one must first identify the specific antigen against which the response is directed. In most cases of autoimmune disease, as we learned in Chapter 12, the autoantigens recognized by T cells are unknown. It will therefore be necessary to carry out extensive testing to identify the correct antigen before one can think of actually treating disease in this way. This could make such treatments very expensive and difficult to establish. A more generic approach to manipulating CD4 T-cell subset balance in ongoing immune responses, such as novel drugs that selectively inhibit responses by the different types of T cells, would undoubtedly be much more useful.

Summary.

Existing treatments for unwanted immune responses, such as allergic reactions, autoimmunity and graft rejection, depend largely on three types of drugs. Anti-inflammatory drugs, of which the most potent are the corticosteroids, are used for all three types of responses. These have a broad spectrum of actions, however, and a correspondingly wide range of toxic side-effects, and their dose must be controlled carefully. They are therefore normally used in combination with either cytotoxic or immunosuppressive drugs. The cytotoxic drugs kill all dividing cells and thereby prevent lymphocyte proliferation but suppress all immune responses indiscriminately and also kill other types of dividing cells. The immunosuppressive drugs act by intervening in the intracellular signaling pathways of T cells and, although they are less generally toxic than the cytotoxic drugs, they also suppress all immune responses indiscriminately. They are also much more expensive than cytotoxic drugs.

Immunosuppressive drugs are now the drugs of choice in the treatment of transplant patients, where they can be used to suppress the immune response to the graft before it has become established. Autoimmune responses are already well established at the time of diagnosis and, in consequence, much more difficult to suppress. They are therefore less responsive to the immunosuppressive drugs and, for that reason, they are usually controlled with a combination of corticosteroids and cytotoxic drugs. In animal experiments attempts have been made to target immunosuppression more specifically with the use of antibodies or of antigenic peptides, or to divert the immune response into a non-pathogenic pathway by administration of cytokines, or by administering antigen through the oral route where a non-pathogenic immune response is likely to be invoked. None of these treatments is yet proven in humans, and most require that the relevant antigen be known. For that reason, and because they are relatively ineffective against established immune responses, the promise of these approaches in animal models may be difficult to realize in a clinical context.

Using the immune response to attack tumors.

Cancer is one of the three leading causes of death in industrialized nations. As treatments for infectious diseases and the prevention of cardiovascular disease continue to improve, and the average life expectancy increases, cancer is likely to become the most common fatal disease in these countries. Cancers are caused by the progressive growth of the progeny of a single transformed cell. Therefore, curing cancer requires that all the malignant cells be removed or destroyed without killing the patient. An attractive way to achieve this would be to induce an immune response against the tumor that would discriminate between the cells of the tumor and their normal cellular counterparts. Immunological approaches to the treatment of cancer have been attempted for over a century with tantalizing but unsustainable results. Experiments in animals have, however, provided evidence for immune responses to tumors and have shown that T cells are a critical mediator of tumor immunity. More recently, advances in our understanding of antigen presentation and the molecules involved in T-cell activation have provided for new immunotherapeutic strategies based on a better molecular understanding of the immune response. These are showing some success in animal models and are now being tested in human patients.

13-10   Some tumors can be recognized and rejected by the immune system.

The experimental study of tumor rejection has generally been based on the use of transplanted tumors. If these bear foreign MHC molecules they are readily recognized and destroyed by the immune system, a fact that was exploited (as we saw in Section 2-23), to develop the first MHC-congenic strains of mice. Specific immunity to tumors must therefore be studied within inbred strains, so that host and tumor can be matched for MHC type. Several such studies have been performed with murine tumors that have been induced experimentally by either carcinogenic chemicals or ultraviolet irradiation. These experimental tumors exhibit a variable pattern of growth when injected into syngeneic recipients. Most tumors, termed 'progressor tumors', grow progressively and eventually kill the host: other tumors, called 'regressor tumors', grow for a period of time and then regress (Fig. 13.10). In animals that have harbored regressor tumors, a second injection with cells from that same tumor produces no tumor growth. Among progressor tumors, there seems to be a spectrum of immunogenicity: injections of irradiated cells that cannot grow and kill the mouse seem to induce varying degrees of protective immunity against a challenge injection of viable

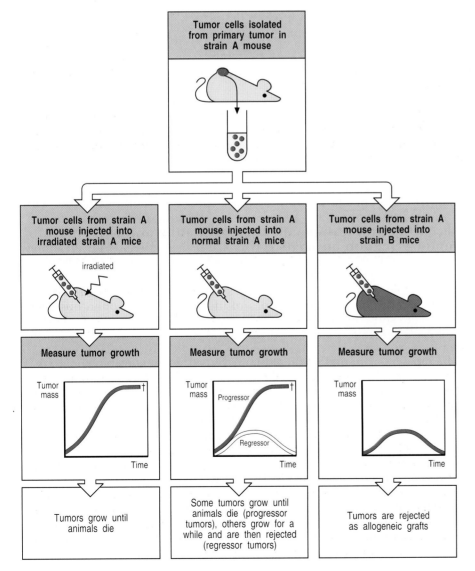

Fig. 13.10   The different growth patterns of transplantable tumors are governed by immune responses. Many tumors will grow progressively in T-cell deficient nude or irradiated mice (left panels). These tumors show two patterns of growth in normal syngeneic recipient mice, progressor or regressor patterns (center panels). The regressor pattern is due to an adaptive immune response to the tumor, and therefore regrafting the same tumor leads to accelerated rejection. These tumors are rejected in allogeneic mice by T cells specific for MHC molecules on the tumor (right panels). † = death of the animal.

Fig. 13.11 Tumor rejection antigens are defined by growth patterns in immunized mice. Mice immunized with an irradiated tumor and challenged with viable cells of the same tumor can reject a lethal dose of that tumor in some cases (left panels). This is the result of an immune response to tumor rejection antigens (TRAs). Some TRAs are unique to a given tumor, while others are shared by tumors of the same type (middle panels) but not by tumors of a different type (right panels).

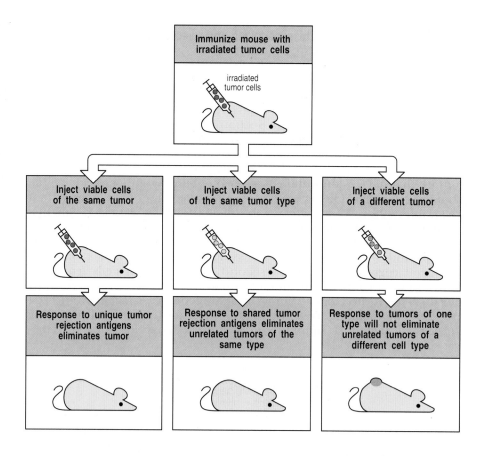

tumor cells at a distant site. These protective effects are not seen in T-cell deficient mice but can be conferred by adoptive transfer of T cells from immune mice, showing the need for T cells to mediate all these effects.

These observations indicate that the tumors express antigenic peptides that can become targets of a tumor-specific T-cell response. The antigens expressed by experimentally induced murine tumors, often termed **tumor-specific transplantation antigens (TSTA)**, or **tumor-rejection antigens (TRA)**, are usually specific for an individual tumor. Thus immunization with irradiated tumor cells from tumor X protects a syngeneic mouse from challenge with live cells from tumor X but not from challenge with a different syngeneic tumor Y, and *vice versa*. Cross-protection between tumors of the same type is often observed, however, showing that some TRAs are shared by tumors of a similar cellular origin (Fig. 13.11).

The molecular identification of tumor rejection antigens has shown that they are peptides of tumor cell proteins that are presented to T cells by MHC molecules. These peptides can become the targets of a tumor-specfic T-cell response because they are not displayed on the surface of normal cells, at least not at levels sufficient to be recognized by T cells (Fig. 13.12). Human tumors are often caused by mutant proteins that may be antigenic, or by proteins whose abnormal patterns of expression may make them targets for tumor rejection (Fig. 13.13). Of these only the melanoma antigens and MUC-1 (mucin-1) on breast or pancreatic tumors have so far been shown to be recognized by autologous T lymphocytes from patients with these tumors. Malignant melanoma is unlike other tumors in that, occasionally, even quite advanced disease shows spontaneous remission. In keeping with this finding, functional melanoma-specific T cells can be propagated from peripheral blood lymphocytes,

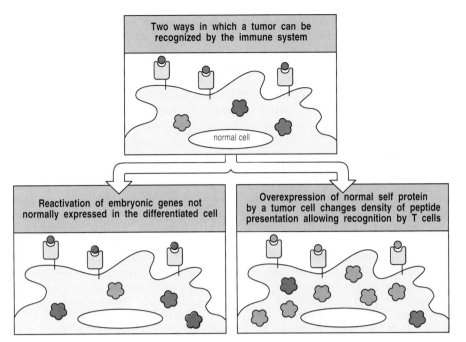

Fig. 13.12 Tumor rejection antigens are peptides of cellular proteins presented by self MHC class I molecules. Tumor rejection antigens (TRAs) are peptides of cellular proteins presented by self MHC class I molecules. TRAs arise mainly in two ways. In some cases, proteins that are normally expressed only in embryonic tissues are re-expressed by the tumor cells (lower left panel). As these proteins are normally expressed at a time when the immune system is not fully developed, T cells are not tolerant of these self antigens and can respond to them as if they were foreign proteins. In other tumors, over-expression of a self protein increases the density of presentation of a normal self peptide on tumor cells (lower right panel). Such peptides are then presented at high enough levels to be recognized by T cells. It is often the case that the same embryonic or self proteins are overexpressed in many tumors of a given type, giving rise to shared TRAs.

Fig. 13.13 There are several proteins that are selectively expressed in human tumors and are therefore candidate tumor-rejection antigens.

Potential tumor-rejection antigens have a variety of origins			
Class of antigen	**Antigen**	**Nature of antigen**	**Tumor type**
Embryonic	MAGE-1 MAGE-3	Normal testicular proteins	Melanoma Breast Glioma
Abnormal post-translational modification	MUC-1	Underglycosylated mucin	Breast Pancreas
Differentiation	Tyrosinase	Enzyme in pathway of melanin synthesis	Melanoma
	Surface Ig	Specific antibody following gene rearrangements in B-cell clone	Lymphoma
Mutated oncogene or tumor-suppressor	Ras	GTP-binding protein; relay in signal transduction pathway	Many tumors
	p53	Cell cycle regulator; tumor supressor gene	Lung Breast Gastrointestinal Brain Hematologic
Fusion protein	BCR-ABL	Fusion protein with tyrosine kinase activity resulting from chromosome translocation t(9;22) (Philadelphia chromosome)	Chronic myeloid leukemia
Oncoviral protein	HPV type 16, E6 and E7 proteins	Viral transforming gene products	Cervical carcinoma

tumor-infiltrating lymphocytes, or draining lymph nodes of patients in whom the melanoma is growing. Interestingly, none of the peptides recognized by these T cells arises from the mutant proto-oncogenes or tumor-suppressor genes that are likely to be responsible for the initial transformation of the cell into a cancer cell, although a few are the products of mutant genes. The rest fall into the two categories already depicted in Fig. 13.12. Antigens of the MAGE family are not expressed in any normal adult tissues with the exception of the testis, which we have learned in Section 12-23 is an immunologically privileged site. They probably represent early developmental antigens re-expressed in the process of tumorigenesis. Only a minority of melanoma patients have T cells reactive with the MAGE family of antigens, indicating that these antigens are either not expressed or not immunogenic in most cases. The most common melanoma antigens are peptides from the enzyme tyrosinase or from three proteins—gp100, MART 1, or gp75. These are differentiation antigens specific to the melanocyte lineage from which melanomas arise. In the case of these antigens, it is likely that over-expression in tumor cells leads to an abnormally high density of specific peptide:MHC complexes and this makes them immunogenic. Although in most cases tumor rejection antigens are presented as peptides complexed with Class I MHC molecules, tyrosinase has been shown to stimulate CD4 T-cell responses in some melanoma patients by being ingested and presented by cells expressing MHC class II.

Tumor rejection antigens (TRAs) shared between most examples of a tumor, and against which tolerance can be broken, represent candidate antigens for tumor vaccines. The MAGE family of antigens are candidates because of their limited tissue distribution and their shared expression by many melanomas. It might seem dangerous to use tumor vaccines based on antigens that are not truly tumor-specific because of the risk of inducing autoimmunity. Often, however, the tissues from which tumors arise are dispensable; the prostate is perhaps the best example of this. In the case of melanoma, however, some melanocyte-specific TRAs are also expressed in certain retinal cells, in the inner ear, in the brain and in the skin. Despite this, melanoma patients receiving immunotherapy with whole tumor cells or tumor-cell extracts, while occasionally developing vitiligo—a destruction of pigmented cells in the skin that correlates well with a good response to the tumor—do not develop abnormalities in the visual, vestibular, and central nervous systems, perhaps because of the low expression of MHC class I molecules in these sites (see Section 4-6).

13-11   Tumors can escape rejection in many ways.

Burnet called the ability of the immune system to detect tumor cells and destroy them **immune surveillance**. However, it is difficult to show that tumors are subject to surveillance by the immune system; after all, cancer is a common disease, and most tumors show little evidence for immunological control. Mice that lack lymphocytes show an incidence of the common tumors that is little different from the incidence of the same tumors in control mice with normal immune systems; the same is true for humans deficient in T cells. The major tumor types that occur with increased frequency in immuno-deficient mice or humans are virus-associated tumors; it can thus be said that immune surveillance is critical for control of virus-associated tumors, while the immune system does not normally respond to the neoantigens derived from the multiple genetic alterations in spontaneously arising tumors.

Mechanisms whereby tumors escape immune recognition		
Low immunogenicity	Antigenic modulation	Tumor-induced immune suppression
No peptide:MHC ligand No adhesion molecules No co-stimulatory molecules	Antibody to tumor cell-surface antigens may induce endocytosis and degradation of the antigen. Immune selection of antigen-loss variants	Factors (eg TGF-β) secreted by tumor cells inhibit T cells directly

Fig. 13.14 Tumors may escape immune surveillance in a variety of ways. First, tumors may have low immunogenicity (left panel). Some tumors do not have peptides of novel proteins that can be presented by MHC molecules, and therefore appear normal to the immune system. Others have lost one or more MHC molecules, and most do not express co-stimulatory proteins, which are required to activate naive T cells. Second, tumors may initially express antigens to which the immune system responds but lose them due to antibody-induced internalization or antigenic variation. When tumors are attacked by cells responding to a particular antigen, any tumor that does not express that antigen will have a selective advantage (center panel). Third, tumors often produce substances, such as TGF-β, that suppress immune responses directly (right panel).

It is not surprising that spontaneously arising tumors are rarely rejected by T cells. It is probable that they usually lack either distinctive antigenic peptides or the adhesion or co-stimulatory molecules necessary to elicit a primary T-cell response. Moreover, there are other mechanisms whereby tumors can avoid or evade immune attack when it occurs (Fig. 13.14). Tumors tend to be genetically unstable, and they can lose their antigens by mutation so that in the event of an immune response escape mutants might be generated. Some tumors, such as colon cancers, lose expression of a particular MHC class I molecule (Fig. 13.15), perhaps through immunoselection by T cells specific for a peptide presented by that MHC class I molecule. In experimental studies, when a tumor loses expression of all MHC class I molecules, it can no longer be recognized by cytotoxic T cells, although it may become susceptible to NK cells (Fig. 13.16). However, tumors that lose only one MHC class I molecule may be able to avoid recognition by specific CD8 cytotoxic T cells while remaining resistant to NK cells, conferring a selective advantage *in vivo*.

Yet another way in which tumors may evade rejection is by making immunosuppressive cytokines. Many tumours make these, although in most cases little is known of their precise nature. Transforming growth factor-β (TGF-β) was first identified in the culture supernatant of a tumor (hence its name) and, as we have seen, tends to suppress inflammatory T-cell responses and cell-mediated immunity, which are needed to control tumor growth. Thus, there are many ways in which tumors avoid recognition and destruction by the immune system.

The goal in the development of cancer vaccines is to break the tolerance of the immune system for antigens expressed mainly or exclusively by the tumor.

13-12	**Monoclonal antibodies to tumor antigens, alone or linked to toxins, can control tumor growth.**

The advent of monoclonal antibodies suggested the possibility of targeting and destroying tumors by making antibodies against tumor-specific

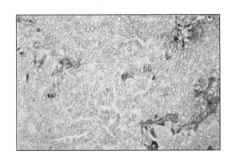

Fig. 13.15 Loss of MHC class I expression in a prostatic carcinoma. Some tumors may evade immune surveillance by loss of expression of MHC class I molecules, preventing their recognition by CD8 T cells. A section of a human prostate cancer, which has been stained using a peroxidase-conjugated antibody to HLA Class I, is shown. The brown stain correlating with HLA class I expression is restricted to infiltrating lymphocytes and tissue stromal cells. The tumor cells that occupy most of the section show no staining. Photograph courtesy of G Stamp.

Fig. 13.16 Tumors that lose expression of all MHC class I molecules as a mechanism of escape from immune surveillance are more susceptible to natural killer (NK) cell killing.
Transplanted tumors that regress are largely controlled by cytotoxic T cells (CTL) (left panels). NK cells have inhibitory receptors that bind MHC class I molecules (see Fig. 9.18), so variants of the tumor that have low MHC class I levels, although they are less sensitive to CD8 cytotoxic T cells, become susceptible to NK cells (center panels). Although *nude* mice lack T cells, they have higher than normal levels of NK cells, and so tumors that are sensitive to NK cells grow less well in *nude* mice than in normal mice. Transfection with MHC class I genes can restore both resistance to NK cells and susceptibility to CD8 cytotoxic T cells (right panels). However tumors that lose only one MHC class I molecule may escape a specific cytotoxic CD8 T-cell response while remaining NK-resistant. The bottom panels show scanning electron micrographs of NK cells attacking leukemia cells. Left panel; shortly after binding to the target cell, the NK cell has put out numerous microvillous extensions and established a broad zone of contact with the leukemia cell. The NK cell is the smaller cell on the left in both photographs. Right panel; 60 minutes after mixing, long microvillous processes can be seen extending from the NK cell (bottom left) to the leukemia cell and there is extensive damage to the leukemia cell membrane; the plasma membrane of the leukemia cell has rolled up and fragmented under the NK cell attack. Photographs courtesy of J C Hiserodt.

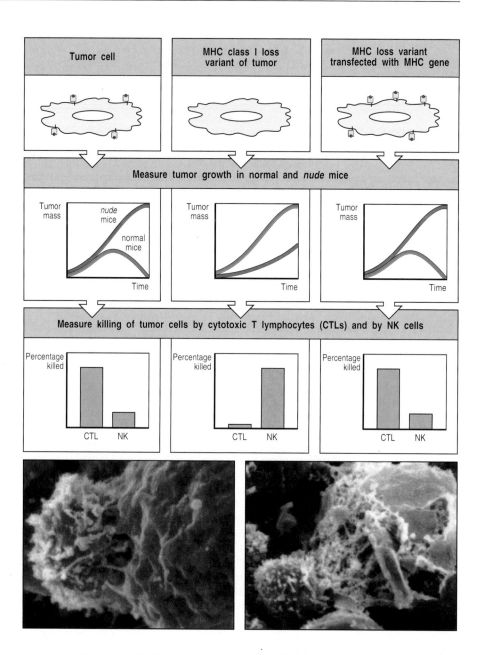

antigens (Fig. 13.17). This depends on finding a tumor-specific antigen that is a cell-surface molecule. To date, there has been limited success using this approach, although, as an adjunct to other therapies, it holds promise. Monoclonal antibodies coupled to a gamma-emitting isotope such as Technetium have also been used to image tumors, for the purpose of diagnosis and monitoring of metastatic disease (Fig. 13.18).

The first reported successful treatment of a tumor with monoclonal antibodies utilized anti-idiotypic antibodies to target B-cell lymphomas whose surface immunoglobulin expressed the specific idiotype. The initial course of treatment usually leads to a remission, but the tumor always reappears in a mutant form that no longer binds to the antibody used for the initial treatment. This case represents a clear example of genetic instability enabling a tumor to evade treatment.

Other problems with tumor-specific or tumor-selective monoclonal antibodies as therapeutic agents include inefficient killing of cells after binding of the monoclonal antibody and inefficient penetration of the antibody into the tumor mass. The first problem can often be

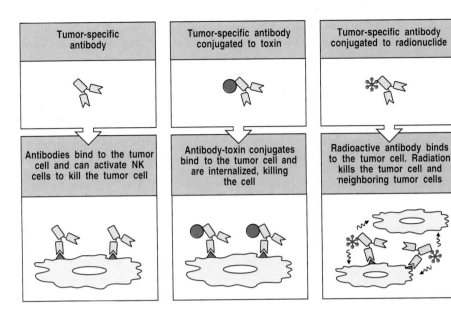

Fig. 13.17 A monoclonal antibody coupled to a toxin chain or a radio-isotope can eliminate or reduce a tumor. Antibodies that recognize tumor-specific antigens can be used in a variety of ways to help eliminate tumors. If they are of the correct isotypes, the antibodies themselves may be able to direct the lysis of the tumor cells by NK cells, activating the NK cells via their Fc receptor (left panels). A more useful strategy may be to couple the antibody to a powerful toxin (center panels). When the antibody binds to the tumor cell and is endocytosed, the toxin is released from the antibody and can kill the tumor cell. If the antibody is coupled to a radionuclide, binding of the antibody to a tumor cell will deliver a dose of radiation sufficient to kill the tumor cell. In addition, nearby tumor cells may also receive a lethal radiation dose, even though they may not bind the antibody.

circumvented by linking the antibody to a toxin, producing a reagent called an **immunotoxin**; two favored toxins are ricin A chain and *Pseudomonas* toxin. Both approaches require the antibody to be internalized to allow the cleavage of the toxin from the antibody in the endocytic compartment (see Fig. 13.17), allowing the toxin chain to penetrate and kill the cell.

Two other approaches using monoclonal antibody conjugates involve linking the antibody molecule to chemotherapeutic drugs such as adriamycin, or to radioisotopes. In the first case, the specificity of the monoclonal antibody for a cell-surface antigen on the tumor concentrates the drug to the site of the tumor. After internalization, the drug is released in the endosomes and exerts its cytostatic or cytotoxic effect. Monoclonal antibodies linked to radionuclides (see Fig. 13.17) concentrate the radioactive source in the tumor site. Both these approaches have the advantage of killing neighboring tumor cells, since the released drug or radioactive emissions can affect cells adjacent to those that actually bind the antibody. Ultimately, combinations of toxin-, drug-, or radionuclide-linked monoclonal antibodies, together with vaccination strategies aimed at inducing T-cell mediated immunity, may provide the most effective cancer immunotherapy.

13-13   Enhancing the immunogenicity of tumors holds promise for cancer therapy.

While antigen-specific vaccines based on dominant shared tumor antigens are, in principle, the ideal approach to T-cell mediated cancer immunotherapy, it may be many decades before the dominant tumor antigens for common cancers can be identified. Even then, it is not clear how widely the relevant epitopes will be shared between tumors, and peptides of TRAs will only be presented by particular MHC alleles. MAGE1 antigens, for example, are only recognized by T cells in melanoma patients expressing the HLA-A1 haplotype.

Thus, the individual patient's tumor removed at surgery may be, in practice, the best source of vaccine antigens. Until recently, most cell-based cancer vaccines have involved mixing either irradiated tumor cells or tumor extracts with bacterial adjuvants such as BCG

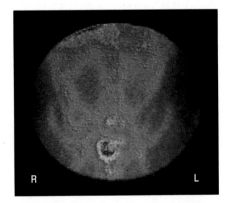

Fig. 13.18 Recurrent colorectal cancer may be detected using a radiolabeled monoclonal antibody to carcino-embryonic antigen. A patient with a possible recurrence of a colorectal cancer was injected intravenously with an [111]Indium-labeled monoclonal antibody to carcinoembryonic antigen. The recurrent tumor is seen as two red spots located in the pelvic region. The blood vessels are faintly outlined by circulating antibody that has not bound to the tumor. Photograph courtesy of A M Peters.

or *Corynebacterium parvum* (see Section 2-4). These adjuvants have generated modest therapeutic results in melanomas but have, in general, been disappointing.

More recently, in experiments in mice, attempts have been made to increase the immunogenicity of tumor cells by introducing genes that encode co-stimulatory molecules or cytokines into the tumor cells. Introducing co-stimulatory molecules is intended to make the tumor itself more immunogenic. The basic scheme of such experiments is as follows (Fig. 13.19): A tumor cell transfected with the gene encoding the co-stimulator molecule B7 (see Section 7-4) is implanted in a syngeneic animal. These B7-positive cells are able to activate naive T cells that recognize TSTAs to become effector T cells able to reject the tumor cells.

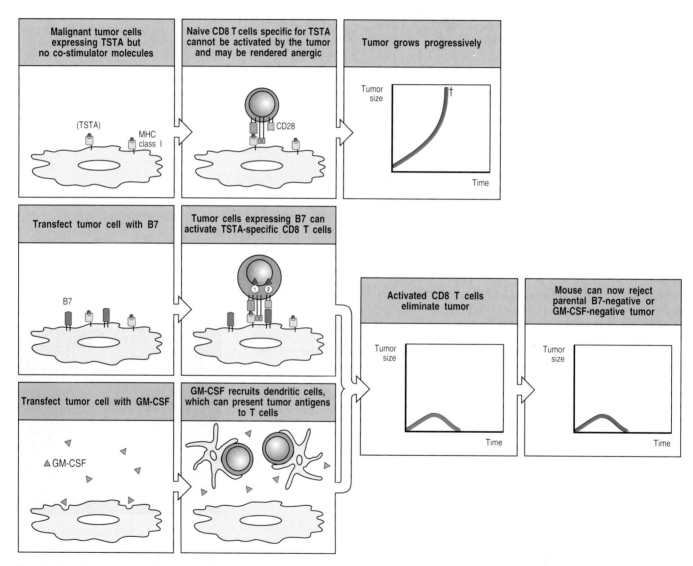

Fig. 13.19   Transfection of tumors with the gene for B7 or GM-CSF enhances tumor immunogenicity. A tumor that does not express co-stimulator molecules will not induce an immune response, even though it may express tumor rejection antigens (TRAs), because naive CD8 T cells specific for the TRA cannot be activated by the tumor. The tumor therefore grows progressively in normal mice (top panels). If such tumor cells are transfected with a co-stimulator molecule, such as B7, TRA-specific CD8 T cells now receive both signal 1 and signal 2 from the same cell (see Section 7-4) and can therefore be activated (center panels). The same effect can be obtained by transfecting the tumor with the gene encoding GM-CSF, which attracts and stimulates the differentiation of the precursors of dendritic cells (bottom panels). Both of these strategies have been tested in mice and shown to elicit memory T cells, although results with GM-CSF are more impressive. Since TRA-specific CD8 cells have now been activated, even the original B7-negative or GM-CSF negative tumor cells can be rejected. † = death of animal.

These effector T cells can recognize the tumor cells whether they express B7 or not; this can be shown by re-implanting non-transfected tumor cells, which are also rejected.

The second strategy, introducing cytokine genes into tumors so that they secrete the relevant cytokine, is aimed at attracting antigen-presenting cells to the tumor and takes advantage of the paracrine nature of cytokines. In mice, the most effective tumor vaccines to date are tumor cells that secrete granulocyte-macrophage colony-stimulating factor (GM-CSF), which attracts hematopoietic precursors to the site and induces their differentiation into dendritic cells. It is believed that these cells process the tumor antigens and migrate to the local lymph nodes where they induce potent anti-tumor responses. The B7-transfected cells appear less potent in inducing anti-tumor responses, perhaps because the bone marrow derived dendritic cells express more of the molecules required to activate naive T cells than do B7-transfected tumor cells (see Fig. 13.19).

Clinical trials are in progress to determine the safety and efficacy of such approaches in human patients. What is not certain is whether people with established cancers can generate sufficient T-cell responses to eliminate all their tumor cells under circumstances where any tumor-specific naive T cells may have been rendered tolerant to the tumor. Moreover, there is always the risk that immunogenic transfectants will elicit an autoimmune response against the normal tissue from which the tumor derived.

Summary.

Tumors represent outgrowths of a single abnormal cell, and animal studies have shown that some tumors elicit specific immune responses that suppress their growth. These seem to be directed at peptides derived from antigens that are either inappropriately expressed or over-expressed in the tumor cells and bound to surface MHC molecules. T-cell deficient individuals, however, do not develop more tumors than normal individuals. This is probably chiefly because most tumors do not make distinctive antigenic proteins and do not express the co-stimulatory molecules necessary to initiate an adaptive immune response. Tumors may also have other means of avoiding or suppressing immune responses. Monoclonal antibodies have been developed for tumor immunotherapy by conjugation to toxins or to cytotoxic drugs or radionuclides, which are thereby delivered at high dose specifically to the tumor cells. More recently, attempts have been made to develop vaccines based on tumor cells taken from patients and made immunogenic by the addition of adjuvants. This approach has been extended in animal experiments to transfection of tumor cells with genes encoding co-stimulatory molecules or cytokines.

Manipulating the immune response to fight infection.

Infection is the leading cause of death in human populations. The two most important contributions to public health in the past 100 years have been sanitation and vaccination, which together, have dramatically reduced deaths from infectious disease. Modern immunology grew from the success of Jenner and Pasteur's vaccination against smallpox and cholera and its greatest triumph has been the global eradication of smallpox, announced by the World Health Organization in 1980. A global campaign to eradicate polio is now underway.

Induced immunity to an infectious agent can be achieved in several ways. One early strategy was to deliberately cause a mild infection using the unmodified pathogen. This was the principle of variolation, in which inoculation of a small amount of dried material from a smallpox pustule would cause a mild infection followed by long-lasting protection against re-infection. However, infection following variolation was not always mild and fatal smallpox ensued in about 3% of cases, which would not meet modern criteria for safety. Jenner's achievement was the realization that infection with a bovine analog of smallpox, vaccinia (from *vacca*—a cow), which caused cowpox, would provide protective immunity against smallpox in humans, without the risk of significant disease. He named the process vaccination and Pasteur, in his honour, extended the term to the stimulation of protection to other infectious agents. Humans are not a natural host of vaccinia, which establishes only a brief and limited subcutaneous infection but which contains antigens that stimulate an immune response that is cross-reactive with smallpox antigens and thereby confers protection from the human disease.

This established the general principles of safe and effective vaccination, and vaccine development in the early part of the 20th century followed two empirical pathways: first the search for **attenuated** organisms with reduced pathogenicity that would stimulate protective immunity; and second, the development of vaccines based on killed organisms and subsequently purified components of organisms that would be as effective as live whole organisms because any live vaccine, including vaccinia, may cause lethal systemic infection in the immunosuppressed.

Immunization is now considered so safe and so important that most states in the USA require all children to be immunized against measles, mumps and polio using live attenuated vaccines, as well as against tetanus, diptheria (which causes scarlet fever) and pertussis (which causes whooping cough) using inactivated toxins or toxoids prepared from these bacteria (see Fig. 1.31). More recently, a vaccine has become available against *Hemophilus B*; the causative agent of meningitis (Fig. 13.20). Impressive as these accomplishments are, there are still many diseases

Fig. 13.20 Childhood vaccination schedules (in red) in the USA.

Current immunization schedule for children (USA)

Vaccine given	2 months	4 months	6 months	15 months	18 months	24 months	4–6 years	14–15 years
Diphtheria-pertussis-tetanus (DPT)	■	■	■		■		■	
Trivalent oral polio (TVOP)	■	■			■		■	
Measles				■				
Rubella				■				
Mumps				■				
Haemophilus B polysaccharide						■		
Diphtheria-tetanus toxoids								■

Some diseases for which effective vaccines are not yet available		
Disease	**Annual mortality**	**Annual incidence**
Malaria	856 000	213 743 000
Schistosomiasis	8000	no numbers available
Worm infestation	22 000	no numbers available
Tuberculosis	1 960 000	6 346 000
Diarrhea	2 946 000	4 073 920 000
Respiratory disease	4 299 000	362 424 000
AIDS	138 000	411 000
Measles*	1 158 000	44 334 000

Fig. 13.21   Diseases for which effective vaccines are still needed. *Current measles vaccines are effective but heat-sensitive, which makes their use difficult in tropical countries. Data from C J L Murray, and A D Lopez. Global Health Statistics: a compendium of incidence, prevalence and mortality estimates for over 200 conditions. Cambridge, Harvard University Press 1996.

for which we lack effective vaccines, as shown in Fig. 13.21. Even where a vaccine such as measles or polio can be used effectively in developed countries, technical and economic problems may prevent its widespread use in developing countries, where mortality from these diseases is still high. The development of vaccines therefore remains an important goal of immunology and the latter half of this century has seen a shift to a more rational approach, based on a detailed molecular understanding of microbial pathogenicity, analysis of the protective host response to pathogenic organisms, and the understanding of the regulation of immune system to generate effective T- and B-lymphocyte responses.

13-14   There are several requirements for an effective vaccine.

The specific requirements for successful vaccination vary according to the nature of the infecting organism. For extracellular organisms, antibody provides the most important adaptive mechanism of host defence, whereas for control of intracellular organisms an effective CD8 T-lymphocyte response is also essential. The ideal vaccination provides host defence at the point of entry of the infectious agent; stimulation of mucosal immunity is therefore an important goal of vaccination against those many organisms that enter through mucosal surfaces.

Effective protective immunity against some organisms requires the presence of pre-existing antibody at the time of exposure to the infection. For example, the clinical manifestations of tetanus and diphtheria are entirely due to the effects of extremely powerful exotoxins, produced respectively by *Clostridium tetani* and *Corynebacterium diphtheriae*. Pre-existing antibody to the bacterial exotoxin is necessary to provide a defense against these diseases. Pre-existing antibodies are also required to protect against some intracellular pathogens, such as the poliomyelitis virus, which infect critical host cells within a short period after entering the body and are not easily controlled by T lymphocytes once intracellular infection is established.

Features of effective vaccines	
Safe	Vaccine must not itself cause illness or death
Protective	Vaccine must protect against illness resulting from exposure to live pathogen
Gives sustained protection	Protection against illness must last for several years
Induces neutralizing antibody	Some pathogens (like poliovirus) infect cells that cannot be replaced (eg neurons). Neutralizing antibody is essential to prevent infection of such cells
Induces protective T cells	Some pathogens, particularly intracellular, are more effectively dealt with by cell-mediated responses
Practical considerations	Low cost-per-dose Biological stability Ease of administration Few side-effects

Fig. 13.22   There are several criteria for an effective vaccine.

Immune responses to infectious agents usually involve antibodies directed at multiple epitopes and only some of these antibodies confer protection. The particular T-cell epitopes recognized may also affect the nature of the response. For example, as we saw in Chapter 10, the predominant epitope recognized by T cells after vaccination with respiratory syncitial virus induces a vigorous inflammatory response but fails to elicit neutralizing antibodies and thus causes pathology without protection. Thus, an effective vaccine must lead to the generation of antibodies and T cells directed at the correct epitopes of the infectious agent. For some of the modern vaccine techniques, in which only one or a few epitopes are used, this consideration is particularly important.

A number of very important additional constraints need to be satisified by a successful vaccine. First, it must be safe. Vaccines must be given to huge numbers of people, relatively few of whom are likely to die of, or sometimes even catch, the disease that the vaccine is designed to prevent, and this means that even a low level of toxicity is unacceptable (Fig. 13.22). Second, the vaccine must be able to produce protective immunity in a very high proportion of the people to whom it is given. Third, since it is impractical to give large or dispersed rural populations regular 'booster' vaccinations, a successful vaccine must generate long-lived immunological memory. This means that both B and T lymphocytes must be primed by the vaccine. Fourth, vaccines must be very cheap if they are to be administered to large populations. Vaccines are one of the most cost-effective measures in health care but this benefit is eroded as the cost-per-dose rises.

An effective vaccination program provides herd immunity—by lowering the number of susceptible members of a population, the natural reservoir of infected individuals in that population falls, reducing the probability of transmission of infection. Thus, even non-vaccinated members of a population may be protected from infection if the majority are vaccinated.

13-15   The history of vaccination against *Bordetella pertussis* illustrates the importance of achieving an effective vaccine that is perceived to be safe.

The history of vaccination against the agent that causes whooping cough, *Bordetella pertussis*, provides a good example of the challenges of developing and disseminating an effective vaccine. At the turn of the 20th century, whooping cough killed approximately 0.5% of American children under the age of 5 years. In the early 1930s, a trial of a killed, whole bacterial cell vaccine, on the Faröe Islands provided evidence of a protective effect. In the USA, systematic use of a whole-cell vaccine, combined with diphtheria and tetanus toxoids (DPT vaccine), since the 1940s resulted in a decline in the annual infection rate from 200 to less than 2 cases per 100 000 of the population. First vaccination with DPT was given typically at the age of 3 months.

Whole-cell pertussis vaccine causes side-effects, typically redness, pain and swelling at the site of the injection; less commonly vaccination is followed by high temperature and persistent crying. Very rarely, fits and a short lived sleepiness or a floppy unresponsive state ensue. During the 1970s, widespread concern developed following several anecdotal observations that encephalitis leading to irreversible brain damage might follow pertussis vaccination very rarely. In Japan, in 1972, approximately 85% of children were given the pertussis vaccine, and less than 300 cases of whooping cough and no deaths were reported.

Following two deaths after vaccination in Japan in 1975, DTP was temporarily suspended and then re-introduced with the first vaccination at 2 years of age rather than 3 months. In 1979 there were approximately 13 000 cases of whooping cough and 41 deaths. The possibility that pertussis vaccine very rarely causes severe brain damage has been studied extensively and expert consensus is that pertussis vaccine is not a primary cause of brain injury. There is no doubt that there is greater morbidity from whooping cough than from the vaccine.

The public and medical perception that whole-cell pertussis vaccination may be unsafe provided a powerful incentive to develop safer pertussis vaccines. Study of the natural immune response to *B. pertussis* showed that infection induced antibodies to four components of the bacterium—pertussis toxin; filamentous hemagglutinin; pertactin; and fimbrial antigens. Immunization of mice with these antigens in purified form protected them against challenge with pertussis. This has led to the development of acellular pertussis vaccines, all of which contain purified pertussis toxoid, that is, toxin inactivated by treatment with hydrogen peroxide. Some also contain one or more of the filamentous hemagglutinin, pertactin, and fimbrial antigens. Current evidence shows that these are probably more effective than whole-cell pertussis vaccine and free of the common minor side-effects of the whole-cell vaccine.

The main messages of the history of pertussis vaccination are: (i) vaccines must be extremely safe and free of side-effects; (ii) the public and medical profession must perceive the vaccine to be safe; and (iii) careful study of the nature of the protective immune response can lead to the design of acellular vaccines that are safer and more effective than whole-cell vaccines.

13-16   Conjugate vaccines have been developed as a result of understanding how T and B cells collaborate in an immune response.

While acellular vaccines are inevitably safer than vaccines based on whole organisms, a fully effective vaccine cannot normally be made from a single isolated constituent of a microorganism, and it is now clear that this is because of the need to activate more than one cell type to initiate an immune response. One consequence of this insight has been the development of **conjugate vaccines**. We have already described briefly one of the most important of these in Section 8-2.

Many bacteria, including *Meningococcus, Pneumococcus and Haemophilus* spp., have an outer capsule composed of polysaccharides that are species- and type-specific for particular strains of bacteria. The most effective defence agains these microorganisms is opsonization of the polysaccharide coat with antibody. The aim of vaccination is therefore to elicit antibodies against the polysaccharide capsules of the bacteria.

Capsular polysaccharides can be harvested from bacterial growth media and because they are T-independent antigens they can be used on their own as vaccines. However, young children under the age of 2 years are not capable of making good T-cell-independent responses and cannot be vaccinated effectively with polysaccharide vaccines. An efficient means of overcoming this problem (see Fig. 8.4) is to chemically conjugate bacterial polysaccharides to protein carriers, which provide peptides for activating T cells and convert a T-cell independent into a T-cell-dependent anti-polysaccharide response. Using this approach, various conjugate vaccines have been developed against *H. influenzae*, an important cause of serious childhood chest infections and meningitis, and these are now widely applied.

| 13-17 | **The use of adjuvants is another important approach to enhancing the immunogenicity of vaccines.** |

Even conjugate vaccines are not usually strongly immunogenic on their own: most require the addition of adjuvants, which we defined in Section 2-4 as substances that enhance immunogenicity of antigens. It is thought that most, if not all adjuvants act on antigen-presenting cells and reflect the importance of these cells in initiating immune responses. *H. influenzae* polysaccharides, for example, can conveniently be conjugated to tetanus toxoid because infants are vaccinated routinely with this protein and their T cells are already primed against it. However, tetanus toxoid is not immunogenic in the absence of adjuvants, and tetanus toxoid vaccines often contain aluminium salts, which bind polyvalently to the toxoid by ionic interactions and selectively stimulate antibody responses. Pertussis toxin, produced by *Bordetella pertussis*, has adjuvant properties in its own right and, when given mixed with tetanus and diphtheria toxoids, not only vaccinates against whooping cough but also acts as an adjuvant for the other two toxoids. This mixture comprises the DTP triple vaccine given to infants in the first year of life.

Several small molecules, for example muramyl dipeptide extracted from the mycobacterial cell wall, also act as adjuvants. Their mechanism of action is, however, unknown. They may act by stimulating the expression of co-stimulatory activity in antigen-presenting cells or by mimicking co-stimulatory signals in T cells. Alternatively, they may enhance uptake of the antigen by dendritic cells that already express co-stimulatory molecules. Other adjuvants stimulate mucosal immune responses, which are particulary important in defense against organisms entering through the digestive or respiratory tract. These adjuvants will be discussed later when we describe strategies for stimulating mucosal immunity.

Yet another approach to enhancing the effectiveness of vaccines is to co-administer cytokines. For example, IL-12 is a cytokine, produced by macrophages and B cells, that stimulates T lymphocytes and NK cells to release interferon-γ and promotes a T$_H$1 response. It has been used as an adjuvant to promote protective immunity against the protozoan parasite *Leishmania major*. Certain strains of mice are susceptible to severe cutaneous and systemic infection by *Leishmania major* and mount an immune response that is predominantly T$_H$2 in type and is ineffective in eliminating the organism. The co-administration of IL-12 with a vaccine containing Leishmania antigens generated a T$_H$1 response and protected these mice against challenge with *L. major*. This use of IL-12 to promote a T$_H$1 response has also proved valuable in reducing the pathogenic consequences of experimental parasitic infection by *Schistosoma mansoni* and is considered in Section 13-23. These are important examples of how an understanding of the regulation of immune responses may allow rational intervention to enhance the effectiveness of vaccines.

| 13-18 | **Live-attenuated viral vaccines are more potent than 'killed' vaccines and may be made safer using recombinant DNA technology.** |

Most anti-viral vaccines currently in use consist of inactivated or live-attenuated viruses. Inactivated, or 'killed' viral vaccines consist of viruses treated so that they are unable to replicate. Live-attenuated virus vaccines are generally far more potent, perhaps because they elicit a greater number of relevant effector mechanisms, including cytotoxic CD8 T cells: inactivated viruses cannot produce proteins in the cytosol, so peptides from the viral antigens cannot be presented by MHC class I molecules and thus cytotoxic CD8 T cells are not generated by these vaccines. Attenuated viral vaccines are now in use for polio, measles, mumps, rubella, and varicella.

The power of this approach is illustrated by the effectiveness of live, attenuated polio vaccines. The Sabin polio vaccine consists of three attenuated polio virus strains and is highly immunogenic. Moreover, just as polio itself can be transmitted by fecal contamination of public swimming pools and other failures of hygeine, the vaccine can be transmitted from one individual to another by the orofecal route. Infection with *Salmonella* likewise stimulates a powerful mucosal and systemic immune response and, as we saw in Section 13-19, has been attenuated for use as a vaccine and carrier of heterologous antigens for presentation to the mucosal immune system.

The rules of mucosal immunity are poorly understood. On the one hand presentation of soluble protein antigens by the oral route often results in tolerance, which is important given the enormous load of food and airborne antigens presented to the gut and respiratory tract. As discussed in Sections 13-9 and 12-22, the capacity to induce tolerance by oral or nasal administration of antigens is being explored as a therapeutic mechanism for reducing unwanted immune responses. On the other hand, the mucosal immune system is capable of responding to and eliminating mucosal infections such as pertussis, cholera and polio. The proteins from these organisms that stimulate immune responses are therefore of special interest. One group of powerfully immunogenic proteins at mucosal surfaces is a series of bacterial toxins that have the property of binding to eukaryotic cells and are protease-resistant. A recent finding of potential practical importance is that certain of these molecules such as the *E.coli* heat-labile toxin and pertussis toxin have adjuvant properties that are retained even when the parent molecule has been engineered to eliminate its toxic activities. These molecules may be used as adjuvants for oral or nasal vaccines. In mice, nasal insufflation of either of these mutant toxins together with tetanus toxoid resulted in the development of protection against lethal challenge with tetanus toxin.

13-23   An important question is whether vaccination can be used therapeutically to control existing chronic infections.

There are many chronic diseases in which infection persists because of a failure of the immune system to eliminate disease. These can be divided into two groups, those infections in which there is an obvious immune response which fails to eliminate the organism, and those in which the infection appears to be invisible to the immune system and evokes a barely detectable immune response.

In the first category, the immune response is often partially responsible for the pathogenic effects of the disease. Infection by the helminth, *Schistosoma mansoni*, is associated with a powerful T_H2-type response, characterized by high IgE levels, circulating and tissue eosinophilia and a harmful fibrotic response to *Schistosoma* ova, leading to hepatic fibrosis. Other common parasites, such as *Plasmodia* and *Leishmania* spp. cause damage because they are not effectively eliminated by the immune response in many patients. Mycobacteria causing tuberculosis and leprosy cause persistent intracellular infection; a T_H1 response helps contain these infections but also causes granuloma formation and tissue necrosis. Among viruses, hepatitis B and hepatitis C infections are commonly followed by persistent viral carriage and hepatic injury, resulting in ultimate death from hepatitis or from hepatoma. HIV infection, as we have seen in Chapter 10, is only followed very rarely by viral clearance and protection against subsequent reinfection.

There is a second category of chronic infection, predominantly viral, in which the immune response fails to clear infection because of relative invisibility of the infectious agent to the immune system. A good example

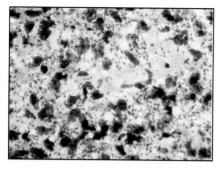

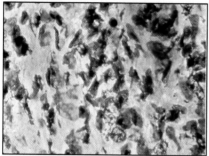

Fig. 13.27   Treatment with anti-IL-4 antibody at the time of infection with *Leishmania major* allows normally susceptible mice to clear the infection. The top panel shows a hematoxylin-eosin stained section through the footpad of a mouse of the Balb/c strain infected with *Leishmania major*. Large numbers of parasites are present in tissue macrophages. The bottom panel shows a similar preparation from a mouse infected in the same experiment but simultaneously treated with a single injection of anti-IL-4 monoclonal antibody. Very few parasites are present. Photographs courtesy of R M Locksley.

of this type of infection is herpes simplex type 2, which is transmitted venereally, becomes latent in nerve tissue, and causes genital herpes, which is frequently recurrent. This appears to be caused by a viral protein, ICP-47, which binds to the TAP complex and inhibits peptide transport in infected cells (see Chapter 4). In the case of genital warts, caused by certain papilloma viruses, very little immune response is evoked.

There are two main immunological approaches to the treatment of chronic infection. One is to try to boost or change the pattern of the host immune response using cytokine therapy. The second is to attempt therapeutic vaccination to see if the host immune response can be super-charged by immunization with antigens from the infectious agent in combination with adjuvant. There has been substantial pharmaceutical investment in therapeutic vaccination but it is too early to know whether the approach will be successful.

Some promise for the cytokine therapy approach comes from the experimental treatment of leprosy: one can clear certain leprosy lesions by injection of cytokines directly into the lesion and cause reversal of the type of leprosy seen. Another example where cytokine therapy has been shown to be effective in treating an established infection depends on combining a cytokine with an anti-parasitic drug. In a proportion of mice infected with *Leishmania* and subsequently treated with a combination of drug therapy and IL-12, the immune response deviated from a T_H2 to a T_H1 pattern and the infection was cleared. In most of the animal studies, however, it seems that the anti-cytokine antibody or the cytokine needs to be present at the first encounter with the antigen in order to modulate the response effectively. For example, in experimental leishmaniasis in the mouse, susceptible BALB/c mice injected with anti-IL-4 antibody at the time of infection clear their infection. However, if administration of anti-IL-4 is delayed by just 1 week, there is progressive growth of the parasite and a dominant T_H2 response (Fig. 13.27).

13-24   Modulation of the immune system may be used to inhibit immunopathological responses to infectious agents.

We have mentioned several times the possibility of modulating immunity by cytokine manipulation of the immune response. This approach is being explored as a means of inhibiting harmful immune responses to a number of important infections. As we have seen in the preceding section, the pathogenesis of the liver fibrosis in schistosomiasis results from the powerful T_H2-type response. The co-adminstration of *S. mansoni* ova together with IL-12 does not protect mice against subsequent infection with *S. mansoni* cercariae but has a striking effect in reducing hepatic granuloma formation and fibrosis in response to ova. IgE levels are reduced, with reduced tissue eosinophilia, and the cytokine response indicating the activation of T_H1 rather than T_H2 cells.

While these results indicate that it may be possible to use a combination of antigen and cytokine to vaccinate against the pathology of diseases for which a fully protective vaccine is unavailable, they do not solve the difficulty of applying this approach in patients whose infection is already established.

13-25   Protective immunity can be induced by injecting DNA encoding microbial antigens and human cytokines into muscle.

The latest development in vaccination has come as a surprise even to the scientists who initially developed the method. The story begins with attempts to use non-replicating bacterial plasmids encoding proteins for

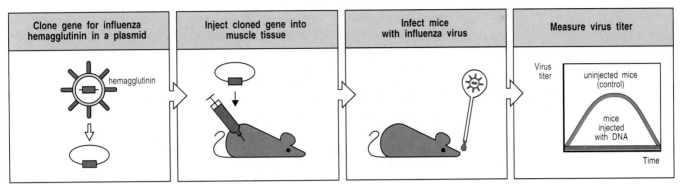

| Clone gene for influenza hemagglutinin in a plasmid | Inject cloned gene into muscle tissue | Infect mice with influenza virus | Measure virus titer |

Fig. 13.28   DNA vaccination by injection of DNA encoding a protective antigen and cytokines directly into muscle. Influenza hemagglutinin contains both B- and T-cell epitopes. When a naked DNA plasmid containing the gene for this protein is injected directly into muscle, a flu-specific immune response consisting of both antibody and cytoxic CD8 T cells results.

The response can be enhanced by including a plasmid encoding GM-CSF. Presumably, the plasmid DNAs are expressed by some of the cells in the muscle tissue into which it was injected, allowing an immune response that involves both antibody and cytotoxic T cells. The details of this process are not yet understood.

gene therapy. When DNA encoding a viral immunogen is injected intramuscularly, it leads to the development of antibody responses and cytotoxic T cells that allow the mice to reject a later challenge with whole virus (Fig. 13.28). This response does not appear to damage the muscle tissue, is safe and effective, and, since it uses only a single microbial gene, it does not carry the risk of active infection. This procedure has been termed 'DNA vaccination'. DNA coated onto minute metal projectiles can be administered by (biological bollistic) gun, so that several metal particles penetrate the skin and enter into the muscle beneath. This technique has been shown to be effective in animals and may be suitable for mass immunization, although it has yet to be tested in humans. Mixing in plasmids that encode cytokines such as GM-CSF allows these immunizations with genes encoding protective antigens to become much more effective, as has been seen earlier in attempts to induce tumor immunity.

It is not yet clear how DNA vaccination actually works. Why is plasmid DNA effectively expressed in muscle tissue? Do the muscle cells elicit the immune response, or do tissue dendritic cells take up the DNA and express it? How do lymphocytes encounter the antigen if it is expressed in muscle cells? How safe is the approach, and how generally applicable will it be?

This intriguing new development may change the face of vaccines more than any other single advance. Or it may be superseded by some other unexpected approach. Few were impressed with Jenner's vaccine when it was introduced nearly 200 years ago, yet attempts to understand how that vaccine works lie at the root of much of the progress in immunology that has been made since then. We clearly have many surprises ahead, and some will surely come from the development of new vaccines.

Summary.

The greatest triumphs of modern immunology have come from vaccination, which has eradicated or virtually eliminated several human diseases. It is the single most successful manipulation of the immune system to date because it takes advantage of its natural specificity and inducibility. Nevertheless, there are many important infectious diseases for which there is still no effective vaccine. While the most effective vaccines are based on live microorganisms, these carry some risk and are potentially lethal to immunosuppressed or immunodeficient individuals. Better techniques for developing live, attentuated vaccines, or vaccines based on immunogenic components of pathogens are therefore sought. Most viral vaccines currently in use are based on live, attenuated microorganisms but many bacterial vaccines are based on components of the microorganism, including components of the toxins that it produces. The immunogenicity of these components may be enhanced by conjugation to a protein. Vaccines based on peptide epitopes are still at an experimental stage and present the problem that they are likely to be specific for polymorphic variants of the MHC molecules to which they must bind, as well as being only very weakly immunogenic. Immunogenicity of vaccines often depends upon adjuvants that may help, directly or indirectly, to activate antigen-presenting cells that are necessary for the initiation of immune responses. The development of oral vaccines is particularly important for stimulating immunity to the many pathogens that enter through the mucosa. Cytokines have been used experimentally as adjuvants to boost the immunogenicity of vaccines or bias the immune response along a specific path.

Summary to Chapter 13.

One of the great future challenges of immunology is the control of the immune response, so that unwanted immune responses can be suppressed and desirable responses elicited. Current methods of suppressing unwanted responses rely, to a great extent, on drugs that suppress adaptive immunity indiscriminately and are thus inherently flawed. We have seen in this book that the immune system can suppress its own responses in an antigen-specific manner and, by studying these endogenous regulatory events, it may be possible to devise strategies to manipulate specific responses, while sparing general immune competence. This should allow the development of new treatments that suppress selectively the responses that lead to allergy, autoimmunity, or the rejection of grafted organs. Similarly, as we understand more about tumors and infectious agents, better strategies to mobilize the immune system against cancer and infection should become possible. To achieve all this, we need to learn more about the induction of immunity and the biology of the immune system, and to apply what we have learned to human disease.

General References

Frontiers in Medicine: Vaccines, *Science* 1994, **265**:1371-1404

Ada, G.: **Vaccination in Third World countries.** *Curr. Opin. Immunol.* 1993, **5**:683-686

Brines, R. (ed.): **Immunopharmacology.** *Immunol. Today* 1993, **14**:241-332.

Klein, G. and Boon, T.: **Tumor immunology: present perspectives.** *Curr. Opin. Immunol.* 1993, **5**:687-692.

Lanzavecchia, A.: **Identifying strategies for immune intervention.** *Science* 1993, **260**:937-944.

Moller, G. (ed.): **Engineered antibody molecules.** *Immunol. Rev.* 1992, **130**:1-212.

Moller, G. (ed.): **Antibodies in disease therapy.** *Immunol. Rev.* 1992, **129**:1-201.

Moller, G. (ed.): **New immunosuppressive drugs.** *Immunol. Rev.* 1993, **136**:1-109.

Moller, G. (ed.): **Tumor immunology.** *Immunol. Rev.* 1995, **145**:1-250.

Plotkin, S.A., and Mortimer, E.A.: *Vaccines*, 2nd edn. Philadelphia, W.B. Saunders Co., 1994

Roth, C., Rochlitz, C., and Kourilsky, P.: **Immune response against tumors.** *Adv. Immunol.* 1994, **57**:281-351.

Waldmann, T.A.: **Monoclonal antibodies in diagnosis and therapy.** *Science* 1991, **252**:1657-1662.

Waldmann, T.A.: **Immune receptors: targets for therapy of leukemia/lymphoma, autoimmune diseases and for the prevention of allograft rejection.** *Ann. Rev. Immunol.* 1992, **10**:675-704.

Section references.

13-1 Corticosteroids are powerful anti-inflammatory drugs that alter the transcription of many genes.

Barnes, P.J. and Adcock, I.: **Anti-inflammatory actions of steroids: molecular mechanisms.** *Trends Pharmacol. Sci.* 1993, **14**:436-441.

Boumpas, D.T., Chrousos, G.P., Wilder, R.L., Cupps, T.R., and Balow, J.E.: **Glucocorticoid therapy for immune-mediated diseases: basic and clinical correlates.** *Ann. Intl. Med.* 1993, **119**:1198-1208.

Cronstein, B.N., Kimmel, S.C., Levin, R.I., Martiniuk, F., and Weissmann, G.: **A mechanism for the antiinflammatory effects of corticosteroids: the glucocorticoid receptor regulates leukocyte adhesion to endothelial cells and expression of endothelial-leukocyte adhesion molecule 1 and intercellular adhesion molecule 1.** *Proc. Natl. Acad. Sci.* 1992, **89**:9991-9995.

Cronstein, B.N., Kimmel, S.C., Levin, R.I., Martiniuk, F., and Weissmann, G.: **Corticosteroids are transcriptional regulators of acute inflammation.** *Trans. Assoc. Am. Physicians* 1992, **105**:25-35.

Cupps, T.R. and Fauci, A.S.: **Corticosteroid-mediated immunoregulation in man.** *Immunol. Rev.* 1982, **65**:133-155.

Schwiebert, L.A., Beck, L.A., Stellato, C., Bickel, C.A., Bochner, B.S., and Schleimer, R.P.: **Glucocorticosteroid inhibition of cytokine production: relevance to antiallergic actions.** *J. Allergy Clin. Immunol.* 1996, **97**:143-152.

13-2 Cytotoxic drugs cause immunosuppression by killing dividing cells and have serious side effects.

Chan, G.L., Canafax, D.M., and Johnson, C.A.: **The therapeutic use of azathioprine in renal transplantation.** *Pharmacotherapy* 1987, **7**:165-177.

Zhu, L.P., Cupps, T.R., Whalen, G., and Fauci, A.S.: **Selective effects of cyclophosphamide therapy on activation, proliferation, and differentiation of human B cells.** *J. Clin. Invest.* 1987, **79**:1082-1090.

13-3 Cyclosporin A, FK506 (tacrolimus), and rapamycin are powerful immunosuppressive agents that interfere with T-cell signaling.

Bierer, B.E., Hollander, G., Fruman, D8., and Burakoff, S.J.: **Cyclosporin A and FK506: molecular mechanisms of immunosuppression and probes for transplantation biology.** *Curr. Opin. Immunol.* 1993, **5**:763-773.

Kunz, J. and Hall, M.N.: **Cyclosporin A, FK506 and rapamycin: more than just immunosuppression.** *Trends Biochem. Sci.* 1993, **18**:334-338.

Schreiber, S.L.: **Chemistry and biology of the immunophilins and their immunosuppressive ligands.** *Science* 1991, **251**:283-287.

Schreiber, S.L. and Crabtree, G.R.: **The mechanism of action of cyclosporin A and FK506.** *Immunol. Today.* 1992, **13**:136-142.

13-4 Immunosuppressive drugs are valuable probes of intracellular signalling pathways in lymphocytes.

Clipstone, N.A. and Crabtree, G.R.: **Identification of calcineurin as a key signalling enzyme in T-lymphocyte activation.** *Nature* 1992, **357**:695-697.

Crabtree, G.R. and Clipstone, N.A.: **Signal transmission between the plasma membrane and nucleus of T lymphocytes.** *Ann. Rev. Biochem.* 1994, **63**:1045-1083.

Dumont, F.J. and Su, Q.: **Mechanism of action of the immunosuppressant rapamycin.** *Life Sci.* 1996, **58**:373-395.

Liu, J., Farmer, J.D.,Jr., Lane, W.S., Friedman, J., Weissman, I., and Schreiber, S.L.: **Calcineurin is a common target of cyclophilin-cyclosporin A and FKBP-FK506 complexes.** *Cell* 1991, **66**:807-815.

Nourse, J., Firpo, E., Flanagan, W.M., Coats, S., Polyak, K., Lee, M.H., Massague, J., Crabtree, G.R., and Roberts, J.M.: **Interleukin-2-mediated elimination of the p27Kip1 cyclin-dependent kinase inhibitor prevented by rapamycin.** *Nature* 1994, **372**:570-573.

Sigal, N.H. and Dumont, F.J.: **Cyclosporin A, FK-506, and rapamycin: pharmacologic probes of lymphocyte signal transduction.** *Ann. Rev. Immunol.* 1992, **10**:519-560.

Spencer, D.M., Wandless, T.J., Schreiber, S.L., and Crabtree, G.R.: **Controlling signal transduction with synthetic ligands.** *Science* 1993, **262**:1019-1024.

13-5 Antibodies to cell-surface molecules have been used to remove specific lymphocyte subsets or to inhibit cell function.

Cobbold, S.P., Qin, S., Leong, L.Y., Martin, G., and Waldmann, H.: **Reprogramming the immune system for peripheral tolerance with CD4 and CD8 monoclonal antibodies.** *Immunol. Rev.* 1992, **129**:165-201.

Waldmann, H. and Cobbold, S.: **The use of monoclonal antibodies to achieve immunological tolerance.** *Immunol. Today* 1993, **14**:247-251.

13-6 Antibodies can be engineered to reduce their immunogenicity in humans.

Winter, G. and Harris, W.J.: **Humanized antibodies.** *Immunol. Today* 1993, **14**:243-246.

Winter, G., Griffiths, A.D., Hawkins, R.E., and Hoogenboom, H.R.: **Making antibodies by phage display technology.** *Ann. Rev. Immunol.* 1994, **12**:433-455.

13-7 Monoclonal antibodies may be used to inhibit allograft rejection.

Charlton, B., Auchincloss, H.,Jr., and Fathman, C.G.: **Mechanisms of transplantation tolerance.** *Ann. Rev. Immunol.* 1994, **12**:707-734.

Chatenoud, L. and Bach, J.F.: **Therapeutic monoclonal antibodies in transplantation.** *Transplant. Proc.* 1993, **25**:473-474.

Fathman, C.G.: **Inhibition of immune induction: the target of current transplantation tolerance strategies.** *Curr. Opin. Immunol.* 1992, **4**:545-547.

Lenschow, D.J., Zeng, Y., Hathcock, K.S., Zuckerman, L.A., Freeman, G., Thistlethwaite, J.R., Gray, G.S., Hodes, R.J., and Bluestone, J.A.: **Inhibition of transplant rejection following treatment with anti-B7-2 and anti-B7-1 antibodies.** *Transplantation* 1995, **60**:1171-1178.

Lenschow, D.J., Zeng, Y., Thistlethwaite, J.R., Montag, A., Brady, W., Gibson, M.G., Linsley, P.S., and Bluestone, J.A.: **Long-term survival of xenogeneic pancreatic islet grafts induced by CTLA4Ig.** *Science* 1992, **257**:789-792.

Qin, S., Cobbold, S.P., Pope, H., Elliott, J., Kioussis, D., Davies, J., and Waldmann, H.: **'Infectious' transplantation tolerance.** *Science* 1993, **259**:974-977.

Waldmann, H., Cobbold, S., and Hale, G.: **What can be done to prevent graft versus host disease?** *Curr. Opin. Immunol.* 1994, **6**:777-783.

Yin, D. and Fathman, C.G.: **Induction of tolerance to heart allografts in high responder rats by combining anti-CD4 with CTLA4Ig.** *J. Immunol.* 1995, **155**:1655-1659.

13-8 Antibodies may be used to alleviate and suppress autoimmune disease.

Adorini, L., Guery, J.C., Rodriguez Tarduchy, G., and Trembleau, S.: **Selective immunosuppression.** *Immunol. Today.* 1993, **14**:285-289.

Chatenoud, L., Thervet, E., Primo, J., and Bach, J.F.: **Anti-CD3 antibody induces long-term remission of overt autoimmunity in nonobese diabetic mice.** *Proc. Natl. Acad. Sci.* 1994, **91**:123-127.

Maini, R.N., Elliott, M.J., Brennan, F.M., Williams, R.O., Chu, C.Q., Paleolog, E., Charles, P.J., Taylor, P.C., and Feldmann, M.: **Monoclonal anti-TNF alpha antibody as a probe of pathogenesis and therapy of rheumatoid disease.** *Immunol. Rev.* 1995, **144**:195-223.

Moreau, T., Thorpe, J., Miller, D., Moseley, I., Hale, G., Waldmann, H., Clayton, D., Wing, M., Scolding, N., and Compston, A.: **Preliminary evidence from magnetic resonance imaging for reduction in disease activity after lymphocyte depletion in multiple sclerosis.** *Lancet* 1994, **344**:298-301.

Riethmuller, G., Rieber, E.P., Kiefersauer, S., Prinz, J., van der Lubbe, P., Meiser, B., Breedveld, F., Eisenburg, J., Kruger, K., Deusch, K., and et al, : **From antilymphocyte serum to therapeutic monoclonal antibodies: first experiences with a chimeric CD4 antibody in the treatment of autoimmune disease.** *Immunol. Rev.* 1992, **129**:81-104.

13-9   Controlled administration of antigen can be used to manipulate the nature of an antigen-specific response.

Adorini, L., Guery, J.C., and Trembleau, S.: **Approaches toward peptide-based immunotherapy of autoimmune diseases.** *Springer Semin. Immunopathol.* 1992, **14**:187-199.

Fairchild, P.J. and Wraith, D.C.: **Peptide-MHC interaction in autoimmunity.** *Curr. Opin. Immunol.* 1992, **4**:748-753.

Metzler, B. and Wraith, D.C.: **Specific immunological non-responsiveness induced by antigens via mucosal surfaces.** *Adv. Exp. Med. Biol.* 1995, **371B**:1243-1244.

Smilek, D.E., Wraith, D.C., Hodgkinson, S., Dwivedy, S., Steinman, L., and McDevitt, H.O.: **A single amino acid change in a myelin basic protein peptide confers the capacity to prevent rather than induce experimental autoimmune encephalomyelitis.** *Proc. Natl. Acad. Sci. 1991*, **88**:9633-9637.

Tisch, R. and McDevitt, H.O.: **Antigen-specific immunotherapy: is it a real possibility to combat T-cell-mediated autoimmunity?** *Proc. Natl. Acad. Sci.* 1994, **91**:437-438.

Weiner, H.L., Mackin, G.A., Matsui, M., Orav, E.J., Khoury, S.J., Dawson, D.M., and Hafler, D.A.: **Double-blind pilot trial of oral tolerization with myelin antigens in multiple sclerosis.** *Science* 1993, **259**:1321-1324.

Weiner, H.L., Friedman, A., Miller, A., Khoury, S.J., al Sabbagh, A., Santos, L., Sayegh, M., Nussenblatt, R.B., Trentham, D.E., and Hafler, D.A.: **Oral tolerance: immunologic mechanisms and treatment of animal and human organ-specific autoimmune diseases by oral administration of autoantigens.** *Ann. Rev. Immunol.* 1994, **12**:809-837.

Wraith, D.C., Smilek, D.E., Mitchell, D.J., Steinman, L., and McDevitt, H.O.: **T cell recognition in experimental autoimmune encephalomyelitis: prospects for immune intervention with synthetic peptides.** *Intl. Rev. Immunol.* 1990, **6**:37-47.

13-10   Some tumors can be recognized and rejected by the immune system.

Boel, P., Wildmann, C., Sensi, M.L., Brasseur, R., Renauld, J.C., Coulie, P., Boon, T., and van der Bruggen, P.: **BAGE: A new gene encoding an antigen recognized on human melanomas by cytolytic T lymphocytes.** *Immunity 1995*, **2**:167-175.

Boon, T., Cerottini, J.C., Van den Eynde, B., van der Bruggen, P., and Van Pel, A.: **Tumor antigens recognized by T lymphocytes.** *Ann. Rev. Immunol.* 1994, **12**:337-365.

Cox, A.L., Skipper, J., Chen, Y., Henderson, R.A., Darrow, T.L., Shabanowitz, J., Engelhard, V.H., Hunt, D.F., and Slingluff, C.L.,Jr.: **Identification of a peptide recognized by five melanoma-specific human cytotoxic T cell lines.** *Science* 1994, **264**:716-719.

Finn, O.J.: **Tumor-rejection antigens recognized by T lymphocytes.** *Curr. Opin. Immunol.* 1993, **5**:701-708.

Slingluff, C.L.,Jr., Hunt, D.F., and Engelhard, V.H.: **Direct analysis of tumor-associated peptide antigens.** *Curr. Opin. Immunol.* 1994, **6**:733-740.

13-11   Tumors can escape rejection in many ways.

Bodmer, W.F., Browning, M.J., Krausa, P., Rowan, A., Bicknell, D.C., and Bodmer, J.G.: **Tumor escape from immune response by variation in HLA expression and other mechanisms.** *Ann. N. Y. Acad. Sci.* 1993, **690**:42-49.

Moller, P. and Hammerling, G.J.: **The role of surface HLA-A,B,C molecules in tumour immunity.** *Cancer Surv.* 1992, **13**:101-127.

Storkus, W.J., Howell, D.N., Salter, R.D., Dawson, J.R., and Cresswell, P.: **NK susceptibility varies inversely with target cell class I HLA antigen expression.** *J. Immunol.* 1987, **138**:1657-1659.

Tada, T., Ohzeki, S., Utsumi, K., Takiuchi, H., Muramatsu, M., Li, X.F., Shimizu, J., Fujiwara, H., and Hamaoka, T.: **Transforming growth factor-beta-induced inhibition of T cell function. Susceptibility difference in T cells of various phenotypes and functions and its relevance to immunosuppression in the tumor-bearing state.** *J. Immunol.* 1991, **146**:1077-1082.

Torre Amione, G., Beauchamp, R.D., Koeppen, H., Park, B.H., Schreiber, H., Moses, H.L., and Rowley, D.A.: **A highly immunogenic tumor transfected with a murine transforming growth factor type beta 1 cDNA escapes immune surveillance.** *Proc. Natl. Acad. Sci. 1990*, **87**:1486-1490.

13-12   Monoclonal antibodies to tumor antigens, alone or linked to toxins, can control tumor growth.

Grossbard, M.L., Press, O.W., Appelbaum, F.R., Bernstein, I.D., and Nadler, L.M.: **Monoclonal antibody-based therapies of leukemia and lymphoma.** *Blood* 1992, **80**:863-878.

Mack, M., Riethmuller, G., and Kufer, P.: **A small bispecific antibody construct expressed as a functional single-chain molecule with high tumor cell cytotoxicity.** *Proc. Natl. Acad. Sci. 1995*, **92**:7021-7025.

Pietersz, G.A., Krauer, K., and McKenzie, I.F.: **The use of monoclonal antibody immunoconjugates in cancer therapy.** *Adv. Exp. Med. Biol.* 1994, **353**:169-179.

Riethmuller, G., Schneider Gadicke, E., and Johnson, J.P.: **Monoclonal antibodies in cancer therapy.** *Curr. Opin. Immunol.* 1993, **5**:732-739.

Senter, P.D.: **Activation of prodrugs by antibody-enzyme conjugates: a new approach to cancer therapy.** *FASEB J.* 1990, **4**:188-193.

Vitetta, E.S. and Uhr, J.W.: **Monoclonal antibodies as agonists: an expanded role for their use in cancer therapy.** *Cancer Res.* 1994, **54**:5301-5309.

13-13   Enhancing the immunogenicity of tumors holds promise for cancer therapy.

Cayeux, S., Beck, C., Aicher, A., Dorken, B., and Blankenstein, T.: **Tumor cells cotransfected with interleukin-7 and B7.1 genes induce CD25 and CD28 on tumor-infiltrating T lymphocytes and are strong vaccines.** *Eur. J. Immunol.* 1995, **25**:2325-2331.

Chen, L., Linsley, P.S., and Hellstrom, K.E.: **Costimulation of T cells for tumor immunity.** *Immunol. Today* 1993, **14**:483-486.

Dranoff, G., Jaffee, E., Lazenby, A., Golumbek, P., Levitsky, H., Brose, K., Jackson, V., Hamada, H., Pardoll, D., and Mulligan, R.C.: **Vaccination with irradiated tumor cells engineered to secrete murine granulocyte-macrophage colony-stimulating factor stimulates potent, specific, and long-lasting anti-tumor immunity.** *Proc. Natl. Acad. Sci. 1993*, **90**:3539-3543.

Leach, D.R., Krummel, M.F., and Allison, J.P.: **Enhancement of antitumor immunity by CTLA-4 blockade**. *Science* 1996, **271**:1734-1736.

Pardoll, D.M.: **New strategies for enhancing the immunogenicity of tumors**. *Curr. Opin. Immunol.* 1993, **5**:719-725.

Pardoll, D.M.: **Paracrine cytokine adjuvants in cancer immunotherapy**. *Ann. Rev. Immunol.* 1995, **13**:399-415.

Townsend, S.E. and Allison, J.P.: **Tumor rejection after direct costimulation of CD8$^+$ T cells by B7-transfected melanoma cells**. *Science* 1993, **259**:368-370.

13-14 There are several requirements for an effective vaccine.

Ada, G.L.: **The immunological principles of vaccination**. *Lancet* 1990, **335**:523-526.

Rabinovich, N.R., McInnes, P., Klein, D.L., and Hall, B.F.: **Vaccine technologies: view to the future**. *Science* 1994, **265**:1401-1404.

Nichol, K.L., Lind, A., Margolis, K.L., Murdoch, M., McFadden, R., Hauge, M., Magnan, S., and Drake, M.: **The effectiveness of vaccination against influenza in healthy, working adults**. *N. Engl. J. Med.* 1995, **333**:889-893.

13-15 The history of vaccination against *Bordetella pertussis* illustrates the importance of achieving an effective vaccine that is perceived to be safe.

Greco, D., Salmaso, S., Mastrantonio, P., Giuliano, M., Tozzi, A.E., Anemona, A., Ciofi degli Atti, M.L., Giammanco, A., Panei, P., Blackwelder, W.C., Klein, D.L., and Wassilak, S.G.: **A controlled trial of two acellular vaccines and one whole-cell vaccine against pertussis. Progetto Pertosse Working Group**. *N. Engl. J. Med.* 1996, **334**:341-348.

Mortimer, E.A.: **Pertussis vaccines**. In Plotkin, S.A., and Mortimer, E.A.: *Vaccines*, 2nd edn. Philadelphia, W.B. Saunders Co., 1994, 91-135.

13-16 Conjugate vaccines have been developed as a result of understanding how T and B cells collaborate in an immune response.

van den Dobbelsteen, G.P. and van Rees, E.P.: **Mucosal immune responses to pneumococcal polysaccharides: implications for vaccination**. *Trends Microbiol.* 1995, **3**:155-159.

Paoletti, L.C., Wessels, M.R., Michon, F., DiFabio, J., Jennings, H.J., and Kasper, D.L.: **Group B Streptococcus type II polysaccharide-tetanus toxoid conjugate vaccine**. *Infect. Immun.* 1992, **60**:4009-4014.

Peltola, H., Kilpi, T., and Anttila, M.: **Rapid disappearance of Haemophilus influenzae type b meningitis after routine childhood immunisation with conjugate vaccines**. *Lancet* 1992, **340**:592-594.

13-17 The use of adjuvants is another important approach to enhancing the immunogenicity of vaccines.

Alving, C.R., Koulchin, V., Glenn, G.M., and Rao, M.: **Liposomes as carriers of peptide antigens: induction of antibodies and cytotoxic T lymphocytes to conjugated and unconjugated peptides**. *Immunol. Rev.* 1995, **145**:5-31.

Audibert, F.M. and Lise, L.D.: **Adjuvants: current status, clinical perspectives and future prospects**. *Immunol. Today.* 1993, **14**:281-284.

Gupta, R.K. and Siber, G.R.: **Adjuvants for human vaccines—current status, problems and future prospects**. *Vaccine* 1995, **13**:1263-1276.

Rhodes, J., Chen, H., Hall, S.R., Beesley, J.E., Jenkins, D.C., Collins, P., and Zheng, B.: **Therapeutic potentiation of the immune system by costimulatory Schiff-base-forming drugs**. *Nature* 1995, **376**:71-75.

Takahashi, H., Takeshita, T., Morein, B., Putney, S., Germain, R.N., and Berzofsky, J.A.: **Induction of CD8$^+$ cytotoxic T cells by immunization with purified HIV-1 envelope protein in ISCOMs**. *Nature* 1990, **344**:873-875.

Vogel, F.R.: **Immunologic adjuvants for modern vaccine formulations**. *Ann. N. Y. Acad. Sci.* 1995, **754**:153-160.

13-18 Live-attenuated viral vaccines are more potent than "killed" vaccines and can now be made safer using recombinant DNA technology.

Connell, N., Stover, C.K., and Jacobs, W.R.,Jr.: **Old microbes with new faces: molecular biology and the design of new vaccines**. *Curr. Opin. Immunol.* 1992, **4**:442-448.

Gilsdorf, J.R.: **Vaccines: moving into the molecular era**. *J. Pediatr.* 1994, **125**:339-344.

Perkus, M.E., Tartaglia, J., and Paoletti, E.: **Poxvirus-based vaccine candidates for cancer, AIDS, and other infectious diseases**. *J. Leuk. Biol.* 1995, **58**:1-13.

13-19 Live-attenuated bacterial vaccines can be developed by selecting non-pathogenic or disabled mutants.

Dougan, G.: **The molecular basis for the virulence of bacterial pathogens: implications for oral vaccine development**. *Microbiology 1994*, **140**:215-224.

Guleria, I., Teitelbaum, R., McAdam, R.A., Kalpana, G., Jacobs, W.R.,Jr., and Bloom, B.R.: **Auxotrophic vaccines for tuberculosis**. *Nat. Med.* 1996, **2**:334-337.

13-20 Attenuated micro-organisms can serve as vectors for vaccination against many pathogens.

Brochier, B., Kieny, M.P., Costy, F., Coppens, P., Bauduin, B., Lecocq, J.P., Languet, B., Chappuis, G., Desmettre, P., Afiademanyo, K., et al, : **Large-scale eradication of rabies using recombinant vaccinia-rabies vaccine**. *Nature* 1991, **354**:520-522.

Chatfield, S., Roberts, M., Londono, P., Cropley, I., Douce, G., and Dougan, G.: **The development of oral vaccines based on live attenuated Salmonella strains**. *FEMS Immunol. Med. Microbiol.* 1993, **7**:1-7.

Chatfield, S.N., Roberts, M., Dougan, G., Hormaeche, C., and Khan, C.M.: **The development of oral vaccines against parasitic diseases utilizing live attenuated Salmonella**. *Parasitology 1995*, **110 Suppl**:S17-S24.

Cirillo, J.D., Stover, C.K., Bloom, B.R., Jacobs, W.R.,Jr., and Barletta, R.G.: **Bacterial vaccine vectors and bacillus Calmette-Guerin**. *Clin. Infect. Dis.* 1995, **20**:1001-1009.

Moss, B.: **Vaccinia and other poxvirus expression vectors**. *Curr. Opin. Biotech.* 1992, **3**:518-522.

13-21 Synthetic peptides of protective antigens can elicit protective immunity.

Berzofsky, J.A.: **Mechanisms of T cell recognition with application to vaccine design**. *Mol. Immunol.* 1991, **28**:217-223.

Berzofsky, J.A.: **Epitope selection and design of synthetic vaccines. Molecular approaches to enhancing immunogenicity and cross-reactivity of engineered vaccines**. *Ann. N. Y. Acad. Sci.* 1993, **690**:256-264.

Hill, A.V., Elvin, J., Willis, A.C., Aidoo, M., Allsopp, C.E., Gotch, F.M., Gao, X.M., Takiguchi, M., Greenwood, B.M., Townsend, A.R., et al.: **Molecular analysis of the association of HLA-B53 and resistance to severe malaria**. *Nature* 1992, **360**:434-439.

Lalvani, A., Aidoo, M., Allsopp, C.E., Plebanski, M., Whittle, H.C., and Hill, A.V.: **An HLA-based approach to the design of a CTL-inducing vaccine against Plasmodium falciparum**. *Res. Immunol.* 1994, **145**:461-468.

13-22 The route of vaccination is an important determinant of success.

Douce, G., Turcotte, C., Cropley, I., Roberts, M., Pizza, M., Domenghini, M., Rappuoli, R., and Dougan, G.: **Mutants of Escherichia coli heat-labile toxin lacking ADP-ribosyltransferase activity act as nontoxic, mucosal adjuvants.** *Proc. Natl. Acad. Sci. 1995,* **92**:1644-1648.

Dougan, G.: **The molecular basis for the virulence of bacterial pathogens: implications for oral vaccine development.** *Microbiology* 1994, **140**:215-224.

Holmgren, J., Czerkinsky, C., Lycke, N., and Svennerholm, A.M.: **Strategies for the induction of immune responses at mucosal surfaces making use of cholera toxin B subunit as immunogen, carrier, and adjuvant.** *Am. J. Trop. Med. Hyg.* 1994, **50**:42-54.

Ivanoff, B., Levine, M.M., and Lambert, P.H.: **Vaccination against typhoid fever: present status.** *Bull. WHO* 1994, **72**:957-971.

Levine, M.M.: **Modern vaccines. Enteric infections.** *Lancet* 1990, **335**:958-961.

Roberts, M., Bacon, A., Rappuoli, R., Pizza, M., Cropley, I., Douce, G., Dougan, G., Marinaro, M., McGhee, J., and Chatfield, S.: **A mutant pertussis toxin molecule that lacks ADP-ribosyltransferase activity, PT-9K/129G, is an effective mucosal adjuvant for intranasally delivered proteins.** *Infect. Immun.* 1995, **63**:2100-2108.

Staats, H.F., Jackson, R.J., Marinaro, M., Takahashi, I., Kiyono, H., and McGhee, J.R.: **Mucosal immunity to infection with implications for vaccine development.** *Curr. Opin. Immunol.* 1994, **6**:572-583.

Takahashi, I., Marinaro, M., Kiyono, H., Jackson, R.J., Nakagawa, I., Fujihashi, K., Hamada, S., Clements, J.D., Bost, K.L., and McGhee, J.R.: **Mechanisms for mucosal immunogenicity and adjuvancy of Escherichia coli labile enterotoxin.** *J. Infect. Dis.* 1996, **173**:627-635.

13-23 An important question is whether vaccination can be used therapeutically to control existing chronic infections.

Burke, R.L.: **Contemporary approaches to vaccination against herpes simplex virus.** *Curr. Top. Microbiol. Immunol.* 1992, **179**:137-158.

Hill, A., Jugovic, P., York, I., Russ, G., Bennink, J., Yewdell, J., Ploegh, H., and Johnson, D.: **Herpes simplex virus turns off the TAP to evade host immunity.** *Nature* 1995, **375**:411-415.

Farrell, H.E., McLean, C.S., Harley, C., Efstathiou, S., Inglis, S., and Minson, A.C.: **Vaccine potential of a herpes simplex virus type 1 mutant with an essential glycoprotein deleted.** *J. Virol.* 1994, **68**:927-932.

Lewandowski, G.A., Lo, D., and Bloom, F.E.: **Interference with major histocompatibility complex class II-restricted antigen presentation in the brain by herpes simplex virus type 1: a possible mechanism of evasion of the immune response.** *Proc. Natl. Acad. Sci. 1993,* **90**:2005-2009.

Modlin, R.L.: **T$_H$1-T$_H$2 paradigm: insights from leprosy.** *J. Invest. Dermatol.* 1994, **102**:828-832.

Reiner, S.L. and Locksley, R.M.: **The regulation of immunity to Leishmania major.** *Ann. Rev. Immunol.* 1995, **13**:151-177.

Stanberry, L.R.: **Herpes simplex virus vaccines as immunotherapeutic agents.** *Trends Microbiol.* 1995, **3**:244-247.

Stanford, J.L.: **The history and future of vaccination and immunotherapy for leprosy.** *Trop. Geog. Med.* 1994, **46**:93-107.

Stanford, J.L. and Grange, J.M.: **The promise of immunotherapy for tuberculosis.** *Respir. Med.* 1994, **88**:3-7.

13-24 Modulation of the immune system may be used to inhibit immunopathological responses to infectious agents.

Afonso, L.C., Scharton, T.M., Vieira, L.Q., Wysocka, M., Trinchieri, G., and Scott, P.: **The adjuvant effect of interleukin-12 in a vaccine against Leishmania major.** *Science* 1994, **263**:235-237.

Biron, C.A. and Gazzinelli, R.T.: **Effects of IL-12 on immune responses to microbial infections: a key mediator in regulating disease outcome.** *Curr. Opin. Immunol.* 1995, **7**:485-496.

Gallin, J.I., Farber, J.M., Holland, S.M., and Nutman, T.B.: **Interferon-gamma in the management of infectious diseases [clinical conference].** *Ann. Intl. Med.* 1995, **123**:216-224.

Grau, G.E. and Modlin, R.L.: **Immune mechanisms in bacterial and parasitic diseases: protective immunity versus pathology.** *Curr. Opin. Immunol.* 1991, **3**:480-485.

Kaplan, G.: **Recent advances in cytokine therapy in leprosy.** *J. Infect. Dis.* 1993, **167 Suppl. 1**:S18-S22.

Locksley, R.M.: **Interleukin-12 in host defense against microbial pathogens.** *Proc. Natl. Acad. Sci. 1993,* **90**:5879-5880.

Murray, H.W.: **Interferon-gamma and host antimicrobial defense: current and future clinical applications.** *Am. J. Med.* 1994, **97**:459-467.

Nabors, G.S., Afonso, L.C., Farrell, J.P., and Scott, P.: **Switch from a type 2 to a type 1 T helper cell response and cure of established Leishmania major infection in mice is induced by combined therapy with interleukin 12 and Pentostam.** *Proc. Natl. Acad. Sci. 1995,* **92**:3142-3146.

Puccetti, P., Romani, L., and Bistoni, F.: **A T$_H$1-T$_H$2-like switch in candidiasis: new perspectives for therapy.** *Trends Microbiol.* 1995, **3**:237-240.

Sher, A., Gazzinelli, R.T., Oswald, I.P., Clerici, M., Kullberg, M., Pearce, E.J., Berzofsky, J.A., Mosmann, T.R., James, S.L., and Morse, H.C.: **Role of T-cell derived cytokines in the downregulation of immune responses in parasitic and retroviral infection.** *Immunol. Rev.* 1992, **127**:183-204.

Wynn, T.A., Cheever, A.W., Jankovic, D., Poindexter, R.W., Caspar, P., Lewis, F.A., and Sher, A.: **An IL-12-based vaccination method for preventing fibrosis induced by schistosome infection.** *Nature* 1995, **376**:594-596.

13-25 Protective immunity can be induced by injecting DNA encoding microbial antigens and human cytokines into muscle.

Donnelly, J.J., Friedman, A., Martinez, D., Montgomery, D.L., Shiver, J.W., Motzel, S.L., Ulmer, J.B., and Liu, M.A.: **Preclinical efficacy of a prototype DNA vaccine: enhanced protection against antigenic drift in influenza virus.** *Nat. Med.* 1995, **1**:583-587.

McDonnell, W.M. and Askari, F.K.: **DNA vaccines.** *N. Engl. J. Med.* 1996, **334**:42-45.

Pardoll, D.M. and Beckerleg, A.M.: **Exposing the immunology of naked DNA vaccines.** *Immunity 1995,* **3**:165-169.

Ulmer, J.B., Donnelly, J.J., Deck, R.R., DeWitt, C.M., and Liu, M.A.: **Immunization against viral proteins with naked DNA.** *Ann. N. Y. Acad. Sci.* 1995, **772**:117-125.

CD antigen	Cellular expression	Molecular weight (kDa)	Functions	Other names	Family relationships
CD54	Hematopoietic and non-hematopoietic cells	75–115	Intercellular adhesion molecule (ICAM)-1, binds CD11a/CD18 integrin (LFA-1) and CD11b/CD18 integrin (Mac-1), receptor for rhinovirus	ICAM-1	Immunoglobulin superfamily
CD55	Hematopoietic and non-hematopoietic cells	60–70	Decay accelerating factor (DAF), binds C3b, disassembles C3/C5 convertase	DAF	CCP superfamily
CD56	NK cells	135–220	Isoform of neural cell adhesion molecule (NCAM), adhesion molecule	NKH-I	Immunoglobulin superfamily
CD57	NK cells, subsets of T cells, B cells, and monocytes		Oligosaccharide, found on many cell-surface glycoproteins	HNK-1, Leu-7	
CD58	Hematopoietic and non-hematopoietic cells	55–70	Leukocyte function-associated antigen-3 (LFA-3), binds CD2, adhesion molecule	LFA-3	Immunoglobulin superfamily
CD59	Hematopoietic and non-hematopoietic cells	19	Binds complement components C8 and C9, blocks assembly of membrane-attack complex	Protectin, Mac inhibitor	
CDw60	T-cell subsets, platelets, monocytes		9-O-acetylated disialyl group present on gangliosides, predominantly ganglioside D3		
CD61	Platelets, megakaryocytes, macrophages	110	Integrin β_3 subunit, associates with CD41 (GPIIb/IIIa) or CD51 (vitronectin receptor)		Integrin β
CD62E	Endothelium	140	Endothelium leukocyte adhesion molecule (ELAM), binds sialyl-Lewis x, mediates rolling interaction of neutrophils on endothelium	ELAM-1, E-selectin	C-type lectin, EGF and CCP superfamily
CD62L	B cells, T cells, monocytes, NK cells	150	Leukocyte adhesion molecule (LAM), binds CD34, GlyCAM, mediates rolling interactions with endothelium	LAM-1, L-selectin, LECAM-1	C-type lectin, EGF and CCP superfamily
CD62P	Platelets, megakaryocytes, endothelium	140	Adhesion molecule, binds PSGL-1, mediates interaction of platelets with endothelial cells, monocytes and rolling interaction of leukocytes on endothelium	P-selectin, PADGEM	C-type lectin, EGF and CCP superfamily
CD63	Activated platelets, monocytes, macrophages	53	Unknown, is lysosomal membrane protein translocated to cell surface after activation	Platelet activation antigen	Transmembrane 4 superfamily
CD64	Monocytes, macrophages	72	High affinity receptor for IgG, binds IgG3>IgG1>IgG4>>>IgG2, mediates phagocytosis, antigen capture, ADCC	FCγRI	Immunoglobulin superfamily
CD65	Myeloid cells		Oligosaccharide component of a ceramide dodecasaccharide		
CD66a	Neutrophils	160–180	Unknown, member of carcinoembryonic antigen (CEA) family (see below)	Biliary glycoprotein-1 (BGP-1)	Immunoglobulin superfamily
CD66b	Granulocytes	95–100	Unknown, member of carcinoembryonic antigen (CEA) family	Previously CD67	Immunoglobulin superfamily

CD antigen	Cellular expression	Molecular weight (kDa)	Functions	Other names	Family relationships
CD66c	Neutrophils, colon carcinoma	90	Unknown, member of carcinoembryonic antigen (CEA) family	Non-specific cross-reacting antigen (NCA)	Immunoglobulin superfamily
CD66d	Neutrophils	30	Unknown, member of carcinoembryonic antigen (CEA) family		Immunoglobulin superfamily
CD66e	Adult colon epithelium, colon carcinoma	180–200	Unknown, member of carcinoembryonic antigen (CEA) family	Carcinoembryonic antigen (CEA)	Immunoglobulin superfamily
CD66f	Unknown		Unknown, member of carcinoembryonic antigen (CEA) family	Pregnancy specific glycoprotein	Immunoglobulin superfamily
CD68	Monocytes, macrophages, neutrophils, basophils, large lymphocytes	110	Unknown	Macrosialin	
CD69	Activated T and B cells, activated macrophages and NK cells	28,32 homodimer	Unknown, early activation antigen	Activation inducer molecule (AIM)	C-type lectin
CD70	Activated T and B cells, and macrophages	75,95,170	Ligand for CD27, may function in co-stimulation of B and T cells	Ki-24	TNF-like
CD71	All proliferating cells, hence activated leukocytes	95 homodimer	Transferrin receptor	T9	
CD72	B cells (not plasma cells)	42 homodimer	Unknown, ligand for CD5	Lyb-2	C-type lectin
CD73	B-cell subsets, T-cell subsets	69	Ecto-5′-nucleotidase, dephosphorylates nucleotides to allow nucleoside uptake		
CD74	B cells, macrophages, monocytes, MHC class II positive cells	33, 35, 41, 43 (alternative initiation and splicing)	MHC class II-associated invariant chain	Ii, Iγ	
CD75	Mature B cells, T-cell subsets		Sialoglycan moiety, ligand for CD22, mediates B cell:B cell adhesion		
CD76	Mature B cells, T-cell subsets		α 2,6 sialylated polylactosamine expressed on glycosphingolipids and glycoproteins		
CD77	Germinal center B cells		Neutral glycosphingolipid (Galα1→4Galβ1→4Glcβ1→ ceramide), binds Shiga toxin, crosslinking induces apoptosis	Globotriaocylcer-amide (Gb₃), P^k blood group	
CDw78	B cells		Unknown	Ba	
CD79α,β	B cells	α: 40–45 β: 37	Components of B-cell antigen receptor analogous to CD3, required for cell-surface expression and signal transduction	Igα, Igβ	Immunoglobulin superfamily
CD80	B-cell subset	60	Co-stimulator, ligand for CD28 and CTLA-4	B7 (now B7.1), BB1	Immunoglobulin superfamily
CD81	Lymphocytes	26	Associates with CD19, CD21 to form B cell co-receptor	Target of antiproliferative antibody (TAPA-1)	Transmembrane 4 superfamily
CD82	Leukocytes	50–53	Unknown	R2	Transmembrane 4 superfamily

CD antigen	Cellular expression	Molecular weight (kDa)	Functions	Other names	Family relationships
CDw84	Monocytes, platelets, circulating B cells	73	Unknown	GR6	
CD85	Monocytes, circulating B cells	120,83	Unknown	GR4	
CD86	Monocytes, activated B cells, dendritic cells	80	Ligand for CD28 and CTLA4	B7.2	Immunoglobulin superfamily
CD87	Granulocytes, monocytes, macrophages, T cells, NK cells, wide variety of non-hematopioetic cell types	35–59	Receptor for urokinase plasminogen activator	uPAR	Ly-6 superfamily
CD88	Polymorphonuclear leukocytes, macrophages, mast cells	43	Receptor for complement component C5a	C5aR	G protein coupled receptor superfamily
CD89	Monocytes, macrophages, granulocytes, neutrophils, B-cell subsets, T-cell subsets	50–70	IgA receptor	FcαR	Immunoglobulin superfamily
CD90	CD34+ prothymocytes (human) thymocytes, T cells (mouse)	18	Unknown	Thy-1	Immunoglobulin superfamily
CD91	Monocytes, many non-hematopoietic cells	515, 85 dimer	α_2-macroglobulin receptor		EGF, LDL receptor superfamily
CDw92	Neutrophils, monocytes, platelets, endothelium	70	Unknown	GR9	
CD93	Neutrophils, monocytes, endothelium	120	Unknown	GR11	
CD94	T-cell subsets, NK cells	43	Unknown	KP43	
CD95	Wide variety of cell lines, in vivo distribution uncertain	43	Binds TNF-like Fas ligand, induces apoptosis	Apo-1, Fas	NGF receptor superfamily
CD96	Activated T cells, NK cells	160	Unknown	T-cell activation increased late expression (TACTILE)	Immunoglobulin superfamily
CD97	Activated B and T cells, monocytes, granulocytes	75–85	Binds CD55	GR1	EGF, G protein coupled receptor superfamily
CD98	T cells, B cells, natural killer cells, granulocytes, all human cell lines	80,45 heterodimer	May be amino-acid transporter	4F2, FRP-1	
CD99	Peripheral blood lymphocytes, thymocytes	32	Unknown	MIC2, E2	
CD100	Hematopoietic cells	150 homodimer	Unknown	GR3	
CD101	Monocytes, granulocytes, dendritic cells, activated T cells	120 homodimer	Unknown	BPC#4	Immunoglobulin superfamily
CD102	Resting lymphocytes, monocytes, vascular endothelial cells (strongest)	55–65	Binds CD11a/CD18 (LFA-1) but not CD11b/CD18 (Mac-1)	ICAM-2	Immunoglobulin superfamily
CD103	Intraepithelial lymphocytes, 2–6% peripheral blood lymphocytes	150,25	α_E integrin	HML-1, α_6, α_E integrin	Integrin α
CD104	CD4− CD8− thymocytes, neuronal, epithelial, and some endothelial cells, Schwann cells, trophoblasts	220	Integrin β_4, associates with CD49f, binds laminins	β_4 integrin	Integrin β
CD105	Endothelial cells, activated monocytes and macrophages, bone-marrow cell subsets	90 homodimer	Binds TGF-β	Endoglin	
CD106	Endothelial cells	100, 110	Adhesion molecule, ligand for VLA-4	VCAM-1	Immunoglobulin superfamily

CD antigen	Cellular expression	Molecular weight (kDa)	Functions	Other names	Family relationships
CD107a	Activated platelets, activated T cells, activated neutrophils, activated endothelium	110	Unknown, is lysosomal membrane protein translocated to the cell surface after activation	Lysosomal associated membrane protein-1 (LAMP-1)	
CD107b	Activated platelets, activated T cells, activated neutrophils, activated endothelium	120	Unknown, is lysosomal membrane protein translocated to the cell surface after activation	LAMP-2	
CDw108	Erythrocytes, circulating lymphocytes, lymphoblasts	80	Unknown	GR2, John Milton-Hagen blood group antigen	
CD109	Activated T cells, activated platelets, vascular endothelium	170	Unknown	Platelet activation factor, GR56	
CD110–CD113	Not yet assigned				
CD114	Granulocytes, monocytes	95, 139	Granulocyte colony stimulating factor (G-CSF) receptor		
CD115	Monocytes, macrophages	150	Macrophage colony stimulating factor (M-CSF) receptor	M-CSFR, c-fms	Immunoglobulin superfamily, tyrosine kinase
CD116	Monocytes, neutrophils, eosinophils, endothelium	70–85	Granulocyte macrophage colony stimulating factor (GM-CSF) receptor α chain	GM-CSFRα	Cytokine receptor superfamily, fibronectin type III superfamily
CD117	Hematopoietic progenitors	145	Stem cell factor (SCF) receptor	c-kit	Immunoglobulin superfamily, tyrosine kinase
CD118	Broad cellular expression		Interferon-α,β receptor	IFN-α,βR	
CD119	Macrophages, monocytes, B cells, endothelium	90–100	Interferon-γ receptor	IFN-γR	
CD120a	Hematopoietic and non-hematopoietic cells, highest on epithelial cells	50–60	TNF receptor, binds both TNF-α and TNF-β	TNFR-I	TNF receptor superfamily
CD120b	Hematopoietic and non-hematopoietic cells, highest on myeloid cells	75–85	TNF receptor, binds both TNF-α and TNF-β	TNFR-II	TNF receptor superfamily
CD121a	Thymocytes, T cells	80	Type I interleukin-1 receptor, binds IL-1α and IL-1β	IL-1R type I	Immunoglobulin superfamily
CDw121b	B cells, macrophages, monocytes	60–70	Type II interleukin-1 receptor, binds IL-1α and IL-1β	IL-1R type II	Immunoglobulin superfamily
CD122	NK cells, resting T-cell subsets, some B-cell lines	75	IL-2 receptor β chain	IL-2Rβ	Cytokine receptor superfamily, fibronectin type III superfamily
CD123	Bone marrow stem cells, granulocytes, monocytes, megakaryocytes	70	IL-3 receptor α chain	IL-3Rα	Cytokine receptor superfamily, fibronectin type III superfamily
CD124	Mature B and T cells, hematopoietic precursor cells	130–150	IL-4 receptor	IL-4R	Cytokine receptor superfamily, fibronectin type III superfamily
CD125	Eosinophils, basophils, activated B cells	55–60	IL-5 receptor	IL-5R	Cytokine receptor superfamily, fibronectin type III superfamily

CD antigen	Cellular expression	Molecular weight (kDa)	Functions	Other names	Family relationships
CD126	Activated B cells and plasma cells (strong), most leukocytes (weak)	80	IL-6 receptor α subunit	IL-6Rα	Immunoglobulin superfamily, cytokine receptor superfamily, fibronectin type III superfamily
CD127	Bone marrow lymphoid precursors, pro-B cells, mature T cells, monocytes	68–79, possibly forms homodimers	IL-7 receptor	IL-7R	Fibronectin type III superfamily
CDw128	Neutrophils, basophils, T-cell subsets	58–67	IL-8 receptor	IL-8R	G protein coupled receptor superfamily
CD129	Not yet assigned				
CD130	Most cell types, strong on activated B cells and plasma cells	130	Common subunit of IL-6, IL-11, oncostatin-M (OSM) and leukemia inhibitory factor (LIF) receptors	IL-6Rβ, IL-11Rβ, OSMRβ, LIFRβ	Immunoglobulin superfamily, cytokine receptor superfamily, fibronectin type III superfamily
CDw131	Myeloid progenitors, granulocytes	140	Common β subunit of IL-3, IL-5, and GM-CSF receptors	IL-3Rβ, IL-5Rβ, GM-CSFRβ	Cytokine receptor superfamily, fibronectin type III superfamily
CD132	B cells, T cells, NK cells, mast cells, neutrophils	64	IL-2 receptor γ chain, common subunit of IL-2, IL-4, IL-7, IL-9, and IL-15 receptors		Cytokine receptor superfamily
CD134	Activated T cells	50	May act as adhesion molecule costimulator	OX40	TNF receptor superfamily
CD135	Multipotential precursors, myelomonocytic and B-cell progenitors	130,155	Growth factor receptor	FLK2, STK-1	Tyrosine kinase
CDw136	Monocytes, epithelial cells, central and peripheral nervous system	180	Chemotaxis, phagocytosis, cell growth and differentiation	MSP-R, RON	Tyrosine kinase
CDw137	T and B lymphocytes, monocytes, some epithelial cells		Co-stimulator of T-cell proliferation	ILA (induced by lymphocyte activation), 4-1BB	TNF receptor superfamily
CD138	B cells		Heparan sulphate proteoglycan, binds collagen type I	Syndecan-1	
CD139	B cells	209,228	Unknown		
CD140a,b	Stromal cells, some endothelial cells	a: 180 b: 180	Platelet derived growth factor (PDGF) receptor α and β chains		
CD141	Vascular endothelial cells	105	Anticoagulant, binds thrombin, the complex then activates protein C	Thrombomodulin, fetomodulin	C-type lectin, EGF
CD142	Epidemal keratinocytes, various epithelial cells, astrocytes, Schwann cells. Absent from cells in direct contact with plasma unless induced by inflammatory mediators	45–47	Major initiating factor of clotting. Binds Factor VIIa; this complex activates Factors VII, IX, and X	Tissue factor, thromboplastin	Fibronectin type III superfamily
CD143	Endothelial cells, except large blood vessels and kidney, epithelial cells of brush borders of kidney and small intestine, neuronal cells, activated macrophages and some T cells. Soluble form in plasma	170–180	Zn^{2+} metallopeptidase, dipeptidyl pedtidase, cleaves angiotensin I and bradykinin from precursor forms	Angiotensin converting enzyme (ACE)	

CD antigen	Cellular expression	Molecular weight (kDa)	Functions	Other names	Family relationships
CD145	Endothelial cells, some stromal cells	25, 90, 110	Unknown		
CD146	Endothelium	130	Potential adhesion molecule, localized at cell:cell junctions	MCAM, MUC18,S-ENDO	Immunoglobulin superfamily
CD147	Leukocytes, red blood cells, platelets, endothelial cells	55–65	Potential adhesion molecule	M6, neurothelin, EMMPRIN, basigin, OX-47	Immunoglobulin superfamily
CD148	Granulocytes, monocytes, dendritic cells, T cells, fibroblasts, nerve cells	240–260	Contact inhibition of cell growth	HPTPη	Fibronectin type III superfamily, protein tyrosine phosphatase
CD151	Platelets, megakaryocytes, epithelial cells, endothelial cells	32	Associates with β1 integrins	PETA-3, SFA-1	Transmembrane 4 superfamily
CD152	Activated T cells	33	Ligand for B7.1 (CD80), B7.2 (CD86); negative regulator of T-cell activation	CTLA-4	Immunoglobulin superfamily
CD153	Activated T cells, activated macrophages, neutrophils, B cells	38–40	Ligand for CD30, may co-stimulate T cells	CD30L	TNF superfamily
CD154	Activated CD4 T cells	28,30,33	Ligand for CD40, inducer of B cell proliferation and activation	CD40L, TRAP, T-BAM, gp39	TNF receptor family
CD155	Monocytes, macrophages, thymocytes, CNS neurons	80–90	Normal function unknown; receptor for poliovirus	Poliovirus receptor	Immunoglobulin superfamily
CD156	Neutrophils, monocytes	69	Unknown, may be involved in leukocyte extravasation	MS2, ADAM 8 (A disintegrin and metalloprotease)	
CD157	Granulocytes, monocytes, bone marrow stromal cells, vascular endothelial cells, follicular dendritic cells	42–45 (50 on monocytes)	ADP-ribosyl cyclase, cyclic ADP-ribose hydrolase	BST-1	
CD158a	NK-cell subsets	50 or 58	Inhibits NK cell cytotoxicity on binding MHC class I molecules	p50.1, p58.1	Immunoglobulin superfamily
CD158b	NK-cell subsets	50 or 58	Inhibits NK cell cytotoxicity on binding HLA-Cw3 and related alleles	p50.2, p58.2	Immunoglobulin superfamily
CD161	NK cells, T cells	44	Regulates NK cytotoxicity	NKRP1	C-type lectin
CD163	Monocytes, macrophages	130	Unknown	M130	
CD166	Activated T cells, thymic epithelium, fibroblasts, neurons	100–105	Ligand for CD6, involved in neurite extension	ALCAM, BEN, DM-GRASP, SC-1	Immunoglobulin superfamily

Appendix II. Cytokines and their receptors.						
Family	Cytokine (alternative names)	Size (no. of amino acids) and form	Receptors (c denotes common subunit)	Producer cells	Actions	Effect of cytokine or receptor knock-out (where known)
Hematopoietins (four-helix bundles)	Epo (erythropoietin)	165, monomer*	EpoR	Kidney	Stimulates erythroid progenitors	
	IL-2 (T-cell growth factor)	133, monomer	CD25 (α), CD122 (β),γc	T cells	T-cell proliferation	IL-2: decreased T-cell proliferation; premature death IL-2Rα: Incomplete T-cell development
	IL-3 (multicolony CSF)	133, monomer	CD123, βc	T cells, thymic epithelial cells	Synergistic action in early hematopoiesis	IL-3: impaired eosinophil development. Bone marrow unresponsive to IL-5, GM-CSF
	IL-4 (BCGF-1, BSF-1)	129, monomer	CD124, γc	T cells, mast cells	B-cell activation, IgE switch	IL-4: decreased IgE synthesis
	IL-5 (BCGF-2)	115, homodimer	CD125, βc	T cells, mast cells	Eosinophil growth, differentiation	IL-5: decreased IgE, IgG1 synthesis; levels of IL-9, IL-10 decreased
	IL-6 (IFN-β2, BSF-2, BCDF)	184, monomer	CD126, CD 130	T cells, macrophages	T- and B-cell growth and differentiation, acute phase protein production	IL-6: decreased acute phase reaction, reduced IgA production
	IL-7	152, monomer*	CD127, γc	Bone marrow stroma	Growth of pre-B cells and pre-T cells	IL-7: Early lymphocyte expansion severely impaired
	IL-9	125, monomer	IL-9R, γc	T cells	Mast cell enhancing activity	
	IL-11	178, monomer	IL-11R, CD130	Stromal fibroblasts	Synergistic action with IL-3 and IL-4 in hematopoiesis	
	IL-13 (P600)	132, monomer	IL-13R, γc	T cells	B-cell growth and differentiation, inhibits macrophage inflammatory cytokine production	
	G-CSF	?, monomer*	G-CSFR	Fibroblasts	Stimulates neutrophil development	
	IL-15 (T-cell growth factor)	114, monomer	IL-15R, γc	T cells	IL-2-like, stimulates growth of intestinal epithelium	
	GM-CSF (granulocyte macrophage colony stimulating family)	127, monomer*	CD116, βc	Macrophages, T cells	Stimulates growth and differentiation of myelomonocytic lineage	
	OSM (OM, oncostatin M)	196, monomer	OMR, CD130	T cells, macrophages	Stimulates Kaposi's sarcoma cells, inhibits melanoma growth	
	LIF (leukemia inhibitory factor)	179, monomer	LIFR, CD130	Bone marrow stroma, fibroblasts	Maintains embryonic stem cells, like IL-6, IL-11, OSM	LIFR: die at or soon after birth; decreased hematopoietic stem cells.
Interferons	IFN-γ	143, monomer	CD119	T cells, natural killer cells	Macrophage activation, increased MHC expression	

* May function as dimers

Family	Cytokine (alternative names)	Size (no. of amino acids) and form	Receptors (c denotes common subunit)	Producer cells	Actions	Effect of cytokine or receptor knock-out (where known)
	IFN-α	166, monomers	CD118	Leukocytes	Anti-viral, increased MHC class I expression	IFN-α: susceptibility to intracellular infection Anti-viral defense impaired
	IFN-β	166, monomer	CD118	Fibroblasts	Anti-viral, increased MHC class I expression	
Immunoglobulin superfamily	B7.1 (CD80)	262, dimer	CD28, CTLA-4	Antigen-presenting cells	Co-stimulation of T-cell responses	CD28: decreased T-cell responses
	B7.2 (B70, CD86)		CD28, CTLA-4	Antigen-presenting cells	Co-stimulation of T-cell responses	B7.2: decreased co-stimulator response to alloantigen CTLA-4: Massive lymphoproliferation, early death
TNF family	TNF-α (cachectin)	157, trimers	p55, p75 CD120a, CD120b	Macrophages, natural killer cells	Local inflammation, endothelial activation	TNF-αR: resistance to septic shock, susceptibility to Listeria
	TNF-β (lymphotoxin, LT, LT-α)	171, trimers	p55, p75 CD120a, CD120b	T cells, B cells	Killing, endothelial activation	TNF-β: absent lymph nodes, decreased antibody, increased IgM
	LT-β	Transmembrane trimerizes with TNF-β		T cells, B cells	Unknown	
	CD40 ligand (CD40L)	Trimers	CD40	T cells, mast cells	B-cell activation, class switching	CD40L: poor antibody response, no class switch, diminished T cell priming
	Fas ligand	Trimers	CD95 (Fas)	T cells, stroma?	Apoptosis, Ca^{2+}-independent cytotoxicity	FasL: lymphoproliferation, autoimmune antibody production
	CD27 ligand	Trimers (?)	CD27	T cells	Stimulates T cell proliferation	
	CD30 ligand	Trimers (?)	CD30	T cells	Stimulates T and B cell proliferation	CD30: Increased thymic size, alloreactivity
	4-1BBL	Trimers (?)	4-1BB	T cells	Co-stimulates T and B cells	
Chemokines	IL-8 (NAP-1)	69–79, dimers	CDw128	Macrophages, others	Chemotactic for neutrophils, T cells	CDw128: lymphoadenopathy, splenomegaly
	MCP-1 (MCAF)	76, monomer(?)		Macrophages, others	Chemotactic for monocytes	
	MIP-1α	66, monomer (?)		Macrophages, others	Chemoattractant for monocytes, T cells, eosinophils	
	MIP-1β	66, monomer (?)		T cells, B cells, monocytes	Chemoattractant for monocytes, T cells	

Family	Cytokine (alternative names)	Size (no. of amino acids) and form	Receptors (c denotes common subunit)	Producer cells	Actions	Effect of cytokine or receptor knock-out (where known)
	RANTES	66, monomer (?)		T cells, platelets	Chemoattractant for monocytes, T cells, eosinophils	
Unassigned	TGF-β	112, homo- and heterotrimers		Chondrocytes, monocytes, T cells	Inhibits cell growth, anti-inflammatory	TGFβ: lethal inflammation
	IL-1α	159, monomer	CD121a	Macrophages, epithelial cells	Fever, T-cell activation, macrophage activation	
	IL-1β	153, monomer	CD121a	Macrophages, epithelial cells	Fever, T-cell activation, macrophage activation	
	IL-1 RA	?, monomer		Macrophages	Binds to but doesn't trigger IL-1 receptor, acts as a natural antagonist of IL-1 function	
	IL-10 (cytokine synthesis inhibitor F)	160, homodimer		T cells, macrophages, Epstein-Barr virus	Potent suppressant of macrophage functions	IL-10: reduced growth, anemia, chronic enterocolitis
	IL-12 (NK cell stimulatory factor)	197 and 306, heterodimer		B cells, macrophages	Activates NK cells, induces CD4 T cell differentiation to T_H1-like cells	
	MIF	115, monomer		T cells, others	Inhibits macrophage migration	

BIOGRAPHIES

Emil von Behring (1854–1917) discovered antitoxin antibodies with Shibasaburo Kitasato.

Baruj Benacerraf (1920–) discovered immune response genes and collaborated in the first demonstration of MHC restriction.

Jules Bordet (1870–1961) discovered complement as a heat-labile component in normal serum that would enhance the anti-microbial potency of specific antibodies.

Frank Macfarlane Burnet (1899–1985) proposed the first generally accepted clonal selection hypothesis of adaptive immunity.

Jean Dausset (1916–) was an early pioneer in the study of the human major histocompatibility complex or HLA.

Peter Doherty (1940–) and **Rolf Zinkernagel** (1944–) showed that antigen recognition by T cells is MHC-restricted, thereby establishing the biological role of the proteins encoded by the major histocompatibility complex and leading to an understanding of antigen processing and its importance in the recognition of antigen by T cells.

Gerald Edelman (1929–) made crucial discoveries about the structure of immunoglobulins, including the first complete sequence of an antibody molecule.

Paul Ehrlich (1854–1915) was an early champion of humoral theories of immunity, and proposed a famous side-chain theory of antibody formation that bears a striking resemblance to current thinking about surface receptors.

James Gowans (1924–) discovered that adaptive immunity is mediated by lymphocytes, focusing the attention of immunologists on these small cells.

Michael Heidelberger (1888–1991) developed the quantitative precipitin assay, ushering in the era of quantitative immunochemistry.

Edward Jenner (1749–1823) described the successful protection of humans against smallpox infection by vaccination with cowpox or vaccinia virus. This founded the field of immunology.

Niels Jerne (1911–1994) developed the hemolytic plaque assay and several important immunological theories, including an early version of clonal selection, a prediction that lymphocyte receptors would be inherently biased to MHC recognition, and the idiotype network.

Shibasaburo Kitasato (1892–1931) discovered antibodies in collaboration with Emil von Behring.

Robert Koch (1843–1910) defined the criteria needed to characterize an infectious disease, known as Koch's postulates.

Georges Köhler (1946–1995) pioneered monoclonal antibody production from hybrid antibody-forming cells with Cesar Milstein.

Karl Landsteiner (1868–1943) discovered the ABO blood group antigens. He also carried out detailed studies of the specificity of antibody binding using haptens as model antigens.

Peter Medawar (1915–1987) used skin grafts to show that tolerance is an acquired characteristic of lymphoid cells, a key feature of clonal selection theory.

Elie Metchnikoff (1845–1916) was the first champion of cellular immunology, focusing his studies on the central role of phagocytes in host defense.

Cesar Milstein (1927–) pioneered monoclonal antibody production with Georges Köhler.

Louis Pasteur (1822–1895) was a French microbiologist and immunologist who validated the concept of immunization first studied by Jenner. He prepared vaccines against chicken cholera and rabies.

Rodney Porter (1920–1985) worked out the polypeptide structure of the antibody molecule, laying the groundwork for its analysis by protein sequencing.

George Snell (1903–1996) worked out the genetics of the murine major histocompatibility complex and generated the congenic strains needed for its biological analysis, laying the groundwork for our current understanding of the role of the MHC in T cell biology.

Susumu Tonegawa (1939–) discovered the somatic recombination of immunological receptor genes that underlies the generation of diversity in human and murine antibodies and T-cell receptors.

GLOSSARY

The **12/23 rule** states that gene segments of immunoglobulin or T-cell receptors can only be joined if one has a recognition signal sequence with 12 base pairs as a spacer, and the other has a 23 base pair spacer.

The **ABO blood group system** antigens are expressed on red blood cells. They are used for typing human blood for transfusion. People naturally form antibodies to the A or B blood group antigens if they do not express them on their red blood cells.

The removal of antibodies specific for one antigen from an antiserum to render it specific for another antigen or antigens is called **absorption**.

α:β T-cell receptor: see **T-cell receptor**.

Accessory cells in adaptive immunity are cells that aid in the response but do not directly mediate specific antigen recognition. They include phagocytes, mast cells, and natural killer cells, and are also known as **accessory effector cells**.

The **acquired immune deficiency syndrome (AIDS)** is a disease caused by infection with the human immunodeficiency virus. AIDS occurs when an infected patient has lost most of his or her CD4 T cells, so that infections with opportunistic pathogens occur.

Acquired immune response: see **adaptive immune response**.

Immunization with antigen is called **active immunization** to distinguish it from the transfer of antibody to a naive individual, which is called passive immunization.

Acute lymphoblastic leukemia is a highly aggressive, undifferentiated form of lymphoid malignancy that is derived from a progenitor cell that is believed to be able to give rise to both lineages of lymphoid cells.

Acute phase proteins are a series of proteins found in the blood shortly after the onset of an infection. These proteins participate in early phases of host defense against infection. An example is the mannose-binding protein.

The **acute phase response** is a change in the blood that occurs during early phases of an infection. It includes the production of acute phase proteins and also of cellular elements.

The **adaptive immune response** or **adaptive immunity** is the response of antigen-specific lymphocytes to antigen, including the development of immunological memory. Adaptive immune responses are generated by clonal selection of lymphocytes. Adaptive immune responses are distinct from innate and non-adaptive phases of immunity, which are not mediated by clonal selection of antigen-specific lymphocytes. Adaptive immune responses are also known as **acquired immune responses**.

The **adenoids** are **mucosal-associated lymphoid tissues** located in the nasal cavity.

The enzyme defect **adenosine deaminase deficiency** leads to the accumulation of toxic purine nucleosides and nucleotides, resulting in the death of most developing lymphocytes within the thymus. It is a common cause of severe combined immunodeficiency.

Adhesion molecules mediate the binding of one cell to other cells or to extracellular matrix proteins. Integrins, selectins, members of the immunoglobulin gene superfamily, and CD44 and related proteins are all adhesion molecules important in the operation of the immune system.

An **adjuvant** is any substance that enhances the immune response to an antigen with which it is mixed.

Adoptive immunity is immunity conferred on a naive or irradiated recipient by transfer of lymphoid cells from an actively immunized donor. This is called **adoptive transfer** or **adoptive immunization**.

Afferent lymphatic vessels drain fluid from the tissues and carry antigens from sites of infection in most parts of the body to the lymph nodes.

Affinity is the strength of binding of one molecule to another at a single site, such as the binding of a monovalent Fab fragment of antibody to a monovalent antigen (also see **avidity**).

Affinity chromatography is the purification of a substance by means of its affinity for another substance immobilized on a solid support; an antigen can be purified by affinity chromatography on a column of specific antibody molecules covalently linked to beads.

Affinity maturation refers to the increase in the affinity of the antibodies produced during the course of a humoral immune response. It is particularly prominent in secondary and subsequent immunizations.

Agammaglobulinemia: see **X-linked agammaglobulinemia**.

Agglutination is the clumping together of particles, usually by antibody molecules binding to antigens on the surfaces of adjacent particles. When the particles are red blood cells, the phenomenon is called hemagglutination.

AIDS: see **acquired immune deficiency syndrome**.

Alleles are variants of a single genetic locus.

Allelic exclusion refers to the expression of immunoglobulin encoded by a single heavy-chain and a single light-chain immunoglobulin constant-region allele on the surface of B cells in heterozygous animals or people. It has come to be used more generally to describe the expression of a single receptor specificity in cells with the potential to express two or more receptors.

Allergens are antigens that elicit hypersensitivity or allergic reactions.

Allergic asthma is constriction of the bronchial tree due to an allergic reaction to inhaled antigen.

An **allergic reaction** is a response to innocuous environmental antigens or allergens due to pre-existing antibody or T cells

There are various immune mechanisms of allergic reactions, but the most common is the binding of allergen to IgE antibody on mast cells that causes asthma, hay fever, and other common allergic reactions.

Allergic rhinitis is an allergic reaction in the nasal mucosa, also known as hay fever, that causes runny nose, sneezing and tears.

Allergy is the symptomatic reaction to a normally innocuous environmental antigen. It results from the interaction between the antigen and antibody or T cells produced by earlier exposure to the same antigen.

Two individuals or two mouse strains that differ at the MHC are said to be **allogeneic**. The term can also be used for allelic differences at other loci (see also **syngeneic**, **xenogeneic**).

Rejection of grafted tissues from unrelated donors usually results from T-cell responses to **allogeneic MHC molecules** expressed by the grafted tissues.

An **allograft** is a graft of tissue from an allogeneic or non-self donor of the same species; such grafts are invariably rejected unless the recipient is immunosuppressed.

Alloreactivity describes the stimulation of T cells by MHC molecules other than self; it marks the recognition of **allogeneic** MHC.

Allotypes are allelic polymorphisms detected by antibodies; in immunology, allotypic differences in immunoglobulin molecules were important in deciphering the genetics of antibodies.

The **altered ligand hypothesis** states that the ligand selecting the T-cell receptor is unable to trigger a mature T cell with the same T-cell receptor. It stands in contrast to the avidity hypothesis, which says that the same exact peptide at different levels can select a T cell either positively or induce deletional tolerance.

T cells respond to agonist peptides by making a variety of cytokines and proliferating; the response to **altered peptide ligands** is different in one or more of these assays.

The **alternative pathway** of complement activation is not triggered by antibody, as is the classical pathway of complement activation, but by the binding of complement protein C3b to the surface of a pathogen; it is therefore a feature of innate immunity. The alternative pathway also amplifies the classical pathway of complement activation.

Anaphylactic shock or **systemic anaphylaxis**, is an allergic reaction to systemically administered antigen that causes circulatory collapse and suffocation due to tracheal swelling. It results from binding of antigen to IgE antibody on connective tissue mast cells throughout the body, leading to the disseminated release of inflammatory mediators .

Anaphylatoxins are small fragments of complement proteins released by cleavage during complement activation. The fragments C5a, C3a, and C4a are all anaphylatoxins, listed in order of decreasing potency *in vivo*. They serve to recruit fluid and inflammatory cells to sites of antigen deposition.

Peptide fragments of antigens are bound to specific MHC class I molecules by **anchor residues** which are amino acid side chains of the peptide that bind into pockets lining the peptide-binding groove of the MHC class I molecule. Each MHC class I molecule binds different patterns of anchor residues called a motif, giving some specificity to peptide binding. Anchor residues are less obvious for peptides that bind to MHC class II molecules.

Anergy is a state of non-responsiveness to antigen. People are said to be **anergic** when they cannot mount delayed-type hypersensitivity reactions to challenge antigens, while T and B cells are said to be anergic when they cannot respond to their specific antigen under optimal conditions of stimulation.

Antagonist peptides are able to inhibit the response of a cloned T-cell line to agonist peptides that are usually closely related in amino acid sequence.

Antibody molecules are plasma proteins that bind specifically to particular molecules known as antigens and are produced in response to immunization with antigen. They bind to and neutralize pathogens or prepare them for uptake and destruction by phagocytes. Each antibody molecule has a unique structure that allows it to bind its specific antigen, but all antibodies have the same overall structure and are known collectively as **immunoglobulins**.

Antibody-dependent cell-mediated cytotoxicity (ADCC) is the killing of antibody-coated target cells by cells with Fc receptors that recognize the Fc region of the bound antibody. Most ADCC is mediated by natural killer (NK) cells that have the Fc receptor FcγRIII or CD16 on their surface.

The **antibody repertoire** describes the total variety of antibodies that an individual can make.

Antigens are molecules that react with antibodies. Their name arises from their ability to **gen**erate **anti**bodies. However, some antigens do not, by themselves, elicit antibody production; only those antigens that can induce antibody production are called **immunogens**.

Antigen:antibody complexes are non-covalently associated groups of antigen and antibody molecules which may vary in size from small, soluble complexes to large, insoluble complexes that precipitate out of solution; they are also known as **immune complexes**.

The **antigen-binding site** or **antigen-combining site** of an antibody is the surface of the antibody molecule that makes physical contact with the antigen. Antigen-binding sites are made up of six hypervariable loops, three from the light-chain variable region and three from the heavy-chain variable region.

Both T and B lymphocytes bear on their surface highly diverse **antigen receptors** capable of recognizing a wide diversity of antigens. Each lymphocyte bears receptors of a single antigen specificity.

An **antigenic determinant** is the portion of an antigenic molecule bound by a given antibody; it is also known as an **epitope**.

Influenza virus varies from year to year by a process of **antigenic drift** in which point mutations of viral genes cause small differences in the structure of viral surface antigens. Periodically, influenza viruses undergo an **antigenic shift** through reassortment of their segmented genome with another influenza virus, changing their surface antigens radically. Such antigenic shift variants are not recognized by individuals immune to influenza, so when antigenic shift variants arise, there is widespread and serious disease.

Many pathogens evade the adaptive immune response by **antigenic variation** in which new antigens are displayed that are not recognized by antibodies or T cells elicited in earlier infections.

Antigen presentation describes the display of antigen as peptide fragments bound to MHC molecules on the surface of a cell; all T cells recognize antigen only when it is presented in this way.

Antigen-presenting cells are highly specialized cells that can process antigens and display their peptide fragments on the cell surface together with molecules required for lymphocyte activation. The main antigen-presenting cells for T cells are dendritic cells, macrophages, and B cells, while the main antigen-presenting cells for B cells are follicular dendritic cells.

Antigen processing is the degradation of proteins into peptides that can bind to MHC molecules for presentation to T cells. All antigens except peptides must be processed into peptides before they can be presented by MHC molecules.

Anti-immunoglobulin antibodies are antibodies to immunoglobulin constant domains, useful for detecting bound antibody molecules in immunoassays and other applications.

An **antiserum** (plural: **antisera**) is the fluid component of clotted blood from an immune individual that contains antibodies against the molecule used for immunization. Antisera contain heterogeneous collections of antibodies, which bind the antigen used for immunization, but each has its own structure, its own epitope on the antigen, and its own set of cross-reactions. This heterogeneity makes each antiserum unique.

Aplastic anemia is a failure of bone marrow stem cells so that formation of all cellular elements of the blood ceases; it can be treated by bone marrow transplantation.

Apoptosis, or **programmed cell death**, is a form of cell death in which the cell activates an internal death program. It is characterized by nuclear DNA degradation, nuclear degeneration and condensation, and the phagocytosis of cell residua. Proliferating cells frequently undergo apoptosis, which is a natural process in development, and proliferating lymphocytes undergo high rates of apoptosis in development and during immune responses. It contrasts with necrosis, death from without, which occurs in situations such as poisoning and anoxia.

The **appendix** is a **gut-associated lymphoid tissue** located at the beginning of the colon.

In this book, we have termed activated effector T cells **armed effector T cells**, because these cells are triggered to perform their effector functions immediately upon contact with cells bearing the peptide:MHC complex for which they are specific. They contrast with memory T cells which need to be activated by antigen-presenting cells before they can mediate effector responses.

The **Arthus reaction** is a skin reaction in which antigen is injected into the dermis and reacts with IgG antibodies in the extracellular spaces, activating complement and phagocytic cells to produce a local inflammatory response.

Ascertainment artefact refers to data that appear to demonstrate some finding, but fail to do so because they are collected from a population which is selected in a biased fashion.

Atopic allergy, or **atopy**, is a condition of increased susceptibility to immediate hypersensitivity usually mediated by IgE antibodies.

Pathogens are said to be **attenuated** when they will grow in their host and induce immunity without producing serious clinical disease.

Antibodies specific for self antigens are called **autoantibodies**.

A graft of tissue from one site to another on the same individual is called an **autograft**.

Diseases in which the pathology is caused by immune responses to self antigens are called **autoimmune diseases**.

Autoimmune hemolytic anemia is a pathological condition with low levels of red blood cells (anemia), due to autoantibodies that bind red blood cell surface antigens and target the red blood cell for destruction.

An adaptive immune response directed at self antigens is called an **autoimmune response**, and likewise, adaptive immunity specific for self antigens is called **autoimmunity**.

In the disease **autoimmune thrombocytopenic purpura**, antibodies to a patients platelets are made. Binding of these antibodies causes the platelets to be taken up by cells with Fc receptors and complement receptors, causing a fall in platelet counts, leading to purpura (bleeding).

Autoreactivity describes immune responses directed at self antigens.

Avidity is the sum total of the strength of binding of two molecules or cells to one another at multiple sites. It is distinct from affinity, which is the strength of binding of one• site on a molecule to its ligand.

The **avidity hypothesis** (formerly called the affinity hypothesis) of T-cell selection in the thymus states that T cells must have a measurable affinity for self MHC molecules in order to mature, but not so great an affinity as to cause activation of the cell when it matures, as this would require that the cell be deleted to maintain self tolerance.

Azathioprine is a potent immunosuppressive drug that is converted to its active form *in vivo* and then kills rapidly proliferating cells, including lymphocytes responding to grafted tissues.

B cells are divided into two classes, known as **B-1 B cells**, also known as CD5 B cells, and **B-2 B cells**, also known as conventional B cells.

The major T cell co-stimulatory molecules are closely related members of the immunoglobulin gene superfamily, called **B7.1** and **B7.2**. They are expressed differently in various antigen presenting cell types, and they may have different consequences for the responding T cells. **B7 molecules** refers to both B7.1 and B7.2.

A **β sheet** is one of the fundamental structural building blocks of proteins, consisting of adjacent, extended strands of amino acids which are bonded together by interactions between backbone amide and carbonyl groups. Along a single strand, amino acid side chains alternate between the two sides of the sheet. β sheets may be parallel, in which case the adjacent strands run in the same direction, or antiparallel, where adjacent strands run in opposite directions. All immunoglobulin domains are made up of antiparallel β sheet structures. A **β strand** is one strand of amino acids in a β sheet. A **β barrel** is another way to describe the structure of the immunoglobulin domain.

Many infectious diseases are caused by **bacteria**, which are prokaryotic microorganisms that exist as many different species and strains. Bacteria can live on body surfaces, in extracellular spaces, in cellular vesicles, or in the cytosol, and different bacterial species cause distinctive infectious diseases.

The **bare lymphocyte syndrome** is an immunodeficiency in which MHC class II molecules are not expressed on cells as a result of one of several different regulatory gene defects. Patients with bare lymphocyte syndrome are severely immunodeficient and have few CD4 T cells.

Basophils are white blood cells containing granules that stain with basic dyes, and which are thought to have a function similar to **mast cells**.

The **B-cell antigen receptor**, or **B-cell receptor**, is a cell surface, transmembrane immunoglobulin molecule associated with the invariant **Igα** and **Igβ** chains in a non-covalent complex.

A complex of CD19, TAPA-1, and CR2 makes up the **B-cell co-receptor**; co-ligation of this complex with the B cell antigen receptor increases responsiveness to antigen by about 100-fold.

The **B-cell corona** in the **spleen** is the zone of the **white pulp** primarily made up of B cells.

B-cell mitogens are substances that cause B cells to proliferate.

B cells, or **B lymphocytes**, are one of the two major classes of lymphocyte. The antigen receptor on B lymphocytes, sometimes called the **B-cell receptor**, is a cell-surface immunoglobulin molecule. Upon activation by antigen, B cells differentiate into cells producing antibody of the same specificity as their initial receptor.

Blk: see tyrosine kinase.

Blood group antigens are surface molecules on red blood cells that are detectable with antibodies from other individuals. The major blood group antigens are called ABO and Rh (Rhesus), and are used in routine blood banking to type blood. There are many other blood group antigens that can be detected in cross-matching.

In transfusion medicine, **blood typing** is used to determine if donor and recipient have the same ABO and Rh blood group antigens. A cross-match, in which serum from the donor is tested on the cells of the recipient, and vice versa, is used to rule out other incompatibilities. Transfusion of incompatible blood causes a transfusion reaction, in which red blood cells are destroyed and the released hemoglobin causes toxicity.

B lymphocytes: see **B cells**.

The **bone marrow** is the site of hematopoiesis, the generation of the cellular elements of blood, including red blood cells, mono-cytes, polymorphonuclear leukocytes, and platelets. The bone marrow is also the site of B-cell development in mammals and the source of stem cells that give rise to T cells upon migration to the thymus. Thus, bone marrow transplantation can restore all the cellular elements of the blood including the cells required for adaptive immunity.

A **bone marrow chimera** is formed by transferring bone marrow from one mouse to an irradiated recipient mouse, so that all of the lymphocytes and blood cells are of donor genetic origin. Bone marrow chimeras have been crucial in elucidating the develop-ment of lymphocytes and other blood cells.

A **booster immunization** is given after a primary immunization, to increase the state of immunity.

The lymphoid cells and organized lymphoid tissues in the resp-iratory tract have been termed the **bronchial-associated lymphoid tissues** or **BALT**. These tissues are very important in the induction of immune responses to inhaled antigens and respira-tory infection.

Bruton's X-linked agammaglobulinemia: see **X-linked agamma-globulinemia**.

The **bursa of Fabricius** is an outpouching of the cloaca found in birds. It is an aggregate of epithelial tissue and lymphoid cells and the site of intense early B-cell proliferation. The bursa of Fabricius is required for B-cell development in birds as its removal (bursectomy) early in life causes absence of B cells in adult birds. An equivalent structure has not been detected in humans, where B-cell development follows a different pathway.

C1 inhibitor (C1INH) is a protein that inhibits the activity of activated complement component C1 by binding to and inactivating its C1r:C1s enzymatic activity. Deficiency in C1INH is the cause of the disease **hereditary angioneurotic edema**, in which spontaneous complement activation causes episodes of epiglottal swelling and suffocation.

The generation of the enzyme **C3/C5 convertase** on the surface of a pathogen or cell is a crucial step in complement activation. The C3/C5 convertase then catalyzes the deposition of large numbers of C3 molecules on the pathogen surface, leading to opsonization and the activation of the effector cascade that causes membrane lesions.

The receptor for the C5a fragment of complement, the **C5a receptor**, is a seven transmembrane spanning receptor that cou-ples to a heterotrimeric G protein.

The cytosolic serine/threonine phosphatase **calcineurin** plays a crucial but undefined role in signaling via the T-cell receptor. The immunosuppressive drugs cyclosporin A and FK506 form com-plexes with cellular proteins called immunophilins that bind and inactivate calcineurin, suppressing T-cell responses.

The protein **calnexin** is an 88 kDa protein found in the endoplasmic reticulum. It binds to partially folded members of the immuno-globulin superfamily of proteins and retains them in the endoplasmic reticulum until folding is completed.

Antibodies or antigens can be measured in various **capture** assays. In these assays, antigens or antibodies are captured by the oppo-site species bound to plastic. When one is measuring the titre of antibody binding to a plate bound antigen, one can either used labelled antigen or anti-immunoglobulin. When one wishes to measure the amount of antigen, as for cytokines or hormones, one can use an antibody which binds to a different epitope.

Carriers are foreign proteins to which small, non-immunogenic antigens, or haptens, can be coupled to render the hapten immuno-genic. *In vivo*, self proteins can also serve as carriers if they are correctly modified by the hapten; this is important in drug allergy.

Caseation necrosis is a form of necrosis seen in the center of large granulomas, such as the granulomas in tuberculosis. The term comes from the white cheesy appearance of the central necrotic area.

CD: see **clusters of differentiation** and Appendix I.

The **CD3 complex** describes a complex of αβ or γδ T cell receptor chains with the invariant subunits, cd3γ,δ, and ε, and the dimeric ζ chains.

CD5 B cells are a class of atypical, self-renewing B cells found mainly in the peritoneal and pleural cavities in adults and which have a far less diverse receptor repertoire than conventional B cells.

CD19:CR2:TAPA-1 complex: see **B cell co-receptor**.

B-cell growth is triggered in part by the binding of **CD40 ligand** expressed on activated helper T cells to **CD40** on the B-cell surface.

CD45 or the leukocyte common antigen is a transmembrane tyrosine phosphatase that is expressed in various isoforms on different T cells. These **isoforms** are commonly denoted by the designation of CD45R followed by the exon whose presence gives rise to distinc-tive antibody binding patterns.

CDRs: see **complementarity determining regions**.

The three complementarity-determining regions, **CDR1**, **CDR2**, and **CDR3** are loops at the end of a V domain in antibodies or T cell receptors that make direct contact with antigen or peptide: MHC respectively.

Cell adhesion molecules (CAMs) are cell-surface proteins that are involved in binding cells together in tissues, and also in less permanent cell–cell interactions.

Cell-mediated immunity, or **cell-mediated immune responses**, describes any adaptive immune response in which antigen specific T cells play the main role. It encompasses all adaptive immunity that cannot be transferred to a naive recipient with serum antibody, the definition of humoral immunity.

Cell-surface immunoglobulin is the B-cell receptor for antigen: see **B cell**.

Cellular immunology is the study of the cellular basis of immunity.

Central lymphoid organs are sites of lymphocyte development. In humans, B lymphocytes develop in bone marrow whereas T lymphocytes develop within the thymus from bone marrow derived progenitors.

Central tolerance is tolerance that is established in lymphocytes developing in central lymphoid organs (cf. **peripheral tolerance**).

Centroblasts are large, rapidly dividing cells found in germinal centers, and are the cells in which somatic hypermutation is believed to occur. Antibody-secreting and memory B cells derive from these cells.

Centrocytes are the small, non-proliferating B cells in germinal centers that derive from centroblasts. They may mature into antibody-secreting plasma cells or memory B cells, or may undergo apoptosis, depending on their receptor's interaction with antigen.

Chediak-Higashi syndrome is a defect in phagocytic cell function, due to unknown causes, in which lysosomes fail to fuse properly with phagosomes and which there is impaired killing of ingested bacteria.

Chemokines are small cytokines that are involved in the migration and activation of cells, especially phagocytic cells and lymphocytes. They play a central part in inflammatory responses.

Chronic granulomatous disease is an immunodeficiency disease in which multiple granulomas form as a result of defective elimination of bacteria by phagocytic cells. It is caused by a defect in the NADPH oxidase system of enzymes that generate the superoxide radical involved in bacterial killing.

The **class II-associated invariant chain peptide**, or **CLIP**, is a peptide of varying length cleaved from the class II invariant chain by proteases. It remains associated with the MHC class II molecule in an unstable form until it is removed by the HLA-DM protein.

Class switching: see **isotype switching**.

Classes: see **isotypes**.

The **classical pathway** of complement activation is the pathway activated by antibody bound to antigen, and involves complement components C1, C4, and C2 in the generation of the C3/C5 convertase (see also **alternative pathway**).

According to clonal selection theory, tolerance to self is due to **clonal deletion**, the elimination of immature lymphocytes upon binding to self antigens. Clonal deletion is the main mechanism of central tolerance and can also occur in peripheral tolerance.

Clonal expansion is the proliferation of antigen-specific lymphocytes in response to antigenic stimulation and precedes their differentiation into effector cells. It is an essential step in adaptive immunity, allowing rare antigen-specific cells to increase in number so that they can effectively combat the pathogen that elicited the response.

The **clonal selection theory** is a central paradigm of adaptive immunity. It states that adaptive immune responses derive from individual antigen-specific lymphocytes that are self-tolerant. These specific lymphocytes proliferate in response to antigen and differentiate into antigen-specific effector cells to eliminate the eliciting pathogen, and memory cells to sustain immunity. The theory was formulated by Sir Macfarlane Burnet and in earlier forms by Niels Jerne and David Talmage.

A **clone** is a population of cells all derived from a common progenitor.

A **cloned T-cell line** is a continuously growing line of T cells derived from a single progenitor. Cloned T cell lines must be stimulated with antigen periodically to maintain growth. They are useful for studying T-cell specificity, growth, and effector functions.

A feature unique to individual cells or members of a clone is said to be **clonotypic**. Thus, a monoclonal antibody that reacts with the receptor on a cloned T cell line is said to be a clonotypic antibody and to recognize its clonotype or the clonotypic receptor of that cell. See **idiotype** and **idiotypic**.

Clusters of differentiation (CD) are groups of monoclonal antibodies that identify the same cell-surface molecule. The cell surface molecule is designated CD (cluster of differentiation) followed by a number (eg. CD1, CD2, etc.). For a current listing of CD see Appendix I.

The expression of a gene is said to be **co-dominant** when both alleles at one locus are expressed in roughly equal amounts in heterozygotes. Most genes show this property, including the highly polymorphic MHC genes.

A **coding joint** is formed by the imprecise joining of a V gene segment to a (D)J gene segment in immunoglobulin or T cell receptor genes.

co-isogenic: see **congenic**.

Collectins are a structurally related family of calcium-dependent sugar-binding proteins or lectins containing collagen-like sequences, to which **mannose-binding protein** belongs.

Immunological receptors manifest two distinct types of **combinatorial diversity** generated by combination of separate units of genetic information. Receptor gene segments are joined in many different combinations to generate diverse receptor chains, and then two different receptor chains (heavy and light in immunoglobulins, α and β or γ and δ in T-cell receptors) are combined to make the antigen recognition site.

Common lymphoid progenitors are stem cells which give rise to all lymphocytes. They are derived from pluripotent **hematopoietic stem cells**.

Common variable immunodeficiency is a relatively common deficiency in antibody production whose pathogenesis is not yet understood. There is a strong association with genes mapping within the MHC.

Competitive binding assays are serological assays in which unknowns are detected and quantitated by their ability to inhibit the binding of a labeled known ligand to its specific antibody.

The **complement** system is a set of plasma proteins that act together to attack extracellular forms of pathogens. Complement can be activated spontaneously on certain pathogens or by antibody binding to the pathogen. The pathogen becomes coated with complement proteins that facilitate pathogen removal by phagocytes and may also kill the pathogen.

Complement receptors (CR) are cell-surface proteins on various cells which recognize and bind complement proteins that have bound a pathogen. Complement receptors on phagocytes allow them to identify pathogens coated with complement proteins for uptake and destruction.

The **complementarity determining regions (CDRs)** of immunological receptors are the parts of the receptor that make contact with specific ligand and determine its specificity. The CDRs are the most variable part of the receptor protein, giving receptors their diversity, and are carried on six loops at the distal end of the receptor's variable domains, three loops coming from each of the two variable domains of the receptor.

Some epitopes on a protein antigen are called **conformational** or **discontinuous epitopes** because they are formed from several separate regions in the primary sequence of a protein by protein folding. Antibodies that bind conformational epitopes only bind native, folded proteins.

Congenic strains of mice are genetically identical at all loci except one. Each strain is generated by the repetitive backcrossing of mice carrying the desired trait onto a strain that provides the genetic background for the set of congenic strains. The most important congenic strains in immunology are the **congenic resistant strains**, developed by George Snell, that differ from each other at the MHC.

Constant regions: see **C regions**.

Contact hypersensitivity is a form of delayed-type hypersensitivity in which T cells respond to antigens that are introduced by contact with the skin. Poison ivy is a contact sensitivity reaction due to T-cell responses to the chemical antigen pentadeca-catechol in poison ivy leaves.

Continuous or **linear epitopes** are antigenic determinants on proteins that are contiguous in the protein sequence and therefore do not require protein folding for antibody to bind. See also **conformational** or **discontinuous epitopes**.

A **convertase** is an enzymatic activity that converts a complement protein into its reactive form by cleaving it. Generation of the C3/C5 convertase is the pivotal event in complement activation.

The **Coombs test** is a test for antibody binding to red blood cells. Red blood cells that are coated with antibody are agglutinated if they are exposed to an anti-immunoglobulin antibody. The Coombs test is important in detecting the non-agglutinating antibodies to red blood cells produced in Rh incompatibility.

Two binding sites are said to demonstrate **cooperativity** in binding to their ligands when the effect of binding to both is greater than the sum of each binding site acting on its own.

A **co-receptor** is a cell-surface protein that increases the sensitivity of the antigen receptor to antigen by binding to associated ligands and participating in signaling for activation. CD4 and CD8 are MHC-binding co-receptors on T cells, while CD19 is part of a complex that makes up a co-receptor on B cells.

Corticosteroids are steroids related to those produced in the adrenal cortex, such as cortisone. Corticosteroids can kill lymphocytes, especially developing thymocytes, inducing apoptotic cell death. They are useful anti-inflammatory and immunosuppressive agents.

The proliferation of lymphocytes requires both antigen binding and the receipt of a **co-stimulatory signal**, usually delivered by a cell-surface molecule on the cell presenting antigen. For T cells, the co-stimulatory signals are B7 and B7.2, related molecules that act on the T-cell surface molecules CD28 and CTLA-4. For B cells, CD40 ligand acting on CD40 serves an analogous role.

Cowpox is the common name of the disease produced by vaccinia virus, used by Edward Jenner in the successful vaccination against smallpox, which is caused by the related variola virus.

C-reactive protein is an acute phase protein that binds to phosphatidylcholine which is a constituent of the C-polysaccharide of the bacterium *Streptococcus pneumoniae*, hence its name. Many other bacteria also have surface phosphatidylcholine that is accessible to C-reactive protein, so C-reactive protein can bind many different bacteria and opsonize them for ready uptake by phagocytes.

The bulk of an antibody molecule consists of **C-regions** or **constant regions**. These are encoded in separate exons, one for each **C-domain**, which is an approximately 110 amino acid block, also known as an **Ig domain**. This is a basic building block of many different proteins, making up what is called the **immunoglobulin gene superfamily**.

Cross-matching is used in blood typing and histocompatibility testing to determine whether donor and recipient have antibodies against each other's cells that might interfere with successful transfusion or grafting.

A **cross-reaction** is the binding of antibody to an antigen not used to elicit that antibody. Thus, if antibody raised against antigen A also binds antigen B, it is said to cross-react with antigen B. The term is used generically to describe the reactivity of antibodies or T cells with more than the eliciting antigen.

CTLA-4: High-affinity receptor for B7 molecules on T cells.

The **cutaneous lymphoid antigen**, or **CLA**, is a molecule that is involved in lymphocyte homing to the skin in humans.

Cutaneous T-cell lymphoma is a malignant growth of T cells that home to the skin.

Cyclophosphamide is an alkylating agent that is used as an immunosuppressive drug. It acts by killing rapidly dividing cells including lymphocytes proliferating in response to antigen.

Cyclosporin A is a potent immunosuppressive drug that inhibits signaling from the T-cell receptor, preventing T-cell activation and effector function. It binds to cyclophilin, and this complex binds to and inactivates the serine/threonine phosphatase **calcineurin**.

Cytokines are proteins made by cells that affect the behavior of other cells. Cytokines made by lymphocytes are often called **lymphokines** or **interleukins** (abbreviated IL), but the generic term cytokine is used in this book and most of the literature. Cytokines act on specific cytokine receptors on the cells they affect. Cytokines and their receptors are listed in Appendix II.

Cytokine receptors are cellular receptors for cytokines. Binding of the cytokine to the cytokine receptor induces new activities in the cell, such as growth, differentiation, or death. Cytokine receptors are listed in Appendix II.

Cytotoxic T cells are T cells that can kill other cells. Most cytotoxic T cells are MHC class I-restricted CD8 T cells, but CD4 T cells can also kill in some cases. Cytotoxic T cells are important in host defense against cytosolic pathogens.

Cytotoxins are proteins made by cytotoxic T cells that participate in the destruction of target cells. **Perforins** and **granzymes** or **fragmentins** are the major defined cytotoxins.

Defective endogenous retroviruses are partial retroviral genomes integrated into host cell DNA and carried as host genes. There are a great many defective endogenous retroviruses in the mouse genome.

Delayed-type hypersensitivity is a form of cell-mediated immunity elicited by antigen in the skin. It is mediated by inflammatory CD4 T cells. It is called delayed-type hypersensitivity because the reaction appears hours to days after antigen is injected, as distinct from immediate hypersensitivity in which skin reactions are seen minutes after antigen injection.

Dendritic cells, also known as **interdigitating reticular cells**, are found in T-cell areas of lymphoid tissues. They have a branched or dendritic morphology and are the most potent stimulators of T-cell responses. Non-lymphoid tissues also contain dendritic cells, but these do not appear to stimulate T-cell responses until they are activated and migrate to lymphoid tissues. The dendritic cell derives from bone marrow precursors. It is distinct from the follicular dendritic cell that presents antigen to B cells.

Dendritic epidermal cells (dEC) are a specialized class of γ:δ T cells found in the skin of mice and some other species, but not humans. All dEC have the same γ:δ T-cell receptor; their function is unknown.

Desensitization is a procedure in which an allergic individual is exposed to increasing doses of allergen in hopes of inhibiting their allergic reactions. It probably involves shifting CD4 T-cell types and thus changing antibody from IgE to IgG.

D gene segments, or **diversity gene segments** are short DNA sequences that join the V and J gene segments in immunoglobulin heavy-chain genes and T-cell receptor β and δ chain genes during the somatic generation of a variable-region exon. See **gene segments**.

Diacylglycerol (DAG) is a product of lipid breakdown, most commonly released from inositol phospholipids by the action of phospholipase C-γ, which produces inositol trisphosphate as well as diacylglycerol. Diacylglycerol production is stimulated by ligation of many receptors. It activates cytosolic protein kinase C which further propagates the signal.

Diapedesis is the movement of blood cells, particularly leukocytes, from the blood across blood vessel walls into tissues.

The **differential signaling hypothesis** is one way to explain the distinction between the processes of positive and negative selection in the thymus during T cell maturation.

Differentiation antigens are proteins detected on some cells by means of specific antibodies. Many differentiation antigens play important functional roles characteristic of the differentiated phenotypes of the cell on which they are expressed, such as cell-surface immunoglobulin on B cells.

DiGeorge syndrome is a recessive genetic immunodeficiency disease in which there is a failure to develop thymic epithelium associated with absent parathyroid glands and large vessel anomalies. It appears to be due to a developmental defect in neural crest cells.

The **direct Coombs test** uses anti-immunoglobulin to agglutinate red blood cells as a way of detecting whether they are coated with antibody *in vivo* due to autoimmunity or maternal anti-fetal immune responses (see **Coombs test, indirect Coombs test**).

Discontinuous epitopes: see **conformational epitopes**.

Diversity gene segments: see **D gene segments**.

A truncated heavy chain known as a **Dμ protein** can be produced during B-cell development as a result of heavy-chain transcription from a previously inactive promoter 5' to the D gene segments.

The genetic defect in scid mice, which cannot rearrange their T or B cell receptor genes, is in the enzyme **DNA-dependent kinase**. This enzyme is part of a complex of proteins that bind to the hairpin ends of double stranded breaks in DNA, that includes the DNA-binding Ku proteins.

The catalytic subunit of the molecule **DNA-dependent protein kinase** is critical for VDJ recombination. Its absence due to mutation leads to the phenotype of the *severe combined immunodeficient* or *scid* mouse.

In tissue grafting experiments, the grafted tissues come from a **donor** and are placed in a **recipient** or **host**.

Double-negative thymocytes are immature T cells within the thymus that lack expression of the two co-receptors, CD4 and CD8, whose selective expression parallels T-cell development. The four main intrathymic T-cell populations are double-negative, double-positive, and CD4 and CD8 single-positive thymocytes.

Double-positive thymocytes are an intermediate stage in T-cell development within the thymus characterized by expression of both the CD4 and the CD8 co-receptor proteins.

The **early induced responses** or **early non-adaptive responses** are a series of host defense responses that are triggered by infectious agents early in infection. They are distinct from innate immunity because there is an inductive phase, and from adaptive immunity in that they do not operate by clonal selection of rare, antigen-specific lymphocytes.

Early pro-B cell: see **pro-B cell**.

The common skin disease **eczema** is mainly seen in children and its etiology is poorly understood.

Effector cells are lymphocytes that can mediate the removal of pathogens from the body without the need for further differentiation, as distinct from naive lymphocytes, which must proliferate and differentiate before they can mediate effector functions, and memory cells which must differentiate and often proliferate before they become effector cells. They are also called **armed effector cells** in this book, to indicate that they can be triggered to effector function by antigen binding alone.

The innate and adaptive immune responses use most of the same **effector mechanisms** to eliminate pathogens.

Lymphocytes leave a lymph node through the **efferent lymphatic vessel**.

Electrophoresis is the movement of molecules in a charged field. In immunology, many forms of electrophoresis are used to separate molecules, especially protein molecules, to determine their charge, size, and subunit composition.

ELISA: see **enzyme-linked immunosorbent assay**.

ELISPOT assay is an adaptation of ELISA in which cells are placed over antibodies or antigens attached to a plastic surface which trap the cells' secreted products. The trapped products are then detected with an enzyme-coupled antibody that cleaves a colorless substrate to make a localized colored spot.

Embryonic stem (ES) cells are continuously growing cells that retain the ability to contribute to all lineages of cells in developing mouse embryos. ES cells can be genetically manipulated in tissue culture and then inserted into mouse blastocysts to generate mutant lines of mice; most often, genes are deleted in ES cells by homologous recombination and the mutant ES cells then used to generate **gene knock-out** mice.

Some bacteria have thick carbohydrate coats that protect them from phagocytosis; these **encapsulated bacteria** can cause extracellular infections and are effectively engulfed and destroyed by phagocytes only if they are first coated with antibody and complement produced in an adaptive immune response.

Some anti-carbohydrate antibodies are called **end-binders** because they bind the ends of oligosaccharide antigens, while others bind the sides of these molecules.

Cytokines that can induce a rise in body temperature are called **endogenous pyrogens**, as distinct from exogenous substances like endotoxin from Gram-negative bacteria that induce fever by triggering endogenous pyrogen synthesis and release.

Endotoxins are bacterial toxins that are only released when the bacterial cell is damaged, as opposed to exotoxins which are secreted bacterial toxins. The most important endotoxin is lipopolysaccharide, a potent inducer of cytokine synthesis found in Gram-negative bacteria.

The **enzyme-linked immunosorbent assay (ELISA)** is a serological assay in which bound antigen or antibody is detected by a linked enzyme that converts a colorless substrate into a colored product. The ELISA assay is widely used in biology and medicine as well as immunology.

Eosinophils are white blood cells thought to be important chiefly in defense against parasitic infections; they are activated by the lymphocytes of the adaptive immune response.

The chemokine **eotaxin** is a C-chemokine that acts specifically on eosinophils.

An **epitope** is a site on an antigen recognized by an antibody; epitopes are also called **antigenic determinants**. A T-cell epitope is a short peptide derived from a protein antigen. It binds to an MHC molecule and is recognized by a particular T cell.

Epitope spreading is shorthand used to describe the phenomenon that responses to autoantigens tend to become more diverse as the response persists.

The **Epstein-Barr virus (EBV)** is a herpes virus that selectively infects human B cells by binding to complement receptor 2 (CR2, also known as CD21). It causes infectious mononucleosis and establishes a life-long latent infection in B cells that is controlled by T cells. Some B cells latently infected with EBV will proliferate *in vitro* to form lymphoblastoid cell lines.

The affinity of an antibody can be determined by **equilibrium dialysis**, a technique in which antibody in a dialysis bag is exposed to varying amounts of a small antigen able to diffuse across the dialysis membrane. The amount of antigen inside and outside the bag at the equilibrium diffusion state is determined by the amount and affinity of the antibody in the bag.

E-rosettes are human T cells which will bind to treated sheep red blood cells; the many red blood cells bound to each T cell give it the appearance of a rosette and increase its buoyant density so that the T cells can be isolated by gradient centrifugation. E-rosetting is often used for isolating human T cells.

Erythroblastosis fetalis is a severe form of Rh hemolytic disease in which maternal anti-Rh antibody enters the fetus and produces a hemolytic anemia so severe that the fetus has mainly immature erythroblasts in the peripheral blood.

E-selectin: see **selectins**.

Experimental allergic encephalomyelitis (EAE) is an inflammatory disease of the central nervous system which develops after mice are immunized with neural antigens in a strong adjuvant.

The movement of cells or fluid from within blood vessels to the surrounding tissues is called **extravasation**.

IgG antibody molecules can be cleaved into three fragments by the enzyme papain. Two of these are called the **Fab fragments** because they are the **F**ragment with specific **a**ntigen **b**inding. The Fab fragment consists of the light chain and the amino-terminal half of the heavy chain held together by an interchain disulfide bond. See also **Fc fragment**.

FACS[R]: see **fluorescence-activated cell sorter**.

Factor P: see **properdin**

Farmer's lung is a hypersensitivity disease caused by the reaction of IgG antibodies with large amounts of an inhaled allergen in the alveolar wall of the lung, causing alveolar wall inflammation and compromising gas exchange.

Fas is another member of the TNF receptor gene family; it is expressed on certain target cells that are susceptible to killing by cells expressing the **Fas ligand**, a member of the TNF family of cytokines and cell surface molecules.

When IgG antibodies are cleaved with the enzyme papain, three fragments are generated. Two are the identical **Fab** fragments and one fragment is called the **Fc** fragment for **F**ragment **c**rystallizable. The Fc fragment comprises the carboxy-terminal halves of the two heavy chains disulfide-bonded to each other by the resid-

ual hinge region. One can also prepare so-called **Fv** or **Fragment variable** either by chemical cleavage, or, more recently, it has been possible to generate similar fragments by genetic engineering: these are called **single chain Fv**.

Fc receptors are receptors for the Fc piece of various immunoglobulin isotypes. They include the **Fcγ** and **Fcε receptors**.

The high affinity **Fcε receptor (FcεRI)** found on mast cells and basophils binds free IgE. When antigen binds this IgE, it can crosslink the FcεRI and cause mast cell activation.

Fcγ receptors, including **FcγRI, RII,** and **RIII** are cell-surface receptors that bind the Fc domain of IgG molecules. Most Fcγ receptors only bind aggregated IgG, allowing them to discriminate bound antibody from free IgG. They are expressed on phagocytes, B lymphocytes, natural killer cells, and follicular dendritic cells. They play a key role in humoral immunity, linking antibody binding to effector cell functions.

When tissue or organ grafts are placed in naive recipients, they are eventually rejected by an immune response. This is called a **first set rejection**, to distinguish it from subsequent responses to grafts from the same or related donors, which are much more intense and are called **second set rejections**.

FK506 or **tacrolimus**, is an immunosuppressive polypeptide drug that inactivates T cells by inhibiting signal transduction from the T-cell receptor. FK506 and cyclosporin A are the most commonly used immunosuppressive drugs in organ transplantation.

Individual cells can be characterized and separated in a machine called a **fluorescence-activated cell sorter (FACS**[R]**)** that measures cell size, granularity, and fluorescence due to bound fluorescent antibodies as single cells pass in a stream past photodetectors. The analysis of single cells in this way is called **flow cytometry** and the instruments that carry out the measurements are called **flow cytometers**.

Lymphoid **follicles** consist of clusters of B cells organized around a dense network of **follicular dendritic cells**, cells of uncertain origin with long, branching processes that make intimate contact with many different B cells. Follicular dendritic cells have non-phagocytic Fc receptors that allow them to hold antigen:antibody complexes on their surface for long periods of time; these play a crucial role in selecting antigen-binding B cells during antibody responses.

Fragmentins or **granzymes** are serine esterases found in the granules of cytotoxic lymphocytes including T cells and natural killer cells. When fragmentins enter the cytosol of other cells they induce apoptosis, inducing nuclear DNA fragmentation into 200 base pair multimers, hence their name.

The variable regions of immunological receptors can be divided into two types of sequence: **framework regions** and **hypervariable regions**. The framework regions are relatively invariant sequences in variable regions that provide a protein scaffold for the hypervariable regions that make contact with antigen.

Fungi are single-cell eukaryotic organisms, yeasts, and molds, that can cause a variety of diseases. Immunity to fungi is complex and involves both humoral and cell-mediated responses.

Fyn: see **tyrosine kinase**.

Most T lymphocytes have α:β heterodimeric T-cell receptors, but the receptor on γ:δ T cells has distinct antigen recognition chains assembled in a **γ:δ heterodimer**. The specificity and function of these cells is uncertain.

Plasma proteins can be separated into albumin and the α, β, and γ globulins on the basis of their electrophoretic mobility. Most antibodies migrate as **γ globulins** (or **gamma globulins**), and patients who lack antibodies are said to have agammaglobulinemia based on the absence of gamma globulins on serum protein electrophoresis.

In birds and rabbits, immunoglobulin receptor diversity is generated mainly by **gene conversion**, in which homologous inactive V gene segments exchange short sequences with an active, rearranged variable-region gene.

Gene knock-out is slang for gene disruption by homologous recombination.

The variable domains of immunological receptors are encoded in **gene segments** that must first undergo somatic recombination to form a complete exon encoding the **variable region**. There are three types of gene segment, **V gene segments** that encode the first 95 amino acids, **D gene segments** that encode about 5 amino acids, and **J gene segments** that form the last 10–15 amino acids of the variable region. There are multiple copies of each type of gene segment in the germline DNA, but only one is expressed in a receptor-bearing lymphocyte.

A gene can be specifically disrupted by a technique known as **gene targeting** or **gene knock-out**. Usually this involves homologous recombination in embryonic stem cells followed by preparation of chimeric mice by blastocyst injection of these cells into the blastocyst.

Gene therapy is the correction of a genetic defect by the introduction of a normal gene into bone marrow or other cell types.

Genetic immunization is a novel technique for inducing adaptive immune responses. Plasmid DNA encoding a protein of interest is injected into muscle, and for unknown reasons is expressed and elicits antibody and T-cell responses to the protein encoded by the DNA.

Germinal centers are sites in secondary lymphoid tissues of intense B-cell proliferation, selection, maturation, and death during antibody responses. Germinal centers form around follicular dendritic cell networks when activated B cells migrate into lymphoid follicles.

Immunological receptor genes are said to be in the **germline configuration** in the DNA of germ cells and in all somatic cells in which somatic recombination has not yet occurred.

Immunological receptors have specificity for antigen because of their diversity of structure. Some of this diversity is due to the inheritance of multiple gene segments that encode variable regions; such diversity is called **germline diversity** and can be distinguished from diversity arising during gene rearrangement or after receptor gene expression, which is somatically generated.

One theory of antibody diversity, the **germline theory**, proposed that each antibody was encoded in a separate germline gene.

GlyCAM-1 is a mucin-like molecule found on the high endothelial venules of lymphoid tissues. It is an important ligand for the **L-selectin** molecule expressed on naive lymphocytes, directing these cells to leave the blood and enter the lymphoid tissues.

Goodpasture's syndrome is an autoimmune disease in which autoantibodies to basement membrane or type IV collagen are produced and cause extensive vasculitis. It is rapidly fatal.

G proteins are proteins that bind GTP and convert it to GDP in the process of cell signal transduction. There are two kinds of G protein, the trimeric (α,β,γ) receptor-associated G proteins, and the small G proteins, like Ras, that act downstream of many transmembrane signaling events.

Tissue and organ grafts between genetically distinct individuals almost always elicit an immune response that causes **graft rejection**, the destruction of the grafted tissue by attacking lymphocytes.

When mature T lymphocytes are injected into a non-identical immuno-incompetent recipient, they can attack the recipient causing a **graft-versus-host (GVH) reaction**; in human patients, mature T cells in allogeneic bone marrow grafts can cause **graft-versus-host disease**.

Granulocyte: another name for **polymorphonuclear leukocyte**.

Granulocyte–macrophage colony-stimulating factor (GM-CSF): is a cytokine involved in the growth and differentiation of myeloid and monocytic lineage cells, including dendritic cells, monocytes and tissue macrophages, and cells of the granulocyte lineage.

granuloma is a site of chronic inflammation usually triggered by persistent infectious agents such as mycobacteria or by a non-degradable foreign body. Granulomas have a central area of macrophages, often fused into multinucleate giant cells, surrounded by T lymphocytes.

Granzymes: another name for **fragmentins**.

Graves' disease is an autoimmune disease in which antibodies to the thyroid-stimulating hormone receptor cause overproduction of thyroid hormone and thus hyperthyroidism.

The **gut-associated lymphoid tissues** or **GALT** are lymphoid tissues closely associated with the gastrointestinal tract, including the palatine tonsils, Peyer's patches, and intraepithelial lymphocytes. The GALT has a distinctive biology related to its exposure to antigens from food and normal intestinal microbial flora.

The major histocompatibility complex of the mouse is called histocompatibility-2 or more commonly **H-2**. Haplotypes are designated by a lower case superscript, as in H-2^b.

Histocompatibility or **H antigens** are intensively studied by immunologists. They can be major histocompatibity complex (**MHC**) or **minor H antigens**. The former are studied *in vivo* by employing various MHC congenic, mutant, or recombinant strains.

A **haplotype** is a linked set of genes associated with one haploid genome. The term is used mainly in connection with the linked genes of the major histocompatibility complex, which are usually inherited as one haplotype from each parent. Some MHC haplotypes are over-represented in the population, a phenomenon known as **linkage disequilibrium**.

Haptens are molecules that can bind antibody but cannot by themselves elicit an adaptive immune response. Haptens must be chemically linked to protein **carriers** to elicit antibody and T-cell responses.

Hashimoto's thyroiditis is an autoimmune disease characterized by high, persistent antibody levels to thyroid-specific antigens which recruit NK cells to the tissue, leading to damage and inflammation.

All immunoglobulin molecules have two types of chain, a **heavy (H) chain** of 50–70 kDa and a light chain of 25 kDa. The basic unit of immunoglobulin consists of two identical heavy and two identical light chains. Heavy chains come in a variety of **heavy-chain classes** or **isotypes**, each of which specifies a distinctive functional activity in the antibody molecule.

Helper CD4 T cells are CD4 T cells that can help B cells make antibody in response to antigenic challenge. The most efficient helper T cells are also known as T$_H$2, cells that make the cytokines IL-4 and IL-5. Some experts refer to all CD4 T cells, regardless of function, as **helper T cells**; we do not accept this usage as function can only be determined in cellular assays, and some CD4 T cells kill the cells they interact with.

A **hemagglutinin** is any substance that causes red blood cells to agglutinate, a process known as **hemagglutination**. The hemagglutinins in human blood are antibodies that recognize the ABO blood group antigens. Influenza and some other viruses have hemagglutinin molecules that must bind to glycoproteins on host cells to initiate the infectious process.

Hematopoiesis is the generation of the cellular elements of blood, including the red blood cells, leukocytes and platelets. These cells all originate from pluripotent **hematopoietic stem cells** whose differentiated progeny divide under the influence of **hematopoietic growth factors.**

A **hematopoietic lineage** is any developmental series of cells that derives from **hematopoietic stem cells** and results in the production of mature blood cells.

Hemolytic disease of the newborn or **erythroblastosis fetalis** is caused by a maternal IgG antibody response to paternal antigens expressed on fetal red blood cells. The usual target of this response is the **Rh blood group antigen**. The maternal IgG antibodies cross the placenta to attack the fetal red blood cells.

The **hemolytic plaque assay** detects antibody-forming cells by the ability of their secreted antibodies to produce a **hemolytic plaque**, an area of localized destruction of a thin layer of red blood cells around each antibody-producing cell. The antibodies secreted by the B cell are trapped by antigens on the red blood cells immediately surrounding it, and then complement is added that is triggered by the bound antibody to lyse the red blood cells.

The gene segments that recombine to form variable domains of immunological receptors are flanked on one or both sides by recombination signal sequences consisting of a seven-nucleotide **heptamer** followed by a spacer of 23 base pairs followed by a nine-nucleotide nonamer. The sequences of heptamer and nonamer are highly conserved for all receptor gene segments. These recombination signal sequences direct somatic recombination of receptor gene segments and are removed during gene segment joining.

Hereditary angioneurotic edema is the clinical name for a genetic deficiency of the C1 inhibitor of the complement system. In the absence of C1 inhibitor, spontaneous activation of the complement system can cause diffuse fluid leakage from blood vessels, the most serious consequence of which is epiglottal swelling leading to suffocation.

Individuals **heterozygous** for a particular gene have two different alleles of that gene.

An excellent model for membranous glomerulonephritis is **Heymann's nephritis**, a disease induced by injecting animals with tubular epithelial tissue.

High endothelial venules (HEV) are specialized venules found in lymphoid tissues. Lymphocytes migrate from blood into lymphoid tissues by attaching to and migrating across the **high endothelial cells** of these vessels.

Tolerance to injected protein antigens occurs at low or high doses of antigen. Tolerance induced by injection of high doses of antigen is called **high-zone tolerance**, while tolerance produced with low doses of antigen is called **low-zone tolerance**.

The **hinge region** of antibody molecules is a flexible domain that joins the Fab arms to the Fc piece. The flexibility of the hinge region in IgG and IgA molecules allows the Fab arms to adopt a wide range of angles, permitting binding to epitopes spaced variable distances apart.

Histamine is a vasoactive amine stored in mast cell granules. Histamine released by antigen binding to IgE molecules on mast cells causes dilation of local blood vessels and smooth muscle contraction, producing some of the symptoms of immediate hypersensitivity reactions. **Anti-histamines** are drugs that counter histamine action.

Histocompatibility is literally the ability of tissues (Greek: *histo*) to get along. It is used in immunology to describe the genetic systems that determine the rejection of tissue and organ grafts that results from immunological recognition of **histocompatibility (H) antigens.**

HIV: see **human immunodeficiency virus.**

HLA, the acronym for **H**uman **L**eukocyte **A**ntigen, is the genetic designation for the human **major histocompatibility complex.** Individual loci are designated by upper case letters, as in HLA-A, and alleles are designated by numbers, as in HLA-A*0201.

The MHC of humans contains an MHC class II like set of genes that encode **HLA-DM** that is involved in the loading of peptides onto MHC class II molecules. An homologous gene in mice is called **H-2M**.

Hodgkin's disease is a malignant disease in which antigen presenting cells that resemble dendritic cells appear to be the transformed cell type. **Hodgkin's lymphoma** is a form of Hodgkin's disease in which lymphocytes predominate, and it has a much better prognosis than the **nodular sclerosis** form of this disease in which the predominant cell type is non-lymphoid.

Cellular genes can be disrupted by **homologous recombination** with copies of the gene into which erroneous sequences have been inserted. When these exogenous DNA fragments are introduced into cells, they recombine selectively with the cellular gene, replacing the functional gene with a non-functional copy.

The **human immunodeficiency virus (HIV)** is the causative agent of the acquired immune deficiency syndrome (AIDS). HIV is a retrovirus of the lentivirus family that selectively infects CD4 T cells, leading to their slow depletion and eventually resulting in immunodeficiency.

Humanization is a term used to describe the production of antibodies with mainly human sequences. The DNA encoding hypervariable loops of mouse monoclonal antibodies or V regions selected in phage display libraries is inserted into the framework regions of human immunoglobulin genes. This allows production of antibodies of a desired specificity that do not cause an immune response in humans treated with them.

Protective immunity can be divided into cell-mediated immunity and **humoral immunity**, specific immunity mediated by antibodies made in a **humoral immune response**. Humoral immunity can be transferred to naive recipients with immune serum containing specific antibody, whereas cell-mediated immunity can only be transferred by specifically immune cells.

Monoclonal antibodies are produced most commonly by hybrid cell lines or **hybridomas**. These are formed by fusing a specific antibody-producing B lymphocyte with a myeloma cell that is selected for its ability to grow in tissue culture and the absence of immunoglobulin chain synthesis.

The response to allogeneic tissue grafts can vary from acceptance to **hyperacute rejection**, which is mediated by antibodies preformed against tissue antigens. The antibodies bind to endothelium and trigger the clotting cascade, leading to an engorged, ischemic graft and rapid loss of the organ.

Repetitive immunization to achieve a heightened state of immunity is called **hyperimmunization**.

Immune responses to innocuous antigens that lead to symptomatic reactions upon re-exposure are called **hypersensitivity reactions**. These can cause **hypersensitivity diseases** if they occur repetitively. This state of heightened reactivity to antigen is called **hypersensitivity**.

The variable regions of immunological receptor chains can be divided into two types of sequence: **hypervariable (HV) regions**, which occur at sites that make contact with antigen and differ extensively from one receptor to the next, and **framework regions** of much less variable sequence that provide the molecular scaffold for V region structure.

ICAM: see **intercellular adhesion molecule**.

Iccosomes are small fragments of membrane coated with immune complexes that fragment off the processes of follicular dendritic cells in lymphoid follicles early in a secondary or subsequent antibody response.

Each immunoglobulin molecule has the potential of binding to a variety of antibodies directed at its unique features or **idiotype**. An idiotype is made up of a series of **idiotopes**.

Lymphocyte receptors can recognize one another through idiotope: anti-idiotope interactions, forming an **idiotypic network** of receptors that may be important for the generation and main-tenance of the repertoire of receptors. The various components of idiotype networks exist, but their functional significance is uncertain.

Ig: standard abbreviation for **immunoglobulin**. Different immuno-globulin isotypes are called **IgM, IgD, IgG, IgA,** and **IgE**.

Ig α, Ig β: see also **B-cell antigen receptor**.

Ig α: The **heavy chain of Immunoglobulin A**.

Ig δ: The **heavy chain of Immunoglobulin D**.

Ig ε: The **heavy chain of Immunoglobulin E**.

Ig γ: The **heavy chain of Immunoglobulin G**.

Ig μ: The **heavy chain of Immunoglobulin M**.

Immature B cells are B cells that have rearranged heavy and light chain V-region genes and express a surface IgM receptor, but have not yet matured sufficiently to express a surface IgD receptor as well.

Hypersensitivity reactions that occur within minutes of exposure to antigen are called **immediate hypersensitivity reactions**; such reactions are antibody mediated, whereas **delayed-type hypersensitivity reactions**, which occur hours to days after anti-gen exposure, are T-cell mediated.

When large amounts of antigen are injected into the blood, they are initially removed slowly by normal catabolic processes that also degrade plasma proteins. However, if the antigen elicits an antibody response, then antigen is removed at an accelerated rate as antigen:antibody complexes, a process known as **immune clearance**.

When antibody reacts with soluble antigen, the binding of antigen by antibody forms **immune complexes**. Larger immune complexes form when sufficient antibody is available; these are readily cleared by the reticuloendothelial system of cells bearing Fc and comple-ment receptors, but small, soluble immune complexes forming when antigen is in excess can deposit in and damage small blood vessels.

Immune deviation is a term used to describe polarization of an immune response to T$_H$1-dominated or T$_H$2-dominated by injection of antigen.

The **immune response** is the response made by the host to defend itself against a pathogen.

An **immune response (Ir) gene defect** is usually, but not always, due to failure to bind an immunogenic peptide, so that no T-cell response is observed.

Immune response (Ir) genes are genetic polymorphisms that control the intensity of the immune response to a particular antigen. Virtually all Ir phenotypes are due to differential binding of peptide fragments of antigen to MHC molecules, especially MHC class II molecules. The term is little used now.

It has been proposed that most tumors that arise are detected and eliminated by **immune surveillance** mediated by lympho-cytes specific for tumor antigens. There is little evidence for the efficacy of this proposed process, but it remains an important concept in tumor immunology.

The **immune system** is the name used to describe the tissues, cells, and molecules involved in adaptive immunity, or sometimes the totality of host defense mechanisms.

Immunity is the ability to resist infection.

Immunization is the deliberate provocation of an adaptive immune response by introducing antigen (see also **active immunization** and **passive immunization**).

Immunobiology is the study of the biological basis for host defense against infection.

Immunoblotting is a term used to describe a common technique in which proteins are displayed by a gel, and the proteins are revealed by probing with specific, labeled antibodies.

Immunodeficiency diseases are a group of inherited or acquired disorders in which some aspect or aspects of host defense are absent or functionally defective.

Immunodiffusion is the detection of antigen or antibody by the formation of an antigen:antibody precipitate in a clear agar gel.

Immunoelectrophoresis is a technique in which antigens are identified by first separating them by electrophoretic mobility and then detecting them by **immunodiffusion**.

Immunofluorescence is a technique for detecting molecules using antibodies labeled with fluorescent dyes. The bound fluorescent antibody can be detected by microscopy, by flow cytometry, or by fluorimetry, depending on the application being used. **Indirect immunofluorescence** uses anti-immunoglobulin antibodies labeled with fluorescent dyes to detect binding of a specific, unlabeled antibody.

Any molecule that can elicit an adaptive immune response upon injection into a person or animal is called an **immunogen**. In practice, only proteins are fully **immunogenic** because only proteins can be recognized by T lymphocytes.

Immunogenetics was originally the analysis of genetic traits by means of antibodies to genetically polymorphic molecules such as blood group antigens or MHC proteins. Immunogenetics now includes the genetic analysis of molecules important in immunology by any technique.

All antibody molecules belong to a family of plasma proteins called **immunoglobulins** and abbreviated **Ig**. Surface immuno-globulin serves as the specific antigen receptor of B lymphocytes.

Many molecules are made up in part or in their entirety of blocks of protein known as **immunoglobulin domains** or **Ig domains** because they were first described in the structure of antibody molecules. Immunoglobulin domains are the characteristic feature of proteins of the immunoglobulin superfamily of proteins that includes antibodies, T-cell receptors, MHC molecules, and many other molecules described in this book. The immunoglobulin domain comprises two β-pleated sheets held together by a disulfide bond, called the **immunoglobulin fold**. There are two main types of immunoglobulin domain, C domains with a three-strand and a four-strand sheet, and V domains with an extra strand in each sheet. Domains less closely related to the canonical Ig domains are sometimes also called **Ig-like domains**.

Immunoglobulin fold: see **immunoglobulin domains**.

Many proteins involved in antigen recognition and cell–cell interaction in the immune and other biological systems are members of a family of genes and proteins called the **immunoglobulin superfamily**, or **Ig superfamily**, because their shared structural and genetic features were first defined in immunoglobulin molecules. All members of the immunoglobulin superfamily have at least one **immunoglobulin domain.**

The detection of antigens in tissues by means of visible products produced by the degradation of a colorless substrate by enzymes linked to antibodies is called **immunohistochemistry**. This technique has the advantage that it can be combined with other special stains viewed in the light microscope, whereas immunofluorescent microscopy requires a special dark-field microscope.

Immunological ignorance describes a form of self tolerance in which reactive lymphocytes and their target antigen are both detectable within an individual yet no autoimmune attack occurs. Most autoimmune diseases probably occur when immunological ignorance is broken.

When an antigen is encountered more than once, the adaptive immune response to each subsequent encounter is speedier and more effective, a crucial feature of protective immunity known as **immunological memory**. Immunological memory is specific and long-lived.

Allogeneic tissue placed in certain sites in the body, such as the brain, does not elicit graft rejection. Such sites are called **immunologically privileged sites**. Immunological privilege results from the effects of both physical barriers to cell and antigen migration and soluble immunosuppressive mediators such as certain cytokines.

Immunology is the study of all aspects of host defense against infection and of adverse consequences of immune responses.

Immunophilins are proteins with peptidyl-prolyl *cis-trans* isomerase activity that bind the immunosuppressive drugs cyclosporin A, FK506, and rapamycin.

Soluble proteins, or membrane proteins solubilized in detergents, can be labeled and then detected by **immunoprecipitation analysis** using specific antibodies. The immunoprecipitated labeled protein is usually detected by SDS-PAGE followed by autoradiography.

The T and B cell antigen receptors are associated with transmembrane molecules with **immunoreceptor tyrosine-based activation motifs (ITAMs)** in their cytoplasmic domains. Each ITAM consists of a pair of YXXL motifs spaced by about 10 amino acids. They are sites of tyrosine phosphorylation and association with tyrosine kinases and other phosphotyrosine binding moieties involved in receptor signaling.

The ability of the immune system to sense and regulate its own responses is called **immunoregulation**.

Compounds that inhibit adaptive immune responses are called **immunosuppressive drugs**. They are used mainly in the treatment of graft rejection and severe autoimmune disease.

Antibodies that are chemically coupled to toxic molecules usually derived from plant or microbial toxins are called **immunotoxins**. The antibody targets the toxin moiety to specific cells. Immunotoxins are being tested as anti-cancer agents and as immuno-suppressive drugs.

The **indirect Coombs test** is a variation of the **direct Coombs test** in which an unknown serum is tested for antibodies to normal red blood cells by first mixing the two and then washing the red blood cells and reacting them with anti-immunoglobulin antibody. If antibody in the unknown serum binds to the red blood cells, agglutination by anti-immunoglobulin occurs.

Indirect immunofluorescence: see **immunofluorescence**.

Macrophages and many other cells have an **inducible NO synthase**, or **iNOS**, that is induced by many different stimuli to activate NO synthesis. This is a major mechanism of host resistance to intracellular infection in mice, and probably in humans as well.

Infectious mononucleosis, or glandular fever, is the term used to describe the common form of infection with the Epstein-Barr virus. It consists of fever, malaise, and swollen lymph nodes.

Inflammation is a general term for the local accumulation of fluid, plasma proteins, and white blood cells that is initiated by physical injury, infection, or a local immune response. This is also known as an **inflammatory response**. Acute inflammation is the term used to describe early and often transient episodes, while chronic inflammation occurs when the infection persists or during autoimmune responses. Many different forms of inflammation are seen in different diseases. The cells that invade tissues undergoing inflammatory responses are often called **inflammatory cells** or an **inflammatory infiltrate**.

Inflammatory CD4 T cells, also known as T_H1, are armed effector T cells that make the cytokines interferon-γ and tumor necrosis factor upon recognition of antigen. Their major function is the activation of macrophages. Some T_H1 also have cytotoxic activity.

Influenza hemagglutinin: see **hemagglutinin.**

The early phases of the host response to infection depend on **innate immunity** in which a variety of **innate resistance mechanisms** recognize and respond to the presence of a pathogen. Innate immunity is present in all individuals at all times, does not increase with repeated exposure to a given pathogen, and does not discriminate between pathogens. It is followed by adaptive immunity mediated by clonal selection of specific lymphocytes and leading to long-term protection from disease.

When inositol phospholipid is cleaved by phospholipase C-γ, it yields **inositol trisphosphate** and diacylglycerol. Inositol trisphosphate releases calcium ions from intracellular stores in the endoplasmic reticulum.

The **instructive model** of T-cell lineage development during differentiation of CD4,CD8 double-positive thymocytes into CD4 or CD8 single-positive lymphocytes. It states that an MHC class II restricted receptor should always give rise to CD4 T cells, and a class I restricted receptor to CD8 T cells, because a different signal is transmitted by co-ligation of CD4 in the former and CD8 in the latter case. It is in contrast to the **stochastic/selection model**, which says that T cells randomly inactivate one or the other co-receptor, and only mature if they can then co-aggregate the co-receptor with the T-cell receptor.

In **insulin-dependent diabetes mellitus**, the β cells of the pancreatic islets of Langerhans are destroyed so that no insulin is produced. The disease is believed to result from an autoimmune attack on the β cells.

The **integrins** are heterodimeric cell-surface proteins involved in cell–cell and cell–matrix interactions. They are important in adhesive interactions between lymphocytes and antigen-presenting cells and in lymphocyte and leukocyte migration into tissues.

The **β_1-integrins** are a family of integrins with shared β_1 chains and distinct α chains that mediate adhesion to other cells and to extracellular matrix proteins. They are also known as the very late antigens (VLA).

The **intercellular adhesion molecules (ICAMs) ICAM-1, ICAM-2, and ICAM-3** are cell-surface molecules that are ligands for the leukocyte integrins and play a crucial role in the binding of lymphocytes and other leukocytes to certain cells, including antigen-presenting cells and endothelial cells. They are members of the immunoglobulin superfamily of proteins.

The **intercrines** are a family of small cytokines, also known as chemokines, that are produced by many cell types and play an important role in leukocyte migration into sites of inflammation. They are listed in Appendix II.

Interdigitating reticular cells: see **dendritic cells**.

Interferons are cytokines that can induce cells to resist viral replication. **Interferon-α (IFN-α)** and **interferon-β (IFN-β)** are produced by leukocytes and fibroblasts respectively, as well as by other cells, while **interferon-γ (IFN-γ)** is a product of inflammatory CD4 T cells, CD8 T cells, and natural killer cells. Interferon-γ has as its primary action the activation of macrophages.

Interleukin, abbreviated **IL**, is a generic term for cytokines produced by leukocytes. We use the more general term cytokine in this book, but the term interleukin is used in the naming of specific cytokines such as interleukin-2 (abbreviated **IL-2**). The interleukins are listed in Appendix II.

The major histocompatibility complex (MHC) class II proteins are assembled in the endoplasmic reticulum with the **invariant chain** (abbreviated **Ii**), which is involved in shielding the MHC class II molecules from binding peptides and in delivering them to cellular vesicles. There Ii is degraded, leaving the MHC class II molecules able to bind peptide fragments of antigen.

ISCOMs are **i**mmune **s**timulatory **com**plexes of antigen held within a lipid matrix that acts as an adjuvant and enables the antigen to be taken up into the cytoplasm after fusion of the lipid with the plasma membrane.

Isoelectric focusing is an electrophoretic technique in which proteins migrate in a pH gradient until they reach the place in the gradient at which their net charge is neutral, their isoelectric point. Uncharged proteins no longer migrate so that each protein is focused at its isoelectric point.

Immunoglobulins are made in several distinct **isotypes** or classes, IgM, IgG, IgD, IgA, and IgE, each of which has a distinct heavy-chain constant region encoded by a distinct constant region gene. The isotype of an antibody determines what effector mechanisms it can engage upon binding antigen.

The first antibodies produced in a humoral immune response are IgM, but activated B cells subsequently undergo **isotype switching** to secrete antibodies of different isotypes: IgG, IgA, and IgE. Isotype switching does not affect antibody specificity significantly, but alters the effector functions an antibody can engage. Isotype switching occurs by a site-specific recombination involving deletion of the intervening DNA.

Cytokine receptors signal via **Janus kinases (JAK)**—tyrosine kinases that are activated by cytokine receptor aggregation. In turn, these kinases phosphorylate proteins known as **STATs**, for **S**ignal **T**ransducers and **A**ctivators of **T**ranscription. These proteins are found in the cytosol normally, but move to the nucleus upon phosphorylation and activate a variety of genes.

The **J gene segments**, or **joining gene segments** are immunological receptor gene segments found some distance 5′ to the C genes. A V and D gene segment must rearrange to a J gene segment to form a complete variable-region exon.

Junctional diversity is diversity in immunological receptors created during the process of joining V, D, and J gene segments.

Killer T cell is another commonly used term for **cytotoxic T cell**.

Kit is a cell-surface receptor found on developing B cells and other developing white blood cells for the **stem cell factor** borne on bone marrow stromal cells. Kit has protein tyrosine kinase activity.

Kupffer cells are phagocytes lining the hepatic sinusoids; they remove debris and dying cells from the blood, but are not known to elicit immune responses.

λ5: see **pre-B-cell recepto**r.

Langerhans' cells are phagocytic dendritic cells found in the epidermis. They can migrate from the epidermis to regional lymph nodes via the lymphatics. In the lymph node they differentiate into dendritic cells.

The **large pre-B cells** have a cell surface **pre-B-cell receptor**, which is lost on the transition to **small pre-B cells**, in which light chain gene rearrangement occurs.

In type 1 immediate hypersensitivity reactions, the **late phase reaction** persists and is resistant to anti-histamine treatment.

Some viruses can enter a cell but not replicate, a state known as **latency**. Latency can be established in various ways; when the virus is reactivated and replicates, it can produce disease.

Late pro-B cell: see pro-B cell.

LCMV: see **lymphocytic choriomeningitis virus**.

The **lectin pathway** of complement activation is initiated by collectins, carbohydrate-binding proteins with collagen-like domains found in serum.

Lentiviruses area group of retroviruses, which includes the human immundeficiency virus (HIV), that cause disease after a long incubation, which may take years to become apparent.

Leprosy is caused by *Mycobacterium leprae* and occurs in a variety of forms. There are two polar forms, **lepromatous leprosy** which is characterized by abundant replication of leprosy bacilli and abundant antibody production without cell-mediated immunity, and **tuberculoid leprosy** in which few organisms are seen in the tissues, there is little or no antibody, but cell-mediated immunity is very active. The other forms of leprosy are intermediate between the polar forms.

Leukemia is the unrestrained proliferation of a malignant white blood cell characterized by very high numbers of the malignant cells in the blood. Leukemias can be lymphocytic, myelocytic, or monocytic.

Leukocyte is a general term for a white blood cell. Leukocytes include lymphocytes, polymorphonuclear leukocytes, and monocytes.

Leukocyte adhesion deficiency is an immunodeficiency disease in which the common β chain of the leukocyte integrins is not produced. This mainly affects the ability of leukocytes to enter sites of infection with extracellular pathogens, so that infections cannot be effectively eradicated.

The **leukocyte common antigen** is found on all leukocytes. It is also known as **CD45** and is a transmembrane tyrosine phosphatase that can be produced in a variety of isoforms depending on the cell type on which it appears.

Leukocyte integrins: see **lymphocyte function-associated antigens**.

Leukocytosis is the presence of increased numbers of leukocytes in the blood. It is commonly seen in acute infection.

LFA-1, LFA-3: see **lymphocyte function-associated antigen**.

The immunoglobulin **light (L) chain** is the smaller of the two chains that make up all immunoglobulins. It consists of one V and one C domain, and is disulfide-bonded to the heavy chain. There are two classes of light chain, known as κ and λ.

Linear epitope: see **continuous epitope**.

Alleles at linked loci within the major histocompatibility complex are said to be in **linkage disequilibrium** if they are inherited together more frequently than predicted from their individual frequencies.

Epitopes recognized by B cells and helper T cells must be physically linked in order for the helper T cell to activate the B cell. This is called **linked recognition**.

Low-zone tolerance: see **high-zone tolerance**.

L-selectin is an adhesion molecule of the selectin family found on lymphocytes. L-selectin binds to CD34 and GlyCAM-1 on high endothelial venules to initiate the migration of naive lymphocytes into lymphoid tissue.

Lyme disease is a chronic infection with *Borrelia burgdorferi*, a spirochete that can evade the immune response.

The **lymphatic system** is the system of lymphoid channels that drains fluid from the periphery via the **thoracic duct** to the blood, including the **lymph nodes**, **Peyers patches**, and other organized lymphoid elements apart from the spleen, which communicates directly with the blood.

Lymphatic vessels or **lymphatics** are thin-walled vessels that carry **lymph**, the extracellular fluid that accumulates in tissues, back through the lymph nodes to the thoracic duct.

Lymph nodes are secondary lymphoid organs where adaptive immune responses are initiated. They are found in many locations where lymphatic vessels come together, delivering antigen to antigen-presenting cells which display it to the many recirculating lymphocytes that migrate through the lymph node. Some of these can recognize the antigen and respond to it, triggering an adaptive immune response.

A **lymphoblast** is a lymphocyte that has enlarged and increased its rate of RNA and protein synthesis.

Lymphocyte function-associated antigen-1 (LFA-1) is one of the **leukocyte integrins**, which are heterodimeric molecules involved in the interaction of leukocytes with other cells, such as endothelial cells and antigen-presenting cells. LFA-1 is particularly important in T-cell adhesion to these cells. The other leukocyte integrins are also known as Mac-1 and gp150,95.

Lymphocyte function-associated antigen-3 (LFA-3) is a molecule found on many cells that is the ligand for CD2 (also known as LFA-2). It is a member of the immunoglobulin superfamily.

All adaptive immune responses are mediated by **lymphocytes**. Lymphocytes have cell-surface receptors for antigen that are encoded in rearranging gene segments. There are two main classes of lymphocyte, B lymphocytes (B cells) and T lymphocytes (T cells), which mediate humoral and cell-mediated immunity respectively. Small lymphocytes have little cytoplasm and condensed nuclear chromatin; upon antigen recognition, the cell enlarges to form a lymphoblast and then proliferates and differentiates into an antigen-specific effector cell.

Lymphocytic choriomeningitis virus (LCMV) is a virus that causes a non-bacterial meningitis in mice and occasionally humans. It is used extensively in experimental studies.

Lymphoid organs are organized tissues characterized by very large numbers of lymphocytes interacting with a non-lymphoid stroma. The primary lymphoid organs, where lymphocytes are generated, are the thymus and bone marrow. The main secondary lymphoid organs, where adaptive immune responses are initiated, are the lymph nodes, spleen, and mucosal-associated lymphoid tissues such as tonsils and Peyer's patches.

Lymphokines are **cytokines** produced by lymphocytes.

Lymphomas are tumors of lymphocytes that grow in lymphoid and other tissues but do not enter the blood in large numbers. There are many types of lymphoma which represent the transformation of various classes of lymphoid cells.

Lymphotoxin (LT, TNF-β): Also known as tumor necrosis factor-β, a cytokine secreated by inflammatory CD4 T cells, which is directly cytotoxic for some cells.

Lyn: see tyrosine kinase.

Macroglobulin describes plasma proteins that are globulins of high molecular weight, including immunoglobulin M (IgM).

Macrophages are large mononuclear phagocytic cells important in innate immunity, in early non-adaptive phases of host defense, as antigen-presenting cells, and as effector cells in humoral and cell-mediated immunity. They are migratory cells deriving from bone marrow precursors and are found in most tissues of the body. They play a critical role in host defense.

Resting macrophages will not destroy certain intracellular bacteria unless the macrophage is activated by a T cell. **Macrophage activation** is important in controlling infection and also causes damage to neighboring tissues.

Macrophage chemoattractant and activating protein is a chemokine and is described in Appendix II.

MadCAM-1 is the mucosal cell adhesion molecule-1 or mucosal addressin that is recognized by the lymphocyte surface proteins L-selectin and VLA-4, allowing specific homing of lymphocytes to mucosal tissues.

Eosinophils can be triggered to release their **major basic protein** which can then act on mast cells to cause their degranulation.

The **major histocompatibility complex (MHC)** is a cluster of genes on human chromosome 6 or mouse chromosome 17 that encodes the **MHC molecules**. These are the **MHC class I molecules** or proteins that present peptides generated in cytosol to CD8 T cells, and the **MHC class II molecules** or proteins that present peptides degraded in cellular vesicles to CD4 T cells. The MHC also encodes proteins involved in antigen processing and host defense. The MHC is the most polymorphic gene cluster in the human genome, having large numbers of alleles at several different loci. Because this polymorphism is usually detected using antibodies or specific T cells, the MHC proteins are often called **major histocompatibility antigens**.

The **mannan-binding lectin** or **MBL** is an acute phase protein also called **mannose-binding protein** that binds to mannose residues. It can opsonize pathogens bearing mannose on their surfaces and can activate the complement system. It has an important role in innate immunity.

The follicular **mantle zone** is a rim of B lymphocytes that surrounds lymphoid follicles. The precise nature and role of mantle zone lymphocytes has not yet been determined.

Mast cells are large cells found in connective tissues throughout the body, most abundantly in the submucosal tissues and the dermis. They contain large granules that store a variety of mediator molecules including the vasoactive amine histamine. Mast cells have high-affinity Fcε receptors (FcεRI) that allow them to bind IgE monomers. Antigen binding to this IgE triggers mast cell degranulation and mast cell activation, producing a local or systemic immediate hypersensitivity reaction. Mast cells play a crucial role in allergic reactions.

Mature B cells are B cells that have acquired surface IgM and IgD and have become able to respond to antigen.

Antigens and pathogens enter the body from the intestines through cells called **M cells**, which are specialized for this function. They are found over the gut-associated lymphoid tissue, or GALT. They are believed to be the primary route by which HIV infects the body.

The **medulla** is usually a central or collecting point of organs. The thymic medulla is the central area of each thymic lobe, rich in bone marrow derived antigen-presenting cells and cells of a distinctive medullary epithelium. The medulla of the lymph node is a site of macrophage and plasma cell concentration through which the lymph flows on its way to the efferent lymphatics.

The **membrane-attack complex** is made up of the terminal complement components which assemble to generate a membrane-spanning hydrophilic pore, damaging the membrane.

Membranous glomerulonephritis is a disease of the kidneys characterized by proteinuria and heavy deposits of antibody and complement.

MHC: see **major histocompatibility complex**.

The MHC contains MHC class I, MHC class II, and **MHC class IB** molecules. The MHC class IB molecules are able to present a restricted set of antigens and are not highly polymorphic like the class I and class II genes.

The **MHC class II compartment**, or **(MIIC)**, is a site in the cell where MHC class II molecules accumulate, encounter HLA-DM, and bind antigenic peptides, before migrating to the surface of the cell.

The protein that activates transcription of MHC class II genes, the **MHC class II transactivator**, or **CIITA**, is defective in the disease **bare lymphocyte syndrome**, a lack of expression of MHC class II gene products on all cells.

Various specialized strains of mice are used to explore the role of MHC polymorphism *in vivo*. These are called **MHC congenic**, meaning that the mice differ only at the MHC complex, **MHC recombinant**, meaning that the mice have a crossover within the MHC, or **MHC mutant**, meaning that they are mutant at one or more loci.

MHC genes are inherited in most cases as an **MHC haplotype**, the set of genes in a haploid genome inherited from one parent. Thus, if the parents are said to be ab or cd, then the offspring will be ac, ad, bc, or bd in most cases.

Antigen recognition by T cells is **MHC restricted**, which means that a given T cell will recognize antigen only when its peptide fragments are bound to a particular MHC molecule. Normally, as T cells are stimulated only in the presence of self MHC molecules, antigen is recognized only as peptides bound to self MHC molecules. However, experimental manipulations can produce T cells that recognize antigen only when its peptide fragments are bound to non-self MHC molecules. Thus, MHC restriction defines T-cell specificity both in terms of the antigen recognized and in terms of the MHC molecule that binds its peptide fragments.

Microorganisms are microscopic organisms, unicellular except for some fungi, which include bacteria, yeasts and other fungi, and protozoa, all of which can cause human disease.

Anti-carbohydrate antibodies can bind either the ends or the middles of polysaccharide chains; the latter antibodies are called **middle-binders.**

Minor histocompatibility antigens, or **minor H antigens**, are peptides of polymorphic cellular proteins bound to MHC molecules that can lead to graft rejection when they are recognized by T cells.

Minor lymphocyte stimulatory (Mls) loci are non-MHC loci that provoke strong primary mixed lymphocyte responses. The Mls loci are endogenous mammary tumor viruses integrated in the mouse genome. They produce their effects by making a viral superantigen encoded in the 3′ long terminal repeat of the integrated virus. The superantigen stimulates a large number of T lymphocytes by binding to the V_β domain of the T-cell receptor.

When lymphocytes from two unrelated individuals are cultured together, the T cells proliferate in a **mixed lymphocyte reaction** to the allogeneic MHC molecules on cells of the other donor. This **mixed lymphocyte culture** is used in testing for histocompatibility.

MMTV: see **mouse mammary tumor virus**.

It has been proposed that infectious agents could provoke autoimmunity by **molecular mimicry**, the induction of antibodies and T cells that react against the pathogen but also cross-react with self antigens.

Monoclonal antibodies are antibodies produced by a single clone of B lymphocytes. Monoclonal antibodies are usually produced by making hybrid antibody-forming cells from fusion of myeloma cells with immune spleen cells.

Monocytes are white blood cells with a bean-shaped nucleus which are precursors to macrophages.

Some antibodies recognize all allelic forms of a polymorphic molecule such as an MHC class I protein; these antibodies are thus said to recognize a **monomorphic** epitope.

Lymphocytes have only one receptor and thus have the property of **monospecificity** in response to antigen.

Mouse mammary tumor virus (MMTV) is a retrovirus that encodes a viral superantigen; integrated copies of related viruses encode the endogenous superantigens known as minor lymphocyte stimulatory loci (Mls).

Mucins are highly glycosylated cell-surface proteins. Mucin-like molecules are bound by L-selectin in lymphocyte homing.

The **mucosal-associated lymphoid tissue** or **MALT**, comprises all lymphoid cells in epithelia and in the lamina propria lying below the body's **mucosal surfaces**. The main sites of mucosal associated lymphoid tissues are the **gut-associated lymphoid tissues**, or **GALT**, and the **bronchial-associated lymphoid tissues**, or **BALT**.

Multiple myeloma is a tumor of plasma cells, almost always first detected as multiple foci in bone marrow. Myeloma cells produce a monoclonal immunoglobulin called a myeloma protein which is detectable in the patient's plasma.

Multiple sclerosis is a neurological disease characterized by focal demyelination in the central nervous system, lymphocytic infiltration in the brain, and a chronic progressive course. It is believed to be an autoimmune disease.

Myasthenia gravis is an autoimmune disease in which autoantibodies to the acetylcholine receptor on skeletal muscle cells cause a block in neuromuscular junctions, leading to progressive weakness and eventually death.

Myeloid progenitors are cells in bone marrow that give rise to the granulocytes and macrophages of the immune system.

Myeloma proteins are the secreted immunoglobulin products of myeloma tumors that are found in the patient's plasma.

Myelopoiesis is the production of monocytes and polymorpho-nuclear leukocytes in bone marrow.

Naive lymphocytes are lymphocytes that have never encountered their specific antigen and thus have never responded to it, as distinct from memory or effector lymphocytes. All lymphocytes leaving the central lymphoid organs are naive lymphocytes, those from the thymus being **naive T cells** and those from bone marrow being **naive B cells**.

Natural killer cells or **NK cells** are non-T, non-B lymphocytes usually having granular morphology, that kill certain tumor cells. NK cells are important in innate immunity to viruses and other intracellular pathogens as well as in **antibody-dependent cell-mediated cytotoxicity (ADCC)**.

Necrosis is the death of cells or tissues due to chemical or physical injury, as opposed to apoptosis, which is a biologically programmed form of cell death. Necrosis leaves extensive cellular debris that needs to be removed by phagocytes, while apoptosis does not.

During intrathymic development, thymocytes that recognize self are deleted from the repertoire, a process known as **negative selection**. Autoreactive B cells undergo a similar process in bone marrow.

Antibodies that can inhibit the infectivity of a virus or the toxicity of a toxin molecule are said to **neutralize** them. Such antibodies are known as **neutralizing antibodies** and the process of inactivation as **neutralization**.

Neutrophils, also known as **neutrophilic polymorphonuclear leukocytes**, are the major class of white blood cell in human peripheral blood. They have a multilobed nucleus and neutrophilic granules. Neutrophils are phagocytes and have an important role in engulfing and killing extracellular pathogens.

The small subset of T cells that expresses the NK1.1 marker, a molecule normally found on NK cells, as well as α:β T cell receptors of a limited variety and usually CD4, the so-called **NK1.1 CD4 T cells,** are the major producers of IL-4 early in the immune response.

NK cells: see **natural killer cells**.

Nodular sclerosis: see **Hodgkin's disease**.

Recombination signal sequences (RSS) consist of a seven nucleotide **heptamer** and a nine-nucleotide **nonamer** of conserved sequence, separated by 12 or 23 nucleotides. RSS forms the target for the site-specific recombinase that joins the gene segments.

When T- and B-cell receptor gene segments rearrange, they often form **non-productive rearrangements** that cannot encode a protein because the coding sequences are in the wrong translational reading frame.

N regions are made up of nucleotides that are inserted into the junctions between gene segments of T-cell receptor and immunoglobulin heavy-chain V-region genes during gene segment joining. These **N-nucleotides** are not encoded in either gene segment, but are inserted by the enzyme terminal deoxynucleotidyl transferase (TdT). They markedly increase the diversity of these receptors.

The *nude* mutation of mice produces hairlessness and defective formation of the thymic stroma, so that nude mice, which are homozygous for this mutation, have no mature T cells.

Oncogenes are genes involved in regulating cell growth. When these genes are defective in structure or expression, they can cause cells to grow continuously to form a tumor.

An **opportunistic pathogen** is a microorganism that causes disease only in individuals with compromised host defense mechanisms, as occurs in AIDS.

Opsonization is the alteration of the surface of a pathogen or other particle so that it can be ingested by phagocytes. Antibody and complement **opsonize** extracellular bacteria for destruction by neutrophils and macrophages.

Organ-specific autoimmune diseases are autoimmune diseases targeted at a particular organ, such as the thyroid in Graves' disease. They contrast with systemic autoimmune diseases that do not show organ specificity.

Original antigenic sin describes the tendency of humans to make antibody responses to those epitopes shared between the original strain of a virus and subsequent related viruses, while ignoring other highly immunogenic epitopes on the second and subsequent viruses.

Lymphocyte subpopulations can be isolated by **panning** on petri dishes coated with monoclonal antibodies against cell-surface markers, to which the lymphocytes bind.

The **paracortical area**, or **paracortex**, is the T cell area of lymph nodes, lying just below the follicular cortex that is primarily B cells.

Parasites are organisms that obtain sustenance from a live host. In medical practice, the term is restricted to worms and protozoa, the subject matter of parasitology.

Paroxysmal nocturnal hemoglobinuria (PNH) is a disease in which complement regulatory proteins are defective, so that complement activation leads to episodes of spontaneous hemolysis.

Partial agonist peptides, or **altered peptide ligands**, are able to stimulate a partial response from a cloned T-cell line, such as induction of cytokine secretion but not proliferation.

Passive hemagglutination is a technique for detecting antibody in which red blood cells are coated with antigen and the antibody is detected by agglutination of the coated red blood cells.

The injection of antibody or immune serum into a naive recipient is called **passive immunization**, as opposed to active immunization, the induction of an immune response by injection of antigen.

Pathogenic microorganisms, or **pathogens**, are microorganisms that can cause disease when they infect a host.

Pathology is the scientific study of disease. The term **pathology** is also used to describe detectable damage to tissues.

Pentadecacatechol is the chemical substance in the leaves of the poison ivy plant that causes the cell-mediated immunity associated with allergy to poison ivy.

Pentraxins are a family of **acute phase proteins** formed of five identical subunits, to which **C-reactive protein** and serum amyloid protein belong.

Perforin is a protein that can polymerize to form the membrane pores that are an important part of the killing mechanism in cell-mediated cytotoxicity. Perforin is produced by cytotoxic T cells and NK cells and is stored in granules that are released by the cell when it contacts a specific target cell.

The **periarteriolar lymphoid sheath (PALS)** is part of the inner region of the white pulp of the spleen, and contains mainly T cells.

Peripheral blood mononuclear cells are lymphocytes and monocytes isolated from peripheral blood, usually by Ficoll Hypaque density centrifugation.

Peripheral lymphoid organs are the lymph nodes, spleen, and mucosal-associated lymphoid tissues where immune responses are induced, as opposed to the central lymphoid organs where lymphocytes develop.

Peripheral tolerance is tolerance acquired by mature lymphocytes in the peripheral tissues, as opposed to central tolerance that is acquired by immature lymphocytes during their development.

Peyer's patches are aggregates of lymphocytes along the small intestine, especially the ileum.

Antibody-like phage can be produced by cloning immunoglobulin V-region genes in filamentous phage, which thus express antigen-binding domains on their surfaces, forming a **phage display library**. Antigen-binding phage can be replicated in bacteria and used like antibodies. This technique is being used to develop novel antibodies of any specificity.

Phagocytosis is the internalization of particulate matter by cells. Usually, the **phagocytic cells** or **phagocytes** are macrophages or neutrophils, and the particles are bacteria that are taken up and destroyed. The ingested material is contained in a vesicle called a **phagosome**, which then fuses with one or more lysosomes to form a **phagolysosome**. The lysosomal enzymes play an important role in pathogen destruction and degradation to small molecules.

Phospholipase C-γ is a key enzyme in signal transduction. It is activated by protein tyrosine kinases that are themselves activated by receptor ligation, and activated phospholipase C-γ cleaves inositol phospholipid into inositol trisphosphate and diacylglycerol.

Plasma is the fluid component of blood containing water, electrolytes, and the plasma proteins.

A **plasmablast** is a B cell in a lymph node that already shows some features of a **plasma cell**.

Plasma cells are terminally differentiated B lymphocytes. Plasma cells are the main antibody-secreting cells of the body. They are found in the medulla of the lymph nodes, in splenic red pulp, and in bone marrow. Malignant plasma cells form multiple tumors in bone marrow and are called **multiple myeloma**.

Platelets are small cell fragments found in the blood and are crucial for blood clotting. They are formed from megakaryocytes.

P-nucleotides are nucleotides found in junctions between gene segments of the rearranged V-region genes of immunological receptors. They are an inverse repeat of the sequence at the end of the adjacent gene segment, being generated from a hairpin intermediate during recombination, and hence are called palindromic or P-nucleotides.

Poison ivy is a plant whose leaves contain pentadecacatechol, a potent contact sensitizing agent and a frequent cause of contact hypersensitivity.

Antigen activates specific lymphocytes while all mitogens, by definition, activate most or all lymphocytes, a process known as **polyclonal activation** because it involves multiple clones of diverse specificity. Such mitogens are known as **polyclonal mitogens**.

The major histocompatibility complex is both **polygenic**, containing several loci encoding proteins of identical function, and **polymorphic**, having multiple alleles at each locus.

The **poly-Ig receptor** binds polymeric immunoglobulins, especially IgA, at the basolateral membrane of epithelia and transports them across the cell where they are released from the apical surface. This transcytotic process transfers IgA from its site of synthesis to its site of action at epithelial surfaces.

The **polymerase chain reaction (PCR)** is a technique for amplifying a specific sequence in DNA by repeated cycles of synthesis driven by pairs of reciprocally oriented primers.

Polymorphism literally means existing in a variety of different shapes. Genetic polymorphism is variability at a gene locus where the variants occur at a frequency of greater than 1%. The major histocompatibility complex is the most polymorphic gene cluster known in humans.

Polymorphonuclear leukocytes are white blood cells with multilobed nuclei and cytoplasmic granules. There are three types of polymorphonuclear leukocytes, the neutrophils with granules that stain with neutral dyes, the eosinophils with granules that stain with eosin, and the basophils with granules that stain with basic dyes.

Some antibodies show **polyspecificity**, the ability to bind to many different antigens.

Only those developing T cells whose receptors can recognize antigens presented by self MHC molecules can mature in the thymus, a process known as **positive selection**. All other developing T cells die before reaching maturity.

During B-cell development, **pre-B cells** are cells that have rearranged their heavy-chain genes but not their light-chain genes.

Pre B-cell receptor: see **surrogate light chain**.

The **precipitin reaction** was the first quantitative technique for measuring antibody production. The amount of antibody is determined from the amount of precipitate obtained with a fixed amount of antigen. The precipitin reaction also can be used to define antigen valence and zones of antibody or antigen excess in mixtures of antigen and antibody.

Prednisone is a synthetic steroid with potent anti-inflammatory and immunosuppressive activity used in treating acute graft rejection and autoimmune disease.

During T-dependent antibody responses, a **primary focus** of B-cell activation forms in the vicinity of the margin between T and B cell areas of lymphoid tissue. Here, the T and B cells interact and B cells can differentiate directly into antibody-forming cells or migrate to lymphoid follicles for further proliferation and differentiation.

Lymphoid tissues contain lymphoid follicles made up of follicular dendritic cells and B lymphocytes. The **primary follicles** contain resting B lymphocytes and are the site at which germinal centers form when they are entered by activated B cells, forming **secondary follicles**

The **primary immune response** is the adaptive immune response to an initial exposure to antigen. **Primary immunization**, also known as **priming**, generates both the primary immune response and immunological memory.

The binding of antibody molecules to antigen is called a **primary interaction**, as distinct from **secondary interactions** in which binding is detected by some associated change such as precipitation of soluble antigen or agglutination of particulate antigen.

One speaks of **priming** when antigen is presented to T or B cells in an immunogenic form; the consequence is priming of cells that can respond as memory cells in a second and subsequent immune response.

During B-cell development **pro-B cells** are cells that have displayed B-cell surface marker proteins but have not yet completed heavy-chain gene rearrangement. They are divided into **early pro-B cells** and **late pro-B cells**.

Professional antigen-presenting cells or **APCs** are cells that normally initiate the responses of naive T cells to antigen. To date, only dendritic cells, macrophages, and B cells have been shown to have this capacity. A professional antigen-presenting cell must be able to display peptide fragments of antigen on appropriate MHC molecules and also have co-stimulatory molecules on its surface.

Progenitors are the more differentiated progeny of stem cells that give rise to distinct subsets of mature blood cells and that lack the self-renewal capacity of true stem cells.

Programmed cell death or **apoptosis** is cell death triggered from within the dying cell. Apoptosis eliminates developing T cells that fail positive or negative selection, excess effector cells, and mature lymphocytes that do not encounter antigen. It plays a critical role in maintaining the numbers of lymphocytes at appropriate levels.

Properdin, or factor P, is a positive regulatory component of the alternative pathway of complement activation. It acts by stabilizing the C3/C5 convertase of the alternative factor (comprising C3b,Bb) on the surface of bacterial cells.

Cytosolic proteins are degraded by a large catalytic multisubunit protease called a **proteasome**. It is thought that peptides that are presented by MHC class I molecules are generated by the action of proteasomes, and two subunits of some proteasomes are encoded in the MHC.

Protective immunity is the resistance to specific infection that follows infection or vaccination.

Protein A is a cell membrane component of *Staphylococcus aureus* which binds to the Fc region of IgG, and is thought to protect the bacteria from IgG antibodies by inhibiting their interactions with complement and Fc receptors. It is useful for purifying IgG antibodies.

Enzymes that add phosphate groups to tyrosine residues are called **protein tyrosine kinases**. These enzymes play crucial roles in signal transduction and regulation of cell growth.

Proto-oncogenes are cellular genes that regulate growth control. When mutated or aberrantly expressed, they can contribute to malignant transformation of cells leading to cancer.

Provirus is the DNA form of a retrovirus when it is integrated into the host cell genome, where it can remain transcriptionally inactive for a long period of time.

P-selectin: see **selectins**.

Purine nucleotide phophorylase deficiency is an enzyme defect that results in severe combined immunodeficiency (SCID). This enzyme is important in purine metabolism, and its deficiency causes accumulation of purine nucleosides which are toxic for developing T cells, causing the immune deficiency.

Many bacteria have large capsules that make them difficult to ingest. Such encapsulated bacteria often produce pus, and so they are called **pyogenic bacteria**.

Radiation bone marrow chimeras are mice that have been heavily irradiated and then reconstituted with bone marrow cells of a different strain of mouse, so that the lymphocytes differ genetically from the environment in which they develop. Such chimeric mice have been important in studying lymphocyte development.

Antigen:antibody interaction can be studied by **radioimmunoassay (RIA)** in which antigen or antibody is labeled with radioactivity. An unlabeled antigen or antibody is attached to a solid support like a plastic surface, and the fraction of the labeled antibody or antigen retained on the surface is determined in order to measure binding.

The recombination activating genes *RAG-1* and *RAG-2* encode the proteins **RAG-1** and **RAG-2** that are critical to receptor gene rearrangement. Mice lacking either of these genes cannot form receptors and are severely immunodeficient.

Rapamycin is an immunosuppressive drug that blocks cytokine action.

IgE antibodies responsible for immediate hypersensitivity reactions were originally called **reagins** or **reaginic antibodies**.

Receptor expression requires variable region gene segment **rearrangement** in developing lymphocytes. Expressed V-region genes are composed of **rearranged** gene segments.

The distinguishing characteristic of lymphocytes is the expression of cell-surface **receptors** for antigen. Each lymphocyte bears a receptor of unique structure generated during lymphocyte development through rearrangement of receptor gene segments to produce a complete gene.

The replacement of a light chain of a self-reactive antigen receptor on immature B cells with a light chain that does not confer autoreactivity is known as **receptor editing**.

Receptor-mediated endocytosis is internalization into endosomes of molecules bound to cell-surface receptors. Antigens bound to B lymphocyte receptors are internalized by this process.

The totality of lymphocyte receptors is known as the lymphocyte **receptor repertoire**. It is made up of many millions of different receptors, with all the receptors on a single lymphocyte being identical in structure.

A **recessive lethal** gene is a gene that is needed for the human or animal to develop to adulthood; when both copies are defective, the human or animal dies *in utero* or early after birth. These are frequent in gene-targeting experiments.

In any situation where cells or tissues are transplanted, they come from a donor and are placed in a **recipient** or host.

Recombination activating genes: see **RAG-1** and **RAG-2**.

Strains of mice derived from intra-strain crosses that have undergone recombination within the MHC are called **recombinant inbred strains**.

Recombination signal sequences (RSS) are short stretches of DNA that flank the gene segments that are rearranged to generate a V-region exon. They always consist of a conserved heptamer and nonamer separated by 12 or 23 base pairs. Gene segments are only joined if one is flanked by an RSS containing a 12 base pair spacer and the other is flanked by an RSS containing a 23 base pair spacer, the **12/23 rule** of gene segment joining.

The non-lymphoid area of the spleen in which red blood cells are broken down is called the **red pulp**.

When neutrophils and macrophages take up opsonized particles, this triggers a metabolic change in the cell called the **respiratory burst**. This leads to the production of a number of mediators.

The virus known as **respiratory scyncytial virus**, or **RSV**, is a human pathogen that is a common cause of severe chest infection in young children, often associated with wheezing.

The **rev** protein is the product of the *rev* gene of the human immunodeficiency virus (HIV). The rev protein promotes the passage of viral RNA from nucleus to cytoplasm during HIV replication.

The enzyme **reverse transcriptase** is an essential component of retroviruses, as it translates the RNA genome into DNA prior to its integration into host cell DNA. Reverse transcriptase also allows RNA sequences to be converted into complementary DNA (cDNA), and so to be cloned, and thus is an essential reagent in molecular biology.

The **Rhesus** or **Rh blood group antigen** is a red cell membrane antigen that is also detectable on the cells of rhesus monkeys.

Anti-Rh antibodies do not agglutinate human red blood cells, so antibody to Rh antigen must be detected using a **Coombs test.**

Rheumatoid arthritis is a common inflammatory joint disease that is probably due to an autoimmune response. The disease is accompanied by the production of **rheumatoid factor**, an IgM anti-IgG antibody that may also be produced in normal immune responses.

The technique of **sandwich ELISA** uses antibody on a surface to trap a protein by binding to one of its epitopes. The trapped protein is then detected by an enzyme-linked antibody specific for a different epitope on the protein's surface. This gives the assay a high degree of specificity.

Scatchard analysis is a mathematical analysis of equilibrium binding that allows affinity and valence of a receptor–ligand interaction to be determined.

SCID, *scid*: see **severe combined immunodeficiency**.

SDS-PAGE is the common abbreviation for polyacrylamide gel electrophoresis (PAGE) of proteins dissolved in the detergent sodium dodecyl sulfate (SDS). This technique is widely used to characterize proteins, especially after labeling and immunoprecipitation.

A **secondary antibody response** is the antibody response induced by a **secondary** or **booster injection** of antigen, or **secondary immunization**. The secondary response starts sooner after antigen injection, reaches higher levels, is of higher affinity than the primary response, and is dominated by IgG antibodies.

Secondary interactions: see **primary interactions**.

When the recipient of a first tissue or organ graft has rejected that graft, a second graft from the same donor is rejected more rapidly and vigorously in what is called a **second set rejection**.

The co-stimulatory signal required for lymphocyte activation is often called a **second signal**, with the first signal coming from binding of antigen by the antigen receptor. Both signals are required to activate most lymphocytes.

The **secretory component** attached to IgA antibodies in body secretions is a fragment of the **poly-Ig receptor** left attached to the IgA after transport across epithelial cells.

A cell is said to be **selected** by antigen when its receptors bind that antigen. If the cell enters proliferation as a result, then this is called clonal selection, and the cell founds a clone; if the cell is killed by binding antigen, this is called negative selection or clonal deletion.

Selectins are a family of cell-surface adhesion molecules of leukocytes and endothelial cells that bind to sugar moieties on specific glycoproteins with mucin-like features.

Tolerance is the failure to respond to an antigen; when that antigen is borne by self tissues, then tolerance is called **self tolerance.** See also: **tolerance.**

Allergic reactions require prior immunization, called **sensitization**, by the allergen that elicits the acute response. Allergic reactions only occur in **sensitized** individuals.

Sepsis is infection of the bloodstream. This is a very serious and frequently fatal condition. Infection of the blood with Gram negative bacteria triggers **septic shock** through the release of the cytokine TNF-α.

A **sequence motif** is a pattern of nucleotides or amino acids shared by different genes or proteins that often have related functions. Sequence motifs observed in peptides that bind a particular MHC glycoprotein are based on the requirements for particular amino acids to achieve binding to that MHC molecule.

Seroconversion is the phase of an infection when antibodies against the infecting agent are first detectable in the blood.

Serology is the use of antibodies to detect and measure antigens using **serological assays**, so called because these assays were originally carried out with **serum**, the fluid component of clotted blood, from immunized individuals.

Serotonin is the principal vasoactive amine found in mast cell granules of rodents.

Serum is the fluid component of clotted blood.

Serum sickness occurs when foreign serum or serum proteins are injected into a person. It is caused by the formation of immune complexes between the injected protein and the antibodies formed against it. It is characterized by fever, arthralgias, and nephritis.

Severe combined immune deficiency or **SCID** is an immune deficiency disease in which neither antibody nor T-cell responses are made. It is usually the result of T-cell deficiencies. The *scid* mutation in mice causes severe combined immune deficiency in mice.

A **signal joint** is formed by the precise joining of recognition signal sequences in the process of somatic recombination that generates T-cell receptor and immunoglobulin genes.

During T-cell maturation in the thymus, mature T cells are detected by the expression of either the CD4 or the CD8 co-receptor and are therefore called **single-positive thymocytes**.

Smallpox is an infectious disease caused by the virus variola that once killed at least 10% of infected people. It has now been eradicated by vaccination.

Small pre-B cells: see **large pre-B cells**.

During B-cell responses to antigen, the V-region genes undergo **somatic hypermutation** to generate variant antibodies, some of which bind with a higher affinity. This allows the affinity of the antibody response to increase. These mutations affect only somatic cells and are not inherited through germline transmission.

Somatic mutation theories of antibody diversity proposed that a single gene encoding all antibody molecules underwent mutation in somatic cells to generate the diversity of secreted antibodies. These are also known as **somatic diversification theories**.

During lymphocyte development, receptor gene segments undergo **somatic recombination** to generate intact V-region exons that encode the variable region of each antibody and T-cell receptor chain. These events occur only in somatic cells and the changes are not inherited.

The **spleen** is an organ containing a red pulp involved in removing senescent blood cells and a white pulp of lymphoid cells that respond to antigens delivered to the spleen by the blood.

Staphylococcal enterotoxins cause food poisoning and also stimulate many T cells by binding to MHC class II molecules and the V$_\beta$ domain of the T-cell receptor; the staphylococcal enterotoxins are thus **superantigens**.

Stem-cell factor (SCF) is a transmembrane protein found on bone marrow stromal cells that binds to **Kit**, a signaling receptor carried on developing B cells and other developing white blood cells.

Superantigens are molecules that stimulate a subset of T cells by binding to MHC class II molecules and V$_\beta$ domains of T-cell receptors, stimulating the activation of T cells expressing particular V$_\beta$ gene segments.

Suppressor T cells are T cells which, when mixed with naive or effector T cells, suppress their activity. The precise nature of suppressor T cells and their modes of antigen recognition and activation remain mysterious.

The membrane-bound immunoglobulin that acts as the antigen receptor on B cells is often known as **surface immunoglobulin**.

During B cell development, the shift from pro-B cells to large pre-B cells is accompanied by the expression of μ heavy chains on their surface in combination with the **surrogate light chain** made up of **VpreB** and **λ5**. Together, this is called the **pre-B-cell receptor**, and it includes Igα and Igβ.

When isotype switching occurs, the active heavy-chain V-region exon undergoes somatic recombination with a 3′ constant-region gene at a **switch region** of DNA. These DNA joints do not need to occur at precise sites, since they occur in intronic DNA. Thus, all switch recombinations are productive.

Syk: see tyrosine kinase.

When one eye is damaged, there is often an autoimmune response that damages the other eye, a syndrome known as **sympathetic ophthalmia**.

A **syngeneic graft** is a graft between two genetically identical individuals. It is accepted as self.

Systemic anaphylaxis is the most dangerous form of immediate hypersensitivity reaction. It involves antigen in the blood stream triggering mast cells all over the body. The activation of these mast cells causes widespread vasodilation, tissue fluid accumulation, epiglottal swelling, and often death.

Systemic autoimmunity or **systemic autoimmune disease** involves the production of antibodies to common self constituents. The major cause of pathology in systemic autoimmunity is deposition of immune complexes. The classical example of a systemic autoimmune disease is **systemic lupus erythematosus**, in which autoantibodies to DNA, RNA, and proteins associated with nucleic acids form immune complexes that damage small blood vessels.

Tacrolimus: see **FK506**.

The transporters associated with antigen processing, or **TAP-1** and **TAP-2**, are ATP-binding cassette proteins involved in transporting short peptides from the cytosol into the lumen of the endoplasmic reticulum. Here, the peptides may bind newly synthesized MHC class I molecules to complete their structure. TAP-1 and TAP-2 are required for proper expression of MHC class I molecules.

Tapasin, or the TAP-associated protein, is a key molecule in assembly of MHC class I molecules; a cell deficient in this protein has only unstable MHC class I molecules on the cell surface.

Effector T cell function is always assayed by changes they produce in antigen-bearing **target cells**. These can be B cells that are activated to produce antibody, macrophages that are activated to kill bacteria or tumor cells, or labeled cells that are killed by cytotoxic T cells.

The **tat** protein is a product of the *tat* gene of human immunodeficiency virus. It is produced when latently infected cells are activated, and it binds to a transcriptional enhancer in the long terminal repeat of the provirus, increasing transcription of the proviral genome.

T-cell antigen receptor: see **T-cell receptor**.

T cells, or **T lymphocytes**, are a subset of lymphocytes defined by their development in the thymus and by heterodimeric receptors associated with the proteins of the CD3 complex. Most T cells have α:β heterodimeric receptors but γ:δ T cells have a γ:δ heterodimeric receptor.

T-cell clones: see **cloned T cell lines**.

T-cell hybrids are formed by fusing a specific, activated T cell with a T-cell lymphoma. The hybrid cells bear the receptor of the specific T cell parent and grow progressively like the lymphoma.

T-cell lines are cultures of T cells grown by repeated cycles of stimulation, usually with antigen and antigen-presenting cells. When single T cells from these lines are propagated, they give rise to **T-cell clones** or **cloned T-cell lines**.

The **T-cell receptor** consists of a disulfide-linked heterodimer of the highly variable **α** and **β chains** expressed at the cell membrane as a complex with the CD3 chains. T cells carrying this type of receptor are often called α:β T cells. An alternative receptor made up of variable γ and δ chains is expressed with CD3 on a subset of T cells.

The complement system can be activated directly or by antibody, but both pathways converge with the activation of the **terminal complement components** which assemble to form the membrane-attack complex.

The enzyme **terminal deoxynucleotidyl transferase (TdT)** inserts non-templated or N-nucleotides into the junctions between gene segments in T-cell receptor and immunoglobulin heavy-chain V-region genes. The N-nucleotides contribute greatly to junctional diversity in V regions.

When antigen is injected a third time, the response elicited is called a **tertiary response** and the injection a **tertiary immunization**.

TH1 cells is an alternative name for inflammatory CD4 T cells.

TH2 cells is an alternative name for helper CD4 T cells.

The term **TH3 cell** has been used to describe unique cells that produce mainly transforming growth factor-β in response to antigen; they develop predominantly in the mucosal immune response to antigens that are presented orally.

The lymph from most of the body, except for the head, neck, and right arm, is gathered in a large lymphatic vessel, the **thoracic duct**, that runs parallel to the aorta through the thorax and drains into the left subclavian vein. The thoracic duct thus returns the lymphatic fluid and lymphocytes back into the peripheral blood circulation.

Surgical removal of the thymus is called **thymectomy**.

The **thymic anlage** is the tissue from which the thymic stroma develops during embryogenesis.

The **thymic cortex** is the outer region of each **thymic lobule** where thymic progenitor cells proliferate, rearrange their T-cell receptor genes, and undergo thymic selection, especially positive selection on **thymic cortical epithelial cells**.

The **thymic stroma** consists of epithelial cells and connective tissue that form the essential microenvironment for T-cell development.

Thymocytes are lymphoid cells found in the thymus. They consist mainly of developing T cells, although a few thymocytes have achieved functional maturity.

The **thymus**, the site of T-cell development, is a lymphoepithelial organ in the anterior superior mediastinum or upper part of the middle of the chest, just behind the breastbone.

Some antigens only elicit responses in animals or people that have T cells; they are called **thymus-dependent** or **TD antigens**. Other antigens can elicit antibody production in the absence of T cells and are called **thymus-independent** or **TI antigens**. There are two types of TI antigen, the **TI-1 antigens** which have intrinsic B-cell activating activity, and the **TI-2 antigens** that appear to activate B cells by having multiple identical epitopes that crosslink the B-cell receptor.

T cell and T lymphocyte are shortened designations for **thymus-dependent T lymphocyte**, the lymphocyte population that does not develop in the absence of a functioning thymus.

During the process of germinal center formation, cells called **tingible body macrophages** appear. These are phagocytic cells engulfing apoptotic B cells, which are produced in large numbers during the height of the germinal center response.

Almost all tissues have resident **tissue dendritic cells** that can take up antigen but only achieve effective co-stimulatory activity if they migrate to local lymphoid organs. Graft rejection is triggered by tissue dendritic cells that migrate from the graft to local lymph nodes to trigger an anti-graft response.

Transplantation of organ or **tissue grafts** such as skin grafts is used medically to repair organ or tissue deficits.

Some autoimmune diseases attack particular tissues, such as connective tissue, resulting in **tissue-specific autoimmune disease**.

An antiserum is said to have a **titer** based on serial dilution to an end point, such as a certain level of color change in an ELISA assay.

T lymphocytes: see **T cells**.

Tolerance is the failure to respond to an antigen. Tolerance to self antigens is an essential feature of the immune system; when tolerance is lost, the immune system can destroy self tissues, as happens in autoimmune disease. See also: **central tolerance**, **peripheral tolerance**, and **self tolerance**.

The palatine **tonsils** that lie on either side of the pharynx are large aggregates of lymphoid cells organized as part of the mucosal or gut-associated immune system.

The recombination activating genes, *RAG-1* and *RAG-2*, seem to be related to **topoisomerases**, enzymes involved in cleaving and sealing DNA molecules to allow DNA replication and repair.

The toxic shock syndrome is caused by a bacterial superantigen, the **toxic shock syndrome toxin-1 (TSST-1)**, which is secreted by *Staphylococcus aureus*. Toxic shock syndrome: See definition of **toxic shock syndrome toxin-1**.

Inactivated toxins called **toxoids** are no longer toxic but retain their immunogenicity so that they can be used for immunization.

The active transport of molecules across epithelial cells is called **transcytosis**. Transcytosis of IgA molecules involves transport across intestinal epithelial cells in vesicles that originate on the baso-lateral surface and fuse with the apical surface in contact with the intestinal lumen.

The insertion of small pieces of DNA into cells is called **transfection**. If the DNA is expressed without integrating into host cell DNA, this is called a transient transfection; if the DNA integrates into host cell DNA, then it replicates whenever host cell DNA is replicated, producing a stable transfection.

Foreign genes can be placed in the mouse genome by **transgenesis**. This generates **transgenic mice** that are used to study the function of the inserted gene, the **transgene**, and the regulation of its expression.

The grafting of organs or tissues from one individual to another is called **transplantation**. The **transplanted organs** or grafts can be rejected by the immune system unless the host is tolerant to the graft antigens or immunosuppressive drugs are used to prevent rejection.

Transporters associated with antigen processing: see **TAP-1** and **TAP-2**.

The **tuberculin test** is a clinical test in which a purified protein derivative (called PPD) of *Mycobacterium tuberculosis*, the causative agent of tuberculosis, is injected subcutaneously. PPD elicits a delayed-type hypersensitivity reaction in individuals who have had tuberculosis or have been immunized against it.

Tuberculoid leprosy; see **leprosy**.

Tumor immunology is the study of host defenses against tumors, usually studied by tumor transplantation. Tumors transplanted into syngeneic recipients can grow progressively or can be rejected through T-cell recognition of **tumor-specific transplantation antigens (TSTA)** or **tumor rejection antigens**. TSTA are peptides of mutant or overexpressed cellular proteins bound to MHC class I molecules on the tumor cell surface.

Tumor necrosis factor-α (TNF-α) is a cytokine that is produced by macrophages and T cells and which has multiple functions in the immune response. It is the defining member of the TNF family of cytokines.

Tumor necrosis factor-β (TNF-β): see **lymphotoxin**.

The TdT-dependent dUTP–biotin nick end labeling or **TUNEL assay** identifies apoptotic cells *in situ* by the characteistic fragmentation of their DNA. Biotin-tagged dUTP added to the free 3′ ends of the DNA fragments by the enzyme TdT can be detected by immunohistochemical staining with enzyme-linked streptavidin.

In **two-dimensional gel electrophoresis**, proteins are separated by isoelectric focusing in one dimension, followed by SDS-PAGE on a slab gel at right-angles to the first dimension. This can separate and identify large numbers of distinct proteins.

Hypersensitivity reactions are classified by mechanism: **type I hypersensitivity reactions** involve IgE antibody triggering of mast cells; **type II hypersensitivity reactions** involve IgG antibodies against cell surface or matrix antigens; **type III hypersensitivity reactions** involve antigen:antibody complexes; and **type IV hypersensitivity reactions** are T-cell mediated.

A **tyrosine kinase** is an enzyme that specifically phosphorylates tyrosine residues in proteins. They are critical in T- and B-cell activation. The kinases that are critical for B-cell activation are **Blk, Fyn, Lyn**, and **Syk**. The tyrosine kinases that are critical for T-cell activation are called **Lck, Fyn**, and **ZAP-70**.

Urticaria is the specific term for hives, which are red, itchy skin welts usually brought on by an allergic reaction.

Vaccination is the deliberate induction of adaptive immunity to a pathogen by injecting a **vaccine**, a dead or attenuated (non-pathogenic) form of the pathogen.

The first effective vaccine was **vaccinia**, a cowpox virus that causes a limited infection in humans which leads to immunity to the human smallpox virus, variola.

The **valence** of an antibody or antigen is the number of different molecules it can combine with at one time.

The **variability** of a protein is a measure of the difference between the amino acid sequences of different variants of that protein. The most variable proteins known are antibodies and T-cell receptors.

Variability plot: see **Wu and Kabat plot**.

Variable gene segments: see **V gene segments**.

The **variable region** or **V region** of an immunological receptor is the most amino-terminal domain which is formed by recombination of V, D, and J gene segments during lymphocyte development.